T0413896

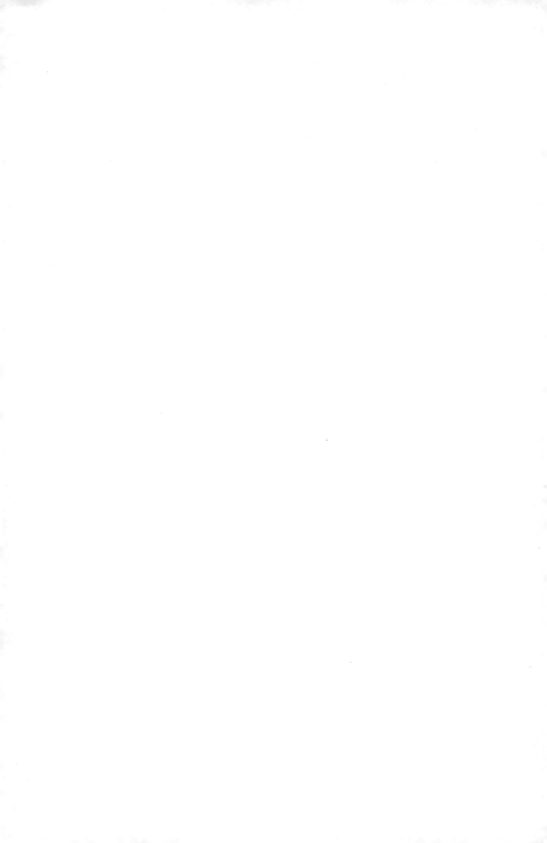

CURRENT CLINICAL ONCOLOGY

Maurie Markman, MD, Series Editor

For further volumes:
http://www.springer.com/series/7631

Thomas F. Gajewski · F. Stephen Hodi
Editors

Targeted Therapeutics in Melanoma

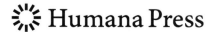 Humana Press

Editors
Thomas F. Gajewski, MD, PhD
Departments of Pathology and Medicine
Section of Hematology/Oncology
University of Chicago
Chicago, IL, USA
tgajewsk@medicine.bsd.uchicago.edu

F. Stephen Hodi, MD
Department of Medical Oncology
Dana-Farber Cancer Institute
and Melanoma Disease Center
Dana-Farber/Brigham
and Women's Cancer Center
Boston, MA, USA
stephen_hodi@dfci.harvard.edu

ISBN 978-1-61779-406-3   e-ISBN 978-1-61779-407-0
DOI 10.1007/978-1-61779-407-0
Springer New York Dordrecht Heidelberg London

Library of Congress Control Number: 2011942473

Printed on acid-free paper

Humana Press is part of Springer Science+Business Media (www.springer.com)

Preface

Cracking the Melanoma Nut

For decades, melanoma has retained a reputation as one of the last major tumor types to lack any therapy shown to improve patient survival in the metastatic setting. The standard chemotherapeutic agent, dacarbazine, was approved in 1976, and the immunotherapeutic agent IL-2 was FDA approved in 1998. However, neither drug traversed the hurdle of a randomized phase III clinical trial. Dozens of chemotherapeutic agents, and more recently signal transduction inhibitors, have been shown to have insignificant clinical activity in phase II clinical trials. Combination chemotherapy has been shown to be no better than single agent dacarbazine, and combined delivery of chemotherapy plus IL-2-based immunotherapy has been reported to offer no additional survival benefit compared to chemotherapy alone. Melanoma also is known to be relatively resistant to standard regimens of ionizing radiation. Based on these facts, it is not difficult to suggest that the traditional empiric oncology drug development paradigm has essentially failed when applied to the treatment of patients with melanoma.

Excitingly, this situation is in the midst of a tremendous change, and that change has been catalyzed by significant advances in fundamental and translational science. Genomic technologies have enabled the identification of driver oncogene mutations in specific kinases that are present in defined subsets of melanoma. These mutated kinases are now targetable with kinase inhibitors which are having potent clinical activity. In addition, tremendous advances in our understanding of immune regulation, with insights derived from analysis of patient material in search for mechanisms of tumor resistance to immune attack, have led to novel therapeutic approaches designed to overcome these barriers and tip the balance toward immune-mediated tumor destruction. While these are still early days, these new discoveries are likely to lead to the FDA approval of several new agents for the treatment of melanoma in 2011 – on the heels of a dry spell of two approvals in 35 years!

This volume, Targeted Therapeutics of Melanoma, aims to present the state-of-the-art information driving the clinical pursuit of agents that target either specific oncogenic pathways that contribute directly to melanoma growth, or immunoregulatory processes that enable tumor escape from immune attack. It is fully anticipated that perseverance to understand additional molecular details of key events that drive melanoma growth will lead to continued development of novel targeted therapies to improve even further the clinical outcome of patients with this disease.

Chicago, IL, USA   Thomas F. Gajewski
Boston, MA, USA   F. Stephen Hodi

Acknowledgments

This book is dedicated to the many basic science, clinical, and translational investigators who continue to devote their time to the challenges of increasing our understanding, and optimizing the treatment for this often dreadful disease. Perhaps more importantly, it is dedicated to the thousands of melanoma patients who enroll in investigational clinical trials, without whom the development of new and effective therapies would not be possible.

Contents

Part I   Advances in Melanoma Biology

1 Molecular Targets and Subtypes in Melanoma.................................   3
   Michael A. Davies

2 Melanoma Genomics   17
   Mohammed Kashani-Sabet

3 Predictive Biomarkers as a Guide to Future Therapy
   Selection in Melanoma..   27
   Thomas F. Gajewski

Part II   Signaling Molecules as Molecular Targets

4 *KIT* as a Therapeutic Target for Melanoma   43
   Nageatte Ibrahim and F. Stephen Hodi

5 Targeted Inhibition of B-Raf...   63
   Paul B. Chapman and Keith Flaherty

6 The Notch and β-Catenin Pathways..................................   77
   John T. Lee and Meenhard Herlyn

7 STAT3 and Src Signaling in Melanoma   89
   Maciej Kujawski, Gregory Cherryholmes,
   Saul J. Priceman, and Hua Yu

8 Targeting the mTOR, PI3K, and AKT Pathways
   in Melanoma   107
   Kim A. Margolin

9 Targeting Apoptotic Pathways in Melanoma   125
   Peter Hersey and Xu Dong Zhang

10   Anti-Angiogenesis Therapy in Melanoma 155
     Daniel S. Chen

Part III   Rational Immunotherapy Approaches in Melanoma

11   Melanoma Antigens Recognized by T Lymphocytes 187
     Nicolas van Baren, Jean-François Baurain,
     Francis Brasseur, and Pierre G. Coulie

12   Melanoma Vaccines 207
     Pedro Romero and Daniel E. Speiser

13   Adoptive Cell Therapy for the Treatment
     of Metastatic Melanoma 233
     Jessica Ann Chacon, Patrick Hwu, and Laszlo G. Radvanyi

14   Anti-CTLA-4 Monoclonal Antibodies 273
     Arvin S. Yang and Jedd D. Wolchok

15   Anti-PD-1 and Anti-B7-H1/PD-L1 Monoclonal Antibodies 291
     Evan J. Lipson, Janis M. Taube, Lieping Chen,
     and Suzanne L. Topalian

16   Treatment of Melanoma with Agonist Immune
     Costimulatory Agents 307
     Andrew Weinberg, Robert H. Vonderheide,
     and Mario Sznol

17   Novel Cytokines for Immunotherapy of Melanoma 333
     Shailender Bhatia and John A. Thompson

18   Modulating the Tumor Microenvironment 353
     Carl E. Ruby and Howard L. Kaufman

Index 371

Contributors

Jean-François Baurain, MD, PhD Centre du Cancer, Cliniques universitaires Saint-Luc, Université catholique de Louvain, Brussels, Belgium

Shailender Bhatia, MD Department of Medicine, Division of Medical Oncology, University of Washington School of Medicine, Fred Hutchinson Cancer Research Center, Seattle Cancer Care Alliance, Seattle, WA, USA

Francis Brasseur, PhD de Duve Institute and Université catholique de Louvain, Brussels, Belgium

Ludwig Institute for Cancer Research, Brussels Branch, Belgium

Jessica Ann Chacon, MSc Department of Melanoma Medical Oncology, Immunology Program of the University of Texas Health Science Center, Graduate School of Biomedical Sciences, The University of Texas M.D. Anderson Cancer Center, Houston, TX, USA

Paul B. Chapman, MD Department of Medicine, Memorial Sloan-Kettering Cancer Center, New York, NY, USA

Daniel S. Chen, MD, PhD Medical Oncology, Stanford University, Stanford, CA, USA

Oncology Clinical Development, Genentech, Inc., South San Francisco, CA, USA

Lieping Chen, MD, PhD Department of Immunobiology, Yale University School of Medicine, New Haven, CT, USA

Gregory Cherryholmes, MSc The Irell and Manella Graduate School of Biological Sciences, Beckman Research Institute and City of Hope Comprehensive Cancer Center, Duarte, CA, USA

Pierre G. Coulie, MD, PhD de Duve Institute and Université catholique de Louvain, Brussels, Belgium

Michael A. Davies, MD, PhD Departments of Melanoma Medical Oncology and Systems Biology, University of Texas M.D. Anderson Cancer Center, Houston, TX, USA

Keith Flaherty, MD Massachusetts General Hospital Cancer Center, Boston, MA, USA

Thomas F. Gajewski, MD, PhD Departments of Pathology and Medicine, Section of Hematology/Oncology, University of Chicago, Chicago, IL, USA

Meenhard Herlyn, DVM Molecular and Cellular Oncogenesis Program, The Wistar Institute, Philadelphia, PA, USA

Peter Hersey Oncology & Immunology Unit, University of Newcastle, Kolling Institute Univesity of Sydney, Room 443, David Maddison Clinical Sciences Building, Cnr King & Watt Streets, Newcastle, NSW, Australia

F. Stephen Hodi, MD Department of Medical Oncology, Dana-Farber Cancer Institute and Melanoma Disease Center, Dana-Farber/Brigham and Women's Cancer Center, Boston, MA, USA

Patrick Hwu, MD Department of Melanoma Medical Oncology, Immunology Program of the University of Texas Health Science Center, Graduate School of Biomedical Sciences, The University of Texas M.D. Anderson Cancer Center, Houston, TX, USA

Nageatte Ibrahim, MD Department of Medical Oncology, Dana-Farber Cancer Institute and Melanoma Disease Center, Dana-Farber/Brigham and Women's Cancer Center, Boston, MA, USA

Mohammed Kashani-Sabet, MD Center for Melanoma Research and Treatment, California Pacific Medical Center Research Institute, San Francisco, CA, USA

Howard L. Kaufman, MD Rush Medical College, Rush University Cancer Center, Rush University Medical Center, Chicago, IL, USA

Maciej Kujawski, PhD Department of Cancer Immunotherapeutics and Tumor Immunology, Beckman Research Institute and City of Hope Comprehensive Cancer Center, Duarte, CA, USA

John T. Lee, PhD Molecular and Cellular Oncogenesis Program, The Wistar Institute, Philadelphia, PA, USA

Evan J. Lipson Department of Oncology, The Johns Hopkins University School of Medicine and the Sidney Kimmel Comprehensive Cancer Cente, Baltimore, MD, USA

Kim A. Margolin, MD Department of Medical Oncology, University of Washington and Seattle Cancer Care Alliance, Seattle, WA, USA

Saul J. Priceman, PhD Department of Cancer Immunotherapeutics and Tumor Immunology, Beckman Research Institute and City of Hope Comprehensive Cancer Center, Duarte, CA, USA

Laszlo G. Radvanyi, PhD Department of Melanoma Medical Oncology, Immunology Program of the University of Texas Health Science Center, Graduate School of Biomedical Sciences, The University of Texas M.D. Anderson Cancer Center, Houston, TX, USA

Pedro Romero, MD Ludwig Center for Cancer Research, University of Lausanne, Lausanne, Switzerland

Carl E. Ruby, PhD Department of General Surgery, Rush University Medical Center, Chicago, IL, USA

Daniel E. Speiser, MD Ludwig Center of the University of Lausanne, Lausanne, Switzerland

Mario Sznol, MD Yale Cancer Center, New Haven, CT, USA

Janis M. Taube, MD Departments of Dermatology and Pathology, Johns Hopkins Hospital, Baltimore, MD, USA

John A. Thompson, MD Department of Medicine, Division of Medical Oncology, University of Washington School of Medicine, Fred Hutchinson Cancer Research Center, Seattle Cancer Care Alliance, Seattle, WA, USA

Suzanne L. Topalian, MD Departments of Surgery and Oncology, The Johns Hopkins University School of Medicine and the Sidney Kimmel Comprehensive Cancer Center, Baltimore, MD, USA

Nicolas van Baren, MD, PhD de Duve Institute and Université catholique de Louvain, Brussels, Belgium

Ludwig Institute for Cancer Research, Brussels Branch, Brussels, Belgium

Centre du Cancer, Unité d'Oncologie Médicale, Cliniques universitaires Saint-Luc, Université catholique de Louvain, Brussels, Belgium

Robert H. Vonderheide, MD, DPhil Abramson Family Cancer Research Institute, University of Pennsylvania School of Medicine, Philadelphia, PA, USA

Andrew Weinberg, PhD Laboratory of Basic Immunology, Robert W. Franz Cancer Research Center, Earle A. Chiles Research Institute, Portland, OR, USA

Jedd D. Wolchok, MD, PhD Department of Medicine, Memorial Sloan-Kettering Cancer Center, New York, NY, USA

Arvin Yang, MD, PhD Oncology Medical Strategy-Ipilimumab,
US Pharmaceuticals Medical, Bristol-Myers Squibb Company,
Plainsboro, NJ, USA

Hua Yu, PhD Department of Cancer Immunotherapeutics
and Tumor Immunology, Beckman Research Institute and City of Hope
Comprehensive Cancer Center, Duarte, CA, USA

Xu Dong Zhang Oncology & Immunology Unit, University of Newcastle,
Kolling Institute Univesity of Sydney, David Maddison Clinical Sciences
Building, Cnr King & Watt Streets, Newcastle, NSW, Australia

Part I
Advances in Melanoma Biology

Chapter 1
Molecular Targets and Subtypes in Melanoma

Michael A. Davies

Abstract Oncology is entering a new era in which patients are being categorized not only by the tissue of origin of their cancer, but also by the molecular character-istics of their tumor. Historically, melanomas have been classified as cutaneous (including superficial spreading, nodular, lentigo maligna, and acral lentiginous subtypes), mucosal, or uveal. Recent molecular analyses have demonstrated that the majority of melanomas harbor one or more genetic alterations in components of key signaling networks. This information is now being integrated with the traditional clinicopathological criteria to develop a more refined system that has both diagnos-tic and therapeutic implications.

Keywords BRAF • NRAS • MEK • MAPK • KIT • PTEN • PI3K • AKT • GNAQ • GNA11 • Mutation • Amplification • Comparative genome hybridization • Targeted therapy • Oncogene addiction • PLX4032 • Imatinib • Acral lentiginous melanoma • Mucosal melanoma • Uveal melanoma • Superficial spreading melanoma • Nodular melanoma • Nevi

Introduction

The treatment of cancer is entering a new era based on an improved understanding of the molecular causes and heterogeneity of this disease. Historically, systemic treatments for patients with advanced cancer have been selected based upon the organ from which the tumor originates (i.e., breast, colon lung). However, both preclinical studies and clinical trials have demonstrated that patients with the same tumor type can exhibit marked molecular differences and subsequently be sensitive

M.A. Davies, MD, PhD (✉)
Departments of Melanoma Medical Oncology and Systems Biology,
University of Texas M.D. Anderson Cancer Center, Houston, TX, USA
e-mail: mdavies@mdanderson.org

T.F. Gajewski and F.S. Hodi (eds.), *Targeted Therapeutics in Melanoma*,
Current Clinical Oncology, DOI 10.1007/978-1-61779-407-0_1,
© Springer Science+Business Media, LLC 2012

(or resistant) to different treatment strategies. For example, the use of antihormonal therapies is clearly beneficial in breast cancer patients whose tumors express the estrogen or progesterone receptor, but they have no benefit in tumors lacking these proteins [4, 36]. More recently, trastuzumab (Hercpetin®) has demonstrated remarkable efficacy in breast cancer patients with amplification of the *HER2/neu* oncogene, but it does not improve outcomes in patients without this genetic event [35, 47]. Thus, the evaluation and treatment for every breast cancer patient critically depends upon the molecular classification of their tumor. There is a clear impetus to identify molecular subtypes in other cancers, particularly based on therapeutic targets.

Melanoma is one of the most aggressive forms of skin cancer. Melanomas have generally been classified on the basis of both clinical and pathologic features of the primary tumor. While melanocytes are present in a number of different tissues in the body, the majority of melanomas arise from melanocytes in the epidermal skin layer. This predominance likely reflects the established causative role of exposure to ultraviolet light in this disease [38]. Cutaneous melanomas are classified into four major subtypes based on clinical presentation and histologic (microscopic) features: superficial spreading, nodular, lentigo maligna, and acral lentiginous [40]. Superficial spreading melanoma represents approximately 70% of cutaneous melanomas, and they generally involve skin regions with intermittent sun exposure. Nodular melanomas comprise 15–25% of melanomas, and they can be associated with a rapid clinical course. Lentigo maligna melanomas (5–10%) are associated with chronic sun exposure, and thus are often located on the head and neck regions. Acral lentiginous melanomas occur on the palms or soles, or beneath the nail beds, and therefore are relatively protected from UV-exposure as compared to the other cutaneous lesions. Acral melanomas represent a small minority of the melanomas that are diagnosed in Caucasians, but they are much more prevalent among the melanomas diagnosed in patients of other ethnicities where sun exposure-related melanomas are comparatively rare. In addition to cutaneous surfaces, melanomas may arise from other sites where melanocytes are present, but where exposure to UV light is much less likely to explain tumorigenesis. Mucosal melanomas arise from mucosal surfaces in the head and neck, the gastrointestinal tract, and the genitourinary tract. Uveal melanomas, which are the most common primary tumors of the eye, arise from melanocytes in the uveal tract (iris, ciliary body, and choroid). While most melanomas are characterized by wide metastatic spread to a variety of organs, the uveal melanomas are distinguished clinically by a high prevalence of metastasis to, and often sole involvement of, the liver.

Patients with advanced melanoma have a very poor prognosis. Multiple trials with chemotherapies, immunotherapies, and combined biochemotherapy regimens have failed to significantly improve outcomes in this disease [58]. Thus, there is a need for new therapeutic approaches for melanoma. One strategy that has proven successful in several other refractory tumors types is "targeted therapy." Targeted therapy refers to the use of inhibitors against molecules and/or pathways that are activated specifically in cancer cells. Targeted therapies have proven successful, and are FDA-approved, in a number of cancer types, including chronic myelogenous leukemia (CML), breast cancer, renal cell carcinoma (RCC), and gastrointestinal stromal tumors (GIST) [11]. In each of these diseases, the successful development of targeted therapy was contingent upon the identification of genetic mutations and the affected pathways in the tumor cells to select rational inhibitors for testing.

It is now clear that the majority of melanomas have genetic mutations that activate kinase signaling pathways. Thus, there is tremendous enthusiasm for the development of targeted therapy approaches for this disease. Interestingly, there is growing evidence that the prevalence of these mutations reflects to some degree the subtypes of melanoma that have been defined based on clinical and pathologic features. This chapter will review these discoveries, and discuss their implications for the development of new therapeutic approaches for this highly aggressive disease.

BRAF

Activation of the RAS-RAF-MEK-MAPK signaling pathway has been implicated in many cancer types [5, 18, 53]. Activation of this pathway in cancer often results from mutations in components of the pathway, or alternatively by stimulation of a variety of upstream mediators (i.e., growth factor receptors). RAS-family GTP-ases, a family of guanine-nucleotide binding proteins embedded in the inner surface of the cell membrane, represent the first component of the pathway (Fig. 1.1). The RAS family includes three isoforms: NRAS, KRAS, and HRAS. Activating signals change the RAS proteins from a GDP-bound state to the active GTP-bound state. The GTP-bound RAS interacts with and activates the serine-threonine protein kinase RAF, which similarly has three isoforms: ARAF, BRAF, and CRAF (RAF1). The kinase cascade signal propagates when activated RAF phosphorylates the MEK

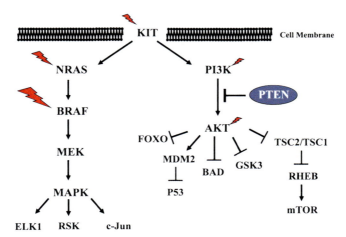

Fig. 1.1 Mutations in kinase signaling pathways in melanoma. *Lightning bolts* indicate genes affected by activating mutations or amplifications; size reflects relative prevalence. *Circle* indicates loss of the PTEN phosphatase

protein kinases (MEK1 and MEK2), thereby activating their serine-threonine protein kinase activity. Activated MEK phosphorylates and activates the p44/42 MAPK serine/threonine protein kinases (ERK1 and ERK2), which is generally referred to as MAPK. The activated MAPK phosphorylates a number of substrates that are the effectors of this pathway, including transcription factors, cytosolic proteins, and other kinases, to promote cell growth and survival.

In 2002, investigators from the Sanger Institute screened a variety of cancer cell lines and tumors for mutations in the *BRAF* gene [10]. While mutations were identified in a small percentage of colon, lung, and ovarian cancers, strikingly over half of the tested melanoma tumors and cell lines had a mutation in the *BRAF* gene. The high prevalence of *BRAF* mutations in melanoma has subsequently been validated in multiple studies. A recent meta-analysis of sequencing results from over 200 studies, including over 2,700 samples, identified a mutation rate of 65% in melanoma cell lines and 42% in uncultured cutaneous melanomas [28]. Mutations in *BRAF* are the most common defined somatic mutation in melanoma.

Over 90% of the identified mutations in *BRAF* affect the valine residue at position 600, and most frequently result in the substitution of a glutamic acid (V600E). The V600E mutation markedly increases the catalytic activity of the BRAF protein, and results in constitutive phosphorylation/activation of MEK and MAPK [10]. The functional importance of the *BRAF V600E* mutation was demonstrated in several early studies, which showed that treatment of melanoma cell lines with this mutation with BRAF siRNA or BRAF inhibitors reduced proliferation and induced cell death [26, 32]. While most studies of the role of *BRAF* mutations in melanoma have focused on the V600E substitution, >50 missense mutations in the gene have been detected in melanoma [28]. In vitro experiments with a spectrum of less common *BRAF* mutations showed that the majority increase the catalytic activity of the BRAF protein (5–700X). However, several of the reported mutations (i.e., G466E, G466V, G596R, D594V) decrease the catalytic activity of BRAF [64]. Interestingly, expression of these low-activity mutant forms still results in increased activation of MEK and MAPK. This pathway activation depends upon interaction of the low-activity mutants with CRAF proteins, whereas the high-activity BRAF mutants activate the pathway independent of CRAF [24, 55].

The initial characterization of the prevalence of *BRAF* mutations was largely conducted in cutaneous melanomas, as they are the most common clinical subtype. In 2005, Dr. Boris Bastian published a seminal paper comparing the molecular characteristics of cutaneous and mucosal melanomas [7]. Based on the hypothesis that tumors arising in the setting of different levels of sun exposure will differ molecularly, the cutaneous tumors in the study were subdivided into three categories: cutaneous melanomas without chronic sun damage (Non-CSD), cutaneous melanomas with chronic sun damage (CSD), and acral lentiginous melanomas. Dr. Bastian's group performed comparative genome hybridization (CGH) to identify regions of copy number gain and loss in these tumor types. Interestingly, the four categories of tumors showed significant differences in the patterns of DNA gain and loss, such that CGH analysis alone was 70% accurate in classifying the tumors. Overall, the acral and mucosal tumors had more regions affected by gain or loss than the cutaneous tumors.

There were also several chromosomal regions that demonstrated significant differences between the Non-CSD and the CSD cutaneous tumors. Having detected significant differences in the copy number analysis, Dr. Bastian went on to sequence the tumors for common mutations. *BRAF* mutations were frequent in the Non-CSD cutaneous melanomas, occurring in 22/40 samples (59%). However, *BRAF* mutations were much less frequent in CSD cutaneous (11%), acral lentiginous (23%), and mucosal melanomas (11%). While this initial study examined a relatively small number of tumors, subsequent studies have generally recapitulated these findings. The meta-analysis of over 203 mutation studies identified an overall *BRAF* mutation rate of 42.5% in cutaneous, 5.6% in mucosal, and 0.8% in uveal melanomas. Among the cutaneous tumors, *BRAF* mutations were common in superficial spreading (53%), spitzoid (33%), and nodular (32%) melanomas, but were less common in acral lentiginous (18.1%) and lentigo maligna (9%) melanomas [28]. Thus, although *BRAF* mutations are the most frequent somatic mutation in melanoma, their prevalence varies widely based on the clinical-pathologic type.

In addition to melanomas, there is evidence that *BRAF* mutations also occur with varying frequency in different types of nevi. Shortly after the initial report of *BRAF* mutations in melanomas, *BRAF* mutations were identified in ~82% of benign nevi [49]. Subsequent studies have demonstrated that common acquired nevi, which represent the majority of nevi and are associated with sun exposure, have a *BRAF* mutation rate (65–87.5%) that is at least as high as that observed in melanoma [31, 50, 54]. A small proportion of nevi develop congenitally; these nevi appear to have a much lower prevalence of *BRAF* mutations (0/32 in one study) [3]. Sptiz nevi, which histologically show high similarity to melanoma, have been reported to have a *BRAF* mutation rate of 5% or less in multiple studies [31, 54]. Blue nevi, which arise in the intradermal layer of the skin, also appear to have a relatively low rate of *BRAF* mutations (12%) [54].

The high prevalence of mutations in common acquired nevi, which have very low malignant potential, suggests that *BRAF* mutations alone cannot fully explain the aggressive nature of melanomas. This hypothesis is supported by functional data testing the transformative potential of the V600E mutant form of BRAF. Studies in human cell lines, zebrafish, and transgenic mice found that expression of the *BRAF V600E* mutation alone failed to fully transform melanocytes [9, 37, 46]. Thus, in addition to identifying critical genetic changes and pathways in melanoma subtypes with a low prevalence of *BRAF* mutations, there is also a need to understand the genetic events that complement *BRAF* mutations to manifest the aggressive behavior of this disease.

NRAS

As described above, mutations in RAS family members are one of the most common activating events in cancer. While mutations in *KRAS* and *HRAS* do not appear to be significant in melanoma, mutations in *NRAS* were identified in melanoma in

1985, well before the discovery of *BRAF* mutations [45]. Similar to BRAF, mutant NRAS activates the RAF-MEK-MAPK signaling pathway. Overall, *NRAS* mutations are present in 14% of human melanoma cell lines and 15–25% of melanoma clinical specimens [15, 28, 42, 59]. The prevalence of *NRAS* mutations varies between different clinical-pathologic types of melanoma, although not as dramatically as observed with *BRAF* mutations. In Dr. Bastian's study of the molecular characteristics of melanoma subtypes, the *NRAS* mutation rate was 22% in Non-CSD cutaneous, 15% in CSD cutaneous, 5% in mucosal, and 10% in acral lentiginous melanomas [7]. The meta-analysis of melanoma mutations studies reported *NRAS* mutations in 26% of cutaneous, 14% of mucosal, and 0.7% of uveal melanomas. Among the cutaneous melanomas, *NRAS* mutations are present in 22% superficial spreading melanoma and 28% nodular melanomas. Lower rates are reported in acral (4%), spitzoid (10%), and lentigo maligna (0/19 samples) melanomas. *NRAS* mutations are also detected in common acquired nevi (6–20%) at a similar rate as has been detected in melanomas [31, 50, 54]. In contrast to *BRAF*, one study identified a very high rate of *NRAS* mutations in congenital nevi [3]. Interestingly, mutational analyses of spitz nevi have reported relatively low rates of *NRAS* mutations, but *HRAS* mutations were identified in 12–29% in these lesions [2, 61].

Similar to *BRAF*, the mutations in *NRAS* are highly conserved. Over 80% of the reported mutations in *NRAS* affect the amino acids at position 12 (i.e., G12D) or 61 (Q61K, Q61R). In melanomas, activating *BRAF* and *NRAS* mutations are almost universally mutually exclusive, although a very small number of tumor and nevi have been identified with both [19, 20, 54]. However, there is more frequent overlap of *NRAS* mutations with low-catalytic activity *BRAF* mutations (i.e., *BRAF D594V*) [24]. While the mutual exclusivity of *BRAF V600E* and *NRAS* mutations supports the hypothesis that both of these events activate MAPK signaling, there is evidence that the mutant NRAS protein activates the pathway in a CRAF-dependent manner [14].

PI3K-AKT Pathway

In addition to activating MEK through a distinct mechanism, the mutant NRAS protein differs from mutant BRAF in its activation of other signaling pathways. One of the pathways critical to the activity of *RAS* is the PI3K-AKT pathway. The PI3K-AKT pathway is one of the most important signaling networks in cancer [63]. PI3K is a lipid kinase that is activated by a variety of stimuli, including growth factor receptors, cell-cell contacts, and RAS family members (Fig. 1.1). Activation of PI3K results in the phosphorylation of phosphatidylinositols at the 3′ position. These phospholipids interact with proteins that have a pleckstrin homology domain, and thereby recruit them to the cell membrane. One such protein is AKT, also known as protein kinase B (PKB). Upon recruitment to the cell membrane AKT, a serine-threonine kinase that normally exists in an inactive state in the cytoplasm, is phosphorylated at two critical residues, Ser473 and Thr308, activating its catalytic activity. The activated AKT molecule translocates to the cytoplasm where it phosphorylates a variety of substrates, including FOXO, GSK3α/β, BAD, TSC2, and MDM2.

Through these and other substrates, activation of AKT regulates a number of processes that contribute to the malignant phenotype, including proliferation, survival, invasion, and angiogenesis [25]. PTEN, a phosphatase that dephosphorylates the 3′ position of phosphatidylinositols, is the major negative regulator of the pathway. Loss of PTEN has been reported in many cancer types, and results in constitutive activation of AKT [68].

The identification of *NRAS* mutations provided the initial evidence for activation of the PI3K-AKT pathway in melanoma. While loss of the *PTEN* gene appears to be frequent in melanoma cell lines, mutations and deletions appear to be much less frequent in patient specimens [21, 66]. However, total loss of PTEN protein expression in the absence of detectable gene deletions or mutations in the gene has also been observed in melanoma, similar to other cancers [39, 69]. Overall, loss of PTEN occurs in 10–30% of melanomas. Loss of PTEN, like *BRAF* mutations, is mutually exclusive with *NRAS* mutation. In contrast, the majority of melanoma tumors and cell lines with PTEN loss also have activating *BRAF* mutations [59]. Genetically, this suggests that the combined presence of mutant BRAF and PTEN loss may be equivalent to *NRAS* mutation. However, a quantitative analysis of AKT activation in melanoma tumors and cell lines demonstrated that loss of PTEN correlated with significantly higher expression of phosphorylated AKT than *NRAS* mutation [12]. The functional significance of PTEN loss in *BRAF*-mutant melanomas is supported by preclinical models. Transgenic mice expressing the BRAF V600E protein develop melanocyte hyperplasia, but they fail to develop invasive lesions. When the *BRAF*-mutant mice were crossed with a strain lacking PTEN, 100% of the mice developed invasive, spontaneously metastatic melanomas [9]. The high rate of *BRAF* mutations in tumors with PTEN loss suggests that activation of the PI3K-AKT pathway most likely occurs with highest frequency in cutaneous melanomas, particularly those without CSD. Consistent with this hypothesis, loss of chromosome 10q, which includes the *PTEN* gene locus, has been detected more frequently in Non-CSD than in CSD cutaneous melanomas [7]. However, there is very little data specifically about PTEN loss, either at the gene or protein level, in other melanoma subtypes. One study has reported complete loss of PTEN protein in 16%, and low expression in 43%, of uveal melanomas [1].

Activating mutations in other components of the PI3K-AKT pathway appear to be quite rare in melanoma. Activating mutations of the catalytic subunit of PI3K, which are detected in up to 20% of breast and colon cancers, have been detected in ~3% of tested samples, and the detected mutations have not involved hotspots commonly involved in other tumor types [8, 41]. Activating mutations of *AKT* homologous to mutations reported in breast, ovarian, and colon cancer have been identified in ~3% of melanomas [13]. Each mutation occurred in a melanoma with a concurrent *BRAF V600E* mutation. Several of the mutations were identified in the AKT3 isoform, which is virtually identical structurally to AKT1 and AKT2, but has a much more restricted pattern of expression in normal adult tissues and cancer. A number of previous studies have demonstrated that AKT3 is the predominant isoform expressed in many melanomas, and may specifically be the predominant isoform that is activated in melanoma metastases [52, 56].

c-KIT

While *BRAF* and *NRAS* mutations appear to be common and functionally significant in cutaneous melanomas, their low prevalence in acral, mucosal, and uveal tumors has spurred investigations to identify other genetic events in these subtypes. In Dr. Bastian's comparative analysis of DNA copy number changes, amplification or copy number gain of the 4q12 region was detected in 18 *BRAF/NRAS* wild-type CSD-cutaneous, acral, and mucosal melanomas, but in none of the non-CSD melanomas [7]. This region includes several genes that have been implicated in cell growth and proliferation, including the v-kit Hardy Zuckerman 4 feline sarcoma viral oncogene homolog *KIT*, the platelet-derived growth factor α receptor *PDGFRA*, and the vascular endothelial growth factor receptor *KDR*. Detailed analysis of the genes in the region identified focal amplification of the *KIT* gene [6]. Further analysis demonstrated that several melanomas had somatic mutations in the *KIT* gene. Overall, *KIT* point mutations or copy number increases were identified in 39% of mucosal, 36% of acral, 28% of CSD-cutaneous, and 0% of non-CSD cutaneous melanomas. Subsequent studies by other groups have validated the high prevalence of *KIT* mutations in acral and mucosal melanomas [65]. These studies have also confirmed the near complete absence of *KIT* alterations in non-CSD cutaneous melanomas, but lower rates have been reported in CSD-cutaneous tumors [22]. To date, no *KIT* mutations have been identified in uveal melanoma [34, 44].

KIT is a receptor tyrosine protein kinase. Upon ligand binding, the activated KIT receptor activates a variety of kinase signaling pathways, including the RAS-RAF-MEK-MAPK and the PI3K-AKT pathways in various cellular settings. Somatic mutations of the *KIT* gene are present in ~80% of GIST [27]. The mutations in the *KIT* gene in GIST affect the regulatory and catalytic domains of the protein, and result in increased KIT activity and signaling. Both in vitro experiments and clinical trials have demonstrated that *KIT* mutations in GIST result in oncogenic addiction to KIT-mediated survival signals, and treatment with KIT inhibitors results in tumor shrinkage and improved survival in the overwhelming majority of patients [11].

The *KIT* mutations detected in melanoma affect the same exons that are affected by mutations in GIST. The discovery of activating *KIT* mutations in melanoma was somewhat surprising, as a number of lines of evidence supported a role for the loss of KIT function in melanoma progression. Immunohistochemical studies have shown that loss of KIT protein expression correlates with melanoma progression [30]. In addition, enforced expression of KIT protein in cell lines inhibited the growth of human melanoma cell lines in vitro and in vivo [30]. Finally, three different phase II trials of the KIT inhibitor imatinib (Gleevec®) reported only a single clinical response among a total of 63 treated patients [33, 60, 67].

The finding that *KIT* aberrations specifically occur in non-cutaneous melanomas suggests that the KIT protein may have a different functional role in acral, mucosal, and CSD-cutaneous melanomas. IHC studies have shown that KIT protein is frequently expressed in acral and mucosal melanomas, particularly in those with *KIT* mutations or amplifications [57]. In addition, several case reports have described impressive clinical responses to various KIT inhibitors in melanoma patients with *KIT* mutations [29, 51]. The responsiveness of melanomas with amplification of the wild-type *KIT* gene is less established, but is currently being investigated in clinical trials restricted to patients with *KIT* gene abnormalities [16].

GNAQ

Less than 1% of uveal melanomas have activating mutations in *BRAF*, *NRAS*, or *KIT*. In 2003, two different groups reported the identification of point mutations in the *GNAQ* gene [43, 62]. *GNAQ* encodes the α-subunit of the G-protein-coupled receptor. In both studies, *GNAQ* point mutations involving the Q209 residue were identified in ~50% of uveal melanomas. In contrast, *GNAQ* mutations were detected in only 1 of 42 cutaneous melanomas, and 0/15 acral melanomas [62]. The Q209 residue that is the site of all of the *GNAQ* mutations reported to date is analogous to the Q61 residue of *NRAS* that is the most common site of mutations in that gene. Expression of the Q209L mutant form of the GNAQ protein resulted in increased activation of MAPK, enhanced anchorage-independent growth, and increased tumorigenicity of melanocytes [62]. Recently, point mutations in another G-protein regulatory subunit, *GNA11*, have been identified in 34% of primary uveal melanomas, and 59% of uveal melanoma metastases [16]. The *GNA11* and *GNAQ* mutations are mutually exclusive. Thus, approximately 80% of uveal melanomas harbor a mutation in one of these subunits, similar to the cumulative frequency of *BRAF* and *NRAS* mutations in cutaneous melanomas. Hopefully an improved understanding of the consequences of these mutations will lead to new, more effective treatments for uveal melanomas.

Conclusions

In the last 10 years, the classification of melanoma has dramatically changed with the identification of targetable mutations in this disease. This is primarily being driven by the selection of specific therapeutics based on the mutations present in a patient's tumor. This strategy has proven to be critical in the use of the mutant-specific BRAF inhibitor PLX4032. While PLX4032 treatment has produced significant tumor shrinkage in the majority of *BRAF*-mutant melanoma patients, no responses were seen in patients without a *BRAF* mutation [17]. Perhaps even more critically, experiments in preclinical models support that treatment of *BRAF*-wild-type tumors with BRAF inhibitors may actually accelerate tumor growth [23]. The clinical experience with PLX4032 emphasizes the need for careful consideration of the molecular characteristics of the tumors in the future development of targeted therapies in this disease. As chromosomal studies indicate that acral and mucosal tumors are characterized by distinct regions of copy number gain and loss, it will be important to determine if *BRAF*-mutant tumors arising from those sites respond differently to BRAF inhibitors relative to the *BRAF*-mutant cutaneous melanomas. In addition to informing decisions about the choice of systemic therapies, it will be important to determine if the presence of the targetable mutations correlates with the risk of disease progression and/or recurrence in localized melanoma. Prognostic significance of the mutations could then be used to guide the appropriate use of aggressive vs. conservative management of localized tumors. Such findings would also emphasize the need to include mutational analysis as an integral part of the classification of every melanoma.

While the discovery and characterization of *BRAF*, *NRAS*, *PTEN*, *KIT*, and *GNAQ* mutations has clearly improved our understanding of melanoma, there remains a tremendous need to gather additional information about the molecular basis of these tumors. The prevalence of *BRAF* and *NRAS* mutations in nevi with low malignant potential indicates that additional molecules and/or pathways must contribute to the pathogenesis of invasive melanoma. The identification of such factors would inform the clinical stratification of premalignant or low-grade lesions. In addition to the need to identify events that complement the known mutations, $\geq 30\%$ of melanoma patients have no detectable mutation in any of the genes described here. The identification and characterization of genetic aberrations in these patients may help illuminate whether the different mutations that occur in melanoma converge on the same pathways and therapeutic targets (i.e., the MAPK pathway), or if they in fact are dependent upon completely distinct pathways and thus novel therapeutic strategies. Recently, the sequencing of the first complete melanoma genome was reported [48]. This study identified over 33,000 somatic changes in the melanoma genome, including 186 missense or truncating mutations in coding regions of DNA, as well as numerous chromosomal rearrangements. These initial findings support the need for similar analyses of additional melanoma genomes to identify recurrent events to prioritize for functional testing. However, the existing data regarding genetic and functional differences in molecules and pathways between different clinical-pathologic melanoma subtypes (i.e. *KIT*) should serve as a reminder of the need to place such studies within the appropriate context.

References

1. Abdel-Rahman MH, Yang Y, Zhou X-P, Craig EL, Davidorf FH, Eng C. High frequency of submicroscopic hemizygous deletion is a major mechanism of loss of expression of PTEN in uveal melanoma. J Clin Oncol. 2006;24:288–95.
2. Bastian BC, LeBoit PE, Pinkel D. Mutations and copy number increase of HRAS in Spitz nevi with distinctive histopathological features. Am J Pathol. 2000;157:967–72.
3. Bauer J, Curtin JA, Pinkel D, Bastian BC. Congenital melanocytic nevi frequently harbor NRAS mutations but no BRAF mutations. J Invest Dermatol. 2007;127:179–82.
4. Buzdar AU. Hormonal therapy in early and advanced breast cancer. Breast J. 2004;10 Suppl 1:S19–21.
5. Colicelli J. Human RAS superfamily proteins and related GTPases. Sci STKE. 2004; 2004(250):RE13.

6. Curtin JA, Busam K, Pinkel D, Bastian BC. Somatic activation of KIT in distinct subtypes of melanoma. J Clin Oncol. 2006;24:4340–6.
7. Curtin JA, Fridlyand J, Kageshita T, Patel HN, Busam KJ, Kutzner H, et al. Distinct sets of genetic alterations in melanoma. N Engl J Med. 2005;353:2135–47.
8. Curtin JA, Stark MS, Pinkel D, Hayward NK, Bastian BC. PI3-kinase subunits are infrequent somatic targets in melanoma. J Invest Dermatol. 2006;126:1660–3.
9. Dankort D, Curley DP, Cartlidge RA, Nelson B, Karnezis AN, Damsky Jr WE, et al. Braf(V600E) cooperates with Pten loss to induce metastatic melanoma. Nat Genet. 2009;41: 544–52.
10. Davies H, Bignell GR, Cox C, Stephens P, Edkins S, Clegg S, et al. Mutations of the BRAF gene in human cancer. Nature. 2002;417:949–54.
11. Davies M, Hennessy B, Mills GB. Point mutations of protein kinases and individualised cancer therapy. Expert Opin Pharmacother. 2006;7:2243–61.
12. Davies MA, Stemke-Hale K, Lin E, Tellez C, Deng W, Gopal YN, et al. Integrated molecular and clinical analysis of AKT activation in metastatic melanoma. Clin Cancer Res. 2009;15: 7538–46.
13. Davies MA, Stemke-Hale K, Tellez C, Calderone TL, Deng W, Prieto VG, et al. A novel AKT3 mutation in melanoma tumours and cell lines. Br J Cancer. 2008;99:1265–8.
14. Dumaz N, Hayward R, Martin J, Ogilvie L, Hedley D, Curtin JA, et al. In melanoma, RAS mutations are accompanied by switching signaling from BRAF to CRAF and disrupted cyclic AMP signaling. Cancer Res. 2006;66:9483–91.
15. Edlundh-Rose EA, Egyhazi SB, Omholt KB, Mansson-Brahme EB, Platz AB, Hansson JB, et al. NRAS and BRAF mutations in melanoma tumours in relation to clinical characteristics: a study based on mutation screening by pyrosequencing. Melanoma Res. 2006;16:471–8.
16. Fisher DE, Barnhill R, Hodi FS, Herlyn M, Merlino G, Medrano E, et al. Melanoma from bench to bedside: meeting report from the 6th international melanoma congress. Pigment Cell Melanoma Res. 2010;23:14–26.
17. Flaherty KT, Puzanov J, Sosman J, Kim K, Ribas A, McArthur G, et al. Phase I study of PLX4032: proof of concept for V600E BRAF mutation as a therapeutic target in human cancer. J Clin Oncol. 2009;27:9000.
18. Giehl K. Oncogenic Ras in tumor progression and metastasis. Biol Chem. 2005;386: 193–205.
19. Goel VK, Lazar AJ, Warneke CL, Redston MS, Haluska FG. Examination of mutations in BRAF, NRAS, and PTEN in primary cutaneous melanoma. J Invest Dermatol. 2006;126: 154–60.
20. Gorden A, Osman I, Gai W, He D, Huang W, Davidson A, et al. Analysis of BRAF and N-RAS mutations in metastatic melanoma tissues. Cancer Res. 2003;63:3955–7.
21. Haluska FG, Tsao H, Wu H, Haluska FS, Lazar A, Goel V. Genetic alterations in signaling pathways in melanoma. Clin Cancer Res. 2006;12:2301s–7.
22. Handolias D, Salemi R, Murray W, Tan A, Liu W, Viros A, et al. Mutations in KIT occur at low frequency in melanomas arising from anatomical sites associated with chronic and intermittent sun exposure. Pigment Cell Melanoma Res. 2010;23:210–5.
23. Hatzivassiliou G, Song K, Yen I, Brandhuber BJ, Anderson DJ, Alvarado R, et al. RAF inhibitors prime wild-type RAF to activate the MAPK pathway and enhance growth. Nature. 2010;464(7287):431–5.
24. Heidorn SJ, Milagre C, Whittaker S, Nourry A, Niculescu-Duvas I, Dhomen N, et al. Kinase-dead BRAF and oncogenic RAS cooperate to drive tumor progression through CRAF. Cell. 2010;140:209–21.
25. Hennessy BT, Smith DL, Ram PT, Lu Y, Mills GB. Exploiting the PI3K/AKT pathway for cancer drug discovery. Nat Rev Drug Discov. 2005;4:988–1004.
26. Hingorani SR, Jacobetz MA, Robertson GP, Herlyn M, Tuveson DA. Suppression of BRAF(V599E) in human melanoma abrogates transformation. Cancer Res. 2003;63:5198–202.
27. Hirota S, Isozaki K, Moriyama Y, Hashimoto K, Nishida T, Ishiguro S, et al. Gain-of-function mutations of c-kit in human gastrointestinal stromal tumors. Science. 1998;279:577–80.

28. Hocker T, Tsao H. Ultraviolet radiation and melanoma: a systematic review and analysis of reported sequence variants. Hum Mutat. 2007;28:578–88.
29. Hodi FS, Friedlander P, Corless CL, Heinrich MC, Mac Rae S, Kruse A, et al. Major response to imatinib mesylate in KIT-mutated melanoma. J Clin Oncol. 2008;26:2046–51.
30. Huang S, Luca M, Gutman M, McConkey DJ, Langley KE, Lyman SD, et al. Enforced c-KIT expression renders highly metastatic human melanoma cells susceptible to stem cell factor-induced apoptosis and inhibits their tumorigenic and metastatic potential. Oncogene. 1996;13: 2339–47.
31. Indsto JO, Kumar S, Wang L, Crotty KA, Arbuckle SM, Mann GJ. Low prevalence of RAS-RAF-activating mutations in Spitz melanocytic nevi compared with other melanocytic lesions. J Cutan Pathol. 2007;34:448–55.
32. Karasarides M, Chiloeches A, Hayward R, Niculescu-Duvaz D, Scanlon I, Friedlos F, et al. B-RAF is a therapeutic target in melanoma. Oncogene. 2004;23:6292–8.
33. Kim KB, Eton O, Davis DW, Frazier ML, McConkey DJ, Diwan AH, et al. Phase II trial of imatinib mesylate in patients with metastatic melanoma. Br J Cancer. 2008;99:734–40.
34. Lefevre G, Glotin AL, Calipel A, Mouriaux F, Tran T, Kherrouche Z, et al. Roles of stem cell factor/c-Kit and effects of Glivec/STI571 in human uveal melanoma cell tumorigenesis. J Biol Chem. 2004;279:31769–79.
35. Mass RD, Press MF, Anderson S, Cobleigh MA, Vogel CL, Dybdal N, et al. Evaluation of clinical outcomes according to HER2 detection by fluorescence in situ hybridization in women with metastatic breast cancer treated with trastuzumab. Clin Breast Cancer. 2005;6:240–6.
36. McGuire WL. Current status of estrogen receptors in human breast cancer. Cancer. 1975;36: 638–44.
37. Michaloglou C, Vredeveld LC, Soengas MS, Denoyelle C, Kuilman T, van der Horst CM, et al. BRAFE600-associated senescence-like cell cycle arrest of human naevi. Nature. 2005;436:720–4.
38. Miller AJ, Mihm Jr MC. Melanoma. N Engl J Med. 2006;355:51–65.
39. Mirmohammadsadegh A, Marini A, Nambiar S, Hassan M, Tannapfel A, Ruzicka T, et al. Epigenetic silencing of the PTEN gene in melanoma. Cancer Res. 2006;66:6546–52.
40. Morton DL, Essner R, Kirkwood JM, Wollman RC. Malignant melanoma. In: Kufe DW, Bast RC, Hait WN, Hong WK, Pollock RE, Weichselbaum RR, Holland JF, Frei E, editors. Cancer medicine. Hamilton: BC Decker Inc.; 2006. p. 1644–62.
41. Omholt K, Krockel D, Ringborg U, Hansson J. Mutations of PIK3CA are rare in cutaneous melanoma. Melanoma Res. 2006;16:197–200.
42. Omholt K, Platz A, Kanter L, Ringborg U, Hansson J. NRAS and BRAF mutations arise early during melanoma pathogenesis and are preserved throughout tumor progression. Clin Cancer Res. 2003;9:6483–8.
43. Onken MD, Worley LA, Long MD, Duan S, Council ML, Bowcock AM, et al. Oncogenic mutations in GNAQ occur early in uveal melanoma. Invest Ophthalmol Vis Sci. 2008;49: 5230–4.
44. Pache M, Glatz K, Bosch D, Dirnhofer S, Mirlacher M, Simon R, et al. Sequence analysis and high-throughput immunohistochemical profiling of KIT (CD 117) expression in uveal melanoma using tissue microarrays. Virchows Arch. 2003;443:741–4.
45. Padua RA, Barrass NC, Currie GA. Activation of N-ras in a human melanoma cell line. Mol Cell Biol. 1985;5:582–5.
46. Patton EE, Widlund HR, Kutok JL, Kopani KR, Amatruda JF, Murphey RD, et al. BRAF mutations are sufficient to promote nevi formation and cooperate with p53 in the genesis of melanoma. Curr Biol. 2005;15:249–54.
47. Piccart-Gebhart MJ, Procter M, Leyland-Jones B, Goldhirsch A, Untch M, Smith I, et al. Trastuzumab after adjuvant chemotherapy in HER2-positive breast cancer. N Engl J Med. 2005;353:1659–72.
48. Pleasance ED, Cheetham RK, Stephens PJ, McBride DJ, Humphray SJ, Greenman CD, et al. A comprehensive catalogue of somatic mutations from a human cancer genome. Nature. 2010;463: 191–6.

49. Pollock PM, Harper UL, Hansen KS, Yudt LM, Stark M, Robbins CM, et al. High frequency of BRAF mutations in nevi. Nat Genet. 2003;33:19–20.
50. Poynter JNA, Elder JTBCI, Fullen DRD, Nair RPB, Soengas MSB, Johnson TMBEF, et al. BRAF and NRAS mutations in melanoma and melanocytic nevi. Melanoma Res. 2006;16: 267–73.
51. Quintas-Cardama A, Lazar AJ, Woodman SE, Kim K, Ross M, Hwu P. Complete response of stage IV anal mucosal melanoma expressing KIT Val560Asp to the multikinase inhibitor sorafenib. Nat Clin Practice Oncol. 2008;5:737–40.
52. Robertson GP. Functional and therapeutic significance of Akt deregulation in malignant melanoma. Cancer Metastasis Rev. 2005;24:273–85.
53. Rubinfeld H, Seger R. The ERK cascade: a prototype of MAPK signaling. Mol Biotechnol. 2005;31:151–74.
54. Saldanha G, Purnell D, Fletcher A, Potter L, Gillies A, Pringle JH. High BRAF mutation frequency does not characterize all melanocytic tumor types. Int J Cancer. 2004;111:705–10.
55. Smalley KS, Xiao M, Villanueva J, Nguyen TK, Flaherty KT, Letrero R, et al. CRAF inhibition induces apoptosis in melanoma cells with non-V600E BRAF mutations. Oncogene. 2009;28:85–94.
56. Stahl JM, Sharma A, Cheung M, Zimmerman M, Cheng JQ, Bosenberg MW, et al. Deregulated Akt3 activity promotes development of malignant melanoma. Cancer Res. 2004;64:7002–10.
57. Torres-Cabala CA, Wang WL, Trent J, Yang D, Chen S, Galbincea J, et al. Correlation between KIT expression and KIT mutation in melanoma: a study of 173 cases with emphasis on the acral-lentiginous/mucosal type. Mod Pathol. 2009;22:1446–56.
58. Tsao H, Atkins MB, Sober AJ. Management of cutaneous melanoma. N Engl J Med. 2004;351:998–1012.
59. Tsao H, Goel V, Wu H, Yang G, Haluska FG. Genetic interaction between NRAS and BRAF mutations and PTEN//MMAC1 inactivation in melanoma. J Investig Dermatol. 2004;122: 337–41.
60. Ugurel S, Hildenbrand R, Zimpfer A, La Rosee P, Paschka P, Sucker A, et al. Lack of clinical efficacy of imatinib in metastatic melanoma. Br J Cancer. 2005;92:1398–405.
61. van Dijk MCRFMD, Bernsen MRP, Ruiter DJP. Analysis of mutations in B-RAF, N-RAS, and H-RAS genes in the differential diagnosis of spitz nevus and spitzoid melanoma. Am J Surg Pathol. 2005;29:1145–51.
62. Van Raamsdonk CD, Bezrookove V, Green G, Bauer J, Gaugler L, O'Brien JM, et al. Frequent somatic mutations of GNAQ in uveal melanoma and blue naevi. Nature. 2009;457:599–602.
63. Vivanco I, Sawyers CL. The phosphatidylinositol 3-Kinase AKT pathway in human cancer. Nat Rev Cancer. 2002;2:489–501.
64. Wan PTC, Garnett MJ, Roe SM, Lee S, Niculescu-Duvaz D, Good VM, et al. Mechanism of activation of the RAF-ERK signaling pathway by oncogenic mutations of B-RAF. Cell. 2004;116:855–67.
65. Woodman S. Targeting KIT in melanoma: a paradigm of molecular medicine and targeted therapeutics. Biochem Pharmacol. 2010;80(5):568–74.
66. Wu H, Goel V, Haluska FG. PTEN signaling pathways in melanoma. Oncogene. 2003;22:3113–22.
67. Wyman K, Atkins MB, Prieto V, Eton O, McDermott DF, Hubbard F, et al. Multicenter phase II trial of high-dose imatinib mesylate in metastatic melanoma: significant toxicity with no clinical efficacy. Cancer. 2006;106:2005–11.
68. Yuan TL, Cantley LC. PI3K pathway alterations in cancer: variations on a theme. Oncogene. 2008;27:5497–510.
69. Zhou XP, Gimm O, Hampel H, Niemann T, Walker MJ, Eng C. Epigenetic PTEN silencing in malignant melanomas without PTEN mutation. Am J Pathol. 2000;157:1123–8.

Chapter 2
Melanoma Genomics

Mohammed Kashani-Sabet

Abstract Remarkably, 10 years have elapsed since the initial paper describing genomic profiles of melanoma (Nature 406:536–540, 2000). Since that initial publication, several additional studies have been published examining the potential utility of gene expression profiling of melanoma using a plethora of different technological platforms, data sets, and tissue collections. These studies have provided significant new insights into several aspects of melanoma biology. These include the development of molecular diagnostics assays based on gene expression profiles that are nearing clinical application. As a result, the time is ripe to review the literature regarding gene expression profiling of melanoma. This review will focus on the insights gained in the transcriptomic analysis of (1) distinct phases of melanoma progression; (2) primary melanoma; and (3) metastatic melanoma.

Keywords Gene expression profiling • Microarray analysis • Biomarkers

Gene Expression Profiling of Distinct Phases of Melanoma Progression

Melanoma is an ideal clinical model to which genomic analyses can be applied to study tumor progression because of the readily defined clinical phases of melanoma progression that have histological correlates. The classical model of melanoma progression, defined by Clark et al. [2], described these successive stages, and has represented an important framework for the identification of novel melanoma progression genes. In this model, benign melanocytic proliferation yields a nevus, which can transform into primary melanoma, beginning in the radial growth phase,

M. Kashani-Sabet, MD (✉)
Center for Melanoma Research and Treatment, California Pacific Medical Center
Research Institute, 475 Brannan Street, San Francisco, CA 94107, USA
e-mail: kashani@cpmcri.org

T.F. Gajewski and F.S. Hodi (eds.), *Targeted Therapeutics in Melanoma*,
Current Clinical Oncology, DOI 10.1007/978-1-61779-407-0_2,
© Springer Science+Business Media, LLC 2012

with a capacity to progress to the vertical growth phase, and culminating in metastatic melanoma. While melanoma development is not absolutely dependent on the progression through each of these distinct phases (e.g., melanomas can develop without the presence of preexisting nevi), the vertical growth phase has been postulated to be required for metastatic competency. While this model of melanoma progression was described several years ago and is well understood, prior to the advent of microarray analysis, one would be hard pressed to identify genes whose differential expression corresponded to any of these phases of melanoma progression. In addition, it is important to note that, while BRAF mutations appear to represent an important event in melanoma progression [3] and appear to represent an attractive target for melanoma therapy [4], the high prevalence of BRAF mutations in nevi suggests that they are selected for early in melanoma development. As a result, BRAF mutations are unable to distinguish between the successive phases in melanoma progression as described by this classical model.

To date, several studies have examined the comparative gene expression profiles of melanoma progression. The first published study by Haqq et al. [5] assigned separate gene expression profiles to these distinct phases of melanoma progression using cDNA microarray analysis. Thus, statistical analysis of microarrays (SAM) was able to distinguish between nevi and primary melanomas, and primary and metastatic melanomas. Intriguingly, microarray analysis of radial vs. vertical growth phase melanoma demonstrated exclusive loss of gene expression in the vertical growth phase, and also showed that the gene expression profile characteristic of radial growth phase melanoma was recapitulated in a subset of metastases. These studies suggested that the gene expression signature for metastasis was present in the radial growth phase, challenging the conventional dogma that radial growth phase melanomas are incapable of metastasis.

In addition, unsupervised hierarchical analysis was able to accurately discriminate between a small number of freshly acquired primary melanomas and nevi. This suggested that gene expression profiles could be useful as an adjunct to the pathological diagnosis of melanoma, which has been shown to be discordant in a relatively high percentage of cases [6]. Recently, five markers derived from that microarray analysis were selected for further validation and incorporation into an immunohistochemical multi-marker assay for melanoma [7]. This multi-marker assay was shown to have a high degree of accuracy in the diagnosis of melanocytic neoplasms, with a specificity of 95% and a sensitivity of 91% in a training set of 534 nevi and primary melanomas, comprising the largest analysis of molecular markers in melanoma to date. Subsequently, the multi-marker assay was subjected to four validation sets with greater relevance to the differential diagnosis of nevus vs. melanoma, and found to accurately diagnose a high percentage of melanomas arising in a nevus, Spitz, and dysplastic nevi. Finally, the multi-marker assay was able to correctly diagnose 75% of misdiagnosed neoplasms, suggesting that these markers could help prevent or correct a high percentage of diagnostic errors using routine histopathology of melanocytic neoplasms. This is one of the first demonstrations of the utility of genomic profiles to resolve a differential diagnosis in the realm of oncology, and one of the first successful validations of gene expression profiles

Table 2.1 Selected validated differentially expressed genes between nevi and primary melanoma

Gene	Platform	Gene bank accession number	References
ARPC2	RNA, IHC	NM_005731	[5, 6]
CDH3	RNA	NM_001793	[6, 7]
FN1	RNA, IHC	NM_212482	[5, 6]
KNSL5	RNA	NM_138555	[6, 7]
PLAB	RNA	NM_004864	[6, 7]
PRAME	RNA	NM_206954	[6, 10]
RGS1	RNA, IHC	NM_002922	[5, 6]
SPP1	RNA, IHC	NM_001040058	[5–7]
WNT2	RNA, IHC	NM_003391	[5, 6]

IHC immunohistochemistry

using immunohistochemical techniques. Following further validation in distinct cohorts, it is anticipated that this assay will be available for clinical use.

Subsequently, additional studies investigating the differential gene expression signature of melanoma progression were reported. Three studies have examined the transition between nevus and melanoma. Talantov et al. [8] analyzed 45 primary melanomas, 18 benign nevi, and 7 normal skin specimens analyzed using the Affymetrix platform. Hierarchical clustering was able to identify a unique signature for melanomas. Among the genes overexpressed in melanomas were SPP1 (osteopontin), PLAB, SEMA3B, NES, MAP3K12, and DUSP4. Intriguingly, several genes were identified that were previously shown to be differentially expressed in the Haqq et al. study [5], including SPP1, PLAB, CDH3, KNSL5, CITED1, CSTB, and PSEN2. Separately, Nambiar et al. [9] profiled 11 congenital nevi, 10 primary and 11 metastatic melanomas using the Affymetrix platform. They also identified gene signatures that distinguished nevi from primary melanomas. Upregulated in melanomas were MAPK1, STAT3, ASK/Dbf4, CCNA1, CCNB1, CCNE2, CXCL1, and MCM4. Among the genes downregulated in melanomas were SPON1 and IL-18.

Finally, Koh et al. [10] used a custom array containing 1,100 selected genes to search for differential gene signatures in a tissue set of 120 lesions. They observed higher expression of PHACTR1, HLA-A, HLA-B, PRAME, and STAT1 in melanomas, with higher expression of PTN, GPX3, FABP7, DLC1, and GSTM2 in nevi. The use of these gene signatures was shown to have concordance rates of 90% for melanoma and 86% for nevi. Thus, it is clear that distinct gene expression profiles exist for nevi vs. melanomas, and that these differential gene signatures can be used to assist in this potentially problematic differential diagnosis. A list of novel diagnostic markers for melanoma consistently appearing in several of these studies appears in Table 2.1.

Additional work has focused on exploring the transition between primary and metastatic melanoma. Jaeger et al. [11] profiled 19 primary and 22 metastatic melanomas using Affymetrix oligonucleotide microarrays, and identified 308 genes with differential expression between primary and metastatic lesions. The upregulated genes included SPP1, CDC6, CDK1, mitosin, and fibronectin, whereas E-cadherin, FGFBP, desmocollins 1 and 3, and CCL27 were downregulated. The differential expression of selected genes in metastatic vs. primary melanomas was validated by immunohistochemical analysis. Using support vector machines, greater than 85% correct classification was achieved between the two types of lesions. Intriguingly, characteristic gene expression profiles were identified in superficial spreading vs. nodular melanomas, and in thin (<1.0 mm) vs. intermediate/thick tumors (>2.0 mm). This is similar to the results identified by Riker et al. [12], who identified a transition point in global transcript profiles, in which melanomas greater than 2 mm in thickness had a gene expression pattern similar to metastases.

Gene Expression Profiles of Primary Melanoma

Due to the paucity of freshly acquired primary melanoma specimens, only a few studies examining the genomic signatures of large numbers of primary melanoma have been performed. In the first study in this category, Winnepenninckx et al. [13] profiled 58 primary melanomas with at least 4 years of follow-up or relapse/death using a pangenomic 44,000 60-mer oligonucleotide microarray. The investigators identified 254 genes that were associated with distant metastasis-free survival, which included genes involved in activating DNA replication origins, e.g., minichromosome maintenance genes and geminin. Twenty-three of these genes were examined at the protein level using immunohistochemical analysis, and found to be associated with overall survival in an independent set. These included MCM3, MCM4, MCM6, KPNA2, and geminin. In a multivariate analysis that included thickness, age, ulceration, and sex, MCM4 and MCM6 were still significantly predictive of overall survival.

Subsequently, the same group of investigators examined whether a gene expression signature correlates with the presence of BRAF mutations in primary cutaneous melanoma [14]. Thus, a cohort of 69 primary melanomas on which global transcript profiles were available was tested for the presence of BRAF mutations. The expression data from these melanomas was analyzed according to BRAF mutational status in 32 melanomas with a BRAF mutation (46%). Two-hundred and nine genes were identified to be differentially expressed in melanomas harboring mutant BRAF, including genes that may be involved in immune responsiveness, such as CD63, MAGE-D2, S100A, and HSP70. In addition, additional genes previously implicated in melanoma progression were identified, including SPP1, CTSB, SERPINE2, and IGFBP2, and in the MITF pathway, such as S100B and MIA-1.

In addition, Alonso et al. [15] examined the gene expression profiles of 34 vertical growth phase melanomas using cDNA microarrays. This tissue set included 21 patients with nodal metastasis vs. 13 without. Supervised analysis of metastasizing melanomas vs. the non-metastasizing group identified 243 differentially expressed genes, of which 206 were upregulated. These included genes involved in numerous cellular pathways, such as cell cycle and apoptosis regulation, epithelial-to-mesenchymal transition, nucleic acid binding, protein synthesis, and metabolism. The prognostic role of SPP1, CDH2, and SPARC on disease-free survival was demonstrated by univariate analysis using immunohistochemical staining.

Table 2.2 Validated molecular prognostic markers for melanoma derived from transcriptomic profiles

Marker	Platform	Outcome parameter	References
RGS1	IHC	RFS, DSS, SLN status	[19, 20]
NCOA3	IHC	RFS, DSS, SLN status	[17, 20]
SPP1	IHC, RNA	RFS, DSS, SLN status	[15, 16, 18, 20]
CDH2	IHC	RFS	[15]
SPARC	IHC	RFS	[15]
MCM4	IHC	OS	[13]
MCM6	IHC	OS	[13]

More recently, Conway et al. [16] performed a profiling analysis of paraffin-embedded primary melanomas using the Illumina DASL array human cancer panel in two distinct cohorts. Intriguingly, SPP1 was identified as the most differentially expressed gene in association with relapse-free survival (RFS) in the first cohort. The association between SPP1 expression and RFS was validated in the second cohort. By multivariate analysis, SPP1 expression level was an independent predictor of RFS when adjusted for age, sex, tumor site, and histological parameters. In addition, the expression of PBX1, BIRC5, and HLF was most strongly correlated with SPP1 expression.

Finally, the prognostic role of several genes identified from the microarray analysis of distinct phases of melanoma progression [5] has been recently demonstrated. From this analysis, three markers (SPP1, NCOA3, and RGS1) were shown to individually predict three outcome parameters for melanoma: sentinel lymph node (SLN) status, RFS, and disease-specific survival (DSS) using immunohistochemical analysis [17–19]. Subsequently, a multi-marker assay incorporating the expression levels of these proteins was examined for its prognostic role in an initial U.S. cohort of 395 patients, and an independent cohort of 141 patients from a distinct population (Germany) [20]. Multi-marker positivity was significantly associated with SLN status and DSS by univariate analysis in the initial cohort. By multivariate analysis, the multi-marker assay remained independently predictive of SLN status and DSS when adjusted for tumor thickness, ulceration, mitotic rate, age, Clark level, gender, and tumor site. In the analysis of DSS, the multi-marker score was the most significant factor predicting DSS, even when SLN status was included as a covariate in the multivariate model. The powerful and independent prognostic impact of the multi-marker assay was separately confirmed using a digital imaging analysis. In the validation cohort, multi-marker positivity was significantly predictive of DSS, and again outperformed routine clinical and histological factors. This is the first demonstration of the prognostic efficacy of a multi-marker assay in melanoma, and the first demonstration of the prognostic efficacy of molecular markers for melanoma in a distinct patient cohort.

Taken together, these results demonstrate the utility of gene expression profiling of primary melanomas, and have identified several novel prognostic markers of melanoma outcome with various degrees of validation (Table 2.2). Intriguingly,

SPP1 has emerged as a common candidate prognostic marker from these profiling studies, whose prognostic impact has now been validated in several distinct cohorts and using different expression platforms.

Gene Expression Profiling of Metastatic Melanoma

Numerous studies of transcriptomic profiling of metastatic melanoma have now been reported. In general, these studies have attempted to either examine various aspects of melanoma biology, or identify potential markers of immune responsiveness. Bittner et al. [1] examined gene signatures of metastatic melanoma using what is now considered an early cDNA microarray platform containing 6,971 unique genes. The authors identified two subtypes of metastatic melanoma, including a dominant cluster, characterized by higher expression of MART-1, CD63, tropomyosin, and WNT5A and reduced expression of fibronectin. This cluster of metastatic melanomas was found to be inversely correlated with uveal melanoma cell lines with increased invasiveness, and showed a trend toward improved survival. Subsequently, Haqq et al. [5] also identified two subtypes of metastatic melanoma, with some overlap in the gene set identified by Bittner et al. The two subtypes were not distinguished by any clinical or histological characteristics or BRAF mutation status, but did differ in that the dominant subgroup exhibited the gene expression signature of vertical growth phase primary melanoma, whereas the second subtype retained the gene signature identified in radial growth phase melanoma. Again, the dominant cluster was associated with an improved prognosis, indicating that radial growth phase metastatic melanoma may be associated with a worse outlook. Together, these studies suggested the prognostic potential of gene expression profiles of metastatic melanoma in small subgroups of patients.

Subsequently, additional studies have extended a number of these observations in larger patient cohorts. John et al. [21] examined genomic profiles of 29 cases of stage III and stage IV melanoma divided into good-prognosis and poor-prognosis subgroups based on time to progression using an oligo-array platform. A predictive score developed using these genes was found to correctly classify nine of ten patients in an independent tissue set, and 12 of 14 patients from a published database. Importantly, this gene signature was developed from a supervised analysis, with no prognostic impact shown for the gene expression profiles.

In addition, Bogunovic et al. [22] examined the combination of gene expression profiles and other markers in the prognostic assessment of metastatic melanoma patients, and identified a group of 266 genes associated with post-recurrence survival. They identified several factors associated with prolonged survival, including mitotic rate of metastatic lesions, an immune response gene signature, and presence of TILs and CD3+ cells. Thus gene signatures can be combined with other histological prognostic factors and/or biomarkers to refine the survival associated with metastatic melanoma.

More recently, Jonsson et al. [23] examined the gene expression profiles of 57 patients with stage IV melanoma using the Illumina Beadarray system, and identified four subtypes of metastatic melanoma by unsupervised hierarchical analysis. These four subtypes were grouped as follows: (1) immune response group (characterized by LCK, IFNGR1, HLA class I antigen, CXCL12, and IL1R1 expression); (2) pigmentation differentiation (characterized by high MITF, TYR, SILV, DCT, and low WNT5A levels); (3) proliferation (characterized by high E2F1, BUB1, and CCNA2 expression), and (4) normal-like (characterized by high KRT10 and 17, KIT, FGFR3, and EGFR levels). In addition, BRAF and NRAS mutational analysis and examination of deletions in the CDKN2A gene were performed. Intriguingly, the proliferative subtype was associated with poor survival, high frequency of CDKN2A deletions, and the absence of BRAF or NRAS wild-type samples. In addition, low expression of the gene set associated with immune response signaling was associated with a significantly worse outcome.

Finally, a few studies have used microarray analysis of metastatic melanoma to identify potential signatures of immune responsiveness. Wang et al. [24] analyzed 63 subcutaneous melanoma metastases using a 6,018 cDNA chip in a cohort of patients undergoing various immunotherapies. Global transcript analysis failed to identify subsets of metastases that were predictive of immune responsiveness. However, 30 genes were associated with response to interleukin-2/vaccine-based therapy, including several in the interferon signaling pathway. In addition, Harlin et al. [25] examined gene expression profiles of metastatic melanoma specimens from patients undergoing peptide-based immunotherapy, and identified a major cluster of samples based on the presence or absence of T-cell associated transcripts. Specifically, six chemokines (CCL2, CCL3, CCL4, CCL5, CXCL9, and CXCL10) were confirmed by protein array or qRT-PCR in tumors that contained T cells, with expression of the corresponding receptors observed on human CD8+ effector T cells. Finally, functional analysis demonstrated that melanoma cell lines with high chemokine expression recruited human CD8+ effector T cells more effectively in xenograft models.

Taken together, transcriptomic profiles of melanoma metastases have resulted in a number of tantalizing observations regarding melanoma biology that still require validation in larger cohorts. Specifically, it will be important to conclusively demonstrate the prognostic impact of gene signatures of melanoma metastases, and to confirm that this is an independent predictor of survival in metastatic melanoma. Since many of the studies have combined specimens from stage III and stage IV patients, the utility of gene expression profiling in distinct subsets of metastatic melanoma patients will need to be demonstrated. It will be important to confirm observations that have suggested divergent survival associated with (1) radial growth phase signature, (2) proliferative signature, and (3) immune responsiveness signature. The ultimate clinical utility of this approach in the setting of metastatic melanoma would require relevance to either (1) identifying high-risk patients for adjuvant therapy trials, (2) identifying patient subsets that may preferentially respond to various systemic therapies, or (3) identifying novel targets for the therapy of metastatic melanoma.

Conclusions

There has been a dramatic increase in the number of genomic analyses of melanoma with the advent of commercially available array platforms and software for bio-statistical analysis. However, these studies are still hampered by the relative paucity of fresh tissue available for analysis, and the lack of coordinated programs for prospective collection of high-quality tissue. While the use of customized array platforms enables the validation of known progression genes, it is still suboptimal for the identification of novel genes in an unbiased manner.

Importantly, however, gene expression profiling efforts in melanoma have enabled novel insights into the biology of melanoma progression. They have resulted in the development of validated multi-marker diagnostic and prognostic markers for primary melanoma. In the setting of metastatic melanoma, further work will be required to conclusively demonstrate the utility of gene expression profiles. In the era of targeted therapy, transcriptomic efforts need to determine relevant gene signatures in the context of the known mutational events in melanoma that can be targeted therapeutically. This may result in the identification of novel pathways for intervention and in the development of rational approaches for combination therapy.

References

1. Bittner M, Meltzer P, Chen Y, et al. Molecular classification of cutaneous malignant melanoma by gene expression profiling. Nature. 2000;406:536–40.
2. Clark WH, Elder DE, Guerry IV D, et al. A study of tumor progression: the precursor lesions of superficial spreading and nodular melanoma. Hum Pathol. 1984;15:1147–65.
3. Davies H, Bignell GR, Cox C, et al. Mutations of the BRAF gene in human cancer. Nature. 2002;417:949–54.
4. Flaherty KT, Puzanov I, Kim KB, et al. Inhibition of mutated, activated BRAF in metastatic melanoma. N Engl J Med. 2010;363:809–19.
5. Haqq C, Nosrati M, Sudilovsky D, et al. The gene expression signatures of melanoma progression. Proc Natl Acad Sci USA. 2005;102:6092–7.
6. Shoo BA, Sagebiel RW, Kashani-Sabet M. Discordance in the histopathologic diagnosis of melanoma at a melanoma referral center. J Am Acad Dermatol. 2010;62:751–6.
7. Kashani-Sabet M, Rangel J, Torabian S, et al. A multi-marker assay to distinguish malignant melanomas from benign nevi. Proc Natl Acad Sci USA. 2009;106:6268–72.
8. Talantov D, Mazumder A, Ju JX, et al. Novel genes associated with malignant melanoma but not benign melanocytic lesions. Clin Cancer Res. 2005;11:7234–42.
9. Nambiar S, Mirmohammadsadegh A, Hassan A, et al. Identification and functional characterization of ASK/Dbf4, a novel cell survival gene in cutaneous melanoma with prognostic relevance. Carcinogenesis. 2007;28:2501–10.
10. Koh SS, Opel ML, Wei JP, et al. Molecular classification of melanomas and nevi using gene expression microarray signatures and formalin-fixed and paraffin-embedded tissue. Mod Pathol. 2009;22:538–46.
11. Jaeger J, Koczan D, Thiesen HJ, et al. Gene expression signatures for tumor progression, tumor subtype, and tumor thickness in laser-microdissected melanoma tissues. Clin Cancer Res. 2007;13:806–15.

12. Riker AI, Enkemann SA, Fodstad O, et al. The gene expression profiles of primary and metastatic melanoma yields a transition point of tumor progression and metastasis. BMC Med Genomics. 2008;1:13.
13. Winnepenninckx V, Lazar V, Michiels S, et al. Gene expression profiling of primary cutaneous melanoma and clinical outcome. J Natl Cancer Inst. 2006;98:472–82.
14. Kannengiesser C, Spatz A, Michiels S, et al. Gene expression signature associated with BRAF mutations in human primary cutaneous melanoma. Mol Oncol. 2008;1:425–30.
15. Alonso SR, Tracey L, Ortiz P, et al. A high-throughput study in melanoma identifies epithelial-mesenchymal transition as a major determinant of metastasis. Cancer Res. 2007;67:3450–60.
16. Conway C, Mitra A, Jewell R, et al. Gene expression profiling of paraffin-embedded primary melanoma using the DASL assay identifies increased osteopontin expression as predictive of reduced relapse-free survival. Clin Cancer Res. 2009;15:6939–46.
17. Rangel J, Torabian S, Shaikh L, et al. Prognostic significance of NCOA3 overexpression in primary cutaneous melanoma. J Clin Oncol. 2006;24:4565–9.
18. Rangel J, Nosrati M, Torabian S, et al. Osteopontin as a molecular prognostic marker for melanoma. Cancer. 2008;112:144–50.
19. Rangel J, Nosrati M, Leong SP, et al. Novel role for RGS1 in melanoma progression. Am J Surg Pathol. 2008;32:1207–12.
20. Kashani-Sabet M, Venna S, Nosrati M, et al. A multimarker prognostic assay for primary cutaneous melanoma. Clin Cancer Res. 2009;15:6987–92.
21. John T, Black MA, Toro TT, et al. Predicting clinical outcome through molecular profiling in stage III melanoma. Clin Cancer Res. 2008;14:5173–80.
22. Bogunovic D, O'Neill DW, Belitskaya-Levy I, et al. Immune profile and mitotic index of metastatic melanoma lesions enhance clinical staging in predicting patient survival. Proc Natl Acad Sci USA. 2009;106:20429–34.
23. Jonsson G, Busch C, Knappskog S, et al. Gene expression profiling-based identification of molecular subtypes in stage IV melanomas with different clinical outcome. Clin Cancer Res. 2010;16:3356–67.
24. Wang E, Miller LD, Ohnmacht GA, et al. Prospective molecular profiling of melanoma metastases suggests classifiers of immune responsiveness. Cancer Res. 2002;62:3581–6.
25. Harlin H, Meng Y, Peterson AC, et al. Chemokine expression in melanoma metastases associated with CD8+ T-cell recruitment. Cancer Res. 2009;69:3077–85.

Chapter 3
Predictive Biomarkers as a Guide to Future Therapy Selection in Melanoma

Thomas F. Gajewski

Abstract It is becoming clear that multiple molecular subtypes of melanoma likely exist that not only define distinct biologic entities, but also may be associated with clinical response to defined therapeutic modalities. For signal transduction inhibitors, activating mutations in B-Raf and c-kit are associated with clinical response to the specific kinase inhibitors PLX4032 and imatinib, respectively. Several other signaling pathways have been found to be constitutively active or mutated in other subsets of melanoma tumors that are potentially targetable with new agents. For immunotherapies, gene expression profiling has revealed a signature that is associated with clinical benefit to melanoma vaccines, with preliminary observations suggesting a correlation with response to other immunotherapy agents as well. Together, these emerging data suggest the evolution of a new paradigm in melanoma therapy in which molecular analysis of the tumor will be utilized to assign the most appropriate therapeutic modality for each individual patient. The anticipated result will be improved therapeutic success, as well as the tools to identify mechanisms of therapeutic resistance.

Keywords Biomarker • B-Raf • c-kit • Immunotherapy • Gene expression profiling • Patient selection

Evidence for Existence of Biologic Subsets of Melanoma

Two FDA approved drugs are available to treat patients with metastatic melanoma, the chemotherapeutic agent dacarbazine (DTIC; approved in 1976) and the immunomodulatory cytokine interleukin-2 (IL-2; approved in 1998). Each of

T.F. Gajewski, MD, PhD (✉)
Departments of Pathology and Medicine, Section of Hematology/Oncology,
University of Chicago, 5841 S. Maryland Avenue, MC2115, Chicago, IL 60637, USA
e-mail: tgajewsk@medicine.bsd.uchicago.edu

T.F. Gajewski and F.S. Hodi (eds.), *Targeted Therapeutics in Melanoma*,
Current Clinical Oncology, DOI 10.1007/978-1-61779-407-0_3,
© Springer Science+Business Media, LLC 2012

these produces response rates of less than 15% in unselected patients. It has been known for almost 20 years that there is minimal cross-resistance between dacarbazine and IL-2 [48] – some patients who progress after treatment with dacarbazine clearly can respond to IL-2, and vice versa. In addition, combination regimens of chemotherapy and cytokines (biochemotherapy designs) appear to show additive but not synergistic activity, with increased response rates but no improvement in overall survival observed in randomized trials [2]. Together, these observations with established agents already suggest that there may be subsets of melanoma patients with biologic characteristics that render them susceptible to the therapeutic effect of one modality (chemotherapy) vs. another (immunotherapy). Still, all histological subtypes of melanoma (superficial spreading, acral lentiginous, nodular, lentigo maligna, and mucosal) have been clinically managed similarly, without evidence for differences in clinical response to these agents based on histological criteria alone.

Molecular evidence pointing to the existence of clinically meaningful subsets of melanoma took a great leap forward with the comparative genomic hybridization and systematic oncogene mutation analyses studies of Bastian and colleagues [10]. In those studies, melanomas arising in a context of sun-damaged skin, non-sun-damaged skin, acral surfaces, or mucosal regions were found to have distinct major molecular aberrations. Specifically, mutations in B-Raf were most frequently found in lesions from non-sun-damaged skin. Amplifications in CCND1 and CDK4 (downstream cell cycle regulators in the Ras pathway) were found in lesions that lacked upstream mutations in N-Ras or B-Raf. In addition, amplifications in the c-kit gene locus were found in a significant proportion of acral and mucosal lesions. Thus, rather than classical histological subcategorization of melanoma lesions, these data began to suggest that molecular subtyping of melanoma may be possible, both to define these subsets biologically, and to consider rational assignment of therapy based on molecular characteristics. The latter is becoming possible as drugs that specifically target receptor tyrosine kinases, downstream kinases, and other signaling molecules are being developed and are undergoing clinical testing. In addition, early evidence is suggesting that a distinct set of molecular features of the tumor microenvironment may predict clinical benefit from new immunotherapy approaches.

Kinase Mutations and Clinical Response to Kinase Inhibitors

B-Raf

The identification of activating mutations in B-Raf as a common genetic alteration in melanoma [13] rapidly led to the hypothesis that kinase inhibitors with activity against B-Raf might have therapeutic utility. Over 90% of B-Raf mutations in melanoma involve a substitution of glutamate for valine at position 600, and over 50% of melanomas carry such a mutation. The first agent with potential inhibitory activity against Raf family kinases, sorafenib, was explored with much enthusiasm in melanoma. It was surprising to many that there was lack of meaningful clinical activity among melanoma patients treated on the phase I/II studies of sorafenib as a single agent [15]. Despite this observation, an unusually high response rate to carboplatin and paclitaxel combined with sorafenib sustained interest in the drug for [18]. These observations led to two phase III trials of carboplatin and paclitaxel with or without sorafenib in patients with metastatic melanoma, either in the first line or in the second line setting. Unfortunately, there were no significant differences in clinical outcome in either study [16, 17]. While these outcomes temporarily dampened enthusiasm for the concept of Raf blockade in this disease, it was also clear that sorafenib was not extremely potent at inhibiting Raf activity. The clinical activity of sorafenib in other cancers, such as renal cell carcinoma, is presumed to be mediated through inhibition of other kinases, including the VEGF receptor tyrosine kinase. Other clinical trials aiming to block Ras pathway signaling at other levels, including farnesyltransferase inhibitors (aiming to target Ras proteins directly) and early MEK inhibitors (targeting the kinase downstream from Raf), also showed disappointing clinical activity in melanoma [22].

However, other small molecule inhibitors with more potent activity against mutant B-Raf had continued in development. PLX4032 was reported to have eightfold greater activity against mutant B-Raf over wild-type Raf, showing inhibition in vitro at nanomolar concentrations. A phase I study with an expansion cohort in melanoma was conducted and recently reported [16, 17]. Of the 48 V600E B-Raf mutated melanoma patients treated at the recommended phase II dose, 34 partial and 3 complete responses were observed. In contrast, the five patients with melanomas expressing wild-type B-Raf had no clinical response. These impressive results have provided the first evidence that an agent targeting a commonly mutated signaling protein in melanoma can exert meaningful clinical activity. Together, these observations suggest that expression of a V600E mutation in B-Raf may be a predictive biomarker for response to PLX4032 in melanoma. Similar results have recently been observed with a second B-Raf inhibitor from Glaxo Smith Kline (GSK2118436).

c-kit

Along with the report by Bastian and colleagues that the c-kit gene is amplified in a subset of melanomas, activating mutations in c-kit have been described. Interestingly, these have been seen in around 30% of tumors from mucosal and acral sites, as well as a minority of patients with melanomas arising out of sun-damaged skin [3, 53]. The spectrum of mutations identified to date parallel those reported in gastrointestinal stromal tumors, which are associated with clinical response to c-kit inhibitors such as imatinib [29]. Based on these observations, imatinib has been investigated clinically in melanoma patients bearing c-kit mutations, and studies with nilotinib and desatinib have recently been initiated. Several case reports have been published

[30, 35, 45, 52], revealing at least 10 clinical responders in total. In contrast, clinical testing of imatinib in unselected melanoma patients revealed minimal clinical activity [32, 66]. Thus, it is very likely that a clinically relevant response rate will be observed in the subset of melanoma patients with tumors that have specific activating mutations in c-kit. This notion is currently being examined systematically in a series of prospective phase II and phase III clinical trials. As such, activating mutations in c-kit will likely be validated as a predictive biomarker for the potential to respond to kinase inhibitors that block activity of c-kit.

New Pathways Showing Heterogeneity Among Individual Melanoma Patients

In addition to mutations that lead to activation of the Ras pathway, other parallel signaling pathways have been found to be constitutively activated in subsets of melanoma tumors and could lead to new therapeutic approaches in selected subgroups of patients. The Notch pathway has been reported to be activated in many melanomas, apparently via ligand and receptor overexpression rather than through mutation [36]. Notch signaling is mediated, in part, through proteolytic cleavage by an enzyme called gamma secretase, which liberates the intracellular domain of Notch to participate in transcriptional regulation. Gamma secretase inhibitors (GSIs) have been developed for clinical exploration as a strategy to inhibit Notch pathway signaling in patients. Results of a phase I study of a GSI were presented at the ASCO 2010 annual meeting, with two melanoma patients showing clinical responses [62]. Phase II studies of this agent in melanoma have been initiated. It will be critical to pursue tumor-based biomarker analysis in these studies to generate the tools with which to identify the potentially responsive patient subpopulation.

Activating mutations in PI3 kinase have been reported in a minor subset of melanomas [11], and the critical negative regulator of PI3 kinase activity, the lipid phosphatase PTEN, is mutated or epigenetically silenced in many melanomas [8, 69]. The recent development of PI3 kinase inhibitors for clinical testing makes it attractive to consider targeting this pathway in this disease. In addition, a total kinome sequencing study in melanoma has recently been published, which has suggested that activating mutations in ErbB4 might be present in a subset of melanomas [43]. As functional activity of ErbB4 can be inhibited by the already available kinase inhibitor lapatinib [4], it is attractive to consider testing of lapatinib in melanoma patients bearing ErbB4 mutant tumors. Mutations in c-met also have been reported in a series of melanoma cell lines [44], and the recent development of agents with inhibitory activity against c-met for clinical testing makes a similar hypothesis attractive for this molecule. However, there has been minimal analysis of primary tumor samples reported, so the fraction of patients with tumors harboring c-met mutations is not clear.

Several additional signaling pathways have been reported to be active in subsets of melanomas, and have been found to be functionally important for melanoma biology, but without pharmacologic agents yet available for pathway inhibition in the clinic. Expression of stabilized β-catenin has been observed in a major subset of melanomas, and β-catenin has been shown to contribute to melanoma development in mouse models [33]. Constitutive phosphorylation of the transcription factor Stat3 also has been identified in a subset of melanomas [37]. In vitro, knockdown of Stat3 has direct antitumor activity, but also induces expression of important immunoregulatory genes, including a subset of chemokines that might mediate lymphocyte trafficking [7]. Therefore, Stat3 inhibitors, if developed, might have two complementary mechanisms of action, and synergy of such agents with other immunotherapeutic agents might be anticipated. Developing novel strategies to inhibit the β-catenin and Stat3 pathways in melanoma therefore should receive significant attention. Once such agents enter clinical trial testing, those studies should incorporate careful tumor-based biomarker analysis to determine whether constitutive activation of the pathway is predictive of clinical response to therapy.

Gene Expression Profiling and Clinical Response to Melanoma Vaccines

The best clinical responses of metastatic melanoma to immunotherapeutic agents such as IL-2, IFN-α2b, and experimental cancer vaccines are around 10–15%. This response in a subset of patients makes it plausible to consider that there is a distinct biologic subset of tumors capable of responding to immunotherapeutic interventions. This notion has been advanced farthest in the context of melanoma vaccines. In early trials, a potential correlation was extensively investigated between clinical response and the magnitude of the specific T cell response induced by the vaccine as measured in the peripheral blood compartment. While such correlations have been observed in some studies, clinical responses have clearly been seen in patients with frequencies of such T cells below the limit of detection using standard assays [9], and conversely, complete lack of clinical benefit has been seen in patients with very high T cell frequencies [50]. This apparent paradox has led several investigators to perform a systematic analysis of tumor biopsy material to probe for factors in the tumor microenvironment that may determine clinical outcome to melanoma vaccines. Using Affymetrix gene expression profiling, clinical benefit was seen in a subset of patients who showed an "inflamed" tumor microenvironment at baseline (Gajewski et al.) [21]. Metastases of this type show expression of an array of chemokines predicted to be capable of recruiting activated T cells into the tumor site. Using an in vivo xenograft model, preferential recruitment of CD8+ effector T cells into human melanomas producing high levels of chemokines was confirmed [27]. These results suggest that one major determining factor for clinical response to melanoma vaccines is whether T cell trafficking into the tumor microenvironment can be supported, which is thought to be necessary to bring activated cytotoxic T cells into contact with tumor cells in order for the latter to be killed.

Two additional independent melanoma vaccine trials have also revealed evidence for an "inflamed" tumor phenotype being associated with clinical benefit from the vaccine. The first is a dendriticcell-based vaccine led by Gerold Schuler's group in Erlangen. They utilized a combination of class I and class II MHC-binding epitopes pulsed onto mature autologous dendritic cells. While strong immune responses were induced in the majority of patients, there was not a clear association between the magnitude of that immune response and clinical benefit. A subset of patients had tumor material available for gene expression profiling. When gene expression data were analyzed according to patient survival, the set of transcripts associated with favorable clinical outcome included a set of chemokines and T cell markers [24]. In a separate study of a MAGE3 protein-based vaccine carried out by GSK-Bio, patients with advanced melanoma were vaccinated and gene expression profiling from pretreatment biopsies was similarly analyzed. Again, favorable clinical outcome was associated with a set of chemokines and T cell transcripts present in the tumor [65]. Thus, although the sample size from each of these studies was relatively small, these results collectively support the notion that an "immune signature" pre-existing in the melanoma microenvironment might be predictive of a positive clinical outcome to melanoma vaccines [20]. This hypothesis is currently being tested in prospective clinical trials of the MAGE3 protein vaccine by GSK-Bio.

It may seem paradoxical that a subset of tumors shows evidence for spontaneous inflammation that includes activated $CD8^+$ T cells, yet those tumors have nonetheless persisted in the face of an ongoing immune response. In a limited number of patients with sufficient fresh tissue for analysis, peptide/HLA-A2 tetramer staining has confirmed that a subset of these T cells in fact recognizes tumor antigens [1, 26, 38, 70]. The reason why these tumors are not rejected spontaneously probably lies at the level of immune suppressive pathways engaged within the tumor microenvironment. Direct ex vivo analysis of $CD8^+$ T cells from melanoma metastases has shown minimal expression of cytotoxic granule proteins and defective cytokine production in response to restimulation with specific antigen, consistent with this notion [1, 26, 38, 70]. As a potential mechanistic explanation, analysis of the inflamed tumor subset has revealed the highest level of expression of defined immune inhibitory factors [19]. These include the tryptophan-catabolizing enzyme indoleamine-2,3-dioxygenase (IDO), which has been implicated in maternal/fetal tolerance [40]; the ligand PD-L1/B7-H1, which engages an inhibitory receptor on activated T cells called PD-1 [14]; and the presence of regulatory T cells expressing the $CD4^+CD25^+FoxP3^+$ phenotype, which have been shown to mediate extrinsic suppression of activated T cells in the tumor setting [42]. In addition to the presence of these three dominant inhibitory mechanisms, these tumors also lack meaningful levels of expression of the T cell costimulatory ligands B7-1 and B7-2. Absence of B7 ligands has been shown to lead to the T cell refractory state called T cell anergy [54, 67], which also likely contributes to T cell hyporesponsiveness in the tumor context.

The characterization of these defined immune inhibitory mechanisms has pointed toward new potential targets for therapeutic intervention. Blockade or reversal of these immune-suppressive pathways should be capable of restoring T cell function and promoting immune-mediated tumor regression in vivo. Indeed, preclinical studies have shown that blockade of IDO with small molecule inhibitors [39, 64], interference with PD-1/PD-L1 interactions with specific monoclonal antibodies or through the use of knockout mice [5, 68], depletion of Tregs by targeting CD25 [58], and reversal of T cell anergy through forced homeostatic proliferation [6] have shown evidence of antitumor activity in defined model systems.

Each of these approaches to block negative regulation is already being translated to the clinic. The IDO inhibitor 1-methyltryptophan is currently undergoing phase I clinical development, and a newer more potent IDO inhibitor has just entered clinical testing [34]. Impressive phase II results with an anti-PD-1 mAb were presented at the 2010 ASCO annual meeting, in which approximately 30% of patients with advanced melanoma, renal cell carcinoma, and non-small-cell lung cancer showed clinical responses [59]. Depletion of Tregs has been pursued with denileukin diftitox [12], an IL-2-diptheria toxin fusion protein, and with daclizumab, an anti-CD25 mAb [47]. Interestingly, clinical responses with Ontak as a single agent have been reported in melanoma [46]. Finally, homeostatic proliferation of T cells, driven by their transfer into lymphopenic hosts, has been found to markedly increase the clinical efficacy of adoptively transferred autologous tumor-infiltrating lymphocytes in melanoma [49]. Together, these observations firmly support the continued study of the tumor microenvironment for clues to improve the effector phase of the antitumor T cell response toward improved tumor rejection in patients.

It seems likely that clinical responses to each of the above maneuvers to counter negative regulatory pathways might be preferentially observed in patients with tumors showing a high level of basal expression of the immune inhibitory mechanism of interest. For example, preliminary biomarker studies in a subset of patients with available tissue have suggested that clinical response to anti-PD-1 mAb may be enriched in the patients with tumors showing high cell surface staining for PD-L1. Similar results might be expected for strategies targeting IDO and Tregs. Therefore, it is hoped that tumor tissue will be banked whenever possible as clinical development of these agents continues, to determine whether a biologic feature of the tumor microenvironment can reproducibly enrich for the potentially responsive patient subpopulation.

While the observations and implications described above have been driven by analysis of the tumor microenvironment in the context of melanoma vaccines, it is critical to understand whether clinical benefit from other immunotherapeutic approaches might also be associated with an "inflamed" melanoma tumor microenvironment phenotype. In fact, preliminary results presented at the ASCO 2009 annual meeting suggest that this may be the case. Atkins and colleagues reported that tumors with expression of a set of chemokines and cytokines were more likely to respond after treatment with IL-2 [57]. In addition, Hamid et al. reported that clinical responses to the anti-CTLA-4 mAb ipilimumab were more likely to occur in patients with tumors expressing several immunoregulatory molecules [25]. Together, these observations suggest that an ongoing dialogue between the tumor and the host immune response might be a prerequisite for clinical benefit to several specific immunotherapeutic interventions, a concept that should be evaluated in more detail through prospective biomarker-driven clinical trials.

Molecular Features Associated with Response to Chemotherapy

There is often excitement surrounding the scientific development of new drugs such as kinase inhibitors and novel mAbs, and biomarker studies can be more compelling to carry out with new agents. However, it may be just as important to identify predictive biomarkers for clinical activity of older therapies, such as chemotherapeutic agents. This is especially important to entertain given the low response rate to chemotherapies such as dacarbazine, which implies that the majority of patients might receive the drug and never derive clinical benefit. Sensitivity vs. resistance to alkylating agents such as dacarbazine or temozolomide might be predicted to be inversely correlated with expression of DNA repair enzymes, such as O^6-methylguanine methyltransferase (MGMT). Indeed, methylation and presumed silencing of the MGMT gene has been shown to be associated with a favorable clinical response of glioblastoma to temozolomide plus radiation [28]. With this experience as a foundation, Tawby et al. recently reported on a study of molecular profiling in melanoma and association with outcome in 21 patients treated with dacarbazine. Using a combination of gene expression profiling and analysis of gene locus methylation status, they identified a 9 gene predictor [61]. Interestingly, some of these genes encode signaling proteins (RasSF4) or immunoregulatory molecules (NKG7). It is noteworthy that MGMT did not emerge as a candidate gene in this study. This is consistent with the lack of added clinical benefit with the addition of the MGMT inhibitor O^6-benzylguanine in melanoma [23], and suggests that alternative resistance mechanisms of melanoma to alkylating agents are likely dominant. Expression of anti-apoptotic proteins such as Mcl-1 is interesting to consider. While still early in development, these initial observations support continued investigation of potential predictive biomarkers for clinical benefit to standard chemotherapeutic agents in this disease.

Biomarkers as a Tool to Determine Mechanisms of Therapeutic Resistance

Once a mechanism-based predictive biomarker has been defined, identification of resistance mechanisms that emerge following an initial response to therapy should, in principle, be facilitated. As a consequence, rapid development of next generation therapies that counter the acquired mechanism of resistance should be catalyzed. This concept is perhaps best exemplified by the studies of patients with chronic myelogenous leukemia (CML) treated with Gleevec, from whom new mutations in the Abl kinase domain were identified rendering the kinase resistant to inhibition by the drug [55, 60]. In melanoma, early results with B-Raf inhibitors have been generated. In contrast to the CML experience, preliminary data have suggested that patients with melanomas expressing B-Raf V600E do not appear to develop new mutations in the B-Raf molecule when resistant disease emerges. Yet, the Ras pathway appears to become reactivated as evidenced by elevated levels of phosphorylated ERK. Analysis of resistant melanoma cell lines and confirmatory evaluations of biopsy material from a subset of treated patients has suggested that genetic alterations that activate the Ras pathway upstream from, or parallel to, B-Raf can occur. Changes described to date have included acquired mutations in N-Ras, and also acquired expression of the PDGFRβ [41]. Understanding these new molecular changes has suggested candidate drugs that could be tested for synergy with B-Raf inhibitors, either to prevent emergence of resistance or to treat resistant disease.

A similar type of analysis is being carried out through longitudinal analysis of tumor biopsy material from patients being treated with immunotherapies. An interesting case at the University of Chicago has been studied in detail in which a patient at baseline was found to display the "inflamed" melanoma gene expression profile, and experienced a clinical response to a melanoma peptide vaccine. This response lasted around 3 years, at which time recurrent tumor was biopsied and reanalyzed by gene expression profiling. The recurrent tumor was found to lack the inflamed signature, and also to lack tumor penetration of $CD8^+$ T cells (Gajewski et al., unpublished observation). This observation suggests that a more aggressive tumor microenvironment can emerge under immune selective pressure, and highlights the need to develop new therapeutic strategies to promote T cell recruitment into metastatic tumor sites.

Predictive Biomarkers from Non-Tumor Tissue: Serum and Germline DNA

All of the analyses described above have been performed using tumor tissue as a source of material for biomarker study. However, it would be very desirable to develop less invasive means by which to determine the potential to respond to a given therapy. One approach being explored involves analysis of serum or plasma obtained prior to treatment, to identify patterns of circulating proteins that might indirectly reflect the biology of the tumor site. An interesting pilot study has been published by Kaufman and colleagues in the context of clinical response to high-dose IL-2, in which high levels of VEGF and fibronectin were found to be inversely correlated with clinical benefit [51]. A second approach is the evaluation of germline genetic polymorphisms, based on the hypothesis that, particularly with immunotherapies, the tumor-host interaction might be greatly influenced by specific differences in immunoregulatory genes. Again in the context of high-dose IL-2, polymorphisms in the gene encoding the chemokine receptor CCR5 have been associated with clinical outcome [63]. It is hoped that the pursuit of these and other blood-based predictive biomarkers will be prospectively evaluated as large phase II and phase III clinical trials of effective agents in melanoma are carried out.

The Evolving Future of Melanoma Therapy

Melanoma has recently earned the designation as "an unlikely poster child for personalized cancer therapy" [56]. It is not difficult to envision that within the next several years, melanoma tumors will be routinely screened for the presence of a panel of specific markers to determine assignment of individual patients to the most appropriate therapeutic approaches (Table 3.1). Indeed, analysis of these markers is now frequently used in academic centers for the majority of new patients presenting with metastatic disease and is on the verge of becoming standard practice. Mutations in B-Raf or c-kit will determine eligibility for treatment with the respective specific kinase inhibitors. The activation status of other signaling pathways may be used to predict benefit to other new targeted agents. Expression of selected tumor antigens (e.g., MAGE-3 or NY-Eso-1) will be utilized to identify patients who are candidates for antigen-specific vaccines. The presence of an "inflamed" tumor microenvironment, anticipated to be characterized using a small gene set analyzed by qRT-PCR much like the OncotypeDx in breast cancer [31], might be utilized to consider patients for a range of immunotherapeutic interventions; and expression of PD-L1, IDO, or presence of intratumoral Tregs might be used to decide on administration of agents targeting those suppressive mechanisms. Having these predictive biomarkers in hand will affect the care of melanoma patients in multiple ways. First, it should lead to a greater likelihood of clinical response with the first therapeutic modality selected for a given patient. This should in turn lead to improved overall survival of this traditionally difficult to treat population. Second, as mentioned above, having a specific molecular pathway that is being targeted should enable identification of escape mechanisms that, when studied, may lead to the more rapid identification of new therapeutic interventions to prevent or overcome resistance.

Table 3.1 Emerging molecular markers that may facilitate patient-specific therapy in melanoma

Molecular biomarker	Therapeutic modality
Ongoing in development	
B-Raf V600E	PLX4032, GSK2118436
Mutant c-kit	Imatinib, nilotinib
MAGE-3+	MAGE-3 protein vaccine
"Inflamed" tumor microenvironment	Vaccines, other immunotherapeutics
Future potential	
Active notch	Gamma secretase inhibitors (GSIs)
Mutant PI3K/PTEN loss	PI3K inhibitors, Akt inhibitors
Mutant c-met	c-met inhibitors
Mutant ErbB4	Lapatinib

Third, characterization of tumors that lack any of these potential predictive biomarkers (e.g., B-Raf and c-kit wild type, absence of inflammatory signature) should proceed at an accelerated pace, to identify new pathways that might be amenable to novel therapeutic approaches. Finally, in order to bring patient-specific therapy into the mainstream, an infrastructure will need to be developed for rapid evaluation of patients' tumors for molecular markers, using validated quality-controlled assays with a rapid turnaround time suitable for the pace of clinical decision making. This will likely involve a combination of molecular diagnostic laboratories at academic oncology centers and commercial laboratories with expertise in specific assay systems, as well as educational programs for updating community oncologists on the rapidly evolving standard practice.

References

1. Appay V, Jandus C, Voelter V, Reynard S, Coupland SE, Rimoldi D, et al. New generation vaccine induces effective melanoma-specific CD8+ T cells in the circulation but not in the tumor site. J Immunol. 2006;177:1670–8.
2. Atkins MB, Hsu J, Lee S, Cohen GI, Flaherty LE, Sosman JA, et al. Phase III trial comparing concurrent biochemotherapy with cisplatin, vinblastine, dacarbazine, interleukin-2, and interferon alfa-2b with cisplatin, vinblastine, and dacarbazine alone in patients with metastatic malignant melanoma (E3695): a trial coordinated by the Eastern Cooperative Oncology Group. J Clin Oncol. 2008;26:5748–54.
3. Beadling C, Jacobson-Dunlop E, Hodi FS, Le C, Warrick A, Patterson J, et al. KIT gene mutations and copy number in melanoma subtypes. Clin Cancer Res. 2008;14:6821–8.
4. Bilancia D, Rosati G, Dinota A, Germano D, Romano R, Manzione L. Lapatinib in breast cancer. Ann Oncol. 2007;18 Suppl 6:vi26–30.
5. Blank C, Brown I, Peterson AC, Spiotto M, Iwai Y, Honjo T, et al. PD-L1/B7H-1 inhibits the effector phase of tumor rejection by T cell receptor (TCR) transgenic CD8+ T cells. Cancer Res. 2004;64:1140–5.
6. Brown IE, Blank C, Kline J, Kacha AK, Gajewski TF. Homeostatic proliferation as an isolated variable reverses CD8+ T cell anergy and promotes tumor rejection. J Immunol. 2006;177: 4521–9.
7. Burdelya L, Kujawski M, Niu G, Zhong B, Wang T, Zhang S, et al. Stat3 activity in melanoma cells affects migration of immune effector cells and nitric oxide-mediated antitumor effects. J Immunol. 2005;174:3925–31.
8. Celebi JT, Shendrik I, Silvers DN, Peacocke M. Identification of PTEN mutations in metastatic melanoma specimens. J Med Genet. 2000;37:653–7.
9. Coulie PG, Karanikas V, Colau D, Lurquin C, Landry C, Marchand M, et al. A monoclonal cytolytic T-lymphocyte response observed in a melanoma patient vaccinated with a tumor-specific antigenic peptide encoded by gene MAGE-3. Proc Natl Acad Sci USA. 2001;21:21.
10. Curtin JA, Fridlyand J, Kageshita T, Patel HN, Busam KJ, Kutzner H, et al. Distinct sets of genetic alterations in melanoma. N Engl J Med. 2005;353:2135–47.
11. Curtin JA, Stark MS, Pinkel D, Hayward NK, Bastian BC. PI3-kinase subunits are infrequent somatic targets in melanoma. J Invest Dermatol. 2006;126:1660–3.
12. Dannull J, Su Z, Rizzieri D, Yang BK, Coleman D, Yancey D, et al. Enhancement of vaccine-mediated antitumor immunity in cancer patients after depletion of regulatory T cells. J Clin Invest. 2005;115:3623–33.
13. Davies H, Bignell GR, Cox C, Stephens P, Edkins S, Clegg S, et al. Mutations of the BRAF gene in human cancer. Nature. 2002;417:949–54.

14. Dong H, Chen L. B7-H1 pathway and its role in the evasion of tumor immunity. J Mol Med. 2003;81:281–7.
15. Eisen T, Ahmad T, Flaherty KT, Gore M, Kaye S, Marais R, et al. Sorafenib in advanced melanoma: a phase II randomised discontinuation trial analysis. Br J Cancer. 2006;95:581–6.
16. Flaherty KT, Lee SJ, Schuchter LM, Flaherty LE, Wright JJ, Leming PD, et al. Final results of E2603: a double-blind, randomized phase III trial comparing carboplatin ©/paclitaxel (P) with or without sorafenib (S) in metastatic melanoma. Clin Oncol. 2010;28:15s. Abstract 8511.
17. Flaherty KT, Puzanov I, Kim KB, Ribas A, McArthur GA, Sosman JA, et al. Inhibition of mutated, activated BRAF in metastatic melanoma. N Engl J Med. 2010;363:809–19.
18. Flaherty KT, Schiller J, Schuchter LM, Liu G, Tuveson DA, Redlinger M, et al. A phase I trial of the oral, multikinase inhibitor sorafenib in combination with carboplatin and paclitaxel. Clin Cancer Res. 2008;14:4836–42.
19. Gajewski TF. Failure at the effector phase: immune barriers at the level of the melanoma tumor microenvironment. Clin Cancer Res. 2007;13:5256–61.
20. Gajewski TF, Louahed J, Brichard VG. Gene signature in melanoma associated with clinical activity: a potential clue to unlock cancer immunotherapy. Cancer J. 2010;16:399–403.
21. Gajewski TF, Meng Y, Harlin H. Chemokines expressed in melanoma metastases associated with T cell infiltration. Journal of Clinical Oncology, 2007 ASCO annual meeting proceedings part I, Vol. 25; 2007, p. 8501.
22. Gajewski TF, Niedzwiecki D, Johnson J, Linette GP, Bucher C, Blaskovich M, et al. Phase II study of the farnesyltransferase inhibitor R115777 in advanced melanoma: CALGB 500104. J Clin Oncol. 2006;24:18S. Abstract 8014.
23. Gajewski TF, Sosman J, Gerson SL, Liu L, Dolan E, Lin S, et al. Phase II trial of the O6-alkylguanine DNA alkyltransferase inhibitor O6-benzylguanine and 1,3-bis(2-chloroethyl)-1-nitrosourea in advanced melanoma. Clin Cancer Res. 2005;11:7861–5.
24. Gajewski TF, Zha Y, Thurner B, Schuler G. Association of gene expression profile in melanoma and survival to a dendritic cell-based vaccine. J Clin Oncol. 2009;27:9002.
25. Hamid O, Chasalow SD, Tsuchihashi Z, Alaparthy S, Galbraith S, Berman D. Association of baseline and on-study tumor biopsy markers with clinical activity in patients with advanced melanoma treated with ipilimumab. J Clin Oncol. 2009;27:Abstract 9008.
26. Harlin H, Kuna TV, Peterson AC, Meng Y, Gajewski TF. Tumor progression despite massive influx of activated CD8(+) T cells in a patient with malignant melanoma ascites. Cancer Immunol Immunother. 2006;55:1185–97.
27. Harlin H, Meng Y, Peterson AC, Zha Y, Tretiakova M, Slingluff C, et al. Chemokine expression in melanoma metastases associated with CD8+ T-cell recruitment. Cancer Res. 2009;69:3077–85.
28. Hegi ME, Diserens AC, Gorlia T, Hamou MF, de Tribolet N, Weller M, et al. MGMT gene silencing and benefit from temozolomide in glioblastoma. N Engl J Med. 2005;352:997–1003.
29. Heinrich MC, Corless CL, Demetri GD, Blanke CD, von Mehren M, Joensuu H, et al. Kinase mutations and imatinib response in patients with metastatic gastrointestinal stromal tumor. J Clin Oncol. 2003;21:4342–9.
30. Hodi FS, Friedlander P, Corless CL, Heinrich MC, Mac Rae S, Kruse A, et al. Major response to imatinib mesylate in KIT-mutated melanoma. J Clin Oncol. 2008;26:2046–51.
31. Kim C, Paik S. Gene-expression-based prognostic assays for breast cancer. Nat Rev Clin Oncol. 2010;7:340–7.
32. Kim KB, Eton O, Davis DW, Frazier ML, McConkey DJ, Diwan AH, et al. Phase II trial of imatinib mesylate in patients with metastatic melanoma. Br J Cancer. 2008;99:734–40.
33. Larue L, Delmas V. The WNT/Beta-catenin pathway in melanoma. Front Biosci. 2006;11: 733–42.
34. Liu X, Shin N, Koblish HK, Yang G, Wang Q, Wang K, et al. Selective inhibition of IDO1 effectively regulates mediators of antitumor immunity. Blood. 2010;115:3520–30.
35. Lutzky J, Bauer J, Bastian BC. Dose-dependent, complete response to imatinib of a metastatic mucosal melanoma with a K642E KIT mutation. Pigment Cell Melanoma Res. 2008;21:492–3.

36. Massi D, Tarantini F, Franchi A, Paglierani M, Di Serio C, Pellerito S, et al. Evidence for differential expression of Notch receptors and their ligands in melanocytic nevi and cutaneous malignant melanoma. Mod Pathol. 2006;19:246–54.
37. Messina JL, Yu H, Riker AI, Munster PN, Jove RL, Daud AI. Activated stat-3 in melanoma. Cancer Control. 2008;15:196–201.
38. Mortarini R, Piris A, Maurichi A, Molla A, Bersani I, Bono A, et al. Lack of terminally differentiated tumor-specific CD8+ T cells at tumor site in spite of antitumor immunity to self-antigens in human metastatic melanoma. Cancer Res. 2003;63:2535–45.
39. Muller AJ, Malachowski WP, Prendergast GC. Indoleamine 2,3-dioxygenase in cancer: targeting pathological immune tolerance with small-molecule inhibitors. Expert Opin Ther Targets. 2005;9:831–49.
40. Munn DH, Zhou M, Attwood JT, Bondarev I, Conway SJ, Marshall B, et al. Prevention of allogeneic fetal rejection by tryptophan catabolism. Science. 1998;281:1191–3.
41. Nazarian R, Shi H, Wang Q, Kong X, Koya RC, Lee H, et al. Melanomas acquire resistance to B-RAF(V600E) inhibition by RTK or N-RAS upregulation. Nature. 2010;468:973–7.
42. Nomura T, Sakaguchi S. Naturally arising CD25+ CD4+ regulatory T cells in tumor immunity. Curr Top Microbiol Immunol. 2005;293:287–302.
43. Prickett TD, Agrawal NS, Wei X, Yates KE, Lin JC, Wunderlich JR, et al. Analysis of the tyrosine kinome in melanoma reveals recurrent mutations in ERBB4. Nat Genet. 2009;41: 1127–32.
44. Puri N, Ahmed S, Janamanchi V, Tretiakova M, Zumba O, Krausz T, et al. c-Met is a potentially new therapeutic target for treatment of human melanoma. Clin Cancer Res. 2007;13:2246–53.
45. Quintas-Cardama A, Lazar AJ, Woodman SE, Kim K, Ross M, Hwu P. Complete response of stage IV anal mucosal melanoma expressing KIT Val560Asp to the multikinase inhibitor sorafenib. Nat Clin Pract Oncol. 2008;5:737–40.
46. Rasku MA, Clem AL, Telang S, Taft B, Gettings K, Gragg H, et al. Transient T cell depletion causes regression of melanoma metastases. J Transl Med. 2008;6:12.
47. Rech AJ, Vonderheide RH. Clinical use of anti-CD25 antibody daclizumab to enhance immune responses to tumor antigen vaccination by targeting regulatory T cells. Ann N Y Acad Sci. 2009;1174:99–106.
48. Richards JM, Gilewski TA, Ramming K, Mitchel B, Doane LL, Vogelzang NJ. Effective chemotherapy for melanoma after treatment with interleukin-2. Cancer. 1992;69:427–9.
49. Rosenberg SA, Dudley ME. Cancer regression in patients with metastatic melanoma after the transfer of autologous antitumor lymphocytes. Proc Natl Acad Sci USA. 2004;101 Suppl 2:14639–45.
50. Rosenberg SA, Sherry RM, Morton KE, Scharfman WJ, Yang JC, Topalian SL, et al. Tumor progression can occur despite the induction of very high levels of self/tumor antigen-specific CD8+ T cells in patients with melanoma. J Immunol. 2005;175:6169–76.
51. Sabatino M, Kim-Schulze S, Panelli MC, Stroncek D, Wang E, Taback B, et al. Serum vascular endothelial growth factor and fibronectin predict clinical response to high-dose interleukin-2 therapy. J Clin Oncol. 2009;27:2645–52.
52. Satzger I, Kuttler U, Volker B, Schenck F, Kapp A, Gutzmer R. Anal mucosal melanoma with KIT-activating mutation and response to imatinib therapy – case report and review of the literature. Dermatology. 2010;220:77–81.
53. Satzger I, Schaefer T, Kuettler U, Broecker V, Voelker B, Ostertag H, et al. Analysis of c-KIT expression and KIT gene mutation in human mucosal melanomas. Br J Cancer. 2008;99: 2065–9.
54. Schwartz RH. T cell anergy. Annu Rev Immunol. 2003;21:305–34.
55. Shah NP, Tran C, Lee FY, Chen P, Norris D, Sawyers CL. Overriding imatinib resistance with a novel ABL kinase inhibitor. Science. 2004;305:399–401.
56. Smalley KS, Sondak VK. Melanoma – an unlikely poster child for personalized cancer therapy. N Engl J Med. 2010;363:876–8.
57. Sullivan RJ, Hoshida Y, Brunet J, Tahan S, Aldridge J, Kwabi C, et al. A single center experience with high-dose IL-2 treatment for patients with advanced melanoma and pilot investigation

of a novel gene expression signature as a predictor of response. J Clin Oncol. 2009;27:15S, Abstract 9003.

58. Sutmuller RP, van Duivenvoorde LM, van Elsas A, Schumacher TN, Wildenberg ME, Allison JP, et al. Synergism of cytotoxic T lymphocyte-associated antigen 4 blockade and depletion of CD25(+) regulatory T cells in antitumor therapy reveals alternative pathways for suppression of autoreactive cytotoxic T lymphocyte responses. J Exp Med. 2001;194:823–32.
59. Sznol M, Powderly JD, Smith DC, Brahmer JR, Drake CG, McDermott DF, et al. Safety and antitumor activity of biweekly MDX-1106 (Anti-PD-1, BMS-936558/ONO-4538) in patients with advanced refractory malignancies. J Clin Oncol. 2010;28:15S. Abstract 2506.
60. Talpaz M, Shah NP, Kantarjian H, Donato N, Nicoll J, Paquette R, et al. Dasatinib in imatinib-resistant Philadelphia chromosome-positive leukemias. N Engl J Med. 2006;354:2531–41.
61. Tawby HA, Buch S, Pancoska P, Lin Y, Saul M, Romkes M, et al. Prediction of response to alkylator-based chemotherapy in metastatic melanoma (MM) using gene expression and promoter methylation signatures. J Clin Oncol. 2010;27:15s. Abstract 9009.
62. Tolcher AW, Mikulski SM, Messersmith WA, Kwak EL, Gibbon D, Boylan J, et al. A phase I study of RO4929097, a novel gamma secretase inhibitor, in patients with advanced solid tumors. J Clin Oncol. 2010;28:15s. Abstract 2502.
63. Ugurel S, Schrama D, Keller G, Schadendorf D, Brocker EB, Houben R, et al. Impact of the CCR5 gene polymorphism on the survival of metastatic melanoma patients receiving immunotherapy. Cancer Immunol Immunother. 2008;57:685–91.
64. Uyttenhove C, Pilotte L, Theate I, Stroobant V, Colau D, Parmentier N, et al. Evidence for a tumoral immune resistance mechanism based on tryptophan degradation by indoleamine 2,3-dioxygenase. Nat Med. 2003;9:1269–74.
65. Vansteenkiste JF, Zielinski M, Dahabreh IJ, Linder A, Lehmann F, Gruselle O. Association of gene expression signature and clinical efficacy of MAGE-A3 antigen-specific cancer immunotherapeutic (ASCI) as adjuvant therapy in resected stage IB/II non-small cell lung cancer (NSCLC). J Clin Oncol. 2008;26:Abstract 7501.
66. Wyman K, Atkins MB, Prieto V, Eton O, McDermott DF, Hubbard F, et al. Multicenter phase II trial of high-dose imatinib mesylate in metastatic melanoma: significant toxicity with no clinical efficacy. Cancer. 2006;106:2005–11.
67. Zha Y, Marks R, Ho AW, Peterson AC, Janardhan S, Brown I, et al. T cell anergy is reversed by active Ras and is regulated by diacylglycerol kinase-alpha. Nat Immunol. 2006;7:1166–73.
68. Zhang L, Gajewski TF, Kline J. PD-1/PD-L1 interactions inhibit antitumor immune responses in a murine acute myeloid leukemia model. Blood. 2009;114:1545–52.
69. Zhou XP, Gimm O, Hampel H, Niemann T, Walker MJ, Eng C. Epigenetic PTEN silencing in malignant melanomas without PTEN mutation. Am J Pathol. 2000;157:1123–8.
70. Zippelius A, Batard P, Rubio-Godoy V, Bioley G, Lienard D, Lejeune F, et al. Effector function of human tumor-specific CD8 T cells in melanoma lesions: a state of local functional tolerance. Cancer Res. 2004;64:2865–73.

Part II
Signaling Molecules as Molecular Targets

Chapter 4
KIT as a Therapeutic Target for Melanoma

Nageatte Ibrahim and F. Stephen Hodi

Abstract We have embarked on an exciting era of targeted therapy in oncology, and in many ways a most exciting one for melanoma. Understanding the fundamental genetic changes that govern the development and growth of melanoma has propelled the field forward. Genetic mutations in *KIT* have proven to be successful targets of several tyrosine kinase inhibitors with demonstrated clinical efficacy in gastrointestinal stromal tumors (GIST). With the identification of mutations and amplifications in *KIT* in melanomas that occur on acral and mucosal surfaces as well as on skin with chronic sun damage, initial reports of treatment with inhibitors in selected patients have suggested promising clinical activity. In this chapter, we review the biology of KIT and its role in melanoma as well report on the current experience with kinase inhibitors in selected melanoma patient populations. We will also outline the ongoing efforts that strive to answer critical questions on efficacy, dosing, and tumor genomics that predict response and suggest mechanisms of resistance.

Keywords KIT • CD117 • Acral melanoma • Mucosal melanoma • Chronic sun-damaged skin • Imatinib • Sunitinib • Nilotinib • Dasatinib • Masatinib

Introduction

The age of targeted therapy is upon us and strides are being made in categorizing melanomas on the basis of their driving oncogenic mutations, with the goal of providing patients with truly personalized medicine. Several mutations in melanoma

N. Ibrahim, MD • F.S. Hodi, MD (✉)
Department of Medical Oncology, Dana-Farber Cancer Institute and Melanoma Disease Center,
Dana-Farber/Brigham and Women's Cancer Center, Boston, MA, USA
e-mail: stephen_hodi@dfci.harvard.edu

T.F. Gajewski and F.S. Hodi (eds.), *Targeted Therapeutics in Melanoma*,
Current Clinical Oncology, DOI 10.1007/978-1-61779-407-0_4,
© Springer Science+Business Media, LLC 2012

have been identified with the hope to exploit these molecular aberrations as effective *drugable* targets (reviewed in Ibrahim and Haluska [42]). The most common mutation in melanoma is BRAF^{V600E}, which occurs in up to 66% of melanomas [14]. Not long after the discovery of BRAF mutations in melanoma, activating mutations and amplification in the *KIT* gene in melanomas originating from mucosal, acral, and skin with chronic sun damage (CSD) were reported with modest frequency [13]. More importantly, for translational relevance, many of the KIT mutations found in these melanomas involve the juxtamembrane position thus predicting sensitivity to inhibition with tyrosine kinase inhibitors (TKIs) such as imatinib. Several case reports have showcased the efficacy of various TKIs in patients with metastatic melanoma with *KIT* mutation/amplification. Clinical trials are underway for selected patients to test the effect of these agents and to better understand the molecular mechanisms associated with response and resistance to such targeted therapy.

KIT as a Proto-Oncogene

The proto-oncogene *KIT* plays a critical role in melanocyte proliferation, migration, and survival. KIT is a type III trans-membrane receptor tyrosine kinase (RTK) that contains five immunoglobulin-like domains in its extracellular portion, a single transmembrane region, an inhibitory cytoplasmic/juxtamembrane domain, and a split cytoplasmic kinase domain separated by a kinase insert segment [84]. Binding of its ligand stem cell factor (SCF) to the extracellular domain results in receptor dimerization, activation of the intracellular tyrosine kinase domain, and finally receptoractivation [50]. The mitogen-activated protein kinase (MAPK), phosphatidylinositol-3'-kinase (PI3K) as well as JAK/signal transducers and activators of transcription (JAK/STAT) are downstream effector pathways of KIT signaling (Fig. 4.1). Such KIT-driven intracellular signaling delineates its critical role in the development of various mammalian cells including melanocytes, hematopoietic progenitor cells, mast cells, primordial germ cells, and intestinal cells of Cajal [22, 29, 63].

Although shown to be essential in melanocyte development, the exact mechanisms for KIT signaling in melanocyte proliferation, migration, differentiation, and survival remain to be elucidated. Inactivating mutations in *KIT* which impair its kinase activity lead to developmental disorders that result in amelanotic congenital patches of white skin associated with human piebaldism and mouse dominant white spotting [26, 27]. Furthermore, KIT inactivation in melanocyte precursors prevents their dispersion and survival [78]. In murine models, mutations in *KIT* or SCF result in animals lacking melanocytes and functional mast cells along with defects in hematopoiesis and germ cell development [23, 24]. This phenotype closely resembles that seen in humans with mutations in MITF (microphthalmia transcription factor), resulting in Waardenburg Syndrome type II [36]. This striking similarity led to the hypothesis that SCF, KIT, and MITF act in a common growth/differentiation pathway. Hemesath et al. demonstrated that the activated protein, c-KIT, phosphorylates MITF through activation of MAPK thereby altering the expression of genes mediating cell lineage commitment, development, and survival [37].

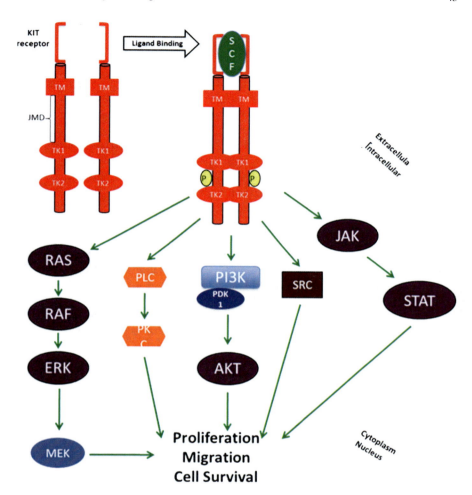

Fig. 4.1 Diagram of c*KIT* signaling pathways. Ligand binding of SCF (stem cell factor) promotes KIT receptor dimerization leading to phosphorylation and activation of the tyrosine kinase domains. Once activated, KIT signals to downstream effector pathways: the RAS-FAR-MEK pathway, the PI3K (phosphoinositol-3 kinase) pathway, and the JAK-STAT pathway. Activated KIT also signal through PLC and SRC leading to cellular proliferation, migration, and survival. *TM* transmembrane; *TK* tyrosine kinase; *JMD* juxtamembrane domain (encoded by exon 11); *JAK* Janus kinase; *STAT* signal transducers and activators of transcription; *Src* short for sarcoma, a tyrosine kinase; *PI3K* phosphoinositol-3 kinase; *PDK1* pyruvate dehydrogenase kinase, isozyme 1; *PLC* phospholipase C; *PKC* protein kinase C; *ERK* extracellular regulated kinase; *MEK* MAP kinase/ERK kinase kinase

The Role of KIT in Cancer

Abnormal activation of KIT via autocrine secretion of SCF has been observed in various cancers such as breast, gynecological, colorectal, small cell lung cancer, and neuroblastoma [9]. The role of KIT in melanoma has been historically controversial. Even though KIT has been shown to be critical for melanocyte development, its expression is frequently lost during progression of melanoma from early to advanced disease [48, 61, 62]. KIT also has antitumor properties as its expression in KIT-negative human melanoma cell lines triggers apoptosis [41]. Alexeev et al. eloquently demonstrated that constitutive activation of the KIT receptor did not result in melanogenesis or proliferation, but promoted migration of melanocytes that was not associated with tumorigenic transformation [2]. This work illustrated the role of KIT in transmitting pro-migration signals, which may antagonize proliferation and tumorigenesis [2]. This may provide an explanation as to why melanocytes lose KIT expression during melanogenesis. KIT is responsible for not only melanocyte migration but also morphology, resulting in spindle-shaped bodies and decreased number of dendrites [2]. These findings were consistent with prior work illustrating how KIT activation can promote melanocyte adhesion and migration on fibronectin, regulate integrin expression, as well as reorganize the cytoskeleton by inducing a rapid increase in actin stress fiber formation [71]. Such observations led to earlier speculation that KIT may function as a tumor suppressor gene, as loss of KIT expression interfered with mobility and proliferative properties in transformed melanocytes.

Bastian et al. set out to identify genetic changes that occur in primary cutaneous melanoma using comparative genomic hybridization (CGH) [5]. In addition to losses and gains of several chromosomes in many of the samples, they observed a small amplification on the proximal 4q region in a subungual melanoma that occurred on the finger [5]. Among potential gene candidates that map to 4q12-13 are platelet-derived growth factor receptor (PDGFR) and KIT. However, the technical resolution at the time was not adequate to sufficiently identify the affected gene. Following up on this initial observation, CGH analysis of chromosomal aberrations in 15 acral melanomas and 15 superficial spreading melanomas (SSM) that were matched for tumor thickness and patient age was performed [4]. Comparisons of gene amplifications in acral melanomas to SSM were made. The most frequently amplified regions occurred at 11q13 (47%), 22q11-13 (40%), and 5p15 (20%) in acral melanomas. These amplifications were believed to occur early in tumorigenesis as supported by the finding of amplifications of 11q13 in 3 of 5 additional cases of acral melanoma in situ. Furthermore, isolated melanocytes with amplifications in the epidermis up to 3 mm beyond the histologically detectable boundary were identified in 5 of 15 invasive acral melanomas. Additional analyses of skin adjacent to acral melanomas using CGH and fluorescent in situ hybridization (FISH) detected melanocytic cells with genetic amplifications in the epidermis in 84% of cases [64]. Further genetic analysis of these cells, termed "field cells," indicated that they were in an early phase of disease preceding melanoma in situ. Tumor thickness was not predictive of the extent of field cells. This is important as it provides a possible explanation for local recurrence of melanoma following complete excision and may even help guide surgical management. This has implications, not only for KIT-driven melanoma, but also potentially for all subtypes. Additional studies are needed to better understand the biology of these field cells and explore the impact of wider surgical margins on recurrence in these patients.

It is now obvious that the role of KIT in melanoma development and propagation is more intricate than initially thought. Although BRAF^{V600E} is the most common mutation in cutaneous melanoma [14], genetic characterization of acral, mucosal, and CSD melanomas revealed rare mutations in BRAF^{V600E} [53]. A paradigm shift in categorizing melanomas based on their anatomic origin provided further opportunity to identify genomic aberrations in melanoma subtypes. A large study of 102 primary melanomas (38 mucosal, 28 acral, 18 CSD skin, and 18 non-CSD skin) utilized CGH to detect DNA copy number aberrations [13]. A narrow amplification on chromosome 4q12 was observed and offered *KIT* as a candidate gene. Mutational analysis of *KIT* in the samples with amplifications detected mutations in three of the seven tumors. Altogether, mutations and/or amplification in *KIT* were discovered in 39% of mucosal, 36% of acral, and 28% of melanomas arising in CSD skin as defined by the presence of pathologic solar elastosis. No aberrations in *KIT* were detected in melanomas occurring on non-CSD skin; these had a high frequency of BRAF^{V600E} mutations. Interestingly, mutations in NRAS or BRAF were almost virtually exclusive of amplifications in KIT, suggesting that certain subtypes of melanomas are dependent on specific genomic aberrations. A separate study of melanoma metastases found a subset to overexpress KIT [6]. Interestingly, and in comparison to other KIT-driven tumors such as gastrointestinal stromal tumors (GIST) [57], approximately one-third of *KIT* mutations found in melanomas involve exon 11 (L576P) [6]. As these mutations occur in the juxtamembrane domain, they are predictive of sensitivity to TKIs, including imatinib, nilotinib, dasatinib, and sunitinib [25].

To better understand the role activating KIT mutations play in melanocytes, Monsel et al. characterized the physiological responses of melanocytes expressing the most frequent KIT mutations in melanoma (K642E, L576P) along with a novel mutation (D576P) that was identified in an acral melanoma [59]. They demonstrated that this activation of the KIT receptor in melanocytes primarily involves the PI3K/Akt pathway rather than the Ras/Raf/Mek/Erk pathway. However, activation of the PI3K pathway alone in cells harboring *KIT* mutations was not sufficient to promote uncontrolled melanocyte growth and melanomagenesis, suggesting that a tissue-specific epigenetic environment is required in vivo. Cooperation with active HIF-1a (hypoxia inducible factor) led to transformation of the KIT mutant melanocytes further suggesting that a hypoxic tissue environment contributes to melanocyte transformation. Furthermore, proliferation of the transformed melanocytes was specifically inhibited by imatinib. The authors speculated that such a strict dependency of *KIT*-mutated cells on the microenvironment might account for the very low frequency (approximately 2%) of *KIT* mutations in cutaneous melanoma [6, 13]. Their work suggests a distinct molecular mechanism for melanocyte transformation as a consequence of a KIT-activating mutation.

KIT Tyrosine Kinase Inhibitors

The identification of *KIT* mutations in melanoma subtypes has direct therapeutic implications. The mutation spectrum of *KIT* in melanoma resembles that of GIST where most mutations occur in exon 11, which encodes the juxtamembrane domain [6]. The juxtamembrane domain of KIT provides a critical auto-inhibitory function that can be disrupted by mutations that change the amino-acid sequence [76]. These mutations lead to constitutive activation of KIT thereby initiating a series of signaling events that result in cellular proliferation [77] and tumor progression. Mutations in the juxtamembrane region predict clinical responsiveness to TKIs [35]. Documented exon 11 mutations in melanoma include point mutations, in-frame deletions, and insertions that result in constitutive activation of the *KIT* receptor [25]. The most common *KIT* mutation in melanoma occurs in exon 11, L576P, with an approximate incidence of 35% across all cases reported to date [25]. Importantly, GIST with exon 11 mutations have been reported to respond well to treatment with imatinib [34]. Mutations in exons 13 (encoding the tyrosine kinase-1) and 17 (encoding the tyrosine kinase-2) are more frequent in melanoma than in GIST. The next most common mutation is K642E in exon 13, with a rate of 16.3% in published melanoma cases [25].

Importantly, the clinical experience with response to different TKIs relevant to the particular *KIT* mutation is not yet mature. Imatinib is a first-generation TKI with activity targeting the Bcr-Abl fusion protein, c-abl, abl-related gene (ARG), PDGFR, and the *KIT* tyrosine kinase receptor [16, 65, 70]. Over 85% of GIST harbor an activating mutation in *KIT* and treatment with imatinib has significantly improved survival in this disease [8, 54]. Clinical experience in patients with GIST indicates that the presence and location of specific mutations in *KIT* can predict sensitivity and resistance patterns to *KIT* inhibitors [34]. One of the first reports testing the efficacy of imatinib in melanoma was its use in patients with ocular melanoma whose tumors were found to express CD117 (*KIT*) by immunohistochemistry (IHC) [19] (Table 4.1). Of the three patients with positive IHC, two had a partial response with a reduction of malignant ascites in one patient and a partial remission of neck lymphadenopathy in the other patient [19]. An additional study of 21 patients with metastatic uveal melanoma revealed strong expression of KIT in 55% of primary uveal melanomas and in 76% of metastases [40]. Twelve patients were subsequently treated with imatinib 600 mg daily. Three patients discontinued therapy early due to significant and obvious disease progression. Of the nine patients who completed more than 8 weeks of treatment, none achieved an objective response. The best clinical outcome was one patient with stable disease for 52 weeks. Evaluation of *KIT* exons 11, 13, 17, and 18 did not reveal any mutations in the 21 cases.

Additional phase II trials of imatinib in unselected patients with metastatic melanoma provided little evidence of clinical benefit [45, 74, 82]. In the study by Ugurel et al., only 2 of 16 patients (one with an acral melanoma and the other with a mucosal melanoma) were representative of the study population that would be most likely to have a *KIT* mutation/amplification [7, 74]. Concluding that *KIT* inhibition was ineffective in melanoma might have been premature in this unselected patient population.

Table 4.1 Case reports of activity of c*KIT* inhibition in melanomas harboring activating mutations in c*KIT*

Melanoma type	No. of patients	*KIT* mutation	Drug/dose	Response	References
Ocular	3	+IHC expression	Imatinib 400 mg/day	2 PR	[19]
Mucosal	1	+IHC expression	Imatinib 400 mg/day	1 PR	[39]
		7 bp duplication in exon 11			
Mucosal	1	K642E in exon 13	Imatinib 400–600 mg/day	1 CR	[52]
		KIT amplification by FISH			
Acral and mucosal	5	Exon 11 mutation in 3 patients; exon 11 amplification in 1 patient; exon 13 mutation in 1 patient	Imatinib 300–800 mg/day	3 PR 2 SD	[11]
Mucosal	1	V560A in exon 11	Sorafenib 800 mg/day	CR (5 months)	[67]
Mucosal	2	L576P in exon 11	Dasatinib 140 mg/day	2 PR	[81]
Acral Mucosal Ocular	2	Exon 13 mutation; deletion exon 11	Dasatinib 140–200 mg/day	2 PR 1 NR	[46]
Mucosal	1	V559A in exon 11	Sunitinib 37.5 mg/day	PR	[85]
Mucosal	1	L576P in exon 11	Imatinib 400 mg/day	SD	[69]
Acral	1	V559A in lung metastasis; WT in primary tumor and regional inguinal node metastasis	Imatinib 400 mg/day	PR of lung; PD of inguinal nodes	[73]
Mucosal	3	21 bp duplication in exon 11; K642E in exon 13; L576P in exon 11	Imatinib 400–600 mg/day	3 PR	[33]
	1	D820Y in exon 17	Sorafenib 400 mg twice daily	1 PR	[33]
Acral	1	K642E in exon 13	Imatinib 400 mg/day	PR	[83]

CR complete response; *PR* partial response; *NR* no response

To date, the clinical activity of imatinib in patients with *KIT*-mutated melanomas has been described in a series of case reports (Table 4.1). In 2008, the first two cases were independently reported by Hodi et al. and Lutzky et al. documenting significant clinical responses to imatinib in metastatic mucosal melanoma [39, 52]. The former report was that of a 79-year-old female with a primary rectal melanoma that exhibited strong CD117 staining by IHC and upon sequencing, found to contain a 7-codon duplication in exon 11 of *KIT* [39]. Following 4 weeks of therapy with imatinib 400 mg daily, PET/CT revealed a marked response in the preexisting metastatic disease with complete resolution of the FDG-avid right epicardial and adrenal masses. The latter report importantly suggested that the responsiveness and durability of response to imatinib was dose-dependent (discussed further in Section "Overcoming Resistance to Tyrosine Kinase Inhibition"). Satzger et al. reported on a 79-year-old female with an anal melanoma with a *KIT*-activating mutation, L576P, in exon 11 who achieved stable disease on 400 mg daily of imatinib [69]. Imatinib was also used to treat a 61-year-old male with a primary acral lentiginous melanoma of the thumb metastatic to the regional axillary lymph nodes and lungs [83]. He had regression of the nodal and lung metastases and a significant decrease in the size of the primary melanoma. A mutation in *KIT* was detected in his primary tumor, K642E, which has also been reported to occur in GIST.

A recent report of four patients with mucosal melanomas containing mutations in *KIT* demonstrated systemic partial responses in all patients. However, it further showcased a potential limitation of therapy, as three of the four patients developed and succumbed to central nervous system (CNS) metastases [33]. Additionally, in this report one patient with a D820Y mutation in exon 17 of *KIT* received sorafenib as this mutation has been shown to be resistant to imatinib therapy in vitro [32]. This presents an important question that remains in targeting *KIT*-mutant melanomas, as to whether specific *KIT* mutations in an individual patient's tumor may have greater susceptibility for clinical responses to one particular *KIT* TKI vs. another. Moreover, it underscores the possibility that the CNS may serve as a sanctuary site for disease relapse and whether TKIs could be effective in treating CNS metastases. Carvajal et al. reported in abstract form five patients with acral and mucosal melanomas containing mutations in either exon 11 or 13 (one patient had amplification of exon 11) who were treated with imatinib [11]. Of the five patients, three achieved a partial response and two had stable disease. Interestingly, heterogeneous mutational status of *KIT* has been reported in one patient with a metastatic melanoma [73]. The 64-year-old woman with a primary acral melanoma of her left great toe had locoregional metastases to inguinal lymph nodes and a large mass obstructing the left main bronchus. She was treated with imatinib 400 mg daily. After 6 weeks of therapy, imaging revealed regression of the pulmonary mass but marked progression of the left lymph node metastasis. Mutation analysis of *KIT* was subsequently performed and revealed only wild-type sequences in the primary tumor and the lymph node. However, a mutation in exon 11, V559A, was detected in the responding lung mass. This case illustrates that genomic heterogeneity in metastatic tumors can exist; the mutational status of a corresponding tumor is highly predictive for treatment outcome, and again echoes that the sole overexpression of *KIT* by IHC may not be suitable for patient selection [40].

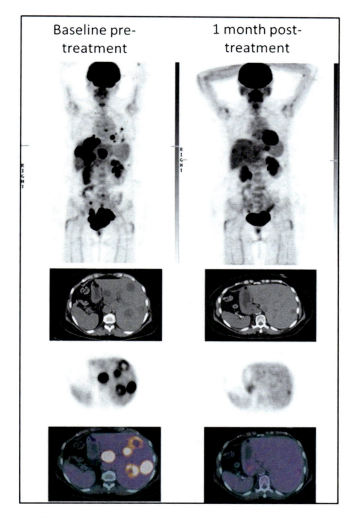

Fig. 4.2 Patient CT images showing response. Dramatic response to treatment with imatinib after 1 month in a patient with an activating KIT mutation

Imatinib is currently being investigated in phase II trials in selected patients with metastatic melanoma occurring on mucosal, acral, or CSD skin that harbor a *KIT* mutation and/or amplification (NCT00881049; NCT00424515). One trial was designed to permit dose escalation from 400 mg daily to 800 mg daily upon disease progression (NCT00424515). The second trial initiated treatment at 800 mg/day and permitted dose reductions. As suggested by case report series, responses can be dramatic with early evidence of activity predicted by PET imaging and can be durable for many months. An example of such a response is depicted in Fig. 4.2.

PET imaging before and after imatinib reveals complete resolution of lung metastases and a dramatic decrease in the hepatic and pelvic metastases. We currently await the mature results of these phase II trials.

Following the appreciation of the importance of *KIT* in driving subsets of melanomas and anecdotal reports of clinical benefits with imatinib, clinical investigation with other *KIT* inhibitors has been initiated in this patient population. These range from case reports with additional agents to the development of phase II trials. Sorafenib is a multi-kinase inhibitor of VEFGR, BRAF (wild-type and V600E mutant), PDGFR-β, *KIT*, and FLT-3 [80]. Single agent activity in melanoma or in combination with chemotherapy has not yielded meaningful responses [3, 18, 20, 21, 55]. A complete response to sorafenib that lasted about 5 months in a patient with a mucosal melanoma with a V560A mutation in exon 11 was reported [67]. Dasatinib is a second-generation inhibitor of BCR-ABL that is 325 times more potent in vitro than imatinib [51] and has been approved in patients with CML who are resistant or intolerant to imatinib [38]. A recent phase III trial comparing dasatinib to imatinib in first-line treatment of chronic-phase CML demonstrated significantly higher and faster rates of cytogenetic and molecular responses indicating that dasatinib may improve the long-term outcomes of these patients [43]. Dasatinib also inhibits EphA2, PDGFR, *KIT*, and Src family kinases. Reports of activity in KIT-driven melanomas have been reported [46, 81]. Currently, an Eastern Cooperative Oncology Group (ECOG) trial is exploring the efficacy of dasatinib in metastatic mucosal and acral melanomas (Table 4.2). Sunitinib is a PDGFR, VEGFR, FGF-2 (FGF-β), *KIT*, FLT-3, RET, and CSF1-R inhibitor that has shown clinical activity in GIST, renal cell carcinoma, neuroendocrine tumors, sarcoma, thyroid cancer, non-small cell lung cancer, and melanoma (reviewed in Chow and Eckhardt [12]). Sunitinib has demonstrated activity in imatinib-resistant GIST harboring a variety of mutations [10, 66]. Zhu et al. reported a partial response of 70% in one patient with a mucosal melanoma containing a V559A mutation in exon 11 [85]. An ongoing phase II trial is evaluating sunitinib in patients with metastatic mucosal or acral melanomas (NCT00577382). The trial is now enrolling its second cohort at a dose of 37.5 mg daily continuous dosing following completion of a cohort of patients treated at 50 mg daily 4 weeks on 2 weeks off. Minor et al. reported in abstract form the preliminary results of their ongoing phase II trial of sunitinib in patients with *KIT* aberrations (amplification or mutation) and at this early point in the trial, *KIT* mutations seem to indicate sensitivity to sunitinib (NCT00631618) [58] (Table 4.2). These trials offer the opportunity to shed insight into the remaining important questions of comparative efficacy between TKIs, differing side effect profiles of various TKIs in this patient population, as well as the significance of dose intensity.

Overcoming Resistance to Tyrosine Kinase Inhibition

It is evident even from the early anecdotal clinical reports that *KIT* mutational status is likely predictive of responses to TKIs in certain subtypes of melanoma. There is

Table 4.2 Clinical trials evaluating *KIT* inhibitors in melanoma subtypes

Drug	Melanoma subtype	c*KIT* mutation	Dose
Imatinib [28]	Acral	Phase II: *KIT* mutation (NCT00424515)	400 mg twice a day
Target: ABL, *c-KIT*, PDGFR	Mucosal		
Indications: first-line in CML and GIST	Chronic sun-damaged skin	Phase II: *KIT* mutation or amplification (NCT00881049) [31]	400–800 mg daily
Major side effects: nausea, fluid retention, diarrhea, bone pain, rash, cytopenias, disturbance of liver function			
Sunitinib [56]	Acral	Phase II: *KIT* status evaluated retrospectively (NCT00577382)	37.5 mg daily
Targets: VEGFR1,2,3, PDGFR-a, PDGFR-b, FGF-2, *c-KIT*, FLT-3, RET, CSF1-R	Mucosal		
	Chronic sun-damaged skin		
Indications: RCC, imatinib-resistant GIST		Phase II: *KIT* mutation or amplification (NCT00631618) [58]	50 mg/day 4 weeks on and 2 weeks off
Major side effects: fatigue, mucositis, hand-foot syndrome, nausea, diarrhea, thrombocytopenia, neutropenia			
Dasatinib [1, 17]	Acral	Phase II: *KIT* mutation and amplification evaluated retrospectively (NCT00700882)	70 mg twice a day
Targets: ABL, EphA2, PDGFR, *c-KIT*, Src family kinases (Src, Lyk, Yes, Fyn)	Mucosal		
	Chronic sun-damaged skin		
Indications: CML first-line. CML resistant to imatinib (except if positive for T351I mutation in BCR-ABL), CML resistant to nilotinib (except for T351I mutations)			
Major side effects: nausea, anorexia, abdominal pain, headache, peripheral edema, pleural effusion, thrombocytopenia			

(continued)

Table 4.2 (continued)

Drug	Melanoma subtype	cKIT mutation	Dose
Nilotinib [44, 68]	Acral	Phase II: patients who have progressed on or were intolerant of another TKI: c-KIT mutation or amplification (NCT00788775)	400 mg twice daily
Targets: ABL, c-KIT, PDGFR	Mucosal		
Indications: CML first-line, imatinib-resistant CML	Chronic sun-damaged skin		
Major side effects: fatigue, rash, pruritis, headache, nausea, neutropenia, thrombocytopenia	Only for phase II trial: CNS metastases, regardless of primary, allowed if KIT mutation is present	Phase III trial of nilotinib vs. DTIC: c-KIT mutations in exons 11, 13, or 17. For exon 17, only Y822D and Y823D allowed (NCT01028222)	
Masatinib [49, 72]		Trials being initiated in Europe	Weight-based dosing
Targets: wild-type c-KIT and its activated form, PDGFRa, PDGFRb, Lyn, FGFR3, the focal adhesion pathway (FAK) pathway			
Indications: phase I and II studies completed in imatinib-resistant and naïve patients with GIST			
Major side effects: rash, neutropenia, asthenia, diarrhea, nausea, edema			

also suggestion that these responses can be self-limited with subsequent evidence for progression with continued therapy. A common mechanism of resistance to TKIs in GIST and CML involves acquiring additional *KIT* exon mutations. The development of new mutations can be subsequently targeted with a different TKI. In addition, resistance to low-dose imatinib can be overcome by dose-escalation with achievement of a superior clinical response in CML and GIST [47]. As previously mentioned, Lutzky et al. reported a dose-dependent complete response to imatinib in a patient with metastatic anal melanoma that harbored a K642E mutation in exon 13 as well as amplification of *KIT* [52]. This patient achieved a complete response on 400 mg daily of imatinib in less than 8 weeks but required a dose reduction due to hematologic side effects. The patient continued to receive 200 mg/day with dose escalation to 200 mg/day alternating with 300 mg/day but had progressive disease 8 weeks later. Imatinib was subsequently increased to 600 mg/day and again a complete response was achieved shortly thereafter. This case demonstrates the complexity of the tumor biology and raises the question as to whether *KIT* amplification in addition to mutational status offer predictive value for response to therapy and which is more influential in overcoming resistance to low-dose tyrosine-kinase inhibition. Furthermore, it highlights the dose-dependent response to imatinib that has been reported in GIST where patients with a suboptimal response and progressive disease on 400–600 mg/day go on to achieve an improved response upon dose escalation to 800 mg/day (reviewed in Gronchi et al. [30]). Additionally, patients with exon 9 mutations had a longer progression-free survival when initially treated with imatinib 800 mg/day compared to patients with exon 11 or no mutations [30]. Again, this raises the question of specific genomic alterations having differing responses to a particular TKI. It can be speculated that tumors harboring *KIT* amplifications may be more prone to developing drug-resistance as they are selected for an escape mechanism to tyrosine-kinase inhibition. As a result, this dose-dependence effect may be reflective of particular mutations and/or amplifications in *KIT*, which is important to better define with further clinical experience.

In order to overcome the mechanisms of resistance that develop following KIT TKI therapy, new generation TKIs have been developed. Nilotinib is a second-generation Bcr-Abl TKI that is effective in patients with imatinib-resistant or intolerant CML in chronic and accelerated phases as well as in imatinib-resistant GIST [44, 60]. It is also an ATP-competitive inhibitor of the protein tyrosine kinase associated with Bcr-Abl. Nilotinib binds to wild-type Bcr-Abl to inhibit the tyrosine kinase activity of the Abl domain with a potency greater than 30 times that of imatinib [44]. It selectively inhibits both wild-type and mutated *KIT* with activity in exon 11 mutations (V560del, V560G), exon 13 mutations (K642E), and double mutants involving exons 11 and exons 13 or 17 [32, 75, 79]. The drug lacks activity in exon 14 mutations (T670I). In addition, nilotinib inhibits FIP1L1-PDGFRα and SCF-induced activation of KIT. Importantly, the side effect profile for nilotinib tends to be less severe and more manageable than those of imatinib, dasatinib, and sunitinib by reports (Table 4.2). A phase II trial is currently underway investigating the efficacy of nilotinib 400 mg twice daily in metastatic melanoma occurring on acral, mucosal, or CSD skin with *KIT* mutations who have developed resistance to or were intolerant of treatment with another TKI (NCT00788775) (Table 4.2). This trial also includes a cohort of patients with CNS metastases with a documented *KIT* mutation. As experience in treating patients with metastatic melanoma with *KIT* inhibitors continues to grow, it is being observed that patients treated with imatinib tend to relapse within the CNS. Therefore, investigating the efficacy of subsequent therapy with TKIs in patients with CNS metastases is paramount in understanding how to best manage these patients. An international, open-label phase III trial was recently launched to compare nilotinib vs. dacarbazine (DTIC) in patients with metastatic melanoma harboring mutations in exons 11, 13, or 17 of *KIT*. The primary endpoint for this trial is progression-free survival (NCT01028222). Only patients with tumors bearing exon 17 mutations Y822D or Y823D will be accepted for this trial (Table 4.2).

Finally, masatinib is a novel TKI with activity against wild-type and activated forms of *KIT*, PDGFRα, PDGFRβ, Lyn, FGFR3, and focal adhesion kinase (FAK) [72]. Due to its superior selectivity for *KIT*, masatinib may exhibit a better safety profile than other kinase inhibitors and can therefore be effective in imatinib-resistant tumors. A phase I study in solid malignancies demonstrated a favorable side effect profile and efficacy in imatinib-resistant patients and allowed for weight-based dosing [72]. Additionally, in a phase II trial in imatinib-naive patients, masatinib had promising clinical activity with tolerable toxicities [49]. Given masatinib's selectivity, its activity in melanomas harboring *KIT* mutations/amplifications is currently being explored (Table 4.2).

As we await the maturity of the phase II clinical trials in *KIT*-mutated melanoma, it is already clear that the next wave in clinical investigation for this melanoma subtype must focus on understanding mechanisms of resistance. Whether melanoma will share the resistance mechanisms seen in CML and GIST or acquire alternate mechanisms such as activation of additional signaling pathways, gene amplification, drug metabolism, or regulation of specific microRNAs is yet to be determined.

Is KIT Amplification or Mutation More Important?

It still remains to be delineated whether *KIT*-activating mutations alone, vs. amplification alone, vs. mutation plus amplification are sufficient for a response to a TKI. While clinical reports thus far have focused on significant responses in patients whose tumors harbor mutations, it will be crucial to understand further the potential for clinical benefit for wild-type amplified tumors as well as whether differences in mutated tumors are influenced by amplification status. In addition, it will be critical to understand the biology that impacts not only response but also the durability of response. Current phase II trials are evaluating the correlation between agent, response, and the amplification/mutational status of *KIT* (Table 4.2). The clinical reports thus far highlight the complexities of intracellular signaling in these melanoma subtypes and demonstrate that clinical efficacy determinations go beyond the tumors' amplification and/or mutational status of *KIT*.

Conclusions

Evaluation of *KIT* mutational status in patients with specific subtypes of metastatic melanoma is an important step in the age of targeted therapeutics. Mutations in *KIT* occur with modest frequencies in melanomas that originate on acral, mucosal, and CSD skin. Activation of *KIT* via either mutation or gene amplification likely contributes to the clinical course of these melanomas. Constitutive activation of mutated *KIT* and the presence of the majority of mutations in the juxtamembrane domain provide potential for therapeutic intervention. To date, there is evidence of clinical effectiveness in genetically selected patients with metastatic melanoma who are treated with *KIT* TKIs. The case reports have documented rapid response to treatment or achievement of stable disease that can last for many months. The mature results of these phase II and III trials with the first- and second-generation *KIT* inhibitors in gnomically selected patients are eagerly awaited. Better understanding of the response to treatment, duration, and sites of disease relapse, as well as the mechanisms of acquired drug resistance will be invaluable in tailoring more effective regimens for patients with *KIT*-mutated/amplified metastatic melanoma. Correlative studies between *KIT* mutational status, *KIT* amplification status, and clinical response will be valuable in this effort. More potent and selective *KIT* inhibitors are now available and their activity in these subtypes of melanomas is also being explored. If the phase II data remain promising, then considerations for adjuvant therapy with *KIT* inhibition in patients with locally advanced disease who have undergone complete surgical resection and lymphadenectomy and found to harbor a *KIT* mutation/amplification would need to be made. Will offering TKIs in the adjuvant setting impact the relapse-free survival in this genetically selected patient population as it has done in patients with GIST [15]? *KIT*-directed therapy in patients whose melanomas are dependent on *KIT* activation is in its early stages of development. The future is sure to bring important insights that will have direct impact on treatment in this subset of melanoma patients.

References

1. Aguilera DG, Tsimberidou AM. Dasatinib in chronic myeloid leukemia: a review. Ther Clin Risk Manag. 2009;5:281–9.
2. Alexeev V, Yoon K. Distinctive role of the cKit receptor tyrosine kinase signaling in mammalian melanocytes. J Invest Dermatol. 2006;126:1102–10.
3. Amaravadi RK, Schuchter LM, McDermott DF, Kramer A, Giles L, Gramlich K, et al. Phase II trial of temozolomide and sorafenib in advanced melanoma patients with or without brain metastases. Clin Cancer Res. 2009;15:7711–8.
4. Bastian BC, Kashani-Sabet M, Hamm H, Godfrey T, Moore II DH, Brocker EB, et al. Gene amplifications characterize acral melanoma and permit the detection of occult tumor cells in the surrounding skin. Cancer Res. 2000;60:1968–73.
5. Bastian BC, LeBoit PE, Hamm H, Brocker EB, Pinkel D. Chromosomal gains and losses in primary cutaneous melanomas detected by comparative genomic hybridization. Cancer Res. 1998;58:2170–5.

6. Beadling C, Jacobson-Dunlop E, Hodi FS, Le C, Warrick A, Patterson J, et al. KIT gene mutations and copy number in melanoma subtypes. Clin Cancer Res. 2008;14:6821–8.
7. Becker JC, Brocker EB, Schadendorf D, Ugurel S. Imatinib in melanoma: a selective treatment option based on KIT mutation status? J Clin Oncol. 2007;25:e9.
8. Blanke CD, Demetri GD, von Mehren M, Heinrich MC, Eisenberg B, Fletcher JA, et al. Long-term results from a randomized phase II trial of standard- versus higher-dose imatinib mesylate for patients with unresectable or metastatic gastrointestinal stromal tumors expressing KIT. J Clin Oncol. 2008;26:620–5.
9. Boissan M, Feger F, Guillosson JJ, Arock M. c-Kit and c-kit mutations in mastocytosis and other hematological diseases. J Leukoc Biol. 2000;67:135–48.
10. Carter TA, Wodicka LM, Shah NP, Velasco AM, Fabian MA, Treiber DK, et al. Inhibition of drug-resistant mutants of ABL, KIT, and EGF receptor kinases. Proc Natl Acad Sci USA. 2005;102:11011–6.
11. Carvajal RD, Chapman PB, Wolchok JD, Cane L, Teitcher JB, Lutzky J, et al. A phase II study of imatinib mesylate (IM) for patients with advanced melanoma harboring somatic alterations of KIT. J Clin Oncol. 2009 ASCO Annual Meeting Proceedings (Post-Meeting Edition) 2009; 27:9001.
12. Chow LQ, Eckhardt SG. Sunitinib: from rational design to clinical efficacy. J Clin Oncol. 2007;25:884–96.
13. Curtin JA, Busam K, Pinkel D, Bastian BC. Somatic activation of KIT in distinct subtypes of melanoma. J Clin Oncol. 2006;24:4340–6.
14. Davies H, Bignell GR, Cox C, Stephens P, Edkins S, Clegg S, et al. Mutations of the BRAF gene in human cancer. Nature. 2002;417:949–54.
15. DeMatteo R, Owzar K, Maki R, Pisters P, Blackstein M, Antonescu C, et al. Adjuvant imatinib mesylate increases recurrence free survival (RFS) in patients with completely resected localized primary gastrointestinal stromal tumor (GIST): North American Intergroup Phase III trial ACOSOG Z9001. J Clin Oncol. 2007;25.
16. Druker BJ, Lydon NB. Lessons learned from the development of an abl tyrosine kinase inhibitor for chronic myelogenous leukemia. J Clin Invest. 2000;105:3–7.
17. Druker BJ, Talpaz M, Resta DJ, Peng B, Buchdunger E, Ford JM, et al. Efficacy and safety of a specific inhibitor of the BCR-ABL tyrosine kinase in chronic myeloid leukemia. N Engl J Med. 2001;344:1031–7.
18. Eisen T, Ahmad T, Flaherty KT, Gore M, Kaye S, Marais R, et al. Sorafenib in advanced melanoma: a phase II randomised discontinuation trial analysis. Br J Cancer. 2006;95:581–6.
19. Fiorentini G, Rossi S, Lanzanova G, Biancalani M, Palomba A, Bernardeschi P, et al. Tyrosine kinase inhibitor imatinib mesylate as anticancer agent for advanced ocular melanoma expressing immunohistochemical C-KIT (CD 117): preliminary results of a compassionate use clinical trial. J Exp Clin Cancer Res. 2003;22:17–20.
20. Flaherty KT, Lee SJ, Schuchter LM, Flaherty LE, Wright JJ, Leming PD, et al. Final results of E2603: a double-blind, randomized phase III trial comparing carboplatin (C)/paclitaxel (P) with or without sorafenib (S) in metastatic melanoma. J Clin Oncol. 2010;(Suppl; abstr 8511):28.
21. Flaherty KT, Schiller J, Schuchter LM, Liu G, Tuveson DA, Redlinger M, et al. A phase I trial of the oral, multikinase inhibitor sorafenib in combination with carboplatin and paclitaxel. Clin Cancer Res. 2008;14:4836–42.
22. Galli SJ, Tsai M, Wershil BK, Tam SY, Costa JJ. Regulation of mouse and human mast cell development, survival and function by stem cell factor, the ligand for the c-kit receptor. Int Arch Allergy Immunol. 1995;107:51–3.
23. Garkavtsev I, Kazarov A, Gudkov A, Riabowol K. Suppression of the novel growth inhibitor p33ING1 promotes neoplastic transformation. Nat Genet. 1996;14:415–20.
24. Garkavtsev I, Riabowol K. Extension of the replicative life span of human diploid fibroblasts by inhibition of the p33ING1 candidate tumor suppressor. Mol Cell Biol. 1997;17:2014–9.
25. Garrido MC, Bastian BC. KIT as a therapeutic target in melanoma. J Invest Dermatol. 2010; 130:20–7.

26. Geissler EN, Ryan MA, Housman DE. The dominant-white spotting (W) locus of the mouse encodes the c-kit proto-oncogene. Cell. 1988;55:185–92.
27. Giebel LB, Spritz RA. Mutation of the KIT (mast/stem cell growth factor receptor) protooncogene in human piebaldism. Proc Natl Acad Sci USA. 1991;88:8696–9.
28. Goldman JM. Initial treatment for patients with CML. Hematol Am Soc Hematol Educ Program. 2009;1:453–60.
29. Grabbe J, Welker P, Dippel E, Czarnetzki BM. Stem cell factor, a novel cutaneous growth factor for mast cells and melanocytes. Arch Dermatol Res. 1994;287:78–84.
30. Gronchi A, Blay JY, Trent JC. The role of high-dose imatinib in the management of patients with gastrointestinal stromal tumor. Cancer. 2010;116:1847–58.
31. Guo J, Si L, Kong Y, Xu XW, Flaherty KT, Corless CL, et al. A phase II study of imatinib for advanced melanoma patients with KIT abberations. J Clin Oncol. 2010;(Suppl; abstr 8527):28.
32. Guo T, Agaram NP, Wong GC, Hom G, D'Adamo D, Maki RG, et al. Sorafenib inhibits the imatinib-resistant KITT670I gatekeeper mutation in gastrointestinal stromal tumor. Clin Cancer Res. 2007;13:4874–81.
33. Handolias D, Hamilton AL, Salemi R, Tan A, Moodie K, Kerr L, et al. Clinical responses observed with imatinib or sorafenib in melanoma patients expressing mutations in KIT. Br J Cancer. 2010;102:1219–23.
34. Heinrich MC, Corless CL, Blanke CD, Demetri GD, Joensuu H, Roberts PJ, et al. Molecular correlates of imatinib resistance in gastrointestinal stromal tumors. J Clin Oncol. 2006;24:4764–74.
35. Heinrich MC, Corless CL, Demetri GD, Blanke CD, von Mehren M, Joensuu H, et al. Kinase mutations and imatinib response in patients with metastatic gastrointestinal stromal tumor. J Clin Oncol. 2003;21:4342–9.
36. Helbing CC, Veillette C, Riabowol K, Johnston RN, Garkavtsev I. A novel candidate tumor suppressor, ING1, is involved in the regulation of apoptosis. Cancer Res. 1997;57:1255–8.
37. Hemesath TJ, Price ER, Takemoto C, Badalian T, Fisher DE. MAP kinase links the transcription factor Microphthalmia to c-Kit signalling in melanocytes. Nature. 1998;391:298–301.
38. Hochhaus A, Baccarani M, Deininger M, Apperley JF, Lipton JH, Goldberg SL, et al. Dasatinib induces durable cytogenetic responses in patients with chronic myelogenous leukemia in chronic phase with resistance or intolerance to imatinib. Leukemia. 2008;22:1200–6.
39. Hodi FS, Friedlander P, Corless CL, Heinrich MC, Mac Rae S, Kruse A, et al. Major response to imatinib mesylate in KIT-mutated melanoma. J Clin Oncol. 2008;26:2046–51.
40. Hofmann UB, Kauczok-Vetter CS, Houben R, Becker JC. Overexpression of the KIT/SCF in uveal melanoma does not translate into clinical efficacy of imatinib mesylate. Clin Cancer Res. 2009;15:324–9.
41. Huang S, Luca M, Gutman M, McConkey DJ, Langley KE, Lyman SD, et al. Enforced c-KIT expression renders highly metastatic human melanoma cells susceptible to stem cell factor-induced apoptosis and inhibits their tumorigenic and metastatic potential. Oncogene. 1996;13:2339–47.
42. Ibrahim N, Haluska FG. Molecular pathogenesis of cutaneous melanocytic neoplasms. Annu Rev Pathol. 2009;4:551–79.
43. Kantarjian H, Shah NP, Hochhaus A, Cortes J, Shah S, Ayala M, et al. Dasatinib versus imatinib in newly diagnosed chronic-phase chronic myeloid leukemia. N Engl J Med. 2010;362: 2260–70.
44. Kantarjian HM, Giles F, Gattermann N, Bhalla K, Alimena G, Palandri F, et al. Nilotinib (formerly AMN107), a highly selective BCR-ABL tyrosine kinase inhibitor, is effective in patients with Philadelphia chromosome-positive chronic myelogenous leukemia in chronic phase following imatinib resistance and intolerance. Blood. 2007;110:3540–6.
45. Kim KB, Eton O, Davis DW, Frazier ML, McConkey DJ, Diwan AH, et al. Phase II trial of imatinib mesylate in patients with metastatic melanoma. Br J Cancer. 2008;99:734–40.
46. Kluger HM, Dudek A, McCann C, Rink L, Ritacco J, Adrada C, et al. A phase II trial of dasatinib in advanced melanoma. J Clin Oncol. 2009;27(Suppl):15.

47. Koh Y, Kim I, Yoon SS, Kim BK, Kim DY, Lee JH, et al. Phase IV study evaluating efficacy of escalated dose of imatinib in chronic myeloid leukemia patients showing suboptimal response to standard dose imatinib. Ann Hematol. 2010;89:725–31.
48. Lassam N, Bickford S. Loss of c-kit expression in cultured melanoma cells. Oncogene. 1992;7:51–6.
49. Le Cesne A, Blay JY, Bui BN, Bouche O, Adenis A, Domont J, et al. Phase II study of oral masitinib mesilate in imatinib-naive patients with locally advanced or metastatic gastro-intestinal stromal tumour (GIST). Eur J Cancer. 2010;46:1344–51.
50. Lev S, Yarden Y, Givol D. Dimerization and activation of the kit receptor by monovalent and bivalent binding of the stem cell factor. J Biol Chem. 1992;267:15970–7.
51. Lombardo LJ, Lee FY, Chen P, Norris D, Barrish JC, Behnia K, et al. Discovery of N-(2-chloro-6-methyl- phenyl)-2-(6-(4-(2-hydroxyethyl)- piperazin-1-yl)-2-methylpyrimidin-4-ylamino)thiazole-5-carboxamide (BMS-354825), a dual Src/Abl kinase inhibitor with potent antitumor activity in preclinical assays. J Med Chem. 2004;47:6658–61.
52. Lutzky J, Bauer J, Bastian BC. Dose-dependent, complete response to imatinib of a metastatic mucosal melanoma with a K642E KIT mutation. Pigment Cell Melanoma Res. 2008;21:492–3.
53. Maldonado JL, Fridlyand J, Patel H, Jain AN, Busam K, Kageshita T, et al. Determinants of BRAF mutations in primary melanomas. J Natl Cancer Inst. 2003;95:1878–90.
54. McAuliffe JC, Lazar AJ, Yang D, Steinert DM, Qiao W, Thall PF, et al. Association of intratumoral vascular endothelial growth factor expression and clinical outcome for patients with gastrointestinal stromal tumors treated with imatinib mesylate. Clin Cancer Res. 2007;13:6727–34.
55. McDermott DF, Sosman JA, Gonzalez R, Hodi FS, Linette GP, Richards J, et al. Double-blind randomized phase II study of the combination of sorafenib and dacarbazine in patients with advanced melanoma: a report from the 11715 Study Group. J Clin Oncol. 2008;26:2178–85.
56. Mena AC, Pulido EG, Guillen-Ponce C. Understanding the molecular-based mechanism of action of the tyrosine kinase inhibitor: sunitinib. Anticancer Drugs. 2010;21 Suppl 1:S3–11.
57. MetaGIST (GSTM-AG). Comparison of two doses of imatinib for the treatment of unresectable or metastatic gastrointestinal stromal tumors: a meta-analysis of 1,640 patients. J Clin Oncol. 2010;28:1247–53.
58. Minor DR, O'Day S, Kashani-Sabet M, Daud A, Salman Z, Bastian B. Sunitinib therapy for metastatic melanomas with KIT aberrations. J Clin Oncol., 2010 ASCO Annual Meeting Proceedings (Post-Meeting Edition) 2010;28:8545.
59. Monsel G, Ortonne N, Bagot M, Bensussan A, Dumaz N. c-Kit mutants require hypoxia-inducible factor 1alpha to transform melanocytes. Oncogene. 2009;29:227–36.
60. Montemurro M, Schoffski P, Reichardt P, Gelderblom H, Schutte J, Hartmann JT, et al. Nilotinib in the treatment of advanced gastrointestinal stromal tumours resistant to both imatinib and sunitinib. Eur J Cancer. 2009;45:2293–7.
61. Montone KT, van Belle P, Elenitsas R, Elder DE. Proto-oncogene c-kit expression in malignant melanoma: protein loss with tumor progression. Mod Pathol. 1997;10:939–44.
62. Natali PG, Nicotra MR, Winkler AB, Cavaliere R, Bigotti A, Ullrich A. Progression of human cutaneous melanoma is associated with loss of expression of c-kit proto-oncogene receptor. Int J Cancer. 1992;52:197–201.
63. Nishikawa S, Kusakabe M, Yoshinaga K, Ogawa M, Hayashi S, Kunisada T, et al. In utero manipulation of coat color formation by a monoclonal anti-c-kit antibody: two distinct waves of c-kit-dependency during melanocyte development. EMBO J. 1991;10:2111–8.
64. North JP, Kageshita T, Pinkel D, LeBoit PE, Bastian BC. Distribution and significance of occult intraepidermal tumor cells surrounding primary melanoma. J Invest Dermatol. 2008;128:2024–30.
65. Okuda K, Weisberg E, Gilliland DG, Griffin JD. ARG tyrosine kinase activity is inhibited by STI571. Blood. 2001;97:2440–8.
66. Prenen H, Cools J, Mentens N, Folens C, Sciot R, Schoffski P, et al. Efficacy of the kinase inhibitor SU11248 against gastrointestinal stromal tumor mutants refractory to imatinib mesylate. Clin Cancer Res. 2006;12:2622–7.

67. Quintas-Cardama A, Lazar AJ, Woodman SE, Kim K, Ross M, Hwu P. Complete response of stage IV anal mucosal melanoma expressing KIT Val560Asp to the multikinase inhibitor sorafenib. Nat Clin Pract Oncol. 2008;5:737–40.
68. Saglio G, Kim DW, Issaragrisil S, le Coutre P, Etienne G, Lobo C, et al. Nilotinib versus imatinib for newly diagnosed chronic myeloid leukemia. N Engl J Med. 2010;362:2251–9.
69. Satzger I, Kuttler U, Volker B, Schenck F, Kapp A, Gutzmer R. Anal mucosal melanoma with KIT-activating mutation and response to imatinib therapy – case report and review of the literature. Dermatology. 2010;220:77–81.
70. Schindler T, Bornmann W, Pellicena P, Miller WT, Clarkson B, Kuriyan J. Structural mechanism for STI-571 inhibition of abelson tyrosine kinase. Science. 2000;289:1938–42.
71. Scott G, Liang H, Luthra D. Stem cell factor regulates the melanocyte cytoskeleton. Pigment Cell Res. 1996;9:134–41.
72. Soria JC, Massard C, Magne N, Bader T, Mansfield CD, Blay JY, et al. Phase 1 dose-escalation study of oral tyrosine kinase inhibitor masitinib in advanced and/or metastatic solid cancers. Eur J Cancer. 2009;45:2333–41.
73. Terheyden P, Houben R, Pajouh P, Thorns C, Zillikens D, Becker JC. Response to imatinib mesylate depends on the presence of the V559A-mutated KIT oncogene. J Invest Dermatol. 2009;130:314–6.
74. Ugurel S, Hildenbrand R, Zimpfer A, La Rosee P, Paschka P, Sucker A, et al. Lack of clinical efficacy of imatinib in metastatic melanoma. Br J Cancer. 2005;92:1398–405.
75. Verstovsek S, Akin C, Manshouri T, Quintas-Cardama A, Huynh L, Manley P, et al. Effects of AMN107, a novel aminopyrimidine tyrosine kinase inhibitor, on human mast cells bearing wild-type or mutated codon 816 c-kit. Leuk Res. 2006;30:1365–70.
76. Wardelmann E, Buttner R, Merkelbach-Bruse S, Schildhaus HU. Mutation analysis of gastrointestinal stromal tumors: increasing significance for risk assessment and effective targeted therapy. Virchows Arch. 2007;451:743–9.
77. Webster JD, Kiupel M, Yuzbasiyan-Gurkan V. Evaluation of the kinase domain of c-KIT in canine cutaneous mast cell tumors. BMC Cancer. 2006;6:85.
78. Wehrle-Haller B, Weston JA. Soluble and cell-bound forms of steel factor activity play distinct roles in melanocyte precursor dispersal and survival on the lateral neural crest migration pathway. Development. 1995;121:731–42.
79. Weisberg E, Manley PW, Breitenstein W, Bruggen J, Cowan-Jacob SW, Ray A, et al. Characterization of AMN107, a selective inhibitor of native and mutant Bcr-Abl. Cancer Cell. 2005;7:129–41.
80. Wilhelm SM, Carter C, Tang L, Wilkie D, McNabola A, Rong H, et al. BAY 43-9006 exhibits broad spectrum oral antitumor activity and targets the RAF/MEK/ERK pathway and receptor tyrosine kinases involved in tumor progression and angiogenesis. Cancer Res. 2004;64:7099–109.
81. Woodman SE, Trent JC, Stemke-Hale K, Lazar AJ, Pricl S, Pavan GM, et al. Activity of dasatinib against L576P KIT mutant melanoma: molecular, cellular, and clinical correlates. Mol Cancer Ther. 2009;8:2079–85.
82. Wyman K, Atkins MB, Prieto V, Eton O, McDermott DF, Hubbard F, et al. Multicenter phase II trial of high-dose imatinib mesylate in metastatic melanoma: significant toxicity with no clinical efficacy. Cancer. 2006;106:2005–11.
83. Yamaguchi M, Harada K, Ando N, Kawamura T, Shibagaki N, Shimada S. Marked response to imatinib mesylate in metastatic acral lentiginous melanoma on the thumb. Clin Exp Dermatol. 2011;36(2):174–7.
84. Yarden Y, Kuang WJ, Yang-Feng T, Coussens L, Munemitsu S, Dull TJ, et al. Human proto-oncogene c-kit: a new cell surface receptor tyrosine kinase for an unidentified ligand. EMBO J. 1987;6:3341–51.
85. Zhu Y, Si L, Kong Y, Chi Z, Yuan X, Cui C, et al. Response to sunitinib in Chinese KIT-mutated metastatic mucosal melanoma. J Clin Oncol. 2009;27(Suppl):e20017.

Chapter 5
Targeted Inhibition of B-Raf

Paul B. Chapman and Keith Flaherty

Abstract The hunt for mutated and activated kinases in cancer has proceeded at an accelerated pace since the successful treatment of chronic myelogenous leukemia with imatinib and with the development of new genomic sequencing technologies. The identification of activating mutations in B-Raf in a major subset of melanomas was first reported in 2002. Basic laboratory experiments confirmed the ability of mutant B-Raf to function as a driver oncogene in vivo. Relatively rapidly, inhibitors that preferentially target the mutated kinase were developed and tested clinically, and these studies revealed that the majority of patients bearing V600E B-Raf mutant melanomas showed a clinical response. Positive results of a randomized phase III clinical trial were released in early 2011. The current phase of this remarkable story is focused upon understanding mechanisms of primary and secondary resistance to B-Raf inhibitors in the clinic.

Keywords BRAF • MAPK • Vemurafenib • MEK • PLX4032

Introduction

The MAPK pathway (Fig. 5.1) is a key signaling pathway in melanoma. Under physiologic conditions, when activated by its ligand, a receptor tyrosine kinase (RTK) activates Ras of which there are three isoforms: NRAS, KRAS, and HRAS, although in melanoma, it appears that most of the signaling is through NRAS. This leads to phosphorylation of the RAF isoforms: ARAF, BRAF, and CRAF. The importance of the MAPK pathway in melanoma is indicated by observations that close to 90% of human melanoma tumors have a mutually exclusive activating mutation in

P.B. Chapman, MD (✉)
Department of Medicine, Memorial Sloan-Kettering Cancer Center, New York, NY, USA
e-mail: chapmanp@mskoc.org

K. Flaherty, MD
Massachusetts General Hospital Cancer Center, Boston, MA, USA

T.F. Gajewski and F.S. Hodi (eds.), *Targeted Therapeutics in Melanoma*,
Current Clinical Oncology, DOI 10.1007/978-1-61779-407-0_5,
© Springer Science+Business Media, LLC 2012

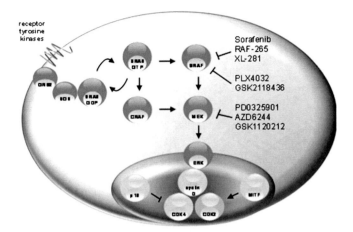

Fig. 5.1 BRAF in the MAP kinase pathway and relation to other genetically altered pathways in melanoma

BRAF, NRAS, or the RTK cKit. Presumably the remaining 10% of melanomas have activating mutations yet to be identified.

This chapter will focus on BRAF mutations which are by far the most common activating mutation in melanoma. Overall, 50–60% of melanomas are found to have an activating mutation in BRAF, most commonly (90–95% of BRAF mutant cases) a glutamic acid substituted for a valine at position 600 (V600E). Alternatively, in a small percentage of cases, lysine, arginine, or aspartic acid is found to be substituted for the valine. While these alternative substitutions are presumed to be activating, much less work has been done on these rare mutations. Therefore, when we discuss BRAF mutations, we will be referring to the V600E mutation.

BRAF mutations appear to be an early event in the development of melanoma. A survey of nevi revealed that BRAF mutations were found at approximately the same frequency as in melanomas [1, 2]. This suggests that BRAF mutations are necessary but not sufficient for transformation of melanocytes. This is supported by observations from transgenic mice. When the V600E BRAF mutation was inserted into the germline of mice under the tyrosinase promoter so that it was only expressed in melanocytic cells, mice developed melanocytic hyperplasia but did not develop melanoma [3]. These observations suggest that mutation in BRAF is an early event in the development of melanoma but not sufficient to transform melanocytes fully. However, as discussed below, clinical experience indicates that melanomas remain addicted to the BRAF mutation and that inhibition of BRAF can lead to dramatic anti-melanoma effects.

The MAPK Pathway

The MAPK pathway is turning out to be far more complex than expected and much is still unknown. However, it appears that engagement of a RTK leads to activation of RAS, reflected by an increase in RAS-GTP. Multiple investigators have shown that the presence of Ras-GTP leads to RAF homo- and heterodimerization [4–6]. When ATP binds to the ATP-binding pocket of one member of dimer pair, it induces a conformational change that leads to activation. At the same time, this leads to transactivation of the other member of the dimer [7, 8].

Activated RAF dimers then phosphorylate MEK1 and MEK2 which phosphorylate and activate ERK. Once activated, ERK has a myriad of targets including transcription factors (notably MITF), kinases, phosphatases, signaling proteins, structural proteins, and others (reviewed in [9]). In addition, pERK induces negative feedback that serves to modulate the output of the MAPK pathway [10]. ERK can directly inhibit CRAF [11, 12] and induces expression of negative regulators such as sprouty (SPRY) proteins [13] and MAP kinase phosphatases (DUSPs) [14]. Sprouty proteins can act inhibit upstream at the level of RAS/RAF; DUSPs can inhibit ERK directly. In BRAF-mutated cells, this feedback suppression is partially disrupted in that Sprouty2 fails to inhibit mutated BRAF [12, 15].

BRAF Mutations in Melanoma

Since the original discovery of BRAF mutations in human malignancies [16], it has become clear that 40–60% of melanomas harbor a BRAF mutation. BRAF mutations are most commonly seen in melanomas that arise at cutaneous sites exposed intermittently to sunlight [17] such as the trunk or extremities. Melanomas arising in chronically sun-exposed skin [17, 18], acral-lentiginous sites [17], mucosal sites [17, 19], harbor BRAF mutations less frequently. Uveal melanomas almost never harbor BRAF mutations [20] although paradoxically, some uveal melanoma cell lines contain BRAF mutations. This may suggest that a small subset of uveal melanomas harbor BRAF mutations and these are more likely to adapt to in vitro culture conditions. Indeed, BRAF-mutated melanomas seem to be generally easier to establish in tissue culture than BRAF wild-type melanoma.

There is some evidence that melanomas harboring BRAF mutations have a worse prognosis than BRAF wild-type melanomas [21, 22], although this correlation has not been seen universally [23]. Larger analyses will be needed to establish whether this correlation can be established.

Preclinical Studies

RAF Inhibition of BRAF Wild-Type Cells Leads to Activation of the MAPK Pathway

Several investigators have reported that the effect of ATP-competitive inhibitors of RAF on normal cells is to *activate* the MAPK pathway [7, 8]. This apparent paradox may be explained by the fact that, in the setting of activated RAS, the RAF kinases

BRAF^{WT} cells

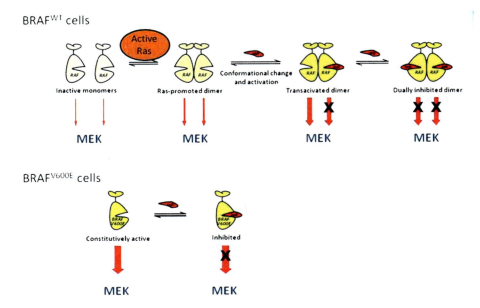

BRAF^{V600E} cells

Fig. 5.2 Model of the effects of RAF inhibitors in the presence of wild-type or mutant BRAF. In the presence of activated RAS, wild-type BRAF forms dimers leading to limited activation. When an ATP-competitive RAF inhibitor is added, it induces a conformational change to the active phosphorylated state that results in transactivation to the partner RAF molecule. This results in marked increase in MEK activation. If a sufficient concentration of RAF inhibitor is present, both partners of the dimer will be blocked resulting in the inhibition of MEK phosphorylation. In cells with mutated BRAF, low RAS activity prevents dimerization and the inhibitor blocks activation of MEK. With permission, from Poulikakos et al. [8]

form homo- and heterodimers [5]. In one model by Poulikakos and colleagues (Fig. 5.2), binding of inhibitor to one RAF ATP-binding domain leads to a conformational change in the partner RAF molecule leading to activation (i.e., transactivation). In this model, the inhibitor is not specific for BRAF but rather binds to all RAF isoforms. This is consistent with the data for the RAF inhibitors described to date, although there is some disagreement in the field [24]. In fact, the model predicts that a highly specific BRAF inhibitor would have similar effects on BRAF wild-type cells.

RAF Inhibition of BRAF-Mutated Melanoma Causes Melanoma Cell Death

In cells with BRAF mutations, the MAPK pathway is dysregulated. Although the precise details are still being worked out, it appears clear that mutated BRAF drives MEK and ERK phosphorylation. This probably leads to feedback inhibition resulting in low Ras-GTP and therefore little RAF dimerization. As a result, In this setting, the cell is being driven by mutated BRAF monomer and binding of a RAF inhibitor leads to decreases in phospho-MEK and phospho-ERK turning off the MAPK pathway in the cell. Other feedback mechanisms serve to further modulate output of the MAPK pathway, but the transcriptional output of the pathway is still increased [25].

Shortly after the V600E BRAF mutation was described in melanoma, several investigators showed that depletion of BRAF using siRNA resulted in apoptosis of BRAF-mutated melanoma but had little effect on cells with wild-type BRAF [26, 27]. This validated mutated BRAF as a target in melanoma and led the development of a variety of RAF inhibitors. None of these molecules are specific for mutated BRAF; they all have activity against other kinases. Even PLX4032 now known as vemurafenib, the RAF inhibitor that we discuss in more detail below and arguably one of the most specific inhibitors of mutated BRAF, also inhibits wild-type BRAF, CRAF, and ARAF [8].

Despite the fact that PLX4032 inhibits all four RAF isoforms (three wild-type as well-mutated BRAF) in vitro, the inhibitory effect of PLX4032 (and other RAF inhibitors) at the cellular level is very specific for cells harboring a BRAF mutation [28]. Cells with wild-type BRAF are not inhibited. As discussed above, this apparent paradox can be understood by the fact that in cells with a BRAF mutation, cells are being driven by monomeric-mutated BRAF rather through the usual signaling through the MAPK pathway that involves RAF homo- and hetero-dimers. Thus, in patients with BRAF-mutated tumor, the specificity of inhibition is not so much due to the specificity of the inhibitor for mutated BRAF over the wild-type isoforms but rather due to the fact that the tumor cell is being driven by BRAF monomer while all normal cells have an intact MAPK pathway. A sufficiently potent RAF inhibitor would be expected to inhibit BRAF-mutated tumor cells at concentrations much lower than required to inhibit wild-type RAF dimers.

Clinical Studies with the RAF Inhibitor PLX4032 (RO5185426)

The first clear evidence that BRAF could be effectively targeted in human melanoma came in the setting of the first-in-human clinical trial of PLX4032. Based on the a priori knowledge of the prevalence of BRAF mutations in melanoma and the selective inhibition of tumor cells that harbor BRAF mutation, the clinical trial was enriched from the outset for patients with metastatic melanoma. As dose escalation proceeded in sequential cohorts, and drug concentrations increased to levels commensurate with those associated with tumor regression in animal models, an increasingly concerted effort was made to screen patients for the presence of a BRAF mutation in their tumor prior to enrollment. This made it possible for tumor responses to be observed at a very early point in the development of this agent (Flaherty et al., NEJM 363:809 2010).

Forty-nine of fifty-five patients enrolled in the dose escalation portion of the PLX4032 trial had metastatic melanoma, and the remaining six patients had metastatic cancers that are also known to harbor BRAF mutations with some frequency (papillary thyroid, colorectal, and ovarian). At a dose of 240 mg twice daily (BID), which was associated with little, if any, toxicity, the first objective response was observed in a patient with V600E BRAF melanoma. As preclinical models did not suggest a plateau in the dose-response relationship, dose escalation continued to a dose of 1,120 mg BID which proved to be intolerable due to severe fatigue, rash, and arthralgia. More manageable degrees of these same toxicities were observed at intermediate doses and responses were observed at each. While the molecular mechanism of these toxicities is not known, when given as a continuous, twice daily therapy, 960 mg BID is the maximum tolerated dose (MTD).

One adverse event that has emerged as a clear consequence of PLX4032 is the development of new nonpigmented lesions within the first few months of therapy (median 2 months). These lesions have typically presented as single lesions, but individual patients have had multiple new lesions appear serially. In all cases, patients have had such lesions excised and PLX4032 treatment continued. Fifteen of patients treated in the dose escalation cohorts developed such lesions, though many of those patients received doses that, in retrospect, induce no other toxicity or evidence of antitumor effect. The first such lesion appeared in a patient treated at 480 mg twice daily for several months. Fifty of these lesions have been reviewed by a central pathologist: 27 were keratoacanthoma (KA), 14 were well-differentiated squamous cell carcinoma with features of KA, 2 were squamous cell carcinoma with some KA features, and 7 were classified as other neoplasia. The natural history of spontaneous KAs, outside of the setting of PLX4032 therapy, suggests that these are entirely benign neoplasms that can spontaneously regress when not treated. It is unclear at this point if the KAs that arise in the setting of PLX4032 share those features, but evidence of invasive squamous cell carcinoma is currently lacking for any of the lesions analyzed to date. The molecular mechanism appears to inudue a pre-existing HRAS mutation in keratinogtes which, when treated with vemurafenib results in by Ref -proliferation. su et al. NEJM 2011 (in press). KAs are known to occur in immunocompromised populations, but no other evidence of immunosuppression has manifested in the PLX4032 trial population. The recently described activation of the MAP kinase pathway by RAF inhibitors, including agents structurally similar to PLX4032, suggests the hypothesis that hyperactivation of the MAP kinase pathway in these lesions might account for their growth [8, 29]. However, more mechanistic studies are needed before concluding that this is the cause.

From 240 to 1120 mg of PLX4032, 16 patients with V600E BRAF were enrolled to the following five dose levels: 240, 360, 480, 720, and 1,120 mg. Eleven of these patients experienced partial responses, and only two patients had tumor growth at the time of initial response assessment. Responses were seen at all sites (skin, lymph node, and visceral), but notably patients with brain metastases that progressive or untreated within a three-month interval before study entry were excluded. The median duration of response was 9 months (range 3.5–20+). Thirty-two additional V600E BRAF melanoma patients were enrolled at the 960 mg BID level to confirm the MTD and gain more insight into efficacy. Seventy-eight percent had previously received therapy for metastatic melanoma; 50% had received two or more.

Fig. 5.3 Immunohistochemistry staining of (**a**) pERK and (**b**) Ki67 of pretreatment and day 15 melanoma tumor samples from a patient treated with 720 mg bid of PLX4032. pERK staining is shown at 10×; Ki67 staining is 40× (Adapted from Puzanov et al. [30])

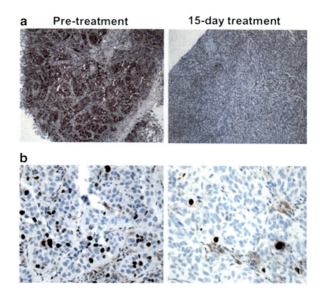

Seventy-five percent of patients had M1c stage IV melanoma indicating that most patients had extensive disease. Twenty-six of thirty-two patients had an objective response; two complete (ORR 81%; 95% CI 67–95%). The median duration response has not been defined, but is currently estimated at greater than 7 months based on relatively immature follow-up of these patients. Survival outcomes are not yet available, as only a minority of patients have succumbed to their disease.

As part of this first-in-human trial, correlative studies were undertaken to determine if treatment with PLX4032 suppressed the MAPK pathway. In selected patients, pretreatment and day 15 tumor biopsies were done and analyzed by immunohistochemistry. Day 15 biopsies generally showed marked decrease in activated ERK as well as proliferation marker Ki67 (Fig. 5.3) [30]. This indicates that this level of MAPK inhibition can be associated with meaningful tumor shrinkage.

A formal phase II trial was recently completed in melanoma patients with a V600E BRAF mutation; 132 patients were treated with 960 mg BID of RG7204. In an initial analysis, 3 CRs and 66 PRs were observed which resulted in a 52% response rate, by intention to treat analysis [1]. In this larger trial, responses were counted only if confirmed durable for at least 1 month, which accounts for the lower response rate compared to the phase I trial. The median duration of response was 6.8 months, similar to what was observed in the phase I extension cohort.

A phase III trial was recently completed in which previously untreated patients with a V600E BRAF mutation were randomized to vemurafenib (PLX4032) or dacarbazine. Ref At the first planned interim analysis, chapman et al. NEJM 364 (20)

:2507–2516,2011 both the overall survival and progression-free survival endpoints had met the prespecified criteria for statistical significance in favor of vemurafenib The hazard ratio for overall survival was 0.37 and for progression free survival was 0.26, both in favour of vemurafenib.

Spectrum of BRAF Inhibitors in Clinical Trials

Since the identification of BRAF mutations, the list of BRAF-targeted therapies has grown substantially in recent years. Sorafenib was the first agent with BRAF among its target kinases to have been tested in a BRAF mutant cancer population, but it failed to show single-agent activity, or consistent efficacy when combined with conventional chemotherapy [31–33]. Notably, sorafenib preferentially binds BRAF in the inactive conformation, unlike PLX4032, which has greater affinity for BRAF in the active conformation. An investigation into sorafenib's ability to inhibit the MAP kinase pathway in human tumors revealed a degree of inhibition far short of that achieved by PLX4032. Given that the dose-limiting toxicities of sorafenib are distinct from PLX4032, it is likely that the non-BRAF targets of sorafenib mediate toxicity and limit the amount of drug that can be delivered. As a consequence the degree of BRAF inhibition at the MTD is insufficient to inhibit BRAF well enough to induce tumor stasis or regression.

Agents with potency and greater selectivity for BRAF than sorafenib have been developed and are in clinical trials currently. This class of therapies share some of the broad-spectrum features of sorafenib, such as potency against CRAF and VEGF receptors. These include RAF-265, which has not yet emerged from phase I testing and XL-281, which has completed phase I and is being evaluated in BRAF mutant cancer populations among others currently. In phase I, few patients enrolled had the types of cancer histologies known to harbor BRAF mutations, and mutation testing was not conducted for those enrolled. With no objective responses observed, it is not clear if the efficacy of this agent has yet been tested. The same properties that limited sorafenib's ability to inhibit BRAF in vivo, remain a concern for these agents until they demonstrate clinical activity at or below their MTD.

At least one additional selective RAF inhibitor, other than PLX4032, has entered clinical trials. This agent, GSK2118436 (GlaxoSmithKline, Philadelphia, PA), was evaluated in a phase I trial that was enriched for melanoma patients and particularly those whose tumors harbored BRAF mutations [34]. Ninety-three patients were enrolled, 82% of whom had V600E BRAF melanoma. Doses ranged from 12 to 200 mg twice daily, with drug concentrations above the preclinical threshold for efficacy being achieved at doses above 70 mg daily. The most common toxicities partly overlapped with those observed with PLX4032, while others were unique. They consisted of dose limiting syncope and generally mild-to-moderate skin changes, headache, nausea, fatigue, vomiting, and low-grade cutaneous squamous cell carcinoma. Among the 15 patients with V600E-mutated melanoma treated at doses ≥150 mg twice daily, 9 experienced a partial response. Although follow-up for this cohort is still immature, it appears that the clinical activity of GSK2118436 may be comparable to PLX4032 reproducing and validating this class of drugs in melanoma tumors with BRAF mutations.

MEK Inhibition as a Strategy for Targeting BRAF Mutant Melanoma

Given that MEK is the only known substrate of BRAF, it is presumed that activating mutations in BRAF have MEK activation as the only direct downstream consequence. Several potent and selective MEK inhibitors have been developed and some have been evaluated in cancer patients harboring V600E BRAF mutations. MEK has several isoforms, but all MEK inhibitors that have progressed beyond phase I trials are selective for MEK-1 and -2. Their selectivity for MEK, compared to other kinases stems partly from the fact that they are allosteric (non-ATP-competitive) inhibitors. These agents include AZD6244 and GSK1120212, for which the most extensive clinical experience exists [35, 36]. Similar MEK inhibitors show relatively selective ability to inhibit the MAP kinase pathway and cell proliferation in cells that harbor activating BRAF mutations rather than RAS mutant cancers and cells that lack either RAS or BRAF mutations [37]. Once the MTD was defined based on dose -limiting rash and diarrhea [38], AZD6244 was evaluated as a single-agent in patients with metastatic melanoma, but without requirement for BRAF mutation at study entry. One hundred patients were enrolled to the AZD6244 arm of a randomized phase II trial, with the control group receiving temozolomide. There were six partial responses in the AZD6244 cohort. Five of these patients had their tumors analyzed for BRAF mutations and all were found to have a BRAF mutation; the sixth patient did not have BRAF mutation testing completed. Overall, 50% of the trial population had BRAF mutations, giving an estimated 12% response rate among the BRAF mutant patients treated with AZD6244. Notably there were no responses among the other patients whose tumors harbored NRAS mutation or lacked BRAF and NRAS mutations.

GSK1120212 has been less extensively evaluated in clinical trials, but appears to be a more active agent when evaluated in patients with BRAF mutant melanoma [36]. In dose escalation studies, rash, diarrhea, and central serous retinopathy were the dose-limiting toxicities. The half-life of GSK1120212 was roughly 4 ½ days, providing very stable exposure when dosed daily after steady-state was achieved. Tumor biopsy data showed reduction of pERK and Ki67 by greater than 90% near the MTD, achieving the desired molecular effect. Among 20 patients with BRAF mutant melanoma (17 with M1c stage), 2 patients had complete responses and 6 had partial response (ORR 40%; 95% CI 19–64%); 2 additional patients had lesser degrees of tumor regression. Response duration has yet to be defined, with all but one patient still responding at the time of the preliminary data presentation.

MEK inhibition is a validated point of intervention for BRAF mutant melanoma, but even GSK1120212 has not achieved the level of clinical activity observed with the two selective RAF inhibitors. Therefore, the question that remains to be answered in the field is to what extent MEK inhibition could complement BRAF inhibitors as they progress further in clinical development. Two rationales for this combination have been proposed. First, the residual activity of BRAF, and thereby the MAP kinase pathway, that persists despite dosing selective RAF inhibitors at their MTD could be targeted with a simultaneous MEK inhibition. There is a desire for preclinical data to be generated, particularly in vivo, to determine if this strategy can further suppress output of the MAP kinase pathway without causing severe toxicity. Second, it is conceivable that mechanisms of resistance to selective RAF inhibition reactivate the MAP kinase pathway and that could be intercepted with MEK inhibition when applied following the emergence of clinical resistance. This hypothesis has been raised in one preclinical study in which resistance was engendered in vitro to a selective RAF inhibitor [39].

Resistance Mechanisms Observed in Clinical Trials

In other cancers for which onco-protein targeted therapy has proven effective, the emergence of resistance in the target protein has been described as a common mechanism of resistance. In the cases of chronic myelogenous leukemia, in which Abl kinase is constitutively activated due to massive overexpression and in gastrointestinal cancer in which activating mutations that are found in the intracellular kinase domain of the KIT receptor, the dominant mechanism of resistance to Abl or KIT kinase inhibitors are gatekeeper mutations that impair binding of the inhibitor and permit continued signaling. In non-small lung cancer harboring activation mutations in the kinase domain of the EGF receptor, approximately 50% of tumors with acquired resistance to EGF receptor kinase inhibitors have a gatekeeper mutation. Thus, in BRAF mutant melanoma, resistance mutations in BRAF were the first focus of molecular investigation in tumors biopsied or resected in patients whose tumors progressed following initial response to therapy. However, to date no gatekeeper mutations have been found and V600E BRAF mutations persist [40, 41]. The observation that V600E BRAF mutations are still present also negates a hypothesis that suggested that metastatic melanoma harbors admixtures of BRAF-mutated and wild-type melanoma cells. If this were true, then one would expect the emergence of a BRAF wild-type clone given that selective RAF inhibitors demonstrate no ability to inhibit the proliferation of BRAF wild-type tumors and may even stimulate their growth [8, 24].

Several distinct mechanisms of acquired resistance have been described through the generation of BRAF inhibitor resistance melanoma cell lines and corroborated in a small number of human tumor samples harvested at the time of disease progression after initial response to PLX4032. One that is arguably, the most straightforward to understand, is the emergence of an activating NRAS mutation with persistence of V600E BRAF [40]. Extensive investigations to identify melanomas that harbor concomitant BRAF and NRAS mutation, in the absence of treatment, have yielded only rare instances where this might be the case. Thus, the emergence of an NRAS mutation in the same tumor in which only a BRAF mutation could be detected from prior therapy suggests that this might be a true treatment-induced change, or that selective pressure from PLX4032 has favored the outgrowth of small subpopulation of melanomas that harbored concomitant BRAF and NRAS mutation at baseline. Mutant NRAS can activate MEK and ERK through CRAF, thus bypassing BRAF blockade [42].

Another genetic alteration has been identified in a single case, namely the deletion of PTEN [41]. PTEN deletions are common in melanoma and are known to facilitate increased PI3K pathway signaling. Thus, it is plausible that the emergence of a PTEN mutation, which could not be identified in the same patient's tumor at baseline could permit upregulated PI3K pathway signaling to mediate resistance. Two separate investigations identified upregulated PDGF receptor beta and insulin growth factor receptor signaling as putative bypass mechanisms through the PI3K pathway. In both cases, genetic alterations in the surface receptors could not be found, but rather increased protein expression (in the case of PDGF receptor) or receptor tyrosine kinase phosphorylation (in the case of IGF receptor). In both of these instances, it is possible that expression of these surface receptors regulated at an epigenetic level or that activation is driven by a autocrine or paracrine signaling loop, in which case, these resistance mechanisms might be predicted to be reversible with removal of the BRAF inhibitor. This possibility has not been explored.

The other mechanism of resistance uncovered from an in vitro resistance model is signaling through COT/TPL2, also known as MAPK38, which has previously been described as a RAF-independent activator of MEK [43]. Upregulation of COT in tumor samples analyzed at the time of disease progression has been demonstrated in two of three cases interrogated. Like NRAS mutation, COT upregulation could restore MEK and ERK signaling in the face of continued BRAF inhibition and provide a bypass mechanism. Like PDGF receptor and IGF receptor, activating mutations in COT have not been described.

It must be emphasized that, aside from NRAS mutations, the other putative mechanisms of resistance have not yet been confirmed by other investigators. Thus, the mechanisms of resistance to BRAF inhibition remain to be defined.

Future Directions for BRAF Inhibitors

The experience with both RAF inhibitors – PLX4032 and GSK2118436 – provides proof of principle that in BRAF-addicted melanomas, inhibition of BRAF results in dramatic antitumor responses. Some of these responses are quite durable but in most patients, tumors will eventually become resistant to BRAF inhibition. In the future, several major questions will need to be answered: why are there so few complete responses? What are the mechanisms of de novo and acquired resistance? What are the long-term effects of MAPK activation in the non-melanoma, BRAF wild-type cells exposed to RAF inhibitor?

Understanding the mechanisms of resistance will point the way to combination regimens aimed at overcoming them. Residual MAP kinase pathway activity could potentially be targeted with MEK or ERK inhibitors, given in combination with RAF inhibitors. Secondary oncogenic pathways that maintain tumor cell survival in the face of effective RAF inhibition can be simultaneously antagonized, such as PI3K pathway inhibitors or CDK4 inhibitors.

As novel therapies emerge that target mediators of cancer phenotypes, such as escape from immune surveillance or angiogenesis, the combination of BRAF inhibition with such approaches warrants consideration. In particular, novel inhibitors of immune checkpoints have shown the ability to improve survival in metastatic melanoma patients [44]. The ability of RAF inhibitors to increase melanocyte-specific antigen expression may provide a basis for these two types of therapy to complement one another [45]. In addition, there is preliminary evidence that a VEGF-targeted monoclonal antibody may enhance the activity of melanoma-directed cytotoxic therapy [46], making this combination worthwhile to evaluate.

With clear evidence that BRAF inhibition represents a point of vulnerability in melanoma, there is hope that understanding the exact molecular consequences of BRAF inhibition and, thus, the basis for building upon these effects will result in more complete and durable responses.

References

1. Wu J, Rosenbaum E, Begum S, Westra WH. Distribution of BRAF T1799A(V600E) mutations across various types of benign nevi: implications for melanocytic tumorigenesis. Am J Dermatopathol. 2007;29(6):534–7.
2. Poynter JN, Elder JT, Fullen DR, et al. BRAF and NRAS mutations in melanoma and melanocytic nevi. Melanoma Res. 2006;16(4):267–73.
3. Dankort D, Curley DP, Cartlidge RA, et al. BrafV600E cooperates with Pten loss to induce metastatic melanoma. Nat Genet. 2009;41(5):544–52.
4. Weber CK, Slupsky JR, Kalmes HA, Rapp UR. Active Ras induces heterodimerization of cRaf and BRaf. Cancer Res. 2001;61(9):3595–8.
5. Rajakulendran T, Sahmi M, Lefrancois M, Sicheri F, Therrien M. A dimerization-dependent mechanism drives RAF catalytic activation. Nature. 2009;461(7263):542–5.
6. Rushworth LK, Hindley AD, O'Neill E, Kolch W. Regulation and role of Raf-1/B-Raf heterodimerization. Mol Cell Biol. 2006;26(6):2262–72.
7. Hatzivassiliou G, Song K, Yen I, et al. RAF inhibitors prime wild-type RAF to activate the MAPK pathway and enhance growth. Nature. 2010;464(7287):431–5.
8. Poulikakos PI, Zhang C, Bollag G, Shokat KM, Rosen N. RAF inhibitors transactivate RAF dimers and ERK signalling in cells with wild-type BRAF. Nature. 2010;464(7287):427–30.
9. Yoon S, Seger R. The extracellular signal-regulated kinase: multiple substrates regulate diverse cellular functions. Growth Factors. 2006;24(1):21–44.
10. Pratilas, Solit. Clin Cancer Res. 2010 (in press).
11. Dougherty MK, Muller J, Ritt DA, et al. Regulation of Raf-1 by direct feedback phosphorylation. Mol Cell. 2005;17(2):215–24.
12. Tsavachidou D, Coleman ML, Athanasiadis G, et al. SPRY2 is an inhibitor of the ras/extracellular signal-regulated kinase pathway in melanocytes and melanoma cells with wild-type BRAF but not with the V599E mutant. Cancer Res. 2004;64(16):5556–9.

13. Kim HJ, Bar-Sagi D. Modulation of signalling by Sprouty: a developing story. Nat Rev Mol Cell Biol. 2004;5(6):441–50.
14. Keyse SM. Dual-specificity MAP kinase phosphatases (MKPs) and cancer. Cancer Metastasis Rev. 2008;27(2):253–61.
15. Brady SC, Coleman ML, Munro J, Feller SM, Morrice NA, Olson MF. Sprouty2 association with B-Raf is regulated by phosphorylation and kinase conformation. Cancer Res. 2009;69(17):6773–81.
16. Davies H, Bignell GR, Cox C, et al. Mutations of the BRAF gene in human cancer. Nature. 2002;417(6892):949–54.
17. Curtin JA, Fridlyand J, Kageshita T, et al. Distinct sets of genetic alterations in melanoma. N Engl J Med. 2005;353(20):2135–47.
18. Cohen Y, Rosenbaum E, Begum S, et al. Exon 15 BRAF mutations are uncommon in melanomas arising in nonsun-exposed sites. Clin Cancer Res. 2004;10(10):3444–7.
19. Edwards RH, Ward MR, Wu H, et al. Absence of BRAF mutations in UV-protected mucosal melanomas. J Med Genet. 2004;41(4):270–2.
20. Edmunds SC, Cree IA, Di Nicolantonio F, Hungerford JL, Hurren JS, Kelsell DP. Absence of BRAF gene mutations in uveal melanomas in contrast to cutaneous melanomas. Br J Cancer. 2003;88(9):1403–5.
21. Kumar R, Angelini S, Czene K, et al. BRAF mutations in metastatic melanoma: a possible association with clinical outcome. Clin Cancer Res. 2003;9(9):3362–8.
22. Houben R, Becker JC, Kappel A, et al. Constitutive activation of the Ras-Raf signaling pathway in metastatic melanoma is associated with poor prognosis. J Carcinog. 2004;3(1):6.
23. Chang D, Panageas K, Osman I, Polsky D, Busam K, Chapman P. Clinical significance of BRAF mutations in metastatic melanoma. J Transl Med. 2004;2(1):46.
24. Heidorn SJ, Milagre C, Whittaker S, et al. Kinase-dead BRAF and oncogenic RAS cooperate to drive tumor progression through CRAF. Cell. 2010;140(2):209–21.
25. Pratilas CA, Taylor BS, Ye Q, et al. (V600E)BRAF is associated with disabled feedback inhibition of RAF-MEK signaling and elevated transcriptional output of the pathway. Proc Natl Acad Sci USA. 2009;106(11):4519–24.
26. Hingorani SR, Jacobetz MA, Robertson GP, Herlyn M, Tuveson DA. Suppression of BRAF(V599E) in human melanoma abrogates transformation. Cancer Res. 2003;63(17): 5198–202.
27. Karasarides M, Chiloeches A, Hayward R, et al. B-RAF is a therapeutic target in melanoma. Oncogene. 2004;23(37):6292–8.
28. Tsai J, Lee JT, Wang W, et al. Discovery of a selective inhibitor of oncogenic B-Raf kinase with potent antimelanoma activity. Proc Natl Acad Sci USA. 2008;105(8):3041–6.
29. Heidorn SJM C, Whittaker S, Nourry A, Niculescu-Duvas I, Dhomen N, Hussain J, et al. Kinase-dead BRAF and oncogenic RAS cooperate to drive tumor progression through CRAF. Cell. 2010;140(2):209–21.
30. Puzanov I, Nathason KL, Chapman PB, Xu X, Sosman JA, McArthur GA, Ribas A, Kim KB, Grippo JF, Flaherty KT. PLX4032, a highly selective V600EBRAF kinase inhibitor: clinical correlation of activity with pharmacokinetic and pharmacodynamic parameters in a phase I trial. J Clin Oncol. 2009;27(15s).
31. Eisen T, Ahmad T, Flaherty KT, et al. Sorafenib in advanced melanoma: a Phase II randomised discontinuation trial analysis. Br J Cancer. 2006;95(5):581–6.
32. Hauschild A, Agarwala SS, Trefzer U, et al. Results of a phase III, randomized, placebo-controlled study of sorafenib in combination with carboplatin and paclitaxel as second-line treatment in patients with unresectable stage III or stage IV melanoma. J Clin Oncol. 2009;27(17): 2823–30.
33. McDermott DF, Sosman JA, Gonzalez R, et al. Double-blind randomized phase II study of the combination of sorafenib and dacarbazine in patients with advanced melanoma: a report from the 11715 Study Group. J Clin Oncol. 2008;26(13):2178–85.
34. Kefford R, Arkenau H, Brown MP, Millward M, Infante JR, Long GV, Ouellet D, Curtis M, Lebowitz PF, Falchook GS. Phase I/II study of GSK2118436, a selective inhibitor of oncogenic

mutant BRAF kinase, in patients with metastatic melanoma and other solid tumors. J Clin Oncol. 2010;28(7s).

35. Dummer RR C, Chapman PB, Sosman JA, Middleton M, Bastholt L, Kemsley K, et al. AZD6244 (ARRY-142886) vs temozolomide (TMZ) in patients (pts) with advanced melanoma: an open-label, randomized, multicenter, phase II study. J Clin Oncol. 2008;26(May 20 suppl):9033.

36. Infante JR, Fecher LA, Nallapareddy S, Gordon MS, Flaherty KT, Cox DS, DeMarini DJ, Morris SR, Burris HA, Messersmith WA. Safety and efficacy results from the first-in-human study of the oral MEK 1/2 inhibitor GSK1120212. J Clin Oncol. 2010;28(7s).

37. Solit DB, Garraway LA, Pratilas CA, et al. BRAF mutation predicts sensitivity to MEK inhibition. Nature. 2006;439(7074):358–62.

38. Adjei AA, Cohen RB, Franklin W, et al. Phase I pharmacokinetic and pharmacodynamic study of the oral, small-molecule mitogen-activated protein kinase kinase 1/2 inhibitor AZD6244 (ARRY-142886) in patients with advanced cancers. J Clin Oncol. 2008;26(13):2139–46.

39. Montagut C, Sharma SV, Shioda T, et al. Elevated CRAF as a potential mechanism of acquired resistance to BRAF inhibition in melanoma. Cancer Res. 2008;68(12):4853–61.

40. Nazarian et al. Nature 2010.

41. Villanueva J et al. Cancer Cell 2010.

42. Dumaz N, Hayward R, Martin J, et al. In melanoma, RAS mutations are accompanied by switching signaling from BRAF to CRAF and disrupted cyclic AMP signaling. Cancer Res. 2006;66(19):9483–91.

43. Johannesen CM, Boehm JS, Kim SY, et al. COT drives resistance to RAF inhibition throught MAP Kinase pathway reactivation. Nature 2010;468:968–72.

44. Hodi FS, O'Day SJ, McDermott DF, et al. Improved survival with ipilimumab in patients with metastatic melanoma. N Engl J Med.2010; 363:711–23.

45. Boni A, Cogdill AP, Dang P, et al. Selective BRAFV600E inhibition enhances T-Cell recognition of melanoma without affecting lymphocyte function. Cancer Res. 2010;70(13):5213–9.

46. O'Day SJ, Kim KB, Sosman JA, et al. 23LBA BEAM: A randomized phase II study evaluating the activity of bevacizumab in combination with carboplatin plus paclitaxel in patients with previously untreated Advanced Melanoma. 2009;7:13.

Chapter 6
The Notch and β-Catenin Pathways

John T. Lee and Meenhard Herlyn

Abstract While central driver mutations in molecules involved in the mitogen-activated protein kinase (MAPK) pathway appear to be involved in the majority of melanomas, concurrent activation of various parallel pathways occurs essentially in all cases. Distinct subsets of melanomas show evidence of activation of a variety of additional signaling cascades; two of these, the Notch and β-catenin pathways, are molecular events first characterized for roles in developmental biology that clearly can participate in malignant transformation. Importantly, therapeutic agents that target these pathways are just entering clinical trial testing. It is anticipated that clinical investigation of these agents, combined with intensive biomarker analysis to identify predictors of response and resistance and also to establish biologically active doses of these agents, may generate new classes of therapeutics with the potential to benefit major subsets of melanoma patients.

Historically, cancer research has focused on the most rapidly dividing cells and the cellular pathways that dictate growth. Those efforts have yielded significant insight into the molecular machinery that drives proliferation in transformed cells; however, it is becoming increasingly apparent that all cancer cells are not the same. Plasticity within the tumor is prevalent and likely contributes to the refractory nature of most cancers to chemotherapy. Thus, studying the molecular circuitry that may confer plasticity to tumor cells may help identify new targets for chemotherapeutic intervention in otherwise resistant cancers.

The Notch and β-catenin signaling pathways are well recognized for their roles in developmental processes. Initial identification and characterization of the biological function of Notch was performed in *Drosophila*, when it was observed to dictate "notch" formation on wing blades. β-catenin was originally described in colorectal tumors [1, 37] and subsequently demonstrated in a variety of stem cell-related processes. The pleiotropic nature of Notch and β-catenin signaling which regu-

J.T. Lee, PhD • M. Herlyn, DVM (✉)
Molecular and Cellular Oncogenesis Program, The Wistar Institute,
3601 Spruce Street, Philadelphia, PA 19104, USA
e-mail: herlynm@wistar.org

T.F. Gajewski and F.S. Hodi (eds.), *Targeted Therapeutics in Melanoma*,
Current Clinical Oncology, DOI 10.1007/978-1-61779-407-0_6,
© Springer Science+Business Media, LLC 2012

lates stem cell maintenance, development, and morphogenesis underscores the multiple phenotypes and resultant plasticity that these pathways control – properties that are equally inherent to advanced melanoma.

Keywords Notch • β-catenin • Wnt • Plasticity • Melanoma • Therapeutics • Gamma secretase inhibitors • RO4929097

Notch Signaling

The Notch signaling cascade is a highly conserved developmental pathway that has functions in an array of biological processes including cellular differentiation, tissue patterning and morphogenesis, and proliferation. There are four known isoforms of Notch (Notch1-4); each is translated as a precursor protein and subsequently cleaved in the golgi apparatus by furin-like convertases [2] before reassembly into a single-pass transmembrane receptor at the plasma membrane. Signaling through Notch is initiated through binding interactions with Notch ligands, namely Jagged and Delta, expressed on adjacent cells. Ligand-receptor interaction triggers dual sequential cleavage events in the Notch receptor to subsequently release intracellular Notch (N_{ic}) for nuclear translocation. First, the metalloprotease TACE (TNF-α converting enzyme; also known as ADAM17) cleaves the extracellular S2 domain of Notch [3], which primes Notch for a secondary cleavage event mediated by the γ-secretase multimer at the intracellular S3 domain. The γ-secretase multimer is composed of several peptides including nicastrin, presenilin1/2, Pen-2, and Aph-1 [4, 5]. After release from the cell membrane, N_{ic} translocates to the nucleus and binds to the transcriptional repressor, CSL (CBF1/RBP-Jκ; Suppressor of Hairless; Lag1), thereby releasing the co-repressor complex. Upon binding to CSL, N_{ic} recruits coactivators such as mastermind-like (MAML) and p300 [6, 7] to initiate expression of Notch target genes (Fig. 6.1a).

The Notch transcriptome includes two primary classes: Hairy/Enhancer of Split (Hes) and Hairy/E (spl)-related (Hey) gene family members. Hes and Hey contain helix-loop-helix domains that determine the hetero- or homodimers that are formed when these family members bind; these dimers subsequently shut down gene expression through interactions with other repressor molecules or by precluding the binding of transcriptional activators to their respective promoters [8]. A number of alternative Notch target genes also include p21, GATA3, cyclin D1, NRARP, c-Myc, and Deltex1 [9].

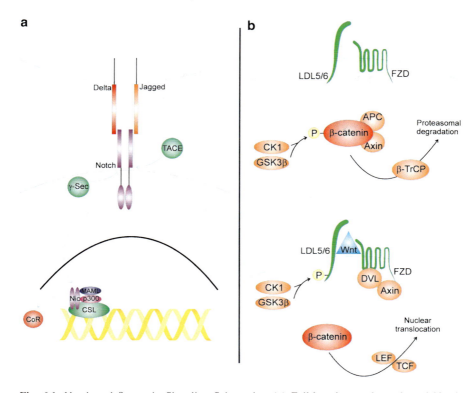

Fig. 6.1 Notch and β-catenin Signaling Schematics. (**a**) Full-length, membrane-bound Notch binds to either Jagged or Delta on an adjacent cell to initiate dual cleavage events; first, TACE (ADAM17) cleaves the extracellular portion of Notch, which is followed by cleavage of the intracellular portion of Notch by the γ-secretase complex (γ-Sec) to release N$_{ic}$ for nuclear translocation. After entering the nuclear, intracellular Notch (N$_{ic}$) displaces corepressor molecules (CoR) from CSL and subsequently associates with coactivators MAML and p300 to upregulate gene expression. See text for more details. (**b**) *Top*: In the absence of Wnt, β-catenin is constantly degraded. Casein kinase-1 (CK1) and glycogen synthase kinase-3 (GSK3β) phosphorylate β-catenin, which is part of the destruction complex also containing adenomatous polyposis coli (APC) and Axin; phosphorylated β-catenin is then ubiquitinated by the E3-ligase, β-TrCP, for proteasomal degradation. *Bottom*: Wnt binds to the frizzled (FZD) receptor, initiating phosphorylation of the LDL-related receptor protein-5/6 (LDL5/6) coreceptor by CK1 and GSK3β. Disheveled (DVL) binds to FZD after phosphorylation of the LDL5/6 coreceptor and recruits Axin to the membrane, releasing it from the destruction complex. β-catenin, now released from the destruction complex, is stabilized and binds to lymphoid enhancer factor (LEF) and/or T-cell factor (TCF) to regulate gene expression in the nuclear department

Notch and Cancer

The Notch signaling pathway was first recognized for its roles in embryonic development, a series of processes that involve rapid proliferation, differentiation, and tissue morphogenesis. More recently, this signaling cascade has been strongly implicated in cancer initiation and progression. In 1991, a chromosomal translocation [t (7, 9)] that placed the Notch1 gene under transcriptional control of the T-cell receptor β locus was discovered in a T-cell acute lymphoblastic leukemia (T-ALL) cell line [10]. The role of Notch in T-ALL was further underscored after it was reported that over 50% of T-ALL patients harbor mutations in Notch1 [11]. Despite a significant role for Notch in T-ALL, there has been no correlation between Notch activity and acute myeloid leukemia (AML), suggesting that Notch activation in nonsolid tumors is not always required for malignant transformation.

Notch signaling is also associated with a variety of solid tumors. Insertional mutagenesis studies provided some of the first evidence that Notch activity is involved in murine mammary cancers [12], although a causal link between Notch signaling and human breast cancer has been less convincing; instead, it appears that Notch may participate with other signaling cascades, such as the Ras pathway, to transduce the signals required to maintain a malignant phenotype [13]. In colorectal tumors, the tumor microenvironment upregulates Notch ligands to enable activation of the pathway [14]; accordingly, inhibition of Notch has been demonstrated to sensitize colon cancer cells to chemotherapies [15]. Similar observations have been made in pancreatic tumors, where Notch inhibition blocks the growth of early pancreatic adenocarcinoma cells and their progression into advanced pancreatic cancer [16]. In glioma, chemical-mediated abrogation of Notch activity renders glioma stem cells susceptible to radiation [17], supporting a prosurvival role for this pathway in yet another solid tumor type.

Interestingly, Notch signaling in the skin can induce either a tumor-suppressive or oncogenic phenotype. When Notch signaling is lost in keratinocytes, basal-cell carcinomas develop [18], indicating that Notch acts as a tumor suppressor protein in this cell type. Conversely, Notch is a potent oncogene in melanocytes, promoting melanomagenesis and activating a number of pathways associated with advanced disease [19–21]. In the lung, Notch signaling can either elicit proliferation [22] or induce apoptosis if under hypoxic conditions [23]. Thus, there is substantial evidence to suggest that cell type and contextual cues from the surrounding microenvironment largely control the phenotypic response to Notch activation.

In pigment-producing cells, Notch is rapidly becoming an interesting player in malignant transformation. The earliest report correlating Notch activity to melanoma came from the Halaban laboratory in 2004 where expression profiling analyses demonstrated that melanomas exhibited heightened levels of Notch pathway activation when compared with nontransformed melanocytes [24]. Supporting immunohistochemical evidence subsequently showed that Notch1 and Notch2, as well as Notch ligands are highly expressed in dysplastic nevi and melanomas [25]. Our own laboratory later investigated the relationship between Notch signaling and melanoma initiation and progression. We demonstrated that activation of Notch is sufficient to transform primary melanocytes [21] and that Notch promotes melanoma progression through distinct interactions with both the PI3K and β-catenin signaling pathways [19, 20]. Other reports have also implicated Notch as an integral effector molecule in the Nodal and PI3K/Akt pathways [26, 27]. Furthermore, chemical and peptide-mediated inhibition of Notch resulted in cell cycle arrest and induction of apoptosis in multiple melanoma cell lines [21, 28]. Collectively, the data describe a thematic role for Notch in the epidemiology of melanoma, whereby Notch activation supports both the initiation and progression of melanoma through a variety of cancer-related signaling pathways.

Targeting Notch in Melanoma

Pharmacological inhibition of Notch has been predominantly pursued through a class of compounds known as γ-secretase inhibitors (GSIs), largely recognized for their therapeutic potential in treating Parkinson's Disease [29]. These compounds inhibit the secondary cleavage event that leads to the generation of intracellular, activated Notch (N_{ic}); consequently, Notch is not released from the membrane to initiate nuclear signaling. GSIs are fairly specific, having few off-target effects, although serious issues have been reported in several trials with gastrointestinal toxicities, likely due to the transformation of proliferative intestinal crypt cells into postmitotic goblet cells [30]. Multiple commercially available "tool compounds" exist for use in preclinical studies, although it is highly advisable that the end-investigator validate the mechanism(s) of action of each individual compound because some of these GSIs are toxic due to the inhibition of proteasomal activities (i.e., Z-Leu-Leu-Nle-CHO), rather than actual inhibition of Notch signaling [31].

RO4929097 is a GSI discovered as a part of the NCI-sponsored Cancer Therapy Evaluation Program (CTEP) that is currently being evaluated in Phase II clinical trials with Stage IV melanoma patients. Preclinical studies with this compound demonstrated reduced proliferative potential both in vitro and in vivo [32]. Phase I trials involving RO4929097 in melanoma patients demonstrated promising antitumor activity (assessed by RECIST), including prolonged stable disease [33]. Related compounds (MK0752, Merck; PF03084014, Pfizer; LY450139, Eli-Lilly; BMS-708163, Bristol-Myers Squibb; GSI136, Wyeth) are all undergoing clinical evaluation for a variety of conditions other than melanoma; it should be expected that successful candidates from those trials will be tested for antitumor efficacy in melanoma in the near future.

β-catenin Signaling

Signaling through the β-catenin pathway is extremely complex due to the exquisite regulation that governs signals being transduced through the pathway [34]. β-catenin signaling is primarily mediated through a well-described pathway known as the canonical Wnt signaling pathway. In the canonical pathway, β-catenin exists in the cytoplasm where it is constitutively degraded by the action of the Axin destruction complex composed of Axin, adenomatous polyposis coli (APC), casein kinase 1

(CK1), and glycogen synthase kinase 3 (GSK3β); here, CK1 and GSK3β sequentially phosphorylate the N-terminal end of β-catenin, which allows subsequent association with an E3 ubiquitin ligase, β-Trcp, to promote proteasomal degradation. The constant degradation of β-catenin by the destruction complex occurs in the absence of Wnt, a ligand responsible for initiating a series of signaling events that eventually stabilize β-catenin. To facilitate β-catenin stabilization, Wnt binds to the Frizzled receptor (FZD) and associates with the coreceptor, LDL-related receptor protein-5/6 (LDL-5/6), which is then phosphorylated by CK1 and GSK3β. Upon phosphorylation of LDL-5/6, disheveled (DVL) is recruited to the membrane to bind FZD. This multimeric complex (Wnt/FZD/LDL-5/6/DVL) subsequently sequesters Axin from the cytosol, thereby releasing it from the destruction complex and stabilizing β-catenin. Thereafter, β-catenin translocates to the nucleus to form complexes with lymphoid enhancer factor (LEF) and/or T-cell factor (TCF) to upregulate appropriate transcriptional targets (Fig. 6.1b).

Nuclear β-catenin, when complexed with TCF/LEF displaces the transcriptional repressor, Groucho, and recruits other coactivators for gene expression. The TCF family of proteins is a high mobility group (HMG) class of proteins that bind to DNA consensus sequences known as Wnt-responsive elements (WRE); upon binding to DNA, these transcriptional factors alter the chromatin structure of the DNA to which they are bound. Other coactivators also exist including Bcl-9, Mediator, p300/CBP, MLL1/2 histone methyltransferases, Swi/Snf chromatin remodelers, and Paf1 [35]. The gene expression profiles initiated through β-catenin-mediated signaling are diverse and can lead to any number of normal biological phenotypes or they may manifest as disease if not appropriately regulated (i.e., cancer).

Wnt/β-catenin and Cancer

Early studies into the Wnt/β-catenin signaling pathway focused on their collective roles in developmental processes. The first connection between Wnt/β-catenin signaling and cancer came from studies in colorectal tumors that connected molecular interactions between the tumor suppressor protein, APC, and β-catenin [36, 37]. In 1998, however, the protooncogene c-Myc was identified as a downstream transcriptional target of the Wnt/β-catenin pathway [38]. Subsequent reports identified additional cancer-related transcriptional targets including Cyclin-D1 [39] and c-Jun [40], among a multitude (>70) of others.

The mechanisms underlying Wnt/β-catenin-mediated tumorigenesis in various tumor types are diverse and worthy of a thorough literature review [34]; given the scope of this short summary, the focus will be directed toward the involvement of this pathway in melanoma. An early report demonstrated that ~25% of melanoma cell lines harbored high levels of stabilized β-catenin through somatic mutations in β-catenin and/or loss of the APC tumor suppressor gene [1], although this conflicted with numerous follow-up analyses showing that mutations in β-catenin are a rare event in melanoma [41]; thus, it is believed that the pathway is activated by means of other somatic mutations in β-catenin. Accordingly, our laboratory reported that β-catenin levels are elevated through cell adhesion interactions in N-cadherin-expressing melanoma cells, resulting in increased migration and survival [42]; relevant studies suggested that paracrine growth factors, namely insulin-like growth factor-1 (IGF1), activate β-catenin in early-stage melanoma cells to promote malignant progression [43]. Murine-based studies showed that β-catenin, when combined with N-Ras activation, leads to the transformation of melanocytes through silencing of the p14^{INK4a} promoter [44].

β-catenin-independent Wnt signaling, otherwise known as "non-canonical" Wnt signaling is also thought to play a significant role in melanoma etiology. For example, Wnt5a was discovered to be highly expressed in a population of melanomas recognized for their invasive phenotype; furthermore, the signaling mediated by Wnt5a was β-catenin-independent and instead channeled through protein kinase C (PKC) [45]; an additional target of Wnt5a was later identified to be STAT3, a transcriptional regulator of several melanoma-associated antigens [46]. Wnt5a was also demonstrated to correlate to poor patient outcome [47]. These data suggest that noncanonical (non-β-catenin) signaling may also represent a means by which melanoma cells may be therapeutically targeted.

It is worth noting that the involvement of β-catenin signaling in melanoma is controversial. Despite the aforementioned studies, there are a number of other reports which suggest that β-catenin signaling in pigmented cells leads to reduced growth potential in both mice and human patients [48]. Accordingly, immunohistochemical-based studies argue that β-catenin expression is actually diminished as melanoma progresses from nevus to metastatic disease [49]. Others have also argued that there is virtually no correlation between activation of β-catenin and a specific cellular event in melanomas [50]. Thus, it will be instrumental to continue exploring the exact role(s) of this molecule in melanoma to avoid future clinical disappointments.

Targeting β-catenin in Melanoma

Pharmacologically targeting β-catenin is a dutiful task, given the diversity with which it is regulated and its vast number of binding partners. Despite this impediment, several inhibitors of the pathway have been discovered and tested in multiple systems for efficacy. Benefits in colorectal cancer have been reported using nonsteroidal antiinflammatory drugs (NSAIDs); this class of compounds functions, in part, by negating TCF/β-catenin signaling by inhibiting prostaglandin E2, an upstream activator of TCF/β-catenin-dependent gene expression [51, 52]. Other small molecules that disrupt TCF/β-catenin [53] or the interaction with alternative coactivators of β-catenin have also been described [54]. A chemical genetic screen later identified a compound antagonist of β-catenin signaling that functions through inhibition of tankyrase, a previously undescribed negative regulator of Axin [55]. Yet another study described the identification of a class of compounds known as inhibitors of Wnt production (IWPs); their mechanism of action is founded upon the inhibition of Porc proteins that otherwise enable Wnt production. Within the same report, the authors identified inhibitors of Wnt response (IWR) compounds that, as described above, stabilize Axin to promote β-catenin degradation [56].

There are virtually no human clinical trials currently underway for modulators of the Wnt/β-catenin pathway in melanoma. A Phase II study in patients with AML involving a GSK3β inhibitor (LY2090314; Eli Lilly) is now recruiting patients to assess its efficacy in this population, where β-catenin levels are a primary determinant in response; such GSK3β inhibitors may also exhibit therapeutic promise in melanomas, based on preclinical data [57].

Perspective

There is little doubt that the MAPK pathway is the preferred target in melanoma therapeutics today. However, there is a deluge of evidence emerging to suggest that inhibition of the MAPK pathway is not enough to elicit long-term, sustained responses in patients [58–61]. Therefore, other pathways will need to be explored to kill the cells that escape MAPK therapeutics and/or are not affected by that class of drugs. These alternative pathways and their molecular intermediates represent the next wave of targeted therapeutics in melanoma.

The Notch and Wnt/β-catenin pathways are renowned for their involvement in embryonic and developmental processes. The cellular plasticity associated with cellular differentiation and tissue morphogenesis is a property that is not unique to embryonic development – cancer cells also share this phenotypic phenomenon. In fact, there are now several studies suggesting that melanomas retain plasticity due to minor subpopulations within the tumor milieu that possess stem cell characteristics, including a slow proliferative index and ability to transdifferentiate into other cell types [62–64]. The signaling pathways that facilitate this cellular plasticity are likely shared between early progenitor and cancer cells; thus, the pathways discussed here are putative culprits for next-generation therapeutics that may be combined with current standards of care (i.e., ipilimumab and/or PLX4032) to achieve enhanced, sustained responses in the clinic.

References

1. Rubinfeld B, Robbins P, El-Gamil M, Albert I, Porfiri E, Polakis P. Stabilization of beta-catenin by genetic defects in melanoma cell lines. Science. 1997;275:1790–2.
2. Blaumueller CM, Qi H, Zagouras P, Artavanis-Tsakonas S. Intracellular cleavage of Notch leads to a heterodimeric receptor on the plasma membrane. Cell. 1997;90:281–91.
3. Brou C, Logeat F, Gupta N, Bessia C, LeBail O, Doedens JR, et al. A novel proteolytic cleavage involved in Notch signaling: the role of the disintegrin-metalloprotease TACE. Mol Cell. 2000;5:207–16.
4. Edbauer D, Winkler E, Regula JT, Pesold B, Steiner H, Haass C. Reconstitution of gamma-secretase activity. Nat Cell Biol. 2003;5:486–8.

5. Saxena MT, Schroeter EH, Mumm JS, Kopan R. Murine notch homologs (N1-4) undergo presenilin-dependent proteolysis. J Biol Chem. 2001;276:40268–73.
6. Wallberg AE, Pedersen K, Lendahl U, Roeder RG. p300 and PCAF act cooperatively to mediate transcriptional activation from chromatin templates by notch intracellular domains in vitro. Mol Cell Biol. 2002;22:7812–9.
7. Wu L, Aster JC, Blacklow SC, Lake R, Artavanis-Tsakonas S, Griffin JD. MAML1, a human homologue of Drosophila mastermind, is a transcriptional co-activator for NOTCH receptors. Nat Genet. 2000;26:484–9.
8. Iso T, Kedes L, Hamamori Y. HES and HERP families: multiple effectors of the Notch signaling pathway. J Cell Physiol. 2003;194:237–55.
9. Yin L, Velazquez OC, Liu ZJ. Notch signaling: emerging molecular targets for cancer therapy. Biochem Pharmacol. 2010;80:690–701.
10. Ellisen LW, Bird J, West DC, Soreng AL, Reynolds TC, Smith SD, et al. TAN-1, the human homolog of the Drosophila notch gene, is broken by chromosomal translocations in T lymphoblastic neoplasms. Cell. 1991;66:649–61.
11. Weng AP, Ferrando AA, Lee W, Morris 4th JP, Silverman LB, Sanchez-Irizarry C, et al. Activating mutations of NOTCH1 in human T cell acute lymphoblastic leukemia. Science. 2004;306:269–71.
12. Gallahan D, Callahan R. Mammary tumorigenesis in feral mice: identification of a new int locus in mouse mammary tumor virus (Czech II)-induced mammary tumors. J Virol. 1987; 61:66–74.
13. Weijzen S, Rizzo P, Braid M, Vaishnav R, Jonkheer SM, Zlobin A, et al. Activation of Notch-1 signaling maintains the neoplastic phenotype in human Ras-transformed cells. Nat Med. 2002;8:979–86.
14. Jubb AM, Turley H, Moeller HC, Steers G, Han C, Li JL, et al. Expression of delta-like ligand 4 (Dll4) and markers of hypoxia in colon cancer. Br J Cancer. 2009;101:1749–57.
15. Meng RD, Shelton CC, Li YM, Qin LX, Notterman D, Paty PB, et al. Gamma-Secretase inhibitors abrogate oxaliplatin-induced activation of the Notch-1 signaling pathway in colon cancer cells resulting in enhanced chemosensitivity. Cancer Res. 2009;69:573–82.
16. Mullendore ME, Koorstra JB, Li YM, Offerhaus GJ, Fan X, Henderson CM, et al. Ligand-dependent Notch signaling is involved in tumor initiation and tumor maintenance in pancreatic cancer. Clin Cancer Res. 2009;15:2291–301.
17. Wang J, Wakeman TP, Lathia JD, Hjelmeland AB, Wang XF, White RR, et al. Notch promotes radioresistance of glioma stem cells. Stem cells. 2009;28:17–28.
18. Nicolas M, Wolfer A, Raj K, Kummer JA, Mill P, van Noort M, et al. Notch1 functions as a tumor suppressor in mouse skin. Nat Genet. 2003;33:416–21.
19. Balint K, Xiao M, Pinnix CC, Soma A, Veres I, Juhasz I, et al. Activation of Notch1 signaling is required for beta-catenin-mediated human primary melanoma progression. J Clin Investig. 2005;115:3166–76.
20. Liu ZJ, Xiao M, Balint K, Smalley KS, Brafford P, Qiu R, et al. Notch1 signaling promotes primary melanoma progression by activating mitogen-activated protein kinase/phosphatidylinositol 3-kinase-Akt pathways and up-regulating N-cadherin expression. Cancer Res. 2006;66:4182–90.
21. Pinnix CC, Lee JT, Liu ZJ, McDaid R, Balint K, Beverly LJ, et al. Active Notch1 confers a transformed phenotype to primary human melanocytes. Cancer Res. 2009;69:5312–20.
22. Konishi J, Kawaguchi KS, Vo H, Haruki N, Gonzalez A, Carbone DP, et al. Gamma-secretase inhibitor prevents Notch3 activation and reduces proliferation in human lung cancers. Cancer Res. 2007;67:8051–7.
23. Chen Y, De Marco MA, Graziani I, Gazdar AF, Strack PR, Miele L, et al. Oxygen concentration determines the biological effects of NOTCH-1 signaling in adenocarcinoma of the lung. Cancer Res. 2007;67:7954–9.

24. Hoek K, Rimm DL, Williams KR, Zhao H, Ariyan S, Lin A, et al. Expression profiling reveals novel pathways in the transformation of melanocytes to melanomas. Cancer Res. 2004;64:5270–82.
25. Massi D, Tarantini F, Franchi A, Paglierani M, Di Serio C, Pellerito S, et al. Evidence for differential expression of Notch receptors and their ligands in melanocytic nevi and cutaneous malignant melanoma. Mod Pathol. 2006;19:246–54.
26. Bedogni B, Warneke JA, Nickoloff BJ, Giaccia AJ, Powell MB. Notch1 is an effector of Akt and hypoxia in melanoma development. J Clin Investig. 2008;118:3660–70.
27. Hardy KM, Kirschmann DA, Seftor EA, Margaryan NV, Postovit LM, Strizzi L, et al. Regulation of the embryonic morphogen Nodal by Notch4 facilitates manifestation of the aggressive melanoma phenotype. Cancer Res. 2010;70:10340–50.
28. Qin JZ, Stennett L, Bacon P, Bodner B, Hendrix MJ, Seftor RE, et al. p53-independent NOXA induction overcomes apoptotic resistance of malignant melanomas. Mol Cancer Ther. 2004; 3:895–902.
29. Bergmans BA, De Strooper B. Gamma-secretases: from cell biology to therapeutic strategies. Lancet Neurol. 2010;9:215–26.
30. van Es JH, van Gijn ME, Riccio O, van den Born M, Vooijs M, Begthel H, et al. Notch/gamma-secretase inhibition turns proliferative cells in intestinal crypts and adenomas into goblet cells. Nature. 2005;435:959–63.
31. Lewis HD, Leveridge M, Strack PR, Haldon CD, O'Neil J, Kim H, et al. Apoptosis in T cell acute lymphoblastic leukemia cells after cell cycle arrest induced by pharmacological inhibition of notch signaling. Chem Biol. 2007;14:209–19.
32. Luistro L, He W, Smith M, Packman K, Vilenchik M, Carvajal D, et al. Preclinical profile of a potent gamma-secretase inhibitor targeting notch signaling with in vivo efficacy and pharmacodynamic properties. Cancer Res. 2009;69:7672–80.
33. Tolcher AW, Mikulski SM, Messersmith WA, Kwak EL, Gibbon D, Boylan JF, Xu ZX, DeMario M, Wheler JJ. A phase I study of RO4929097, a novel gamma secretase inhibitor, in patients with advanced solid tumors. J Clin Oncol 2010;28 (suppl; abstr 2502).
34. Klaus A, Birchmeier W. Wnt signalling and its impact on development and cancer. Nature reviews. 2008;8:387–98.
35. MacDonald BT, Tamai K, He X. Wnt/beta-catenin signaling: components, mechanisms, and diseases. Dev Cell. 2009;17:9–26.
36. Rubinfeld B, Souza B, Albert I, Muller O, Chamberlain SH, Masiarz FR, et al. Association of the APC gene product with beta-catenin. Science. 1993;262:1731–4.
37. Su LK, Vogelstein B, Kinzler KW. Association of the APC tumor suppressor protein with catenins. Science. 1993;262:1734–7.
38. He TC, Sparks AB, Rago C, Hermeking H, Zawel L, da Costa LT, et al. Identification of c-MYC as a target of the APC pathway. Science. 1998;281:1509–12.
39. Rimerman RA, Gellert-Randleman A, Diehl JA. Wnt1 and MEK1 cooperate to promote cyclin D1 accumulation and cellular transformation. J Biol Chem. 2000;275:14736–42.
40. Mann B, Gelos M, Siedow A, Hanski ML, Gratchev A, Ilyas M, et al. Target genes of beta-catenin-T cell-factor/lymphoid-enhancer-factor signaling in human colorectal carcinomas. Proc Natl Acad Sci USA. 1999;96:1603–8.
41. Pollock PM, Hayward N. Mutations in exon 3 of the beta-catenin gene are rare in melanoma cell lines. Melanoma Res. 2002;12:183–6.
42. Li G, Satyamoorthy K, Herlyn M. N-cadherin-mediated intercellular interactions promote survival and migration of melanoma cells. Cancer Res. 2001;61:3819–25.
43. Satyamoorthy K, Li G, Vaidya B, Patel D, Herlyn M. Insulin-like growth factor-1 induces survival and growth of biologically early melanoma cells through both the mitogen-activated protein kinase and beta-catenin pathways. Cancer Res. 2001;61:7318–24.
44. Delmas V, Beermann F, Martinozzi S, Carreira S, Ackermann J, Kumasaka M, et al. Beta-catenin induces immortalization of melanocytes by suppressing p16INK4a expression and cooperates with N-Ras in melanoma development. Genes Dev. 2007;21:2923–35.

45. Weeraratna AT, Jiang Y, Hostetter G, Rosenblatt K, Duray P, Bittner M, et al. Wnt5a signaling directly affects cell motility and invasion of metastatic melanoma. Cancer Cell. 2002;1:279–88.
46. Dissanayake SK, Olkhanud PB, O'Connell MP, Carter A, French AD, Camilli TC, et al. Wnt5A regulates expression of tumor-associated antigens in melanoma via changes in signal transducers and activators of transcription 3 phosphorylation. Cancer Res. 2008;68:10205–14.
47. Da Forno PD, Pringle JH, Hutchinson P, Osborn J, Huang Q, Potter L, et al. WNT5A expression increases during melanoma progression and correlates with outcome. Clin Cancer Res. 2008;14:5825–32.
48. Chien AJ, Moore EC, Lonsdorf AS, Kulikauskas RM, Rothberg BG, Berger AJ, et al. Activated Wnt/beta-catenin signaling in melanoma is associated with decreased proliferation in patient tumors and a murine melanoma model. Proc Natl Acad Sci USA. 2009;106:1193–8.
49. Kageshita T, Hamby CV, Ishihara T, Matsumoto K, Saida T, Ono T. Loss of beta-catenin expression associated with disease progression in malignant melanoma. Br J Dermatol. 2001; 145:210–6.
50. Larue L, Delmas V. The WNT/Beta-catenin pathway in melanoma. Front Biosci. 2006;11: 733–42.
51. Castellone MD, Teramoto H, Williams BO, Druey KM, Gutkind JS. Prostaglandin E2 promotes colon cancer cell growth through a Gs-axin-beta-catenin signaling axis. Science. 2005;310:1504–10.
52. Shao J, Jung C, Liu C, Sheng H. Prostaglandin E2 Stimulates the beta-catenin/T cell factor-dependent transcription in colon cancer. J Biol Chem. 2005;280:26565–72.
53. Lepourcelet M, Chen YN, France DS, Wang H, Crews P, Petersen F, et al. Small-molecule antagonists of the oncogenic Tcf/beta-catenin protein complex. Cancer Cell. 2004;5:91–102.
54. Emami KH, Nguyen C, Ma H, Kim DH, Jeong KW, Eguchi M, et al. A small molecule inhibitor of beta-catenin/CREB-binding protein transcription [corrected]. Proc Natl Acad Sci USA. 2004;101:12682–7.
55. Huang SM, Mishina YM, Liu S, Cheung A, Stegmeier F, Michaud GA, et al. Tankyrase inhibition stabilizes axin and antagonizes Wnt signalling. Nature. 2009;461:614–20.
56. Chen B, Dodge ME, Tang W, Lu J, Ma Z, Fan CW, et al. Small molecule-mediated disruption of Wnt-dependent signaling in tissue regeneration and cancer. Nat Chem Biol. 2009;5:100–7.
57. Smalley KS, Contractor R, Haass NK, Kulp AN, Atilla-Gokcumen GE, Williams DS, et al. An organometallic protein kinase inhibitor pharmacologically activates p53 and induces apoptosis in human melanoma cells. Cancer Res. 2007;67:209–17.
58. Corcoran RB, Dias-Santagata D, Bergethon K, Iafrate AJ, Settleman J, Engelman JA. BRAF gene amplification can promote acquired resistance to MEK inhibitors in cancer cells harboring the BRAF V600E mutation. Science signaling 3, ra84. 2010.
59. Johannessen CM, Boehm JS, Kim SY, Thomas SR, Wardwell L, Johnson LA, et al. COT drives resistance to RAF inhibition through MAP kinase pathway reactivation. Nature. 2010;468: 968–72.
60. Nazarian R, Shi H, Wang Q, Kong X, Koya RC, Lee H, et al. Melanomas acquire resistance to B-RAF(V600E) inhibition by RTK or N-RAS upregulation. Nature. 2010;468:973–7.
61. Villanueva J, Vultur A, Lee JT, Somasundaram R, Fukunaga-Kalabis M, Cipolla AK, et al. Acquired resistance to BRAF inhibitors mediated by a RAF kinase switch in melanoma can be overcome by cotargeting MEK and IGF-1R/PI3K. Cancer Cell. 2010;18:683–95.
62. Boiko AD, Razorenova OV, van de Rijn M, Swetter SM, Johnson DL, Ly DP, et al. Human melanoma-initiating cells express neural crest nerve growth factor receptor CD271. Nature. 2010;466:133–7.
63. Held MA, Curley DP, Dankort D, McMahon M, Muthusamy V, Bosenberg MW. Characterization of melanoma cells capable of propagating tumors from a single cell. Cancer Res. 2010;70: 388–97.
64. Roesch A, Fukunaga-Kalabis M, Schmidt EC, Zabierowski SE, Brafford PA, Vultur A, et al. A temporarily distinct subpopulation of slow-cycling melanoma cells is required for continuous tumor growth. Cell. 2010;141:583–94.

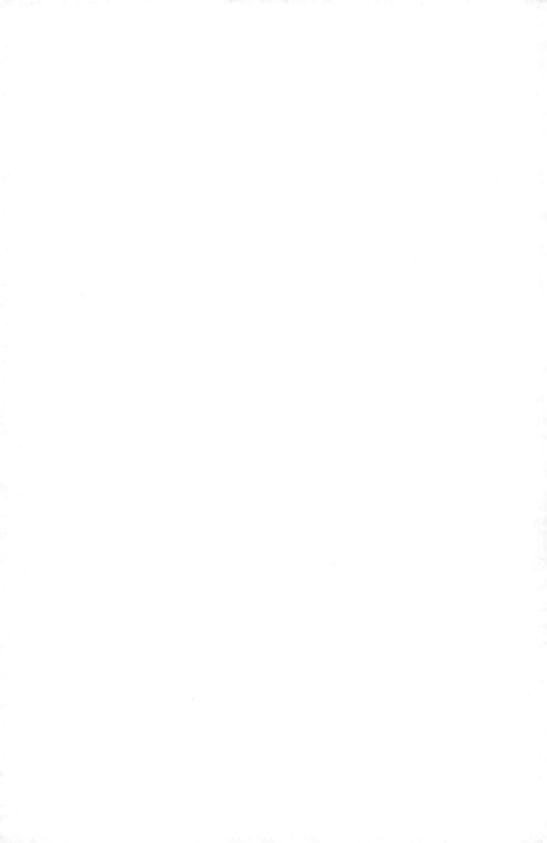

Chapter 7
STAT3 and Src Signaling in Melanoma

**Maciej Kujawski, Gregory Cherryholmes, Saul J. Priceman,
and Hua Yu**

Abstract Several tyrosine kinase signaling pathways play a critical role for melanoma
development and progression. Signal Transducer and Activator of Transcription
(STAT) family proteins function both as cytoplasmic signal-transducing molecules as
well as nuclear transcription factors. A member of the STAT family proteins, STAT3,
is a point of convergence for numerous tyrosine kinases frequently activated in human
cancers. In melanoma tumor cells, Src tyrosine kinase has been shown to be involved
in melanoma oncogenicity, in part by activating STAT3. Many other tyrosine kinases,
such as Janus kinases (JAKs), epidermal growth factor receptor (EGFR), Her2/Neu,
and basic fibroblast growth factor receptor (bFGFR), are also known markers of
malignant melanoma and activators of STAT3. By virtue of its ability to regulate
expression of numerous genes important for proliferation, survival, invasion, and
immunosuppression, STAT3 has emerged as a key target for melanoma therapy. While
direct STAT3 inhibitors for clinical use are still under development, several tyrosine
kinase inhibitors available in the clinic may serve as effective therapeutics for melanoma, especially in conjunction with other promising therapeutic strategies.

Keywords Melanoma • Stat3 • Src • Tumor survival • Proliferation • Metastasis
• Immune evasion • Targeted therapy

M. Kujawski, PhD • S.J. Priceman, PhD • H. Yu, PhD (✉)
Department of Cancer Immunotherapeutics and Tumor Immunology,
Beckman Research Institute and City of Hope Comprehensive Cancer Center,
Duarte, CA 91010, USA

G. Cherryholmes, MSc
The Irell and Manella Graduate School of Biological Sciences, Beckman Research Institute
and City of Hope Comprehensive Cancer Center, Duarte, CA 91010, USA

T.F. Gajewski and F.S. Hodi (eds.), *Targeted Therapeutics in Melanoma*,
Current Clinical Oncology, DOI 10.1007/978-1-61779-407-0_7,
© Springer Science+Business Media, LLC 2012

Introduction

The Signal Transducer and Activator of Transcription (STAT) family of proteins function both as cytoplasmic signal-transducing molecules as well as nuclear transcription factors [132]. Activation of STATs is mediated by either receptor-associated kinases, such as Janus kinases (JAKs), or nonreceptor oncogenic tyrosine kinases, including Src and BCR-ABL (Abelson leukemia protein). These activated kinases phosphorylate monomeric latent STAT proteins, which mediates cytosolic dimerization and nuclear translocation, where they regulate target gene expression (Fig. 7.1).

Like all the STAT family members, STAT3 is tightly controlled in normal cells. The mechanisms that regulate STAT3 activity include dephosphorylation of receptors and STAT dimers by protein tyrosine phosphatases (PTPases); interaction with one of the protein inhibitors of activated STAT (PIAS); and feedback inhibition of JAK/STAT pathway by suppressor of cytokine signaling (SOCS) proteins [39, 66]. However, the dysregulation of autocrine or paracrine stimulation of cytokine and growth factor receptors, observed in the many cancers, results in constitutive and uncontrolled activation of STAT3.

The first direct evidence that STAT3 signaling contributes to oncogenesis emerged in the mid-1990s, when STAT3 was found to be constitutively activate in Src-transformed fibroblasts [131]. After this finding, several studies further confirmed the interactions between Src and STAT3 in oncogenesis [6, 110]. STAT3 as an oncogene was also formally demonstrated using the constitutively active mutant STAT3C, which was capable of transforming fibroblasts [7]. The remainder of this chapter is further devoted to the important roles of STAT3 and Src in the malignant phenotype of melanoma and emphasize STAT3 and Src as attractive targets for melanoma therapy.

STAT3 and Src Signaling in Melanoma

The importance of STAT proteins, and in particular STAT3, in the development of melanoma has been well documented. STAT3 has been shown to be constitutively active in human melanoma cell lines and in primary tumor tissues compared with normal skin [85]. This overactivation may be partially explained by the association of Src kinases to STAT3 in melanoma cells [85]. Src-related kinase family members can be activated by both receptor-dependent and receptor-independent pathways [16, 44]. In the receptor-independent mechanism of Src activation, STAT activity may be regulated by a constitutively activated, cytoplasmic form of Src kinase, known as c-Src. In addition to c-Src, other members of the Src family have been implicated in tumorigenesis. RaLP, a novel member of the Src family, is involved in the migration of metastatic melanoma cells, although the cell signaling pathways it utilizes have yet to be unraveled [22]. Another member of the Src family, FYN, is found overexpressed in melanoma and other solid cancers, yet its precise role during cancer development remains to be clarified [100].

When interacting with signaling proteins such as focal adhesin kinase (FAK) and p130CAS, Src regulates melanoma cell adhesion, motility, and migration, which

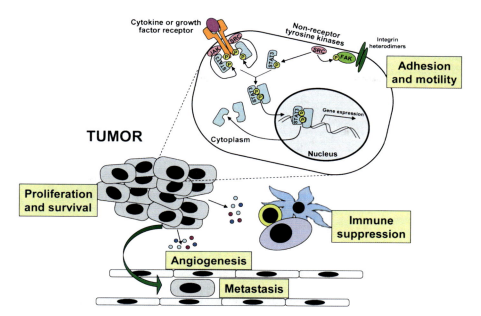

Fig. 7.1 Persistent STAT3 activation in melanoma tumor cells is mediated by both receptor and nonreceptor tyrosine kinases, such as Src and Janus kinases (JAKs) tyrosine kinases. Activated kinases phosphorylate monomeric latent STAT3 protein, leading to its cytosolic dimerization and nuclear translocation, and target gene expression. Src tyrosine kinase, by interacting with other signaling proteins such as Focal Adhesion Kinase (FAK), regulates melanoma cells adhesion, motility, and migration. STAT3-regulated factors contribute to creation of the tumor microenvironment characterized by increased angiogenesis, metastasis, and suppression of antitumor immune responses. Targeting STAT3 directly or indirectly through tyrosine kinase inhibitors, therefore, holds promise for melanoma therapy

can be mediated through STAT3 activation [5, 8, 79]. While the constitutively active form of Src is able to regulate STAT3 directly, the increase in expression or activation of growth factor receptors may also be responsible for both Src and STAT3 activation [51, 78]. Many upstream mediators of STAT3 activation and Src signaling, such as epidermal growth factor receptor (EGFR), Her2/Neu, and basic fibroblast growth factor receptor (bFGFR), are known markers of malignant melanoma [94, 99], further indicating an association between STAT3 and Src during melanoma pathogenesis. It is, however, important to note that growth factor and cytokine-mediated STAT3 activation in many cancers including melanoma may also work independently of Src activation [132–134].

IL-6 and other IL-6-type cytokines, such as oncostatin M, are among the classical STAT3 mediators that use receptor-dependent mechanisms for STAT3 activation [39]. As with multiple myeloma and prostate cancer, IL-6 can also activate STAT3 in melanoma [72]. Melanoma progression in the metastatic stages may be connected to possible loss of oncostatin M receptor beta [69] or activation of RAS-RAF, MAPK-ERK kinase (MEK)-extracellular regulated kinase (ERK) 1/2 signaling pathways [17, 118]. It is well established that overactivation of STAT3 promotes expression of many genes critical for melanoma tumor cell proliferation, survival, invasion, and metastasis [132–134]. STAT3 may also contribute to melanoma tumorigenesis by regulating other transcription factors. It has been demonstrated that constitutively active STAT3 in human cancer cells, including melanoma, is essential for prolonged nuclear retention of NF-κB through RelA acetylation [73]. This STAT3-mediated prolonged nuclear retention of NF-κB may explain why overactivation of both STAT3 and NF-κB in tumor cells can regulate expression of overlapping prosurvival, proangiogenic, and immunomodulatory genes [34]. While additional studies are warranted to fully understand the NF-κB/STAT3 signaling pathway cross talk and their cooperative roles during melanoma progression, the connection between STAT3 activity and other major signaling pathways, such as NF-κB, further validates the importance of STAT3 in oncogenesis.

STAT3/Src Regulation of Tumor Cell Growth

The critical role of STAT3 signaling in the survival of tumor cells was first shown in multiple myeloma. In multiple myeloma cells, constitutively activated STAT3 regulates the expression of the antiapoptotic B-cell lymphoma/leukemia-2 (BCL2) family gene BCL-XL [11]. Blocking STAT3 in multiple myeloma cells downregulates BCL-XL expression, leading to increased apoptosis. Furthermore, specific inhibition of STAT3 or Src kinase activity in head and neck squamous cell carcinoma inhibits BCL-XL expression and induces apoptosis [31, 51]. In melanoma cells, BCL-XL and another member of the BCL2 family, MCL-1, are both downregulated by inhibition of c-Src kinase or STAT3 transcriptional activity [85]. STAT3 also regulates survivin expression [2, 33] and targeting survivin in melanoma cells results in growth arrest and increased apoptosis [35]. Moreover, BCL-XL and MCL-1 are associated with metastatic progression of melanoma, and their expression positively correlates with STAT3 activation [136], thereby strengthening the link between STAT3 and melanoma progression. However, STAT3's role in inhibiting apoptosis goes beyond promoting expression of antiapoptotic proteins. Activation of STAT3 in melanoma also suppresses expression of proapoptotic proteins, such as TRAIL and p53, thereby adding to the regulation of apoptosis by STAT3 [45, 46, 89].

STAT3 and Src Activity Promote Angiogenesis and Metastasis in Melanoma

As with most solid tumors, angiogenesis is required for melanoma growth beyond 2 mm, the limit of efficient nutrient diffusion. In addition, the metastatic spread of melanoma cells requires tumor blood vasculature. As a result of the highly proliferative nature of solid tumors, access to sufficient oxygen and nutrients is often depleted, resulting in hypoxia. Tumor cells respond to reduced oxygen conditions by upregulating factors that regulate the development and maintenance of tumor blood vasculature. In melanoma, hypoxic stress induces activation of numerous factors, in particular the α subunit of hypoxia inducible factor 1 (HIF-1α) [103]. Regulation of HIF-1α occurs posttranslationally by modification of its stability in the cytoplasm [103]. HIF-1α is also transcriptionally regulated, especially in the tumor microenvironment [86]. Both Src and STAT3 have been demonstrated to regulate the RNA and protein levels of HIF1α [49, 88, 128]. In addition to regulating HIF1α, STAT3 can also directly regulate transcription of important genes involved in tumor angiogenesis, including VEGF, bFGF, and MMP-2, many of which have been demonstrated in melanoma cells [86, 88, 118, 123, 124]. Inhibition of STAT3 by siRNA or small-molecule inhibition in melanoma cells showed reduces expression of both HIF-1α and VEGF, induced by multiple oncogenic growth signaling pathways involving Src, EGFR, Her2/Neu, and IL-6R [126]. The existence of multifactor axes involving STAT3, Src, and HIF-1α-mediated regulation of VEGF and tumor angiogenesis has been also described in pancreatic and prostate cancers [32].

STAT3 signaling also appears to be critical for tumor metastasis in melanoma. Multiple biological processes are responsible for tumor metastasis, including epithelial–mesenchymal transition (EMT), migration of tumor cells, tumor cell extravasation, seeding within the premetastatic niche, and subsequent survival and growth of tumors at the secondary site. EMT is one of the key steps involved in tumor metastasis. TGFβ and VEGF, known activators of STAT3 signaling, seem to play a major role in EMT [93, 130]. In AML-12 murine hepatocytes, TGFβ1 induces EMT and is associated with the activation of STAT3 through protein kinase A (PKA) [130]. In the L3.6pl human pancreatic cancer cell line, upregulation of VEGFR-1 can alter the cellular phenotype towards metastasis, which is associated with an increase in the expression of transcription factors involved in EMT transition, namely Snail, Twist, and Slug [127]. Importantly, many of the factors involved in EMT are regulated by STAT3 [3, 13, 121]. Other studies have demonstrated an important role for IL-6 in the induction of EMT in human breast carcinoma through inhibition of the epithelial marker E-cadherin and induction of mesenchymal markers including Vimentin, N-cadherin, Snail, and Twist [107]. Moreover, activation of STAT3 by IL-6, Src, or EGFR signaling in breast carcinoma induces Twist expression, which promotes metastasis and negatively regulates expression of E-cadherin [13, 75]. Moreover, constitutive expression of Twist in breast cancer cells causes production of IL-6 and potent autocrine activation of STAT3 [107].

STAT3 may also play an important role in EMT transition and metastasis of melanoma. STAT3 is known to regulate expression of WNT5A [52], which is an important mediator of melanoma cell motility as well as EMT [19, 117]. Furthermore, Twist is one of the primary EMT regulators overexpressed in melanoma cell lines when compared to normal melanocytes [42]. Together, these observations, directly and indirectly, implicate STAT3 signaling during EMT in melanoma.

Tumor cells must possess high migratory potential to invade distant organs. Several factors have been demonstrated to increase migratory capacity of melanoma cells. Mda-9/Syntenin regulates cell motility and invasion through physical interaction with c-Src in melanoma cells [5, 109]. Furthermore, tensin-3 phosphorylation by Src signaling in advanced lung cancer, breast cancer, and melanoma contributes to cell migration [96]. Pharmacologic inhibition of Src family kinases with the dual Src/Abl kinase inhibitor dasatinib blocks migration and invasion of human melanoma cells in vitro [8]. Src has recently been found to contribute to resistance of migrating tumor cells to anoikis – apoptosis caused by detachment of cells from their extracellular matrix (ECM) [101, 120]. Tumor cell adhesion to blood vessel endothelium and subsequent transendothelial migration within the circulation are critical components of the metastasis cascade. Src was shown to be strongly involved in vascular permeability [15] as well as in transendothelial migration of a human melanoma cell line [95]. Therefore, Src can play a vital role in extravasation during melanoma metastasis, which may act in concert with or independently of STAT3 activation.

STAT3 Signaling in Tumor-Associated Immune Cells: Their Role in Melanoma Development

The tumor microenvironment plays an important role in promoting tumor development. Tumor-associated stromal cells consist of a diverse population of immune cells, fibroblasts, and endothelial cells. Aberrant STAT3 activation is seen not only in tumor cells but also in stromal cells, which may contribute to their tumor-promoting activity [134, 135]. There is growing evidence that tumor cells may alter antitumor immune cells to support tumor growth [134], and that STAT3 is involved in cross talk between tumor cells and immune cells, thus augmenting tumor-induced immunosuppression [133]. STAT3 activity in tumors can negatively regulate expression of several Th-1 immunostimulatory cytokines and chemokines that are important for immune-mediated tumor growth inhibition, such as IL-12, TNF, IFN-γ, IFN-β, CXCL10, and CCL5 [40, 60, 62, 114]. By contrast, elevated STAT3 activity in tumor cells can upregulate expression of immunosuppressive factors, such as IL-10 and TGFβ [53, 116]. Furthermore, known STAT3 activators such as IL-6, IL-10, and VEGF contribute to suppression of dendritic cell (DC) maturation, an event necessary for proper antigen presentation to T-cells [26, 114]. In human melanoma cells with mutated BRAF, STAT3 is required for production of IL-6, IL-10, and VEGF, which inhibits expression of immune-stimulating molecules such as IL-12 and TNF by DCs [108]. Involvement of IL-10 in immune evasion of melanoma patients has also been explored. Tumorigenic ABCB5$^+$ malignant melanoma initiating cells (MMICs), isolated directly from tumor tissues, can elicit IL-10 synthesis when cocultured with peripheral blood mononuclear cells (PBMCs), resulting in induction of CD4$^+$CD25$^+$FoxP3$^+$ regulatory T-cells [102]. Moreover, patients with metastatic melanoma have been found to have increased levels of the STAT3-mediated VEGF production. This tumor-driven VEGF secretion may be responsible for Th-2 inflammation in patients characterized by elevations of the Th-2-promoting cytokines IL-4, IL-5, IL-10, and IL-13 [84].

STAT3 activity in tumors also affects other members of innate immunity, namely, macrophages, neutrophils, and NK cells. In mouse melanoma models, STAT3 activation affects migration of neutrophils and macrophages as well as nitric oxide synthesis by macrophages, thus blocking an antitumor immune response [9]. Moreover, intrinsic STAT3 activity in both tumor-infiltrating neutrophils and NK cells is inhibitory of their antitumor cytotoxic activity [60]. STAT3 signaling in the tumor microenvironment also directly regulates the balance of two major immune factors produced by myeloid cells, IL-23 and IL-12 [62]. These related yet opposing factors are important in regulating pro- and antitumor innate and adaptive immune responses [71].

Another group of important tumor-infiltrating immune cells are myeloid-derived suppressor cells (MDSCs). MDSCs represent a heterogeneous population of myeloid cells at different stages of maturation found both in tumor-bearing mice and in cancer patients [27]. It has been recently shown that myeloid cells with immunosuppressive properties accumulate both in mononuclear and polymorphonuclear fractions of circulating blood leukocytes of patients with melanoma and colon cancer [77]. One of the main functions of MDSCs in the tumor environment is suppression of antitumor T-cell-mediated immune response. This MDSC-mediated T-cell suppression involves several mechanisms, including synthesis of reactive oxygen species, arginase-mediated depletion of arginine, and inhibition of $CD8^+$ T-cell antigen recognition [82]. Accumulation of MDSCs in tumor-bearing animals can be contributed by STAT3-induced upregulation of the myeloid-related protein S100A9 [14]. Furthermore, STAT3 in the tumor microenvironment can mediate multidirectional cross talk among tumor cells, myeloid cells, and endothelial cells in the tumor site, contributing to tumor angiogenesis [67]. MDSCs and macrophages isolated from mouse melanomas secreted angiogenic factors including VEGF and bFGF, and induce angiogenesis by activation of STAT3.

In addition to the suppressive effects of MDSCs, T-cell-mediated antitumor effects are suppressed by tumor cells and myeloid cells through induction of regulatory T-cells (Tregs) [137]. Infiltration of Tregs is associated with progression of many human tumor types, including melanoma [28, 137]. In human melanoma, $FOXP3^+$ Tregs can be linked to immune tolerance early during melanoma development, thus favoring melanoma growth [81]. While their accumulation in tumors as a prognostic factor needs further investigation [70], targeting Tregs in melanoma patients to overcome immunosuppression and enhance antitumor immunotherapy is a desirable therapeutic strategy [54]. Recent evidence suggests an important role for STAT3 signaling in melanoma Tregs. A new STAT3 signaling pathway inhibitor has been shown to enhance T-cell-mediated cytotoxicity against melanoma cells through inhibition of Tregs [58]. Moreover, the same small-molecule inhibitor of STAT3 has antitumor efficacy in a mouse intracerebral melanoma model, in part by inhibition of Tregs [56]. Tyrosine kinase inhibitors such as sunitinib (SU011248), which inhibits STAT3 at relatively high concentrations [125, 128], can also reduce MDSCs and tumor-infiltrating Tregs in patients with renal cell carcinoma [23, 55], as well as in various mouse tumor models [90, 125]. Sunitinib can also drastically enhance the antitumor effects of adoptive T-cell therapy, which is associated with a reduction in tumor-infiltrating Tregs in a mouse melanoma model [68].

Another mechanism of tumor immune evasion involves decreasing the amount of tumor-associated antigens, thus preventing efficient cytotoxic T-cell response. It has recently been shown that Wnt5A inhibits expression of melanoma antigens through STAT3 activation [18]. STAT3 activation reduced expression of PAX3 and subsequent MITF expression, which regulate melanosomal antigen expression.

Treatment of Melanoma by STAT3-Targeted Therapy

One of the currently available therapies for the treatment of patients with melanoma is interferon-alpha-2b (IFNα2b). One important aspect of IFNα2b treatment is the role it plays in STAT3 regulation. STAT3 has been suggested as a biomarker for progression in atypical nevi of patients with melanoma, and the ratio of phospho-STAT1 and phospho-STAT3 in melanoma appears to be an important predicator for IFNα2b response [115, 117]. On the contrary, dysregulation of STAT3 may diminish the therapeutic efficacy of IFNα2b therapy. In fact, defects in the JAK/STAT pathway are found in some IFNα-resistant malignant melanomas [91]. In addition, IFNα2b may cause hyper-activation of STAT3 and further push tumor progression in certain melanoma subtypes [43]. In cases such as these, IFNa2b treatment in conjunction with STAT3 inhibition may enhance antitumor efficacy against brain metastatic melanoma [57].

Immunotherapy has shown promise for melanoma therapy. One such approach is the use of CpG oligonucleotides or other agonists of Toll-like receptors (TLRs) to stimulate antitumor immune responses [65]. Although CpG oligonucleotides/TLR9 agonists have been used in treating melanoma [92], the efficacy of such therapy needs further improvement. While CpG treatment may effectively mediate antitumor immune response, the activation of STAT3 during this response may act as a negative regulator of the Th-1 antitumor response [59, 60]. As a proof of principle, injection of a single dose of CpG oligonucleotides into melanoma tumor-bearing mice lacking the *Stat3* gene in hematopoietic cells caused rapid eradication of large B16 melanoma tumors [59]. Recently, a novel siRNA delivery platform has been developed by physically linking the CpG oligonucleotide with STAT3 siRNA [61]. The CpG-STAT3 siRNA conjugate not only facilitates targeted delivery of siRNA into immune cells, but also stimulates immune activation while blocking a key immunosuppressive checkpoint [30, 61]. Activation of the immune system by administration of immunostimulatory CpG oligonucleotides in conjunction with STAT3 inhibition may be a viable approach for melanoma therapy. Nevertheless, as these studies have been performed using mouse-optimized CpG, the efficacy of human-optimized CpG oligonucleotides in targeted siRNA delivery and gene silencing awaits further studies.

Inhibition of STAT3 Activation in Melanoma
via Small-Molecule Inhibitors

Several small-molecule drugs that target Src and other STAT3-activating kinases may have implications for the treatment of melanoma. Indirubin and dasatinib demonstrate the link of STAT3 and Src in various cancers. Derivatives of indirubin inhibited antiapoptotic proteins and reduced both Src and STAT3 tyrosine phosphorylation [83]. Dasatinib (known to target BCR-ABL, Src-Focal Kinases, PDGFR, and c-KIT) can reduce the invasive and tumorigenic properties in established human melanoma cell lines in vitro [8]. Dasatinib may also target endothelial and myeloid populations, disrupting the tumor microenvironment that promotes tumor progression [74]. Src inhibitor saracatinib tested in Phase II study in patients with advanced melanoma had minimal clinical activity as a single agent in metastatic melanoma but combination therapies still might hold promise for treating melanoma [29]. Interestingly, while resveratrol is a well-known inhibitor of the mTOR pathway, it has been recently shown to target the Src-STAT3 signaling complex [63] and induce TRAIL-mediated apoptosis by decreasing NF-κB and STAT3 activation [45]. Increased TRAIL expression by STAT3 inhibition in melanoma cells also has been shown [87]. Thus, the biological significance of Src and STAT3 signaling during melanoma development has generated increased interest in the clinical evaluation of Src- and STAT3-directed therapies.

Since STAT3 may be activated by Src-independent pathways, STAT3 inhibition via targeting receptor-dependent kinases is also an important strategy for melanoma therapy. Imatinib mesylate is one such kinase inhibitor, which targets the STAT3 activators PDGFR and BCR-ABL [122]. Like resveratrol, imatinib induces TRAIL-mediated apoptosis in melanoma [37], which could result from inhibition of STAT3 activation [87]. However, the treatment of unselected melanoma patients in clinical trials using imatinib has not demonstrated significant efficacy [113, 122]. On the contrary, imatinib can target melanoma subpopulation that express a gain-of-function mutation for the protein KIT [41, 47, 76] and therefore may be used in combination with other kinase inhibitors for effective therapy. In addition to imatinib, sunitinib is in clinical trials for various stages of melanoma [12, 97]. Sunitinib has been shown to reverse the immunosuppressive effects of tumor-associated immune cells in human renal cell carcinoma [23, 55, 80] and mouse tumor models [125]. This inhibition, as shown in mouse renal cell carcinoma, is at least partially mediated by downregulation of STAT3 activity [125]. In addition to the well-established studies in renal cell carcinoma, sunitinib is currently in Phase II clinical trials for the treatment of patients with Stage IV uveal melanoma [12]. Sorafenib has also been shown to inhibit STAT3 in medulloblastoma [129]. Although sorafenib is originally used as a RAF inhibitor, it may also inhibit VEGFR, PDGFR-β, and c-KIT [21, 105, 119]. While sorafenib is already approved by the FDA for the treatment of renal cell carcinoma [50], it was also used in clinical trials for the treatment of advanced melanoma [20]. Silibinin has also been shown to directly affect the constitutive activation of STAT3 in the prostate cancer cell line DU145 [1] and may have antitumor effects against melanoma [106]. Axitinib, a drug that is in Phase II clinical trials for renal cell carcinoma [98], is also being tested in advanced stages of melanoma [25].

Inhibitors of JAK kinases, well-known activators of STATs, may also be used to treat melanoma. For instance, JSI-124 (cucurbitacin I) inhibits highly metastatic murine melanoma tumor growth in vivo by blocking JAK-mediated STAT3 activation [4]. Furthermore, JAK inhibition by AG490 and PP2 decreases melanoma STAT3 activation and growth/viability [64]. WP1066, another small-molecule inhibitor of the JAK/STAT3 pathway, can also effectively initiate antitumor immunity in metastatic sites of melanoma in the brain using mouse models [56]. Other JAK inhibitors may also hold promise and have yet to be studied in melanoma. For instance,

JAK2 inhibitor AZD1480 has been shown to inhibit constitutive STAT3 activity in prostate, breast, and ovarian cancer cell lines and in SCID tumor models [38].

One important aspect/drawback of targeting STAT3 through tyrosine kinase inhibitors, including Src inhibitors, is that prolonged inhibition of a particular tyrosine kinase(s) can lead to activation of alternative pathways [104]. As reported in several cases, inhibition of the tyrosine kinases can initially inhibit STAT3 activity, but eventually activates STAT3, promoting tumor growth [10, 48]. Blocking STAT3 and the tyrosine kinase(s) simultaneously can overcome such feedback loops and enhance antitumor effects. Owing to lack of its own enzymatic activities, transcription factors, such as STAT3, are difficult to target [134]. Nevertheless, several promising direct STAT3 inhibitors have been developed over the years [24, 36, 111, 112, 135]. It is only a matter of time before clinically suitable small-molecule STAT3-specific inhibitors will be available.

Conclusions

As a signal transducer, STAT3 is a common point of convergence for numerous tyrosine kinases frequently activated in human cancers. One such oncogenic kinase is Src. In the case of melanoma, Src has been shown to activate STAT3 at least in some patient tumor samples and tumor cell lines. A major reason that STAT3 is critical for oncogenesis in diverse cancers, including melanoma, is because it is a transcription factor that regulates expression of many genes crucial for survival, proliferation, angiogenesis, invasion, and immunosuppression. However, as a target for cancer therapy, STAT3 proves difficult to directly inhibit compared with tyrosine kinases such as Src. This is due to the lack of intrinsic enzymatic activity of transcription factors. Nevertheless, many tyrosine kinase inhibitors, including but not limited to Src inhibitors, can reduce STAT3 activity in tumors. On the contrary, long-term inhibition of some tyrosine kinases has been shown to activate alternative oncogenic pathways, some of which in turn activate STAT3, leading to cancer-promoting activity. These observations suggest the importance of targeting STAT3 directly through either small-molecule drugs or siRNA. The emergence of several selective STAT3 inhibitors that disrupt either STAT3 dimerization or DNA binding suggests that it is possible to directly target STAT3 for future cancer therapy. Because STAT3 is a critical checkpoint for antitumor immune responses, targeting STAT3 has the unique potential to broadly alter the tumor microenvironment to benefit immunotherapeutic approaches.

References

1. Agarwal C, Tyagi A, Kaur M, Agarwal R. Silibinin inhibits constitutive activation of Stat3, and causes caspase activation and apoptotic death of human prostate carcinoma DU145 cells. Carcinogenesis. 2007;28:1463.
2. Aoki Y, Feldman GM, Tosato G. Inhibition of STAT3 signaling induces apoptosis and decreases survivin expression in primary effusion lymphoma. Blood. 2003;101:1535–42.

3. Azare J, Leslie K, Al-Ahmadie H, Gerald W, Weinreb PH, Violette SM, et al. Constitutively activated Stat3 induces tumorigenesis and enhances cell motility of prostate epithelial cells through integrin beta 6. Mol Cell Biol. 2007;27:4444–53.

4. Blaskovich MA, Sun J, Cantor A, Turkson J, Jove R, Sebti SM. Discovery of JSI-124 (cucur-bitacin I), a selective Janus kinase/signal transducer and activator of transcription 3 signaling pathway inhibitor with potent antitumor activity against human and murine cancer cells in mice. Cancer Res. 2003;63:1270.

5. Boukerche H, Su ZZ, Prevot C, Sarkar D, Fisher PB. mda-9/Syntenin promotes metastasis in human melanoma cells by activating c-Src. Proc Natl Acad Sci USA. 2008;105:15914–9.

6. Bromberg JF, Horvath CM, Besser D, Lathem WW, Darnell Jr JE. Stat3 activation is required for cellular transformation by v-src. Mol Cell Biol. 1998;18:2553–8.

7. Bromberg JF, Wrzeszczynska MH, Devgan G, Zhao Y, Pestell RG, Albanese C, et al. Stat3 as an oncogene. Cell. 1999;98:295–303.

8. Buettner R, Mesa T, Vultur A, Lee F, Jove R. Inhibition of Src family kinases with dasatinib blocks migration and invasion of human melanoma cells. Mol Cancer Res. 2008;6:1766–74.

9. Burdelya L, Kujawski M, Niu G, Zhong B, Wang T, Zhang S, et al. Stat3 activity in mela-noma cells affects migration of immune effector cells and nitric oxide-mediated antitumor effects. J Immunol. 2005;174:3925–31.

10. Byers LA, Sen B, Saigal B, Diao L, Wang J, Nanjundan M, et al. Reciprocal regulation of c-Src and STAT3 in non-small cell lung cancer. Clin Cancer Res. 2009;15:6852–61.

11. Catlett-Falcone R, Landowski TH, Oshiro MM, Turkson J, Levitzki A, Savino R, et al. Constitutive activation of Stat3 signaling confers resistance to apoptosis in human U266 myeloma cells. Immunity. 1999;10:105–15.

12. Chan KR, Gundala S, Laudadio M, Mastrangelo M, Yamamoto A, Sato T. A pilot study using sunitinib malate as therapy in patients with stage IV uveal melanoma. J Clin Oncol. 2008; 26:9047.

13. Cheng GZ, Zhang WZ, Sun M, Wang Q, Coppola D, Mansour M, et al. Twist is transcription-ally induced by activation of STAT3 and mediates STAT3 oncogenic function. J Biol Chem. 2008;283:14665–73.

14. Cheng P, Corzo CA, Luetteke N, Yu B, Nagaraj S, Bui MM, et al. Inhibition of dendritic cell differentiation and accumulation of myeloid-derived suppressor cells in cancer is regulated by S100A9 protein. J Exp Med. 2008;205:2235–49.

15. Criscuoli ML, Nguyen M, Eliceiri BP. Tumor metastasis but not tumor growth is dependent on Src-mediated vascular permeability. Blood. 2005;105:1508–14.

16. Danial NN, Rothman P. JAK-STAT signaling activated by Abl oncogenes. Oncogene. 2000;19:2523–31.

17. Dhomen N, Reis-Filho JS, da Rocha Dias S, Hayward R, Savage K, Delmas V, et al. Oncogenic Braf induces melanocyte senescence and melanoma in mice. Cancer Cell. 2009;15:294–303.

18. Dissanayake SK, Olkhanud PB, O'Connell MP, Carter A, French AD, Camilli TC, et al. Wnt5A regulates expression of tumor-associated antigens in melanoma via changes in signal transduc-ers and activators of transcription 3 phosphorylation. Cancer Res. 2008;68:10205–14.

19. Dissanayake SK, Wade M, Johnson CE, O'Connell MP, Leotlela PD, French AD, et al. The Wnt5A/protein kinase C pathway mediates motility in melanoma cells via the inhibition of metastasis suppressors and initiation of an epithelial to mesenchymal transition. J Biol Chem. 2007;282:17259–71.

20. Eisen T, Ahmad T, Flaherty KT, Gore M, Kaye S, Marais R, et al. Sorafenib in advanced mela-noma: a phase II randomised discontinuation trial analysis. Br J Cancer. 2006;95:581–6.

21. Fabian MA, Biggs WH, Treiber DK, Atteridge CE, Azimioara MD, Benedetti MG, et al. A small molecule–kinase interaction map for clinical kinase inhibitors. Nat Biotechnol. 2005;23:329–36.

22. Fagiani E, Giardina G, Luzi L, Cesaroni M, Quarto M, Capra M, et al. RaLP, a new member of the Src homology and collagen family, regulates cell migration and tumor growth of meta-static melanomas. Cancer Res. 2007;67:3064.

23. Finke JH, Rini B, Ireland J, Rayman P, Richmond A, Golshayan A, et al. Sunitinib reverses type-1 immune suppression and decreases T-regulatory cells in renal cell carcinoma patients. Clin Cancer Res. 2008;14:6674.
24. Fletcher S, Singh J, Zhang X, Yue P, Page BDG, Sharmeen S, et al. Disruption of transcriptionally active Stat3 dimers with non-phosphorylated, salicylic acid-based small molecules: potent in vitro and tumor cell activities. ChemBioChem. 2009;10:1959–64.
25. Fruehauf JP, Lutzky J, McDermott DF, Brown CK, Pithavala YK, Bycott PW, et al. Axitinib (AG-013736) in patients with metastatic melanoma: a phase II study. J Clin Oncol. 2008; 26:484.
26. Gabrilovich D. Mechanisms and functional significance of tumour-induced dendritic-cell defects. Nat Rev Immunol. 2004;4:941–52.
27. Gabrilovich DI, Nagaraj S. Myeloid-derived suppressor cells as regulators of the immune system. Nat Rev Immunol. 2009;9:162–74.
28. Gajewski TF. Failure at the effector phase: immune barriers at the level of the melanoma tumor microenvironment. Clin Cancer Res. 2007;13:5256–61.
29. Gajewski TF, Zha Y, Clark J. Phase II study of the src family kinase inhibitor saracatinib (AZD0530) in metastatic melanoma. J Clin Oncol. 2010;28:8562.
30. Gantier MP, Williams BRG. siRNA delivery not Toll-free. Nat Biotechnol. 2009;27:911–2.
31. Grandis JR, Drenning SD, Zeng Q, Watkins SC, Melhem MF, Endo S, et al. Constitutive activation of Stat3 signaling abrogates apoptosis in squamous cell carcinogenesis in vivo. Proc Natl Acad Sci USA. 2000;97:4227–32.
32. Gray MJ, Zhang J, Ellis LM, Semenza GL, Evans DB, Watowich SS, et al. HIF-1alpha, STAT3, CBP/p300 and Ref-1/APE are components of a transcriptional complex that regulates Src-dependent hypoxia-induced expression of VEGF in pancreatic and prostate carcinomas. Oncogene. 2005;24:3110–20.
33. Gritsko T, Williams A, Turkson J, Kaneko S, Bowman T, Huang M, et al. Persistent activation of stat3 signaling induces survivin gene expression and confers resistance to apoptosis in human breast cancer cells. Clin Cancer Res. 2006;12:11.
34. Grivennikov SI, Karin M. Dangerous liaisons: STAT3 and NF-kappaB collaboration and crosstalk in cancer. Cytokine Growth Factor Rev. 2009;21:11–9.
35. Grossman D, Kim PJ, Schechner JS, Altieri DC. Inhibition of melanoma tumor growth in vivo by survivin targeting. Proc Natl Acad Sci USA. 2001;98:635–40.
36. Gunning PT, Glenn MP, Siddiquee KAZ, Katt WP, Masson E, Sebti SM, et al. Targeting protein-protein interactions: suppression of Stat3 dimerization with rationally designed small-molecule, nonpeptidic SH2 domain binders. Chembiochem. 2008;9:2800.
37. Hamai A, Richon C, Meslin F, Faure F, Kauffmann A, Lecluse Y, et al. Imatinib enhances human melanoma cell susceptibility to TRAIL-induced cell death: relationship to Bcl-2 family and caspase activation. Oncogene. 2006;25:7618–34.
38. Hedvat M, Huszar D, Herrmann A, Gozgit JM, Schroeder A, Sheehy A, et al. The JAK2 inhibitor AZD1480 potently blocks Stat3 signaling and oncogenesis in solid tumors. Cancer Cell. 2009;16:487–97.
39. Heinrich PC, Behrmann I, Haan S, Hermanns HM, Muller-Newen G, Schaper F. Principles of interleukin (IL)-6-type cytokine signalling and its regulation. Biochem J. 2003;374:1–20.
40. Ho HH, Ivashkiv LB. Role of STAT3 in type I interferon responses. Negative regulation of STAT1-dependent inflammatory gene activation. J Biol Chem. 2006;281:14111–8.
41. Hodi FS, Friedlander P, Corless CL, Heinrich MC, Mac Rae S, Kruse A, et al. Major response to imatinib mesylate in KIT-mutated melanoma. J Clin Oncol. 2008;26:2046–51.
42. Hoek K, Rimm DL, Williams KR, Zhao H, Ariyan S, Lin A, et al. Expression profiling reveals novel pathways in the transformation of melanocytes to melanomas. Cancer Res. 2004;64:5270–82.
43. Humpolikova-Adámková L, Kovařík J, Dusek L, Lauerová L, Boudn V, Fait V, et al. Interferon-alpha treatment may negatively influence disease progression in melanoma patients by hyperactivation of STAT3 protein. Eur J Cancer. 2009;45:1315–23.
44. Irby RB, Yeatman TJ. Role of Src expression and activation in human cancer. Oncogene. 2000;19:5636–42.

45. Ivanov VN, Partridge MA, Johnson GE, Huang SXL, Zhou H, Hei TK. Resveratrol sensitizes melanomas to TRAIL through modulation of antiapoptotic gene expression. Exp Cell Res. 2008;314:1163–76.
46. Ivanov VN, Zhou H, Partridge MA, Hei TK. Inhibition of ataxia telangiectasia mutated kinase activity enhances TRAIL-mediated apoptosis in human melanoma cells. Cancer Res. 2009;69:3510.
47. Jiang X, Zhou J, Yuen NK, Corless CL, Heinrich MC, Fletcher JA, et al. Imatinib targeting of KIT-mutant oncoprotein in melanoma. Clin Cancer Res. 2008;14:7726.
48. Johnson FM, Saigal B, Tran H, Donato NJ. Abrogation of signal transducer and activator of transcription 3 reactivation after Src kinase inhibition results in synergistic antitumor effects. Clin Cancer Res. 2007;13:4233.
49. Jung JE, Lee HG, Cho IH, Chung DH, Yoon SH, Yang YM, et al. STAT3 is a potential modulator of HIF-1-mediated VEGF expression in human renal carcinoma cells. FASEB J. 2005; 19:1296–8.
50. Kane RC, Farrell AT, Saber H, Tang S, Williams G, Jee JM, et al. Sorafenib for the treatment of advanced renal cell carcinoma. Clin Cancer Res. 2006;12:7271.
51. Karni R, Jove R, Levitzki A. Inhibition of pp 60c-Src reduces Bcl-XL expression and reverses the transformed phenotype of cells overexpressing EGF and HER-2 receptors. Oncogene. 1999;18:4654–62.
52. Katoh M, Katoh M. STAT3-induced WNT5A signaling loop in embryonic stem cells, adult normal tissues, chronic persistent inflammation, rheumatoid arthritis and cancer (review). Int J Mol Med. 2007;19:273–8.
53. Kinjyo I, Inoue H, Hamano S, Fukuyama S, Yoshimura T, Koga K, et al. Loss of SOCS3 in T helper cells resulted in reduced immune responses and hyperproduction of interleukin 10 and transforming growth factor-beta 1. J Exp Med. 2006;203:1021–31.
54. Kirkwood JM, Tarhini AA, Panelli MC, Moschos SJ, Zarour HM, Butterfield LH, et al. Next generation of immunotherapy for melanoma. J Clin Oncol. 2008;26:3445–55.
55. Ko JS, Zea AH, Rini BI, Ireland JL, Elson P, Cohen P, et al. Sunitinib mediates reversal of myeloid-derived suppressor cell accumulation in renal cell carcinoma patients. Clin Cancer Res. 2009;15:2148.
56. Kong LY, Abou-Ghazal MK, Wei J, Chakraborty A, Sun W, Qiao W, et al. A novel inhibitor of signal transducers and activators of transcription 3 activation is efficacious against established central nervous system melanoma and inhibits regulatory T cells. Clin Cancer Res. 2008;14:5759–68.
57. Kong LY, Gelbard A, Wei J, Reina-Ortiz C, Wang Y, Yang EC, et al. Inhibition of p-STAT3 enhances IFN-efficacy against metastatic melanoma in a murine model. Clin Cancer Res. 2010;16:2550.
58. Kong LY, Wei J, Sharma AK, Barr J, Abou-Ghazal MK, Fokt I, et al. A novel phosphorylated STAT3 inhibitor enhances T cell cytotoxicity against melanoma through inhibition of regulatory T cells. Cancer Immunol Immunother. 2009;58:1023–32.
59. Kortylewski M, Kujawski M, Herrmann A, Yang C, Wang L, Liu Y, et al. Toll-like receptor 9 activation of signal transducer and activator of transcription 3 constrains its agonist-based immunotherapy. Cancer Res. 2009;69:2497.
60. Kortylewski M, Kujawski M, Wang T, Wei S, Zhang S, Pilon-Thomas S, et al. Inhibiting Stat3 signaling in the hematopoietic system elicits multicomponent antitumor immunity. Nat Med. 2005;11:1314–21.
61. Kortylewski M, Swiderski P, Herrmann A, Wang L, Kowolik C, Kujawski M, et al. In vivo delivery of siRNA to immune cells by conjugation to a TLR9 agonist enhances antitumor immune responses. Nat Biotechnol. 2009;27:925–32.
62. Kortylewski M, Xin H, Kujawski M, Lee H, Liu Y, Harris T, et al. Regulation of the IL-23 and IL-12 balance by Stat3 signaling in the tumor microenvironment. Cancer Cell. 2009;15: 114–23.
63. Kotha A, Sekharam M, Cilenti L, Siddiquee K, Khaled A, Zervos AS, et al. Resveratrol inhibits Src and Stat3 signaling and induces the apoptosis of malignant cells containing activated Stat3 protein. Mol Cancer Therap. 2006;5:621.

64. Kreis S, Munz GA, Haan S, Heinrich PC, Behrmann I. Cell density-dependent increase of constitutive signal transducers and activators of transcription 3 activity in melanoma cells is mediated by Janus kinases. Mol Cancer Res. 2007;5:1331.
65. Krieg AM. Toll-like receptor 9 (TLR9) agonists in the treatment of cancer. Oncogene. 2008;27:161–7.
66. Kubo M, Hanada T, Yoshimura A. Suppressors of cytokine signaling and immunity. Nat Immunol. 2003;4:1169–76.
67. Kujawski M, Kortylewski M, Lee H, Herrmann A, Kay H, Yu H. Stat3 mediates myeloid cell-dependent tumor angiogenesis in mice. J Clin Invest. 2008;118:3367–77.
68. Kujawski M, Zhang C, Herrmann A, Reckamp K, Scuto A, Jensen M, et al. Targeting Stat3 in adoptively transferred T cells promotes their in vivo expansion and antitumor effects. Cancer Res. 2010;70:9599–610.
69. Lacreusette A, Nguyen JM, Pandolfino MC, Khammari A, Dreno B, Jacques Y, et al. Loss of oncostatin M receptor beta in metastatic melanoma cells. Oncogene. 2007;26:881–92.
70. Ladanyi A, Mohos A, Somlai B, Liszkay G, Gilde K, Fejos Z, et al. FOXP3(+) cell density in primary tumor has no prognostic impact in patients with cutaneous malignant melanoma. Pathol Oncol Res. 2010;3:303–9.
71. Langowski JL, Zhang X, Wu L, Mattson JD, Chen T, Smith K, et al. IL-23 promotes tumour incidence and growth. Nature. 2006;442:461–5.
72. Lazar-Molnar E, Hegyesi H, Toth S, Falus A. Autocrine and paracrine regulation by cytokines and growth factors in melanoma. Cytokine. 2000;12:547–54.
73. Lee H, Herrmann A, Deng JH, Kujawski M, Niu G, Li Z, et al. Persistently activated Stat3 maintains constitutive NF-kappaB activity in tumors. Cancer Cell. 2009;15:283–93.
74. Liang W, Kujawski M, Wu J, Lu J, Herrmann A, Loera S, et al. Antitumor activity of targeting SRC kinases in endothelial and myeloid cell compartments of the tumor microenvironment. Clin Cancer Res. 2010;16:924–35.
75. Lo HW, Hsu SC, Xia W, Cao X, Shih JY, Wei Y, et al. Epidermal growth factor receptor cooperates with signal transducer and activator of transcription 3 to induce epithelial-mesenchymal transition in cancer cells via up-regulation of TWIST gene expression. Cancer Res. 2007;67:9066–76.
76. Lutzky J, Bauer J, Bastian BC. Dose-dependent, complete response to imatinib of a metastatic mucosal melanoma with a K642E KIT mutation. Pigment Cell Melanoma Res. 2008;21:492–3.
77. Mandruzzato S, Solito S, Falisi E, Francescato S, Chiarion-Sileni V, Mocellin S, et al. IL4Ralpha+myeloid-derived suppressor cell expansion in cancer patients. J Immunol. 2009;182:6562–8.
78. Megeney LA, Perry RL, LeCouter JE, Rudnicki MA. bFGF and LIF signaling activates STAT3 in proliferating myoblasts. Dev Genet. 1996;19:139–45.
79. Mirmohammadsadegh A, Hassan M, Bardenheuer W, Marini A, Gustrau A, Nambiar S, et al. STAT5 phosphorylation in malignant melanoma is important for survival and is mediated through SRC and JAK1 kinases. J Invest Dermatol. 2006;126:2272–80.
80. Motzer RJ, Michaelson MD, Redman BG, Hudes GR, Wilding G, Figlin RA, et al. Activity of SU11248, a multitargeted inhibitor of vascular endothelial growth factor receptor and platelet-derived growth factor receptor, in patients with metastatic renal cell carcinoma. J Clin Oncol. 2006;24:16–24.
81. Mourmouras V, Fimiani M, Rubegni P, Epistolato MC, Malagnino V, Cardone C, et al. Evaluation of tumour-infiltrating CD4+CD25+FOXP3+ regulatory T cells in human cutaneous benign and atypical naevi, melanomas and melanoma metastases. Br J Dermatol. 2007;157:531–9.
82. Nagaraj S, Gupta K, Pisarev V, Kinarsky L, Sherman S, Kang L, et al. Altered recognition of antigen is a mechanism of CD8+ T cell tolerance in cancer. Nat Med. 2007;13:828–35.
83. Nam S, Buettner R, Turkson J, Kim D, Cheng JQ, Muehlbeyer S, et al. Indirubin derivatives inhibit Stat3 signaling and induce apoptosis in human cancer cells. Proc Natl Acad Sci USA. 2005;102:5998.

84. Nevala WK, Vachon CM, Leontovich AA, Scott CG, Thompson MA, Markovic SN. Evidence of systemic Th2-driven chronic inflammation in patients with metastatic melanoma. Clin Cancer Res. 2009;15:1931–9.
85. Niu G, Bowman T, Huang M, Shivers S, Reintgen D, Daud A, et al. Roles of activated Src and Stat3 signaling in melanoma tumor cell growth. Oncogene. 2002;21:7001–10.
86. Niu G, Briggs J, Deng J, Ma Y, Lee H, Kortylewski M, et al. Signal transducer and activator of transcription 3 is required for hypoxia-inducible factor-1alpha RNA expression in both tumor cells and tumor-associated myeloid cells. Mol Cancer Res. 2008;6:1099–105.
87. Niu G, Shain KH, Huang M, Ravi R, Bedi A, Dalton WS, et al. Overexpression of a dominant-negative signal transducer and activator of transcription 3 variant in tumor cells leads to production of soluble factors that induce apoptosis and cell cycle arrest. Cancer Res. 2001;61:3276.
88. Niu G, Wright KL, Huang M, Song L, Haura E, Turkson J, et al. Constitutive Stat3 activity up-regulates VEGF expression and tumor angiogenesis. Oncogene. 2002;21:2000–8.
89. Niu G, Wright KL, Ma Y, Wright GM, Huang M, Irby R, et al. Role of Stat3 in regulating p53 expression and function. Mol Cell Biol. 2005;25:7432–40.
90. Ozao-Choy J, Ma G, Kao J, Wang GX, Meseck M, Sung M, et al. The novel role of tyrosine kinase inhibitor in the reversal of immune suppression and modulation of tumor microenvironment for immune-based cancer therapies. Cancer Res. 2009;69:2514–22.
91. Pansky A, Hildebrand P, Fasler-Kan E, Baselgia L, Ketterer S, Beglinger C, et al. Defective Jak-STAT signal transduction pathway in melanoma cells resistant to growth inhibition by interferon. Int J Cancer. 2000;85:720–5.
92. Pashenkov M, Goass G, Wagner C, Harmann M, Jandl T, Moser A, et al. Phase II trial of a toll-like receptor 9-activating oligonucleotide in patients with metastatic melanoma. J Clin Oncol. 2006;24:5716–24.
93. Peinado H, Quintanilla M, Cano A. Transforming growth factor beta-1 induces snail transcription factor in epithelial cell lines: mechanisms for epithelial mesenchymal transitions. J Biol Chem. 2003;278:21113–23.
94. Potti A, Moazzam N, Langness E, Sholes K, Tendulkar K, Koch M, et al. Immunohistochemical determination of HER-2/neu, c-Kit (CD117), and vascular endothelial growth factor (VEGF) overexpression in malignant melanoma. J Cancer Res Clin Oncol. 2004;130:80–6.
95. Qi J, Wang J, Romanyuk O, Siu CH. Involvement of Src family kinases in N-cadherin phosphorylation and beta-catenin dissociation during transendothelial migration of melanoma cells. Mol Biol Cell. 2006;17:1261–72.
96. Qian X, Li G, Vass WC, Papageorge A, Walker RC, Asnaghi L, et al. The Tensin-3 protein, including its SH2 domain, is phosphorylated by Src and contributes to tumorigenesis and metastasis. Cancer Cell. 2009;16:246–58.
97. Rini BI, Garcia JA, Cooney MM, Elson P, Tyler A, Beatty K, et al. A phase I study of sunitinib plus bevacizumab in advanced solid tumors. Clin Cancer Res. 2009;15:6277–83.
98. Rixe O, Bukowski RM, Michaelson MD, Wilding G, Hudes GR, Bolte O, et al. Axitinib treatment in patients with cytokine-refractory metastatic renal-cell cancer: a phase II study. Lancet Oncol. 2007;8:975–84.
99. Rofstad EK, Halsor EF. Vascular endothelial growth factor, interleukin 8, platelet-derived endothelial cell growth factor, and basic fibroblast growth factor promote angiogenesis and metastasis in human melanoma xenografts. Cancer Res. 2000;60:4932.
100. Saito YD, Jensen AR, Salgia R, Posadas EM. Fyn: a novel molecular target in cancer. Cancer. 2010;116:1629–37.
101. Sakuma Y, Takeuchi T, Nakamura Y, Yoshihara M, Matsukuma S, Nakayama H, et al. Lung adenocarcinoma cells floating in lymphatic vessels resist anoikis by expressing phosphorylated Src. J Pathol. 2010;220:574–85.
102. Schatton T, Schutte U, Frank NY, Zhan Q, Hoerning A, Robles SC, et al. Modulation of T-cell activation by malignant melanoma initiating cells. Cancer Res. 2010;70:697–708.
103. Semenza GL. Targeting HIF-1 for cancer therapy. Nat Rev Cancer. 2003;3:721–32.

104. Sen B, Saigal B, Parikh N, Gallick G, Johnson FM. Sustained Src inhibition results in signal transducer and activator of transcription 3 (STAT3) activation and cancer cell survival via altered Janus-activated kinase-STAT3 binding. Cancer Res. 2009;69:1958–65.
105. Shojaei F, Ferrara N. Role of the microenvironment in tumor growth and in refractoriness/resistance to anti-angiogenic therapies. Drug Resist Update. 2008;11:219–30.
106. Singh RP, Agarwal R. Mechanisms and preclinical efficacy of silibinin in preventing skin cancer. Eur J Cancer. 2005;41:1969–79.
107. Sullivan NJ, Sasser AK, Axel AE, Vesuna F, Raman V, Ramirez N, et al. Interleukin-6 induces an epithelial-mesenchymal transition phenotype in human breast cancer cells. Oncogene. 2009;28:2940–7.
108. Sumimoto H, Imabayashi F, Iwata T, Kawakami Y. The BRAF-MAPK signaling pathway is essential for cancer-immune evasion in human melanoma cells. J Exp Med. 2006;203:1651–6.
109. Summy JM, Gallick GE. Src family kinases in tumor progression and metastasis. Cancer Metastasis Rev. 2003;22:337–58.
110. Turkson J, Bowman T, Garcia R, Caldenhoven E, De Groot RP, Jove R. Stat3 activation by Src induces specific gene regulation and is required for cell transformation. Mol Cell Biol. 1998;18:2545–52.
111. Turkson J, Zhang S, Mora LB, Burns A, Sebti S, Jove R. A novel platinum compound inhibits constitutive Stat3 signaling and induces cell cycle arrest and apoptosis of malignant cells. J Biol Chem. 2005;280:32979–88.
112. Turkson J, Zhang S, Palmer J, Kay H, Stanko J, Mora LB, et al. Inhibition of constitutive signal transducer and activator of transcription 3 activation by novel platinum complexes with potent antitumor activity. Mol Cancer Therap. 2004;3:1533–42.
113. Ugurel S, Hildenbrand R, Zimpfer A, La Rosee P, Paschka P, Sucker A, et al. Lack of clinical efficacy of imatinib in metastatic melanoma. Br J Cancer. 2005;92:1398–405.
114. Wang T, Niu G, Kortylewski M, Burdelya L, Shain K, Zhang S, et al. Regulation of the innate and adaptive immune responses by Stat-3 signaling in tumor cells. Nat Med. 2004;10:48–54.
115. Wang W, Edington H, Rao U, Jukic D, Land S, Wang H, et al. Impact of IFN [alpha] upon the balance of Stat1/Stat3 in vivo in the spectrum of melanocytic progression from nevus to melanoma. J Immunother. 2006;29:642.
116. Wang W, Edington HD, Jukic DM, Rao UN, Land SR, Kirkwood JM. Impact of IFNalpha2b upon pSTAT3 and the MEK/ERK MAPK pathway in melanoma. Cancer Immunol Immunother. 2008;57:1315–21.
117. Weeraratna AT, Jiang Y, Hostetter G, Rosenblatt K, Duray P, Bittner M, et al. Wnt5a signaling directly affects cell motility and invasion of metastatic melanoma. Cancer Cell. 2002;1:279–88.
118. Wei D, Le X, Zheng L, Wang L, Frey JA, Gao AC, et al. Stat3 activation regulates the expression of vascular endothelial growth factor and human pancreatic cancer angiogenesis and metastasis. Oncogene. 2003;22:319–29.
119. Wilhelm SM, Carter C, Tang LY, Wilkie D, McNabola A, Rong H, et al. BAY 43-9006 exhibits broad spectrum oral antitumor activity and targets the RAF/MEK/ERK pathway and receptor tyrosine kinases involved in tumor progression and angiogenesis. Cancer Res. 2004;64:7099.
120. Windham TC, Parikh NU, Siwak DR, Summy JM, McConkey DJ, Kraker AJ, et al. Src activation regulates anoikis in human colon tumor cell lines. Oncogene. 2002;21:7797–807.
121. Wu Y, Diab I, Zhang X, Izmailova ES, Zehner ZE. Stat3 enhances vimentin gene expression by binding to the antisilencer element and interacting with the repressor protein, ZBP-89. Oncogene. 2004;23:168–78.
122. Wyman K, Atkins MB, Prieto V, Eton O, McDermott DF, Hubbard F, et al. Multicenter phase II trial of high-dose imatinib mesylate in metastatic melanoma. Cancer. 2006;106:2005–11.
123. Xie T, Wei D, Liu M, Gao AC, Ali-Osman F, Sawaya R, et al. Stat3 activation regulates the expression of matrix metalloproteinase-2 and tumor invasion and metastasis. Oncogene. 2004;23:3550–60.

124. Xie TX, Huang FJ, Aldape KD, Kang SH, Liu M, Gershenwald JE, et al. Activation of stat3 in human melanoma promotes brain metastasis. Cancer Res. 2006;66:3188–96.
125. Xin H, Zhang C, Herrmann A, Du Y, Figlin R, Yu H. Sunitinib inhibition of Stat3 induces renal cell carcinoma tumor cell apoptosis and reduces immunosuppressive cells. Cancer Res. 2009;69:2506–13.
126. Xu Q, Briggs J, Park S, Niu G, Kortylewski M, Zhang S, et al. Targeting Stat3 blocks both HIF-1 and VEGF expression induced by multiple oncogenic growth signaling pathways. Oncogene. 2005;24:5552–60.
127. Yang AD, Camp ER, Fan F, Shen L, Gray MJ, Liu W, et al. Vascular endothelial growth factor receptor-1 activation mediates epithelial to mesenchymal transition in human pancreatic carcinoma cells. Cancer Res. 2006;66:46–51.
128. Yang F, Jove V, Xin H, Hedvat M, Van Meter TE, Yu H. Sunitinib induces apoptosis and growth arrest of medulloblastoma tumor cells by inhibiting STAT3 and AKT signaling pathways. Mol Cancer Res. 2010;8:35–45.
129. Yang F, Van Meter TE, Buettner R, Hedvat M, Liang W, Kowolik CM, et al. Sorafenib inhibits signal transducer and activator of transcription 3 signaling associated with growth arrest and apoptosis of medulloblastomas. Mol Cancer Therap. 2008;7:3519.
130. Yang Y, Pan X, Lei W, Wang J, Shi J, Li F, et al. Regulation of transforming growth factor-beta 1-induced apoptosis and epithelial-to-mesenchymal transition by protein kinase A and signal transducers and activators of transcription 3. Cancer Res. 2006;66:8617–24.
131. Yu CL, Meyer DJ, Campbell GS, Larner AC, Carter-Su C, Schwartz J, et al. Enhanced DNA-binding activity of a Stat3-related protein in cells transformed by the Src oncoprotein. Science. 1995;269:81–3.
132. Yu H, Jove R. The STATs of cancer – new molecular targets come of age. Nat Rev Cancer. 2004;4:97–105.
133. Yu H, Kortylewski M, Pardoll D. Crosstalk between cancer and immune cells: role of STAT3 in the tumour microenvironment. Nat Rev Immunol. 2007;7:41–51.
134. Yu H, Pardoll D, Jove R. STATs in cancer inflammation and immunity: a leading role for STAT3. Nat Rev Cancer. 2009;9:798–809.
135. Zhang X, Yue P, Fletcher S, Zhao W, Gunning PT, Turkson J. A novel small-molecule disrupts Stat3 SH2 domain-phosphotyrosine interactions and Stat3-dependent tumor processes. Biochem Pharmacol. 2010;79(10):1398–409.
136. Zhuang L, Lee CS, Scolyer RA, McCarthy SW, Zhang XD, Thompson JF, et al. Mcl-1, Bcl-XL and Stat3 expression are associated with progression of melanoma whereas Bcl-2, AP-2 and MITF levels decrease during progression of melanoma. Mod Pathol. 2007;20:416–26.
137. Zou W. Regulatory T cells, tumour immunity and immunotherapy. Nat Rev Immunol. 2006;6: 295–307.

Chapter 8
Targeting the mTOR, PI3K, and AKT Pathways in Melanoma

Kim A. Margolin

Abstract A comprehensive analysis of critical oncogenic signaling pathways in melanoma is leading to new therapeutic approaches for the treatment of this disease. The present chapter addresses the pathways that communicate signals from membrane receptors and selected other intracellular processes that lead to the activation of the mammalian target of rapamycin (mTOR) and its downstream substrates. mTOR exists in two distinct, but related, molecular complexes that control a multitude of cellular processes and intercellular interactions, the normal function of which is to regulate cell metabolism, growth and proliferation, apoptosis, and interactions with the microenvironment. In malignancy, abnormal activation of these pathways either directly or indirectly through other oncogenic signals gives rise to increased proliferation and cell growth, resistance to cell death, and other metabolic and intercellular alterations that are characteristic of the transformed phenotype. Current understanding of mTOR activity, its control by other molecules, and its role in various aspects of malignancy, including preclinical and current clinical data regarding its therapeutic targeting by pharmacologic agents, will be detailed in this chapter.

Keywords • mTor • AKT • PI_3K • Molecular pathway

mTor Overview: Normal Functions and Genetic Alterations of Importance in Melanoma

mTOR-C1: This serine-threonine kinase complex of proteins – mTOR, raptor, and LST8 – is aptly named for its prototypical pharmacologic inhibitor rapamycin, which binds the FKBP12 domain of mTOR [28] mTOR-C1, stimulated by RHEB

K.A. Margolin (✉)
Department of Medical Oncology, University of Washington
and Seattle Cancer Care Alliance, Seattle, WA 98109, USA
e-mail: kmargoli@seattlecca.org

T.F. Gajewski and F.S. Hodi (eds.), *Targeted Therapeutics in Melanoma*,
Current Clinical Oncology, DOI 10.1007/978-1-61779-407-0_8,
© Springer Science+Business Media, LLC 2012

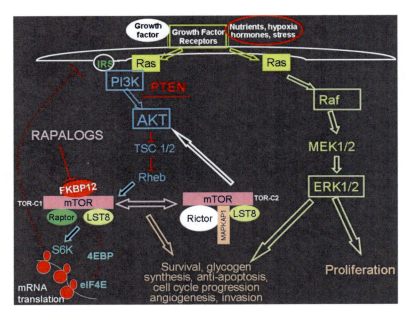

Fig. 8.1 Schematic of the major signaling pathways that interact with PI3K and mTOR. The term "rapalogs" refers to drugs which are functionally similar to rapamycin and inhibit mTOR

(Ras homologue enriched in brain) (which in turn is controlled by inhibition by the complex of the tumor suppressors tuberous sclerosis complex1 and 2, TSC1 and TSC2) possesses pleiotropic activities linking the cellular micro-environment with a series of molecular pathways that control coordinated aspects of protein translation. In the normal balance between the extracellular milieu and cellular and nuclear events, cell membrane receptors responding to a wide variety of mediators in the micro-environment transmit signals that can protect the cell from conditions of limited oxygen or nutrient supply (e.g., controlling apoptosis, limiting energy consumption, and limiting proliferation). Conversely, in the presence of nutrient-rich and oxygen-sufficient conditions, mTOR-C1 activity phosphorylates specific ribosomal and translation factors that control the translation of specific mRNAs encoding proteins involved in cell-cycle progression, cell proliferation, resistance to apoptosis, and glucose metabolism (see Fig. 8.1).

mTOR-C2: A second mTOR complex, mTOR-C2, has a complementary role in "completing" the activation of AKT by phosphorylating it at Ser473 [17, 33]. mTOR-C2 contains the identical multidomain mTOR molecule in association with RICTOR, LST8 and MAPKAP2 [50]. Important feedback loops that regulate the balance of cellular functions controlled by AKT and mTOR through complex interactions with TSC2 may explain the activation of AKT that results from pharmacologic inhibition of mTOR, particularly by agents that are selective for mTOR-C1. These alterations of the feedback loops result in resistance to mTOR inhibition in selected malignant cells and may also paradoxically increase survival of cancer cells by enhancing angiogenesis via the upregulation by PI3K/AKT signaling in response to vascular endothelial growth factor (VEGF) [17].

Mutations in the mTOR gene have not been identified in cancer, but genetic alterations of upstream elements including loss of function of phosphatase and tensin homolog deleted on chromosome 10 (PTEN) are common [35] and result in downstream AKT overexpression and increased activity of the target translation-controlling factors ribosomal S6K1 and 4EIF-BP/EIF4E. Other mutations, including alterations of PI3K subunits and AKT isoforms, have been reported in occasional cell lines or patient samples [7, 11], but may provide clues to the molecular pathogenesis of specific oncogenic changes and inform the design of therapeutic agents.

Upstream Effectors of mTOR Activation: PTEN, PI3K, and AKT

PTEN is a protein phosphatase that can dephosphorylate focal adhesion kinase (FAK) and Src homology collagen (SHC) as well as members of the MAPK pathway, resulting in its contribution to normal control of cell adhesion, spreading, and migration. PTEN also has lipid phosphatase activity that may predominate over its protein phosphatase activities, with negative control of PI3K and downstream AKT tightly regulating processes of cell growth, survival, and apoptosis [5, 29, 50].

Loss of PTEN function occurs early in melanomagenesis and appears to contribute to a self-perpetuating process of serial genetic alterations that promote more aggressive cell phenotypes. It has been hypothesized that chromosome 10 deletion, resulting in loss of PTEN expression, causes increased activation of AKT3 (see below), which provides a survival and growth advantage in concert with other elements of the microenvironment that provide anti-apoptotic signals [30]. The details of these other pathways in melanomagenesis and their potential as therapeutic targets are detailed elsewhere in this volume, but will be addressed here with respect to their interactions with the PI3K/AKT/mTOR pathways.

Phosphatidyl inositol 3 kinase (PI3K) is the term used for a group of cellular lipid kinases that phosphorylate substrate phosphatidyl inositides at the 3′ hydroxy position. The resulting phosphorylated second messenger lipid molecules recruit AKT to the cell membrane. The control of PI3Ks by signals from the microenvironment are mediated through activation by G-protein-coupled receptors and RAS and its effectors, the latter being activated either by mutation or by upstream signals that drive oncogenesis through activation of the AKT pathway as well as the MAP kinase pathway [48].

AKT is a serine-threonine kinase that plays a pivotal role in the balance between cell survival and apoptosis [39]. Apart from its activation of mTOR via phosphorylation and thus inactivation of the negative mTOR regulator TSC2 [35], activated AKT also phosphorylates the pro-apoptotic molecules BAD and pro-caspase-9 to inhibit apoptosis and activates the transcription factor NF-κB, resulting in increased expression of anti-apoptotic and pro-survival genes. Phosphorylation of mdm2 leads to inhibition of p53-mediated apoptosis and negative regulation of forkhead transcription factors, resulting in reduced production of other cell-death-promoting proteins [5]. AKT activation leads to the phosphorylation and monoubiquitination of the checkpoint kinase Chk1, causing genomic instability and double-stranded DNA breaks that contribute to carcinogenesis [30]. In addition to its role in promoting cell growth, survival, and anti-apoptosis, AKT also stimulates pro-angiogenic pathways in endothelial cells, mediating another important element of the tumor microenvironment that may provide a therapeutic target in melanoma and other malignancies.

mTOR Complexes and Downstream Events: Control of Transcription

The activation of mTOR-C1 complexes by AKT and PI3K occurs via the phosphorylation of TSC2, which leads to activation of RHEB and then mTOR-C1, the complex that phosphorylates ribosomal S6 kinase and the inhibitor of eukaryotic initiation factor 4E-BP1. The resulting release from inhibition of eukaryotic initiation factor eIF4E and the activity of ribosomal S6 protein leads to preferential translation of mRNA encoding proteins that support the transformed phenotype, including cell growth and proliferation, protection from apoptosis, and angiogenesis. Feedback inhibition of mTOR-C1 by TSC1-TSC2 complex and PRAS40 controls its activity in normal cell physiology [35].

mTOR-C2 is a complex of mTOR, rictor, mLST8, mSIN1, and protor-1 that is activated by growth factors and itself phosphorylates PKC-α and AKT in addition to regulating the cytoskeleton [44]. Tight forward and feedback control of these complex interactions is provided by phosphorylation of several proteins at different sites under different conditions. mTOR-C2 function probably contributes to control of the cytoskeleton and cell migration [35]. There is also convergence of this pathway with the MAPK pathway, in which downstream ERK activates mTOR-C1 and inhibits BAD, further promoting the downstream consequences of mTOR pathway activation in cancer cells [14].

The expression of phosphorylated 4E-BP1 is widespread in melanoma and was associated with unfavorable survival outcomes in multivariate analysis of 47 patients with advanced melanoma [41]. A recent study of mTOR signaling in 30 uveal and 8 conjunctival melanoma specimens showed that conjunctival melanomas, similar to cutaneous primaries, usually had low levels of PTEN and correspondingly elevated levels of phosphorylated downstream molecules of the mTOR pathway. Uveal primaries, in contrast, did not demonstrate mTOR pathway activation or BRAF or NRAS mutations but increased expression of MAPK signaling likely due to the frequent expression of one of 2 recently-reported RAS-like mutations (GNAQ and GNA11) that also activate the MAPK pathway [51].

The strategies to date for targeting one or more of the PI3K family members upstream of mTOR have taken advantage of investigation into structure-function design principles [53]. Current drug development efforts directed toward agents that inhibit both PI3K and mTOR, based on structural similarities at the active site of their catalytic subunits, are of interest because of the loss of activation of AKT by mTOR-C2 during inhibition of mTOR-C1. AKT inhibition has not yet been explored to the same extent as inhibition of PI3K and mTOR but may have promise in selected tumors. While the need to inhibit broadly either by multi-target inhibition or using complementary or synergistic drug combinations is evident, success must be balanced against the loss of tumor specificity associated with broadening of the therapeutic targets that can cause toxicities to normal organs and compromise of the favorable therapeutic index often characteristic of narrow-spectrum targeted inhibitors. In addition, drugs that target these enzymes may have unusual toxicities that are based on their molecular mechanisms and target specificities. For example, the control of insulin signaling by PI3K subunits explains the resistance to insulin resulting from inhibition of PI3K, an important potential toxicity of drugs that interfere in these pathways [5]. This phenomenon has been shown in a rodent model to be due to the inhibition of the peripheral action of insulin causing diminished glucose uptake, increased gluconeogenesis, and hepatic glycogenolysis [6].

Mutations and Gene Alterations that Lead to Activation of Signaling Via mTOR

mTOR is activated in the majority of melanomas, as evidenced by the mTOR-dependent phosphorylation of S6K, and may represent activation by either the upstream PI3K/AKT system or via activation through elements of the MAPK pathway. For example, in a recent study of 107 human melanomas and six established melanoma cell lines, approximately 80% of tumors showed strongly positive immunohistochemical staining for phospho-S6K, while cells isolated from benign nevi were either negative or only weakly positive. Rapamycin-inhibited phosphorylation of S6K in all cell lines as well as the proliferation of three cell lines tested in this study. Further, an inhibitor of farnesyl transferase, which blocks the activation of mTOR by RHEB, also inhibited the growth of melanoma cell lines with activated mTOR [21].

mTOR is directly activated by RHEB in a farnesylation-dependent manner. NRAS mutations, occurring in 15% of melanomas [13], can activate both pathways, while loss or attenuation of PTEN activity via chromosome 10 loss (particularly prevalent in melanoma), promoter methylation, or post-translational modification can all remove the negative control exerted by normal PTEN on its downstream pathway starting with PI3K and AKT [30]. Mutations of AKT have recently been identified in melanoma as well as several other solid tumor types and may account for tumorigenic activation of this pathway in the absence of other genetic mutations [10]. Activation of the PI3K/AKT/mTOR pathway more indirectly by other oncogenic signal transduction through cell growth factor receptors (e.g., NRAS signaling and c-kit) [47] provides further evidence for the potential value of developing cancer therapies that interrupt one or more elements of the PI3K/AKT/mTOR pathway. The complexities and heterogeneities of these pathways and their molecular alterations in different malignancies raise the challenge that therapeutic strategies that have been highly effective in selected tumors may be of little value in others.

Loss of PTEN function is commonly seen in combination with BRAF mutation in cutaneous melanoma cells and is also characteristic of benign nevi [24]. The latter alone is not sufficient to fully transform melanocytes to express the malignant phenotype, and in fact, the unchecked high activity of V600E BRAF alone promotes the development of nevi, but the level of activity of the MAPK pathway may need to be lowered to support full progression to the malignant melanoma phenotype. Cooperation between AKT3 and mutant BRAF has been shown to promote this final transformation to malignancy, and inhibition of either enzyme in cell lines from melanomas driven by these two pathways can reduce the malignant characteristics of anchorage-independent growth and tumor development, with even greater inhibition when both pathways are inhibited [3]. Cells with mutated NRAS, by contrast, do not feature BRAF mutations because mutated NRAS alone is sufficient to fully transform melanocytes by activating both the MAPK and the PI3K/AKT pathways. Studies in a large series of human melanoma cell lines demonstrated that cells with mutated BRAF, which usually have loss of PTEN function, demonstrate greater activation of AKT than cells with NRAS mutations that activate both pathways further upstream [11].

Activated AKT expression has been evaluated in a clinicopathologic study of 292 cases including normal and dysplastic nevi, and primary and metastatic melanomas and shown to be present in increasing percentage across this spectrum. A multivariate analysis applied to the 170 cases of primary melanoma suggested that strong phospho-AKT expression correlated inversely with overall and disease-specific survival [8]. A fraction of melanomas arising in mucosal and acral sites have been shown to carry a mutation of the KIT oncogene that encodes a receptor responsive to stem cell factor in normal physiology (hematopoiesis and other organogenesis). While a number of currently available kinase inhibitors target the KIT receptor in addition to other related signal transduction pathways (e.g., imatinib, dasatinib and others), their use in melanoma has been promising only in the fraction of patients bearing KIT mutations. Nevertheless, KIT signaling can also activate PI3K, promoting mTOR pathway signaling, so the development of combinations based on this molecular interplay may also have therapeutic potential [19]. Additional genetic alterations such as p53 and/or Rb via loss of the suppressor p16ink4a may be necessary for melanomagenesis in different subgroups of melanoma [1].

Successful targeting of mTOR in preclinical models and in the clinic for selected other malignancies suggested that this pathway is an important therapeutic target, particularly when PTEN loss of function is the source of pathway activation, but also when the pathway is activated by mutations of PI3K or AKT [35]. However, single-agent inhibition of mTOR using FKBP12-binding drugs like the rapalogs have had variable activity against tumors that are driven in part by mTOR activation. Normal feedback inhibition by mTOR of the expression of insulin receptor substrate (IRS-1) is lost when blocked by inhibitors of mTOR-C1 activity, leading to upregulation of AKT and hyperactivation of the pathway, thus overcoming the block and abrogating the antitumor effects of mTOR blockade. When mTOR inhibition is combined with inhibitors of the IGF-1 receptor, however, malignant cell proliferation can be more effectively blocked [40]. This approach, along with others more clinically developed, as detailed later in this chapter, may have promise for the treatment of malignancies in which the activation of PI3K/AKT/mTOR is an important but not the sole pathway driving the tumor [2, 49].

Therapeutic Targeting of PI3K, AKT and mTOR in Melanoma: Single Agent Therapy and Potential for Effective Combinations

While inhibitors of several enzymes have been developed and are currently in various phases of clinical investigation, only the inhibitors of mTOR-C1 have completed clinical testing all the way through Phase III trials and become commercially available. The rapalogs temsirolimus and everolimus had sufficient single-agent activity in renal cancer to meet the Food and Drug Administration's criteria for approval, and temsirolimus has also been approved for mantle cell lymphoma [16]. Other promising data support further study of these agents in low-grade neuroendocrine cancers and possibly endometrial cancer [9]. Unfortunately, even in those tumors that have shown responsiveness to mTOR inhibition, the clinical impact has been modest, evidenced by cytostatic effects and prolonged disease stabilization without substantial objective responses except in mantle cell lymphoma and with the question of substantial survival benefit remaining to be demonstrated. Combination of mTOR pathway inhibitors with cytotoxic agents may hold greater promise; in a recent preclinical investigation, blockade of signaling down the PI3K/AKT/mTOR pathway using one of three different inhibitors added to either cisplatin or temozolomide markedly enhanced growth inhibition and induced apoptosis of several melanoma cell lines compared with most of the single agents [49], and the data for such combinations in other malignancies are summarized elsewhere [9].

For the treatment of advanced melanoma, temsirolimus was tested in a Phase II trial of 33 patients with a good performance status and normal organ function. In this study, completed by the California Cancer Consortium, 11 patients had received one prior cytotoxic regimen for advanced disease, and 14 had received one or more prior biological response modifier regimen for adjuvant and or advanced disease. Only one patient experienced a transient partial response in soft tissue metastatic disease, and the pre-specified primary objective of progression-free survival for a median of at least 4 months was not achieved [31]. In view of this negative study, enthusiasm for clinical testing of the promising preclinical data for combinations with chemotherapy (especially cisplatin, a nonmyelosuppressive drug with the favorable preclinical data detailed above and modest activity in melanoma) has been low. Considering the complex molecular controls of tumor cell sensitivity and resistance to PI3K/AKT/mTOR pathway blockade, the design of optimal combinations of inhibitors plus cytotoxic agents will await more convincing proof of principle for target validation and achievement of the desired therapeutic endpoints (e.g., Phase 0 studies).

While the challenges to combining cytotoxic agents with inhibitors of the mTOR and related pathways remain to be overcome, the nature of preclinical and clinical investigation of targeted agents provided information about pathway interactions to justify the testing of carefully selected combinations. Most of these studies represent additive blockade of sequential steps in a linear molecular pathway (vertical blockade) or inhibition of a step in two parallel pathways (horizontal blockade) that is designed in similar fashion to the traditional principles of combination chemotherapy for hematologic malignancies and solid tumors. The same principles also apply to the choice of agents to minimize toxicities, which requires that the agents have minimal overlap of toxicities that will allow them to be combined at doses close to their individual maximum tolerated doses. Alternative strategies include the design of combinations directed at overcoming resistance (such strategies may be identical in the case of the targeted agents, while in the case of chemotherapy they have been disappointing, due to the poor therapeutic index encountered when agents that prevent or reverse resistance are combined with cytotoxic agents). Another question raised by the availability of growing numbers of targeted agents for clinical investigation is whether drugs with broad target specificity are superior or inferior to those with a more narrow target specificity given as single agents or in combination. It is rare to discover a tumor that is uniquely driven by a single molecular alteration common to nearly all patients with the disease (e.g., chronic myelogenous leukemia and the product of the bcr-abl translocation or gastrointestinal stromal tumor driven by mutated c-kit, both of which achieve substantial and prolonged remissions with single agent imatinib). Thus, it seems that the ideal targeted therapy for most malignancies will consist of combinations of two or more drugs that allow each agent and its target to be independently manipulated to achieve the optimal therapeutic index.

In order to design optimal combinations or better single agents to effectively target the PI3K/AKT/mTOR pathway, it will be necessary to address the challenge posed by the interactions with other pathways that vary with the biology of the malignancy and, for melanoma, are directly related to the molecular oncogenesis of the multiple melanoma subtypes. While the presence of both BRAF V600E and PTEN mutations that markedly upregulate the MAPK and mTOR pathways, respectively, characterizes the most common subtype of melanoma, several other variations exist with unique molecular characteristics that may feature varying degrees of direct or indirect mTOR activation and thus potential sensitivity to its inhibition. For example, a fraction of tumors arising in mucosal surfaces or acral sites have constitutive activation of the KIT receptor for stem cell factor due to mutation or amplification of its gene and may be sensitive to inhibition with imatinib and other drugs that block the active site of this molecule (detailed in Chap. 4). Another variant, uveal melanoma arising in one of the several pigmented tissues of the eyes, has recently been demonstrated to be dependent on mutations in one of two related G-proteins related to RAS that may activate MAPK but are not sensitive to the drugs that were developed to target the V600E-activating mutation of BRAF [51].

Preclinical data were used in support of developing early combinations of targeted inhibitors that included mTOR blockade with rapalogs. Sorafenib plus rapamycin showed at least additive antitumor effects, accompanied by downregulation of the anti-apoptotic proteins Bcl-2 and Mcl-1 when tested against six melanoma cell lines [26], and in a separate report, the same drugs showed greater activity against melanoma cell lines carrying the BRAF V600E mutation than against wild type cells, while demonstrating inhibition of downstream targets (ERK for sorafenib, S6K1 and 4EBP1 for rapamycin) [36]. Additional drugs with similar mechanisms were studied in the more physiologic setting of cell line monolayers and regenerating human skin spiked with melanoma cells. These studies showed potent antitumor effects despite low and variable activity for any of the single agents [34] and further justified the design of clinical studies, (including the consideration of combinations of drugs with demonstrated low single-agent activity). In addition to the targeting of mTOR plus MAPK pathways, which is a logical approach in melanomas based on their common presence in the most common subtype of cutaneous melanoma, other targets were explored based on the extensive network of interactions involving mTOR and its up- and downstream elements. For example, melanoma cells that produce VEGF have recently been shown to be partially inhibited by blockade of VEGFR2, presumably due to a co-dependence on vascular proliferation in the microenvironment. However, an alternative explanation was provided by the results of recent studies that showed bevacizumab in combination with rapamycin had a more potent cytotoxic effect against melanoma cells expressing VEGF than against cells that did not express VEGF, supporting the presence of an autocrine proliferation loop in melanoma cells that can be targeted effectively by this combination [37].

Multi-kinase inhibitors that target more than one enzyme along the PI3K/AKT/mTOR pathway – for example, the dual PI3K and mTOR inhibitors – have recently shown great promise in preclinical investigations and are now ready for testing in the clinic. The preclinical observations with these drugs against melanoma cell lines included direct inhibition of cell growth and cell cycle-promoting molecules without the induction of significant apoptosis. Controls included a pan-class I PI3K inhibitor and rapamycin, each of which resulted in minor reduction of cell proliferation. In a mouse melanoma tumor model, these inhibitors of both PI3K and mTOR efficiently attenuated tumor growth at primary and lymph node metastatic sites with no obvious toxicity. The observation that neovascularization was also blocked, with resulting tumor necrosis, provided support for a dual cellular target effect of these drugs in vivo as both direct antitumor and indirect anti-angiogenesis agents [33].

Clinical Results of Combinations Based on Inhibition of PI3K/AKT/mTOR Pathway

The clinical testing of combinations containing an mTOR pathway inhibitor (temsirolimus) plus sorafenib, which at the time was believed to be a potent inhibitor of BRAF and the MAPK pathway, required careful attention to combined toxicities that were assessed in Phase I trials using a range of doses for each agent, given on their standard schedules. It was initially expected that the relative lack of myelosuppression and their predominantly non-overlapping toxicities would permit the use of combination doses at or near the Phase II recommended doses for each single agent. However, enhanced toxicities of combination therapy that did not appear to be due to pharmacokinetic interactions were reported in these Phase I trials, including mucocutaneous (skin rash, hand-foot syndrome, diarrhea), constitutional (fatigue), and metabolic (hyperlipidemia, hyperglycemia) toxicities. The initiation of a Phase II randomized design of two molecularly targeted combinations for advanced melanoma, solicited by the National Cancer Institute's Cancer Therapy Evaluation Program and designed by the Southwest Oncology Group, had to await the completion of a Phase I trial of each combination – and these enhanced toxicities not only delayed the opening of the trial but demonstrated the need to reduce the doses used in combination to well below those used for single agent therapy. The first Phase I trial was a broad-histology study that included only five melanoma patients with no objective responses or prolonged stabilization of disease [43]. The second trial included only melanoma patients, and 10 of 23 experienced prolonged stable diseases between 2 and 8 months in duration [22].

Patients in this Phase II trial were unselected for molecular type prior to protocol enrollment but had tissue available for later analysis. Treatment consisted of sorafenib 200 mg twice daily, the recommended Phase II dose from Phase I that is only 50% the single agent recommended dose, and temsirolimus 25 mg per week, the standard dose for the approved indications but tenfold lower than the dose previously tested as a single agent in melanoma [31]. Sixty-four patients with cutaneous melanoma who had not received any prior therapy for advanced disease were treated with this combination. Because it was expected to produce cytostatic effects rather than major tumor regressions, assessment of the activity of the combination was based on progression-free survival rather than partial and complete responses measured by traditional RECIST criteria used by the cooperative groups for cytotoxic agents. [32]. The results of this 2-arm study were disappointing but not surprising. Despite the exclusion of patients with the traditionally most unfavorable characteristics – metastases from ocular and mucosal primary sites, patients exposed to any prior systemic therapy and those with a history of brain metastases – there were very few objective responses (three partial responses among 63 patients), and the median progression-free (4 months) and overall (median 7 months) survivals were comparable to those of a large series of prior SWOG studies considered "negative" for benefit [23].

Because this study was performed in parallel with several other molecularly targeted combinations provided by CTEP for other malignancies, the possibility of further investigating target pathways in the tumors that were collected at a central tissue bank as a part of this study will be addressed across multiple tumor types that will provide additional insight into differences and similarities across the spectrum of malignancies. Further, during the time required for completion of the Phase I studies and the subsequent completion of the Phase II SWOG trial, additional data regarding the drugs used in this combination provided additional insight into the limited potential for these particular agents to provide effective antitumor activity in melanoma. In particular, it became clear that sorafenib is not a very good inhibitor of wild-type or mutated BRAF, but has a multiplicity of targets including cellular receptors for fibroblast growth factor, VEGF, and platelet-derived growth factor [20]. The implications of these targets may be widely differing with the molecular pathogenesis of different malignancies, and thus the potential for additive or synergistic combinations with other drugs is difficult to predict. Indeed, melanomas not driven by mutated BRAF are not only resistant to BRAF inhibitors but may experience growth promotion by these drugs [25]. Other limitations included the observation that temsirolimus is in most cells and experimental conditions a more potent inhibitor of mTOR-C1 than of mTOR-C2, so its use in tumors that are driven by this pathway may lead to the mTOR-C2-mediated upregulation of AKT with resistance or escape from control by the inhibition of mTOR.

Unique Toxicity Spectrum of mTOR Inhibitors: Experience with the Rapalogs Temsirolimus and Everolimus

It has become abundantly clear that small molecule and even macromolecule inhibitors of cellular signaling, such as growth factor and growth factor receptor antibodies, are associated with a spectrum of toxicities distinct from those of traditional cytotoxic agents. In fact, some of the features of this group of drugs more closely resemble those occurring with chemotherapies that target metabolic pathways (e.g., pyrimidine or purine analogs like capecitabine and methotrexate) than those that directly target nucleic acid structure/function or the cell-division apparatus (such as alkylating agents, topoisomerase inhibitors, demethylating agents, vinca alkaloids or taxanes). Common to the kinase inhibitors are various mucocutaneous toxicities that include skin rash, irritation that often involves the palms and soles, stomatitis, and diarrhea. Hypothyroidism and myocardial suppression as well as fatigue are further evidence of the subtle but potentially dose- or "duration-limiting" toxicities of these drugs. In the case of the rapalogs temsirolimus and everolimus, the relatively unique spectrum of toxicities may be attributable to the pleiotropic cellular and extracellular functions of the molecules in these pathways. The impact of mTOR-C1 inhibition on glycemic control was detailed earlier in this chapter and is a common clinical finding that may not be optimally managed according to standard diabetic therapy due in part to the distinct mechanisms of hyperglycemia caused by intervention in this pathway [6]. In an animal model, a combination of fasting and low carbohydrate diet was a more effective approach and may be considered in conjunction with other standard medical management in clinical practice. Dyslipidemias are also common with rapalogs, and management to date has been based on standard therapies used for common lipid disorders, like management of common dyslipidemias resulting from the use of rapamycin-based regimens for immunosuppression of recipients of solid organ or hematopoietic cell transplants. Mild to moderate cytopenias are less common but sometimes require dose or schedule adjustments. The precise mechanisms are unknown but again most likely represent additional off-target effects such as inhibition of molecular pathways required for normal hematopoiesis.

Clinical guidance regarding the long list of drug interactions that may further complicate the management of cancer patients receiving mTOR inhibitors has emerged from their use in the post-transplant setting where many patients are on other drugs that interact with the metabolism and clearance of the rapalogs. Even more unique to this class of agents and presumably resulting more directly from some of the specific molecular targets are the rare but life-threatening inflammatory syndromes, particularly interstitial pneumonitis, that have been reported in variable numbers and percentages of patients and may be multifactorial, based on duration, dose, and underlying risk factors. The possibility has been raised that altered immune networks during rapalog therapy also contribute to an autoimmune component of this syndrome. Since interstitial pneumonitis, which has variable clinical and radiographic features, may be asymptomatic, some of the studies suggesting higher incidence were based on CT findings alone. The point at which intervention is required (reduction or discontinuation of therapy, or if symptomatic, treatment with glucocorticosteroids) remains to be further studied [12]. Acute infusion reactions (urticaria, fever, bronchospasm, hypotension) also occur occasionally with Temsirolimus, possibly resulting from a disturbance of the interactions among inflammatory cells and the cytokines that control their function, and it is recommended that patients receiving Temsirolimus be premedicated with an H1 anti-histamine [46].

Pharmacodynamics and Biomarkers of Activity and Resistance

Most of the work on developing molecular markers of effective mTOR pathway inhibition or the study of intrinsic and acquired resistance has focused on the most downstream elements, such as ribosomal S6K1 and 4EBP1/EIF-4E. Target inhibition in tumors and in selected accessible normal tissue has been correlated in limited studies with exposure using different doses and schedules, while the clinical correlation of target inhibition with outcomes has been more elusive due to the enormous complexity of pathways and molecular heterogeneity both within and across tumor types. More practical approaches include the application of functional imaging in assessing treatment with mTOR inhibitors. To date, the only data addressing this modality were reported from a study of 34 rapamycin-treated patients who had tumor assessable by ^{18}F-FDG-PET. The positive and negative predictive values of the PET scan were both very low, leading the authors to conclude that this modality does not provide valuable functional imaging for the early assessment of response or progression in cancer patients receiving mTOR inhibitors. However, close correlation of PET positivity with tumors expressing activated AKT raised the possibility that this form of functional imaging could be used to look for tumors with persistent AKT activation during mTOR inhibitor therapy, which could have implications for treatment decisions and design of combination therapies [29]. At least as important as reliable pharmacodynamic parameters to assess ongoing therapy will be the identification of predictive markers of benefit that can be used to pre-select patients likely to benefit from single agent or combination therapies and to avoid the toxicities and delay associated with ineffective therapy in the case of those with predicted treatment resistance.

Long-Term Therapy Considerations and Potential Immunosuppression

The mTOR inhibitor rapamycin is currently used as part of the immunosuppressive regimen for recipients of solid organ transplants and for the treatment and prevention of graft-versus-host disease in recipients of hematopoietic cell transplants. The quest to develop rapamycin analogs with antitumor activity but without immunosuppressive effects led to temsirolimus and then the oral agent everolimus, both rapalogs that preferentially block mTOR-C1 more than mTOR-C2 and are less immunosuppressive when used intermittently (as for cancer therapy) than continuously. Lack of important immunosuppression by either of these agents was initially confirmed in animal studies and has generally been corroborated by the data from clinical trials. Nevertheless, recent data suggest that although opportunistic infections are uncommon in patients receiving these drugs for the treatment of malignancy, an increased incidence of bacterial infection has been reported, even in the absence of neutropenia. [16, 18, 36]. It is likely that with more effective agents and/or combinations, additional insight into the mechanisms and incidence of infection risk will be elucidated and potentially avoided. Nevertheless, it will be important to continue surveillance for risks of immunosuppression as more potent PI3K/AKT/mTOR pathway inhibitors are tested in the clinic, since better drugs are likely to be used over more prolonged intervals and thus reveal previously unknown cumulative toxicities.

These same principles will also require consideration for combination therapies that include blockade of the PI3K/AKT/mTOR pathway and an immunotherapeutic element such as cytokine, vaccine, antibodies or lymphocyte-based therapy such as adoptive T cell clones or expanded tumor-infiltrating lymphocytes. It is clear that combining modalities will require careful attention to scheduling, dosing, and sequencing details that may dramatically affect the immunologic and clinical outcomes. For example, a recent study in a murine melanoma model demonstrated that combined therapy with sorafenib and the dual PI3K/mTOR inhibitor PI-103 showed in vitro synergy against melanoma cell lines while producing immunosuppression, tumor resistance to apoptosis, and enhanced in vivo survival of experimental melanoma in immunocompetent mice [27]. However, a number of recent reports suggest that in some settings, blockade of the PI3K/AKT/mTOR pathway can have favorable immunotherapeutic results. For example, mTOR inhibition with rapamycin was shown to enhance Th1 polarization of helper T lymphocytes by its interactions with glycogen synthase kinase (GSK3) in the regulation of interleukin-12 expression in dendritic cells [42]. A favorable impact of mTOR inhibition on immunotherapy strategies is also supported by recent data showing that activated AKT signaling in melanoma cells confers "immunoresistance," presumably due to its impact on anti-apoptotic molecules, and this resistance is reversed with rapamycin, rendering the cells sensitive to killing by antigen-specific cytotoxic T cells [15]. Finally, mTOR activity can also determine directly the fate of CD8 cytotoxic T cells by regulating the expression of specific transcription factors (enhancing T-bet for effector cells and suppressing eomesodermin for memory cells). Reversal of this effect with rapamycin, leading to increased numbers of antigen-specific memory CD8 cells, showed promise in a murine model of ovarian cancer that may have immediate applicability to melanoma [45]. A large and growing number of other observations on the effects of inhibiting this pathway on a wide variety of immunologic endpoints is provided in a recent review [50].

Conclusions

The spectrum of opportunities for therapeutic intervention against one or more elements of the mTOR-related pathways is enormous and potentially growing as the complex regulation and interactions among molecular species in the pathogenesis of malignancy are elucidated. Co-dependence of angiogenesis, the immune environment, and tumor biology as well as pharmacogenetic characteristics of the patient all contribute complexity to this quest for the ideal cancer therapy or component of a combination or combined-modality approach. Moving away from the constraints imposed by the currently-available rapalogs has led to the discovery of small molecule inhibitors of the active site of mTOR that, unlike the rapalogs, are not sterically limited to the macromolecular structure of the mTOR complex and can therefore inhibit mTOR activity in both complexes 1 and 2 [4]. While these agents, and others to follow, may prove more active alone or in combinations (see the Table 8.1 for current combinations under investigation), it will once again be necessary to perform carefully-designed clinical trials directed at safety and efficacy, including attention to the metabolic, immunologic and angiogenic aspects of their actions. Meanwhile, proof of the principle that inhibition of the mTOR pathway is a viable option worthy of further development is clearly provided in the case of renal cancer and mantle cell lymphoma, where the single agents are approved for clinical use, and for low-grade neuroendocrine, endometrial and sarcomas where promising activity has also been demonstrated [9].

Table 8.1 Current clinical trials of mTOR-targeted agents in combination with other cancer therapeutics

Agent in combination	Rapalog	
	Everolimus	Sirolimus
Cytotoxic chemotherapy		
Nanoparticle-bound Paclitaxel		Solid tumors, Phase I
Paclitaxel combinations	Breast cancer adjuvant therapy, Phase III	
Capecitabine	Metastatic breast CA, Phase I	
Gemcitabine	Advanced pancreas CA	
Gemcitabine + Cisplatin		Advanced transitional cell CA of urothelium[a]
Pemetrexed		Non-small cell lung CA
Topotecan	Advanced endometrial CA	
Irinotecan + Cetuximab	Colorectal CA, Phase I/ randomized Phase II	
Non-cytotoxic agents		
Vorinostat		Advanced solid tumors
Panobinostat	Hematologic malignancies	
Rituximab	Relapsed lymphoma	
Radiation therapy		Rectal cancer
Tivozanib		Advanced renal cancer[a]
Sorafenib	Relapsed lymphoma, myeloma	

[a]Combination with temsirolimus
Source: http://clinicaltrials.gov (5/6/2010)

References

1. Bennett DC. Human melanocyte senescence and melanoma susceptibility genes. Oncogene. 2003;22:3063–9.
2. Carracedo A, Ma L, Teruya-Feldstein J, Rojo F, Salmena L, Alimonti A, et al. Inhibition of mTORC1 leads to MAPK pathway activation through a PI3K-dependent feedback loop in human cancer. J Clin Invest. 2008;118:3065–74.
3. Cheung M, Sharma A, Madhunapantula SV, Robertson GP. Akt3 and mutant V600E B-Raf cooperate to promote early melanoma development. Cancer Res. 2008;68:3429–39.
4. Chresta CM, Davies BR, Hickson I, Harding T, Cosulich S, Critchlow SE, et al. AZD8055 is a potent, selective, and orally bioavailable ATP-competitive mammalian target of rapamycin kinase inhibitor with in vitro and in vivo antitumor activity. Cancer Res. 2010;70:288–98.
5. Courtney KD, Corcoran RB, Engelman JA. The PI3K pathway as drug target in human cancer. J Clin Oncol. 2010;28:1075–83.
6. Crouthamel MC, Kahana JA, Korenchuk S, Zhang SY, Sundaresan G, Eberwein DJ, et al. Mechanism and management of AKT inhibitor-induced hyperglycemia. Clin Cancer Res. 2009;15:217–25.
7. Curtin JA, Stark MS, Pinkel D, Hayward NK, Bastian BC. PI3-kinase subunits are infrequent somatic targets in melanoma. J Invest Dermatol. 2006;126:1660–3.
8. Dai DL, Martinka M, Li G. Prognostic significance of activated Akt expression in melanoma: a clinicopathologic study of 292 cases. J Clin Oncol. 2005;23:1473–82.
9. Dancey J. mTOR signaling and drug development in cancer. Nat Rev Clin Oncol. 2010;7: 209–19.

10. Davies MA, Stemke-Hale K, Tellez C, Calderone TL, Deng W, Prieto VG, et al. A novel AKT3 mutation in melanoma tumours and cell lines. Br J Cancer. 2008;99:1265–8.
11. Davies MA, Stemke-Hale K, Lin E, Tellez C, Deng W, Gopal YN, et al. Integrated molecular and clinical analysis of AKT activation in metastatic melanoma. Clin Cancer Res. 2009;15:7538–46.
12. Duran I, Siu LL, Oza AM, Chung TB, Sturgeon J, Townsley CA, et al. Characterisation of the lung toxicity of the cell cycle inhibitor temsirolimus. Eur J Cancer. 2006;42:1875–80.
13. Goel VK, Lazar AJ, Warneke CL, Redston MS, Haluska FG. Examination of mutations in BRAF, NRAS, and PTEN in primary cutaneous melanoma. J Invest Dermatol. 2006;126: 154–60.
14. Gossage L, Eisen T. Targeting multiple kinase pathways: a change in paradigm. Clin Cancer Res. 2010;16:1973–8.
15. Hahnel PS, Thaler S, Antunes E, Huber C, Theobald M, Schuler M. Targeting AKT signaling sensitizes cancer to cellular immunotherapy. Cancer Res. 2008;68:3899–906.
16. Hess G, Herbrecht R, Romaguera J, Verhoef G, Crump M, Gisselbrecht C, et al. Phase III study to evaluate temsirolimus compared with investigator's choice therapy for the treatment of relapsed or refractory mantle cell lymphoma. J Clin Oncol. 2009;27:3822–9.
17. Houghton PJ. Everolimus. Clin Cancer Res. 2010;16:1368–72.
18. Hudes G, Carducci M, Tomczak P, Dutcher J, Figlin R, Kapoor A, et al. Temsirolimus, interferon alfa, or both for advanced renal-cell carcinoma. N Engl J Med. 2007;356:2271–81.
19. Jiang X, Zhou J, Yuen NK, Corless CL, Heinrich MC, Fletcher JA, et al. Imatinib targeting of KIT-mutant oncoprotein in melanoma. Clin Cancer Res. 2008;14:7726–32.
20. Jilaveanu L, Zito C, Lee SJ, Nathanson KL, Camp RL, Rimm DL, et al. Expression of sorafenib targets in melanoma patients treated with carboplatin, paclitaxel and sorafenib. Clin Cancer Res. 2009;15:1076–85.
21. Karbowniczek M, Spittle CS, Morrison T, Wu H, Henske EP. mTOR is activated in the majority of malignant melanomas. J Invest Dermatol. 2008;128:980–7.
22. Kim K, Davies MA, Papadopoulos NE, et al. Phase I/II study of the combination of sorafenib and temsirolimus in patients with metastatic melanoma [Abstract 9026]. Proc Am Soc Clin Oncol. 2009;27.
23. Korn EL, Liu PY, Lee SJ, Chapman JA, Niedzwiecki D, Suman VJ, et al. Meta-analysis of phase II cooperative group trials in metastatic stage IV melanoma to determine progression-free and overall survival benchmarks for future phase II trials. J Clin Oncol. 2008;26:527–34.
24. Kumar R, Angelini S, Snellman E, Hemminki K. BRAF mutations are common somatic events in melanocytic nevi. J Invest Dermatol. 2004;122:342–8.
25. Kwong LN, Chin L. The brothers RAF. Cell. 2010;140:180–2.
26. Lasithiotakis KG, Sinnberg TW, Schittek B, Flaherty KT, Kulms D, Maczey E, et al. Combined inhibition of MAPK and mTOR signaling inhibits growth, induces cell death, and abrogates invasive growth of melanoma cells. J Invest Dermatol. 2008;128:2013–23.
27. Lopez-Fauqued M, Gil R, Grueso J, Hernandez-Losa J, Pujol A, Moline T, et al. The dual PI3K/mTOR inhibitor PI-103 promotes immunosuppression, in vivo tumor growth and increases survival of sorafenib-treated melanoma cells. Int J Cancer. 2010;126:1549–61.
28. Ma XM, Blenis J. Molecular mechanisms of mTOR-mediated translational control. Nat Rev Mol Cell Biol. 2009;10:307–18.
29. Ma WW, Jacene H, Song D, Vilardell F, Messersmith WA, Laheru D, et al. [18F]fluorodeoxy-glucose positron emission tomography correlates with Akt pathway activity but is not predictive of clinical outcome during mTOR inhibitor therapy. J Clin Oncol. 2009;27:2697–704.
30. Madhunapantula SV, Robertson GP. The PTEN-AKT3 signaling cascade as a therapeutic target in melanoma. Pigment Cell Melanoma Res. 2009;22:400–19.
31. Margolin K, Longmate J, Baratta T, Synold T, Christensen S, Weber J, et al. CCI-779 in metastatic melanoma: a phase II trial of the California Cancer Consortium. Cancer. 2005;104:1045–8.
32. Margolin KA, Moon J, Flaherty LE, Lao CD, Akerley WL, Sosman JA, Kirkwood JM, Sondak VK. Randomized phase II trial of sorafenib (SO) with temsirolimus (TEM) or tipifarnib (TIPI) in metastatic melanoma: Southwest Oncology Group Trial S0438 [Abstract 8502] ASCO. 2010.

33. Marone R, Erhart D, Mertz AC, Bohnacker T, Schnell C, Cmiljanovic V, et al. Targeting melanoma with dual phosphoinositide 3-kinase/mammalian target of rapamycin inhibitors. Mol Cancer Res. 2009;7:601–13.
34. Meier F, Busch S, Lasithiotakis K, Kulms D, Garbe C, Maczey E, et al. Combined targeting of MAPK and AKT signalling pathways is a promising strategy for melanoma treatment. Br J Dermatol. 2007;156:1204–13.
35. Meric-Bernstam F, Gonzalez-Angulo AM. Targeting the mTOR signaling network for cancer therapy. J Clin Oncol. 2009;27:2278–87.
36. Molhoek KR, Brautigan DL, Slingluff Jr CL. Synergistic inhibition of human melanoma proliferation by combination treatment with B-Raf inhibitor BAY43-9006 and mTOR inhibitor Rapamycin. J Transl Med. 2005;3:39.
37. Molhoek KR, Griesemann H, Shu J, Gershenwald JE, Brautigan DL, Slingluff Jr CL. Human melanoma cytolysis by combined inhibition of mammalian target of rapamycin and vascular endothelial growth factor/vascular endothelial growth factor receptor-2. Cancer Res. 2008;68:4392–7.
38. Motzer RJ, Escudier B, Oudard S, Hutson TE, Porta C, Bracarda S, et al. Efficacy of everolimus in advanced renal cell carcinoma: a double-blind, randomised, placebo-controlled phase III trial. Lancet. 2008;372:449–56.
39. Nicholson KM, Anderson NG. The protein kinase B/Akt signalling pathway in human malignancy. Cell Signal. 2002;14:381–95.
40. O'Reilly KE, Rojo F, She QB, Solit D, Mills GB, Smith D, et al. mTOR inhibition induces upstream receptor tyrosine kinase signaling and activates Akt. Cancer Res. 2006;66:1500–8.
41. O'Reilly KE, Warycha M, Davies MA, Rodrik V, Zhou XK, Yee H, et al. Phosphorylated 4E-BP1 is associated with poor survival in melanoma. Clin Cancer Res. 2009;15:2872–8.
42. Ohtani M, Nagai S, Kondo S, Mizuno S, Nakamura K, Tanabe M, et al. Mammalian target of rapamycin and glycogen synthase kinase 3 differentially regulate lipopolysaccharide-induced interleukin-12 production in dendritic cells. Blood. 2008;112:635–43.
43. Patnaik A, Ricart A, Cooper J, et al. A phase I, pharmacokinetic and pharmacodynamic study of sorafenib (S), a multi-targeted kinase inhibitor in combination with temsirolimus (T), an mTOR inhibitor in patients with advanced solid malignancies [Abstract 3512]. Proc Am Soc Clin Oncol. 2007;25S:141s.
44. Populo H, Soares P, Rocha AS, Silva P, Lopes JM. Evaluation of the mTOR pathway in ocular (uvea and conjunctiva) melanoma. Melanoma Res. 2010;20:107–17.
45. Rao RR, Li Q, Odunsi K, Shrikant PA. The mTOR kinase determines effector versus memory CD8+ T cell fate by regulating the expression of transcription factors T-bet and Eomesodermin. Immunity. 2010;32:67–78.
46. Raymond E, Alexandre J, Faivre S, Vera K, Materman E, Boni J, et al. Safety and pharmacokinetics of escalated doses of weekly intravenous infusion of CCI-779, a novel mTOR inhibitor, in patients with cancer. J Clin Oncol. 2004;22:2336–47.
47. Roskoski Jr R. Structure and regulation of Kit protein-tyrosine kinase–the stem cell factor receptor. Biochem Biophys Res Commun. 2005;338:1307–15.
48. Shaw RJ, Cantley LC. Ras, PI(3)K and mTOR signalling controls tumour cell growth. Nature. 2006;441:424–30.
49. Sinnberg T, Lasithiotakis K, Niessner H, Schittek B, Flaherty KT, Kulms D, et al. Inhibition of PI3K-AKT-mTOR signaling sensitizes melanoma cells to cisplatin and temozolomide. J Invest Dermatol. 2009;129:1500–15.
50. Thomson AW, Turnquist HR, Raimondi G. Immunoregulatory functions of mTOR inhibition. Nat Rev Immunol. 2009;9:324–37.
51. Van Raamsdonk CD, Bezrookove V, Green G, Bauer J, Gaugler L, O'Brien JM, et al. Frequent somatic mutations of GNAQ in uveal melanoma and blue naevi. Nature. 2009;457:599–602.
52. Werzowa J, Cejka D, Fuereder T, Dekrout B, Thallinger C, Pehamberger H, et al. Suppression of mTOR complex 2-dependent AKT phosphorylation in melanoma cells by combined treatment with rapamycin and LY294002. Br J Dermatol. 2009;160:955–64.
53. Workman P, Clarke PA, Raynaud FI, van Montfort RL. Drugging the PI3 kinome: from chemical tools to drugs in the clinic. Cancer Res. 2010;70:2146–57.

Chapter 9
Targeting Apoptotic Pathways in Melanoma

Peter Hersey and Xu Dong Zhang

Abstract Impairment of cell death is a key property of cancer cells. It follows that irrespective of the target of new therapies cell survival mechanisms will need to be overcome for the treatment to be effective. Considerable information is now available about the mechanisms responsible for cancer cell survival. These center largely on the Bcl-2 protein family and the inhibitor of apoptosis proteins. They are regulated by complex pathways that are often initiated by the oncogenic process. A number of new treatments that target the anti- and proapoptotic proteins are at various stages of development and evaluation. In addition, there is an ever-increasing number of agents that target signal pathways involved in regulation of these protein families and which may have potent apoptosis-inducing activities. Complex feedback mechanisms initiated by these treatments as well as the inherent variability of melanoma cells are obstacles that remain to be overcome. Nevertheless, they would appear to be an essential component of future treatment strategies against melanoma.

Keywords Melanoma • Apoptosis • Bcl-2 family • BH3 mimetics • Inhibitors of apoptosis proteins combination treatment

Introduction

Modern anticancer strategies are increasingly focused on rationally designed drugs which target pathways believed to be involved in tumorigenesis. Irrespective of whether anticancer strategies are based on nonspecific or targeted agents, their effectiveness depends on overcoming one of the basic properties of cancer cells, i.e., resistance to

P. Hersey (✉) • X.D. Zhang
Oncology & Immunology Unit, University of Newcastle, Kolling Institute Univesity of Sydney, Room 443, David Maddison Clinical Sciences Building, Cnr King & Watt Streets, Newcastle, NSW 2300, Australia
e-mail: peter.hersey@melanoma.org.au; xu.zhang@newcastle.edu.au

T.F. Gajewski and F.S. Hodi (eds.), *Targeted Therapeutics in Melanoma*, Current Clinical Oncology, DOI 10.1007/978-1-61779-407-0_9, © Springer Science+Business Media, LLC 2012 induction of apoptosis [59]. The discovery that impairment of apoptosis was essential in tumorigenesis came from studies showing that a protein called B cell lymphoma 2 (Bcl-2) was overexpressed in most human follicular lymphomas due to translocation of the gene on chromosome 18 to chromosome 14 at a site where it becomes driven by the promoter for immunoglobulin heavy chains [147]. Vaux et al. [154] demonstrated that Bcl-2 was not involved in proliferation of tumor cells but prolonged their survival. Tumorigenesis was facilitated when the cell cycle was disrupted by expression of oncogenes such as c-Myc (Strasser et al. [137]; reviewed in [2]). Since these seminal studies, there has been a marked increase in knowledge about apoptosis and cell death pathways and their regulation in cancer cells to the extent that targeting resistance pathways in cancer cells is now a realistic aim in targeted therapy approaches.

There are two major pathways that can lead to apoptosis in mammalian cells. One is the "intrinsic" or mitochondrial cell death pathway that is regulated by members of Bcl-2 protein family. Resistance to this pathway is believed to be the result of selection that has allowed the cancer cell to survive the stresses placed on the cell during neoplastic transformation such as dysregulated cell division, impaired energy production, and DNA damage. The other pathway is the extrinsic pathway that is activated when ligands of the tumor necrosis factor (TNF) family interact with death receptors (DR) of the TNF receptor family. This pathway is part of adaptive immunity responses, and apoptosis is mediated by the formation of death-inducing signaling complexes (DISC) on the cytosolic side of the receptors consisting of the DR, an adaptor protein, and proteases of the caspase family. The latter is usually caspase 8 (or 10), which when activated can directly activate the effector caspases 3, 6, and 7 by proteolytic cleavage. More commonly, activation of caspase 8 in solid cancers results in activation of the mitochondrial pathway by caspase 8-mediated cleavage and activation of the proapoptotic Bid protein [181].

Both pathways converge at the level of effector caspase activation where another level of regulation is mediated by members of the inhibitor of apoptosis protein (IAP) family. These proteins (particularly XIAP) are able to bind to and inhibit caspase 9, 3, and 7. This interaction can in turn be inhibited by antagonists released from the mitochondria such as Smac/DIABLO, which bind to XIAP. As reviewed below, other members of the IAP family may have functions upstream of mitochondria at the level of death receptors.

In the sections below we update current information about the cell death resistance pathways in melanoma and how these may be targeted by drugs in use or in development.

Bcl-2 Protein Family-Regulated Apoptosis

A number of excellent reviews have documented the members of the Bcl-2 family, their structure, and role in regulation of apoptosis [2, 19, 91, 172]. In brief, there are three classes of Bcl-2 proteins. One class inhibits apoptosis and includes Bcl-2, Bcl-XL, Mcl-1, Bcl-W, A1, and less commonly Bcl-13. They all share four Bcl-2 homology (BH) domains (BH1–BH4) except Mcl-1 which contains only three BH

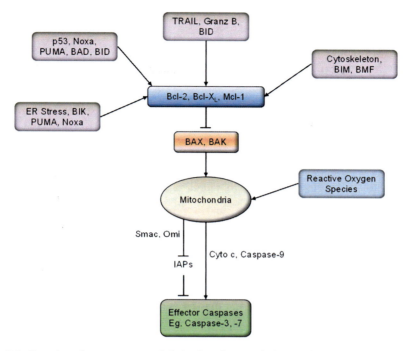

Fig. 9.1 Overview of current concepts in induction of apoptosis through the mitochondrial pathway. Apoptosis is initiated when the proapoptotic BH3 damage sensors increase in response to various signals. They then bind to the antiapoptotic Bcl-2 family proteins and displace the proapoptotic Bax and Bak, allowing them to bind to and permeabilize the outer mitochondrial membrane (OMM), so releasing aptogenic molecules. The role of caspase 2 in induction of apoptosis remains controversial and is omitted from discussion [87]. Similarly, the mechanism by which reactive oxygen species induce apoptosis is poorly defined and not discussed

domains. They all promote survival of cancer cells and are associated with resistance to drugs. Bcl-2 is located in the endoplasmic reticulum, nuclear envelope, and outer mitochondrial membrane (OMM) by its hydrophobic C terminal domain. By contrast, Bcl-XL and Mcl-1 are predominantly cytosolic and translocate to mitochondria during apoptosis (Fig. 9.1). Mcl-1 may be partially bound to mitochondria via Bak bound to mitochondria.

The second class of Bcl-2 proteins Bax, Bak, and Bok promotes apoptosis and has three BH3 domains, hence they are often referred to as multidomain proapoptotic proteins. They are essential for apoptosis due to their interaction with the OMM. This interaction is normally prevented by binding to the antiapoptotic proteins. The C terminal end of Bax fits into a hydrophobic pocket formed by the three BH3 domains and as a consequence Bax is located predominantly in the cytosol. Bak is believed to be located predominantly on the OMM, where it is bound to Mcl-1 and Bcl-XL perhaps due to displacement of the C terminal end of Bak by Mcl-1 and Bcl-XL. Upon activation Bax (and Bok) translocates to mitochondria and the N terminus undergoes a conformational change which is believed to be responsible for oligomerization and insertion into the OMM. Bak is believed to undergo similar oligomerization and OMM insertion. These changes result in release of proapoptotic proteins from the intermembrane space in mitochondria such as cytochrome C, DIABLO, the protease Omi, apoptosis-inducing factor (AIF), and endonuclease G. Cytochrome C and DIABLO appear to be particularly important for activation of caspases.

The third class of Bcl-2 proteins contains only BH3 domains and acts as sensors of cell damage. They have, with the exception of Bid, divergent structures compared to other members of the Bcl-2 family. There are eight members of the BH3 only family of proteins: Bid, Bim, Noxa, PUMA, DP5, Bik, Bad, and Bmf. They are believed to induce apoptosis predominantly by binding to the antiapoptotic Bcl-2 proteins so releasing Bax, Bak (and Bok) and allowing them to bind to the OMM. This is referred to as the "neutralization model." It is possible that some BH3-only proteins such as Bid, Bim, and PUMA may directly activate Bax and Bak but this remains a controversial area of research. It is possible that at low concentrations of BH3 proteins they are bound by antiapoptotic proteins and at high concentrations Bid or Bim may activate Bax and Bak directly (Activation model) [19, 58, 116]. Bim, Bid, and PUMA bind avidly to all the antiapoptotic proteins whereas Noxa binds only to Mcl-1 and A1, and Bad to Bcl-2, Bcl-XL, and Bcl-W. This variation in specificity has important implications in selection of treatments for cancers where Mcl-1 appears the main antiapoptotic protein.

Most of the BH3-only proteins are believed to be located in the cytosol. The main exceptions are BimEL, which is located in microtubules where it is bound to the dynein complex, and Bik, which is predominantly localized in the endoplasmic reticulum (ER) [18]. Certain BH3 proteins are predominantly localized in certain tissues, e.g., DP5/Hrk is found mainly in neuronal tissues [21].

Regulation of the Bcl-2 Antiapoptotic Family in Melanoma

In addition to variation in expression between tissues, it is evident that expression of the Bcl-2 family may also change during progression of tumors. This is illustrated particularly by studies on melanoma where Bcl-2 is overexpressed in melanocytes, nevi, and thin primary melanoma but expression decreased in thick primary and metastatic melanoma [185]. This was particularly evident in lymph nodes, suggesting that signaling from environmental influences may play a role in its expression. In contrast to Bcl-2, as shown in Fig. 9.2a and b, the levels of Mcl-1 and Bcl-XL were relatively low in primary melanoma but increased with progression of the disease.

The factors regulating the antiapoptotic proteins are as yet incompletely understood. The microphthalmia-associated transcription factor (MITF) is believed to be responsible for differentiation and survival of melanocytes [112] and a key factor in regulation of Bcl-2. There was a positive correlation between MITF and Bcl-2 expression in studies on sections from melanoma [185]. MITF is regulated through c-kit and c-kit is downregulated in most melanoma cells [74]. This may therefore play some role in the decreased levels of Bcl-2 via decreased activation of MITF.

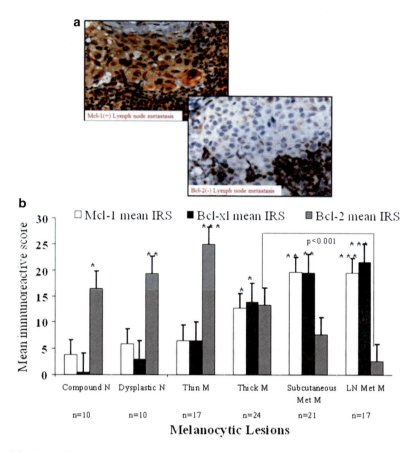

Fig. 9.2 Loss of Bcl-2 expression with melanoma progression. (**a**) Serial sections of a melanoma metastasis in a regional lymph node showing strong staining of melanoma cells for Mcl-1 but no detectable Bcl-2. The lymphocytes stained strongly for Bcl-2 [185]. (**b**) Bcl-2 is expressed at high levels in naevi and thin melanoma but decreases in thick primary melanoma and metastases

Another transcription factor regulating Bcl-2 (and c-kit) is AP-2 [95]. This was previously shown to be lost in progression of melanoma, and loss of AP-2 was associated with short OS and DFS [84]. Reports by others have suggested that translocation of AP-2 from the cytoplasm to the nucleus is disrupted during melanoma progression and is a crucial event in the development of melanoma [12]. Immunohistochemical studies showed a strong positive correlation between AP-2 and Bcl-2 but a negative correlation with Mcl-1 and Bcl-XL [185]. A positive correlation was shown in melanoma between pStat3 and Bcl-XL expression [185] but it is highly likely that other transcription factors, such as NF-κB, are also involved in regulation of Bcl-XL [5].

Mcl-1 expression in melanoma sections was weakly associated with activated Stat3 [185] but Stat3 was regarded as a critical transcriptional activator of Mcl-1, Bcl-XL, and survivin [81]. Although Bax, Bak, Bcl-2, and Bcl-XL are relatively stable with long half-lives, Mcl-1 is relatively labile. This is largely due to ubiquitination by the HECT E3 ligase MULE which targets the protein for degradation in proteasomes [184]. This process is increased by glycogen synthase kinase-mediated phosphorylation of serine 159 in Mcl-1 [109]. It is stabilized by the deubiquitinating (DUB) enzyme USP9X which promotes tumor cell survival [131]. It was considered that drugs targeting USP9X may have a therapeutic role. In addition, Mcl-1 may be ubiquitinated by the E3 ring cullin complex including the substrate-binding adaptor protein Fbw7 (SCF) which has been reported to be lost in certain cancers and to promote tumorigenesis. Upregulation of Mcl-1 is a major factor in protection of melanoma cells from apoptosis during ER stress and in allowing melanoma cells to adapt to ER stress conditions [63]. The transcription factor involved appears to be Ets-1 [30].

Regulation of the Bcl-2 Proapoptotic Family by the Two Key Tumor Suppressors, Retinoblastoma Protein (Rb) and p53

The pRB/E2F pathway is perturbed in the majority of melanomas, either by mutation or loss of CDKN2A/p16 which inhibits CDK4/6, mutation of CDK4 (R24C) or increased copy number of cyclin D1 [11, 23]. This allows the E2F family of transcription factors to induce proliferation of cells but may also induce proapoptotic BH3-only proteins such as PUMA, Noxa, Bim, and Hrk/DP5 [68, 125]. Feedback regulation of the transcription of these proteins may be mediated by methyltransferases, such as the EZH2 histone methylase, which antagonizes Bim expression [171]. Apoptosis signal regulating kinase (ASK1) is also a target of E2F and acts to inhibit Rb activity [140]. It may be responsible in part for histone deacetylase inhibitor-mediated upregulation of Bim and apoptosis reported by us and others [50, 178].

p53 is one of the best characterized tumor suppressors and is encoded by the TP53 gene. Inactivating mutations in p53 occur in more than 50% of human cancers; however, they are uncommon in melanoma. Wild-type p53 was detected in tissue sections in approximately 20–50% of melanoma [37, 167]. p53 induces apoptosis primarily by transcription-dependent mechanisms [125]. In addition, it can induce apoptosis independently of its transcriptional activity by acting directly on pro- and antiapoptotic Bcl-2 family proteins and/or the OMM [60]. A number of proapoptotic proteins are transcriptionally upregulated by p53 and play important roles in p53-mediated apoptosis. These include the BH3-only protein PUMA, Noxa, Bid and Bad, the multidomain Bcl-2 family protein Bax, Apaf-1, the death receptor Fas, and TRAIL-R2 (Fig. 9.3).

Despite its apoptosis-inducing role being well established in normal and many types of cancer cells, induction of p53 or overexpression of wild-type p53 in melanoma cells that harbor endogenous wild-type p53 does not induce apoptosis. One possible explanation for this is that downstream proapoptotic targets of p53 are dysregulated. The expression of PUMA has been shown to decrease with melanoma progression, but activation of p53 by nutlin-3a, which is a small molecule antagonist

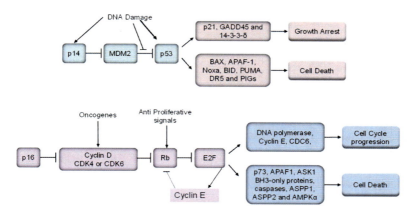

Fig. 9.3 Regulation of apoptosis by the two key tumor suppressors, p53 and Rb (adapted from [125]). P14, p53-induced gene, apoptosis-stimulating protein of p53 (ASPP)

of MDM2, results in upregulation of PUMA along with Noxa and p53 without induction of apoptosis [146].

In circumstances where p53 may be inactivated, E2F1 may have similar roles to p53 in induction of apoptosis via induction of p73 and so act as a backup to p53 (reviewed in [125]). E2F1 transcriptionally upregulates p73 which interacts with similar target genes to p53 (reviewed in [102, 175]). In particular, as well as Bim, Noxa, DP5, and PUMA, the proapoptotic p53 co-factors apoptosis-stimulating p53 proteins (ASPP1 and ASPP2) and tumor protein 53-induced nuclear protein 1 (TP53INP1) are also upregulated by E2F1, so favoring apoptosis.

Extensive crosstalk between E2F and p53 has been identified. E2F was reported to upregulate CDKN2A/ARF (p14) and thereby activate p53 by ARF-mediated inhibition of MDM2. ARF in turn can act as a feedback inhibitor of E2F1. p53 also downregulates CDKN2A/p14 in cells where it is not mutated or lost, so completing the feedback cycles [64]. The extent to which these feedback mechanisms inhibit apoptosis in melanoma remains to be investigated.

Additional Transcription Factors Regulating BH3-Only Proteins

Bim is known to be regulated by the FOXO3A transcription factor, which in turn is regulated by the P13K/Akt pathway. Inhibition of the latter results in dephosphorylation of FOXO3A, entry into the nucleus, and upregulation of Bim [47]. In certain cell types, ER stress may result in upregulation of Bim by induction of the transcription factor CCAAT/enhancer-binding protein homologous protein (CHOP) [128]. Noxa may also be upregulated by c-Myc and HIF-1α ([119]; see also [19]).

Targeting the Bcl-2 Antiapoptotic Proteins

Once it became evident that cancer cells depended on antiapoptotic proteins for survival, a number of strategies were developed to inhibit their activity. One of these was to use antisense oligonucleotides to knockdown expression of Bcl-2 [10] and other antiapoptotic proteins such as Mcl-1 [141]. The most studied of these was the "Genasense" 18mer antisense oligonucleotide against Bcl-2 produced by Genta. A phase I/II study in 14 patients showed that 10 of 12 patients had a reduction in Bcl-2 in their melanoma by day 4, amounting to a median of 40% reduction [75]. In view of this result, a large randomized study was commenced in July 2001 and 771 patients accrued over approximately a 2-year period. The overall survival (OS) of patients in each group (9.1 vs. 7.9 months) did not reach statistical significance (Hazard ratio 0.89, $p = 0.184$). The secondary end points in the trial – progression free survival (PFS) (74 vs. 49 days) and overall response rate (ORR) (11.7% vs. 6.8%) – were statistically significant [10]. The difference in the PFS was not considered clinically significant and the drug was not approved by the FDA. In view of this Genta (8/07) conducted a second randomized trial (AGENDA Trial) in a more favorable group of 315 patients with low LDH. This was because most of the benefit seen in the first trial was in patients with low LDH [10]. The initial results released in October 2009 did not show significant differences in PFS or OS but a final analysis will be conducted after a longer follow-up (http://www.clinicaltrials.gov/NCT00518895).

An alternative approach (see Table 9.1) was to antagonize the function of the antiapoptotic proteins rather than reducing their levels. Screening of a number of natural compounds identified Antimycin A [148] and Gossypol as inhibitors of Bcl-XL and Bcl-2. Gossypol [9] is found in cotton seeds. It has shown activity in vitro against a number of different cancers alone or in combination with other agents [88, 176]. Clinical studies with gossypol (AT-101) are being sponsored by Ascenta Therapeutics in patients with prostate cancer [105] and small cell carcinoma of the lung [66]. A synthetic derivative, apogossypol, was found to be less toxic than gossypol and to have better pharmacodynamics. A further derivative of apogossypol, B179D10, was chosen as a lead compound for further study [166].

Table 9.1 Targeting Bcl-2 family proteins	Antisense	Oblimersen (Genasense)	[10]
	Natural compounds	Antimycin A	[148]
		Gossypol	[9]
		Apogossypol	[166]
	Chemicals	HA14-1	[134]
		BH31-1	[28]
		SAHBs	[49, 159]
	BH3 mimetics	TW-37	[155, 160, 163]
		Obatoclax	[107, 121]
		ABT-737 (ABT-263)	[120, 145]

TW-37 is another gossypol derivative that was modeled on the structure of the Bim BH3 domain and shown to bind with high affinity to Bcl-2, Bcl-XL, and Mcl-1 [115, 155]. A chemical library screen of organic compounds identified HA14-1 by its ability to bind to Bcl-2 or by its ability to disrupt Bcl-XL/Bak complexes (BH3I-1). Some question marks remain over the specificity of these compounds as studies in Bax/Bak knockout cells suggested that apoptosis induction was largely due to off-target effects [157].

Another approach has been the synthesis of hydrocarbon-stapled BH3 helices which are BH3 peptides that are modified to become cell permeable and protease resistant [stabilized α helix of Bcl-2 domains (SAHBs)]. A Bim SAHB was able to induce oligomerization of Bax [49]. Previous studies on a Bid SAHB showed direct activation of Bax and induction of cell death [159]. Whether inhibitory peptides against Mcl-1 are amenable to this approach is not known [94].

BH3 Mimetics

A third strategy is based on providing drugs that mimic the BH3 proapoptotic proteins and so avoid the need to induce their expression in vivo. TW-37 mentioned above is one such compound. A second is Obatoclax, which was shown to release Bak from Mcl-1 and Bim from Bcl-2 and Mcl-1 [90]. It was particularly effective in blocking the interaction between Bak and Mcl-1 in melanoma cells [118]. It also was reported to synergize with bortezomib [124] and to activate Bax in Cholangiocarcinoma cells [136]. It was shown to overcome ER stress-induced apoptosis [79], and has effects on cell cycle arrest that appear independent of effects on apoptosis [143]. This agent is under evaluation in hematological malignancies [130] and solid cancers [121]. Toxicities have mainly been neurologic and similar to alcohol toxicity.

Arguably, the most promising BH3 mimetic to date is ABT-737 and its orally active form ABT-263 [145] developed by Abbott and described by Oltersdorf et al. [120]. It binds with high affinity to Bcl-2, Bcl-XL, and Bcl-W but only weakly to Mcl-1 and A1. This specificity is similar to that of Bad. ABT-737 mainly acts as a sensitizer to allow activator BH3-only proteins to trigger Bax- and Bak-mediated mitochondrial pathway-induced apoptosis [89, 120]. It has monotherapy activity against CLL, ALL, AML, and lymphoma [69, 157] and enhances the response to chemotherapy in vivo [1].

The main limitation of considering this drug in melanoma is its ineffectiveness against Mcl-1, which is the main antiapoptotic protein in melanoma [78, 185]. Nevertheless, if Mcl-1 is neutralized it may induce apoptosis in melanoma and other cancers where Mcl-1 is high [17, 149]. Drug combinations with ABT-737 that are effective against melanoma in vitro include proteasome inhibitors [114] and the standard chemotherapy agents, dacarbazine and fotemustine. Killing by imiquimod was sensitized by ABT-737 [164]. Cragg et al. [22] reported that induction of apoptosis in melanoma by MEK inhibitors was potentiated by ABT-737. Taken together these studies indicated that two conditions need to be met for ABT-737 to kill cells. First, BH3 activators of Bax and Bak such as Bid and Bim are needed. Second, Mcl-1 (and A1) needs to be at sufficiently low levels to allow MOMP to occur [14, 20, 29]. Unexpected effects seen in clinical studies with ABT-263 include thrombocytopenia [83, 177].

Regulation of Apoptosis by the RAS/RAF/MEK/ERK Pathway

The RAS/RAF/MEK/ERK pathway is normally activated by external factors through a number of receptors including tyrosine kinase (TK) receptors for autocrine and hormonal growth factors, and G protein-coupled receptors such as melanocortin receptors. In melanoma it is mainly activated constitutively by acquisition of activating mutations in BRAF in approximately 50% of cases [25] or its upstream activator NRAS in approximately 20% of cases [57]. Other mutations that result in constitutive activation of the pathway are in the G protein α subunit GNAQ in uveal melanoma and blue naevi [150] and in the KIT receptor TK gene [8]. Mutations in the ERBB4 receptor were reported in 19% of metastatic melanoma [126]. ETV1 on chromosome 7p was also reported to be a candidate oncogene downstream of BRAF [73].

The most common mutation in BRAF is of valine at position 600 to glutamic acid (V600E). This substitution can transform immortalized melanocytes [168] and melanoma cell proliferation and survival [56]. Transfection into melanocytes resulted primarily in senescence [113] and dysfunction of p53 was needed for transformation [173]. Similarly, studies in fish also showed that p53 deficiency was needed for development of melanoma [123]. Studies in mice transgenic for V600E in melanocytes showed that BRAF V600E expression alone resulted primarily in naevi, and loss of CDKN2A was needed for development of melanoma [54]. Furthermore, inactivation of PTEN was needed for progression to metastatic disease [24].

Traditionally, the RAS/RAF/MEK/ERK pathway has been linked to cell cycle reentry but it is now clear that it has a central role in cell survival and inhibition of apoptosis, as summarized in Table 9.2. One antiapoptotic mechanism involves phosphorylation of the proapoptotic BH3-only protein Bim [7]. The latter is produced as at least three splice variants referred to as Bim extra long (EL), long (L), and short (S). BimEL is phosphorylated at up to four sites (Serine 55, 65, 73 and Thr112) and this inhibits binding to the Bcl-2 antiapoptotic proteins as well as targeting it for ubiquitination and proteasome degradation. BimL is also believed to have a phosphorylation and ubiquitination site. Ubiquitination may involve Elongin B/C-Cullin2 E3 ligase complex [3]. Both EL and L bind to dynein light chains (DLC) in microtubules and may be released by chemotherapy or by activation of Jun N terminal kinase (JNK), which phosphorylates the DLC binding site [97]. BimS is of particular interest in that it is believed to bind directly to mitochondria perhaps in association with Bax [165]. It is not phosphorylated by ERK but the latter pathway downregulates mRNA for the Bim gene. As discussed below, it may also have a crucial role in suppression of BimS splicing.

Table 9.2 The ERK1/2 pathway blocks apoptosis at multiple sites

Inhibits BimEL by phosphorylation Ser69 and other sites [7, 13]
Phosphorylates Bad indirectly via RSK [7]
Repression of Bmf translocation [151]
Induces Mcl-1 [7, 162]
Induces GRP78 (GRP78 binds Bik, caspase 4) [77, 78]
Induces IL-8 and upregulation of ICAM [98]
Increases HIF-1α expression [99]

Bad may also be phosphorylated on Ser112 by ribosomal protein S6 kinase (RSK), which in turn is activated by ERK1/2 and results in binding of Bad to the cytosolic protein 14-3-3 [133]. Similarly, mRNA for the proapoptotic Bmf BH3 protein is downregulated by activation of ERK. By contrast, ERK1/2 can upregulate Bcl-2, Bcl-XL, and Mcl-1 [151]. This may in part be due to activation of CREB (cyclic AMP element binding) as the antiapoptotic proteins are known to have CREB-binding sites in their promoters. Mcl-1 degradation may also be inhibited by ERK1/2 phosphorylation of the PEST site in the N terminus of Mcl-1 [7].

In addition to these effects on the Bcl-2 family, activation of the ERK pathway may inhibit apoptosis by less direct pathways. One of these is by activation of the ER stress response, which results in upregulation of glucose-regulated protein 78 (GRP78). The latter is a chaperone protein which binds caspase 4 in melanoma cells [67] and possibly to Bik as described in breast carcinoma cells [46]. The second mechanism may involve suppression of the LKB1-AMPK signaling pathway, which is involved in upregulation of glucose intake and glycolysis and in blocking cell growth during low energy states [183]. Inhibitors of BRAF V600E were shown to upregulate the AMPK pathway and thereby inhibit mTOR and growth of melanoma cells. This was associated with increased sensitivity to apoptosis by as yet poorly understood mechanisms [38].

Agents Targeting the RAS/RAF/MEK/ERK Pathway

Development of agents against proteins in this pathway has been of much interest and includes those against RAS, RAF, and MEK, as shown in Table 9.3. Inhibition of RAS using farnesyltransferase (FT) inhibitors has so far not had therapeutic effects perhaps due to lack of specificity for RAS [48]. Nevertheless, this class of drugs may be effective in combination with other agents, as shown for the combination of SCH66336 with cisplatin [135].

In view of these results most attention has focused on inhibition of the RAF proteins which exist in a complex of A, B, and CRAF on the inner aspect of the cell membrane [168]. Much work has shown that BRAF is frequently activated by mutation in exon 15 which circumvents the need for RAS–GTP binding, frees it from negative regulation and its membrane location. The first agent to be tested was sorafenib, which targets a number of kinases including BRAF albeit with low activity

Table 9.3 RAS/RAF/MEK signal pathway inhibitors

Agent	Class of inhibitor	Target protein(s)	References
Sorafenib	Multikinase inhibitor	CRAF; BRAF; VEGF-2, -3; PDGF; Flt-3; c-kit	[4, 40, 65, 111]
Tanespimycin (KOS-953, 17-AGG)	Hsp90 inhibitor	Hsp90 (client proteins, BRAF, Akt, others)	[85]
RAF-265	Multikinase inhibitor	Mutant BRAF, VEGFR-2	[39]
XL281	All RAF Kinases	A, B, and CRAF	[117]
PLX4032, PLX4720	Selective BRAF kinase inhibitor	Mutant BRAF	[144]
GSK2118436	Selective BRAF kinase inhibitor	Mutant BRAF	http://www.gsk-clinical-studyregistrar.com
PD0325901	Non-ATP-competitive specific MEK inhibitor	MEK1, 2	[39]
AZD6244 (Selumetinib)	Non-ATP-competitive specific MEK inhibitor	MEK1, 2	[32, 33]
ARRY-162	Non-ATP-competitive specific MEK inhibitor	MEK1, 2	http://Arraybiopharma.com/productpipeline
XL518	Non-ATP-competitive specific MEK inhibitor	MEK1, 2	[117]
GSK1120212	Non-ATP-competitive specific MEK inhibitor	MEK1, 2	[52]
Tipifarnib (R115777)	Farnesyl transferase inhibitor	Prenylated proteins	[42, 63]
SCH66336	Farnesyl transferase inhibitor	Prenylated proteins	[135]

against the latter. It was found to have low single-agent activity against melanoma [41, 139] and did not potentiate the effects of carboplatin/paclitaxel in randomized phase II [65] or III (ECOG 2603) studies (http://pharmaprojects.com/news/3004). Encouraging results from a randomized phase II study with dacarbazine are as yet untested in a randomized phase III trial [110].

The development of BRAF inhibitors with high selectivity for the mutated protein [144] has resulted in very favorable responses in phase I studies where partial responses were seen in approximately 70% of 38 patients treated at adequate doses with the PLX4032/NP22657 drug. By contrast, PLX4032 had no effects on patients with wild-type BRAF melanoma and was reported to activate ERK and enhance the proliferation of melanoma cells with wild-type BRAF [62]. A second drug with similar potency has been developed by GlaxoSmithKline (GSK2118436) and again has been associated with rapid induction of PRs in phase I studies in melanoma (unreported data). The results of a phase II study with PLX4032/NP22657 on approximately 130 patients are awaited. Both agents have been associated with development of squamous cell carcinoma (SCC)/keratoacanthomas in approximately 20% of patients. Whether these drugs may induce new melanoma has been considered but is unknown [106].

RAF-265 (Novartis Pharmaceuticals) inhibits VEGF receptor 2 and melanoma cells with mutated BRAF or NRAS. Initial reports suggest it is not as effective as the selective inhibitors of mutated BRAF. XL281 (Exelixis, Inc.) is a potent inhibitor of all three RAF kinases. Initial studies were disappointing in that there was considerable toxicity and induction of SCCs [117].

Available evidence suggests that MEK is the only downstream target of BRAF so that inhibitors of MEK might be expected to have similar efficacy to the selective BRAF inhibitors. PD0325901 is a potent inhibitor of MEK but clinical trials were stopped due to induction of retinal vein thrombosis. AZD6244 is also a potent inhibitor that remains under clinical evaluation. It was found to be equivalent to Temozolomide in a phase II trial in patients with melanoma [32]. Other potent MEK inhibitors in clinical trials include ARRY-162, XL518, and GSK1120212.

Tanespimycin (KOS-953), an inhibitor of heat shock protein 90 (Hsp90), targets proteins protected (chaperoned) by Hsp90. This includes RAF, Akt, and other signal pathway proteins. The drug was tested in a phase II study in previously treated stage IV melanoma patients and administered twice weekly for 2 out of 3 weeks. Results from a treatment of 14 patients met the criteria for further evaluation in the second stage of the trial [85].

Inhibitor of Apoptosis Proteins in Melanoma

The IAPs are an evolutionary conserved family of proteins characterized by expression of one to three copies of baculovirus IAP repeat (BIR) domains. There are eight members of the family in humans; BIRC1, cIAP, cIAP2, XIAP, Survivin ML-IAP, Livin, ILP2, and Bruce. The structure and function of the IAPs have been well described in recent reviews [31, 92]. Practically, all the IAPs are able to bind to caspases but XIAP appears the most potent. Caspase 3 is inhibited by the linker region between BIR1 and BIR2 domains and Caspase 9 by binding to the BIR3 domains. Caspase 7 is inhibited by binding to BIR2 and the linker region between BIR1 and BIR2. IAP1 and IAP2 are able to bind caspases but are weak inhibitors. The BIR domains in cIAP and cIAP2 are considered possibly more important in interaction with TRAF1 and TRAF2 interactions at the TNF receptor (TNF-R). The IAP1, IAP2, and XIAP proteins have RING domains that mediate E3 ligase activity and which promote ubiquitination and degradation of Caspase 3 and 7 [92].

IAP1 and IAP2 appear more important in regulating NF-κB activation in response to TNF-α or DNA damage/viruses or alternative NF-κB activation as seen in lymphoid cells in response to CD40L. The cIAPs and TRAF proteins form a complex with the

TRAF proteins, acting as adaptors to activate NF-κB and the MAPK p38 and JNK pathways. They also appear to be associated with ubiquitination of the receptor-interacting protein (RIP) and inhibition of apoptosis [92]. The cIAPs are powerful inhibitors of TNF-α-induced apoptosis by activation of NF-κB signaling as well as inhibition of RIP and MAPK apoptotic pathways.

Several studies have shown overexpression of IAPs in melanoma. This was particularly evident in melanoma cell lines [36, 181]. Emanuel et al. [36] reported that XIAP was not detected in sections of naevi or in situ melanoma but was detectable in 24% of thin melanoma <1 mm in thickness and 73% of thick melanoma. Chen et al. [16] also showed significant upregulation of cIAP1, cIAP2, XIAP, survivin and ML-IAP in melanoma compared to naevi. ML-IAP (livin) was preferentially expressed in melanoma lines and was distinguished by only having one BIR domain [158]. The IAPs are generally thought to be regulated by NF-κB. ML-IAP may however be principally regulated by MITF, as shown by siRNA knockdown studies [34].

Negative Regulation of IAPs by Smac/DIABLO, Omi, and XAF1

Smac/DIABLO (second mitochondria-derived activator of caspases, direct IAP-binding protein with low PI) is a 25-kDa mitochondrial protein that promotes apoptosis through its ability to antagonize IAP-mediated caspase inhibition once released into the cytoplasm. Smac can bind many different IAPs (i.e., XIAP, cIAP1, cIAP2, and survivin), and its cytosolic presence provides a substantial contribution to the apoptotic response. Smac is able to interact with IAPs by binding to BIR2 and BIR3 domains, but not to BIR1; its amino terminal segment appears to be indispensable in this interaction with the various BIR domains, particularly for BIR3.

In addition to simply binding and inhibiting IAPs, Smac and its monovalent or bivalent mimetics may alter levels of certain IAPs. For example, IAP antagonists enhance auto-ubiquitination of cIAP1 and cIAP2 and result in proteasomal degradation of these two inhibitors of apoptosis. However, levels of other molecules such as XIAP remain unchanged until apoptosis is induced and caspases such as 3 and 8 are activated. Degradation of cIAP1 and cIAP2 requires the presence of BIR2 and BIR3 domains for IAP antagonist binding, and also of the RING domain for ubiquitin E3 ligase activity.

Somewhat surprisingly [153], Smac and Smac mimetics activate NF-κB by recruiting RIPK1 to TNF-R1, resulting in phosphorylation and proteasomal degradation of IκB, which would otherwise inhibit nuclear translocation of NF-κB. IAP antagonists also disinhibit NF-κB by preventing cIAP degradation of NIK. Increased levels of NIK activate NF-κB through the noncanonical pathway. Thus, NF-κB activation increases with IAP antagonists in a dose-dependent manner and results in increased TNF-α production. The proapoptotic effects of IAP antagonists

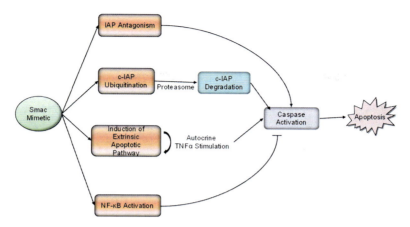

Fig. 9.4 Potential effects of Smac mimetics in melanoma. Smac mimetics may have multiple functions such as inhibition of IAPs and increasing their degradation and induction of the extrinsic pathway to apoptosis. By contrast, they may activate NF-κB and reduce apoptotic pathways

depend specifically on functional TNF-α death receptors, as opposed to other death receptors such as DR5 or Fas [15]. Apoptosis via this pathway involves FADD and activation of caspase 8. The various effects of the Smac mimetics are shown in Fig. 9.4.

Smac Mimetics in Cancer Therapy

A number of peptide mimetics of Smac have been used in experimental in vitro and animal model studies, as reviewed elsewhere [15]. This included inhibition of ML-IAP with a single BIR domain [44]. Antisense strategies (AS) include clinical studies with a second generation AS against XIAP, AEG35156. Phase I studies showed clinical activity against lymphoma, melanoma, and breast carcinoma [27]. Similarly, AS against survivin (LY2181308) are in phase II studies sponsored by Eli Lilly.

As shown in Table 9.4, small molecule Smac mimetics are in various stages of development by a number of pharmaceutical companies. These include Genentech (Compound C, Compound 8), Novartis (LCL161), Ascenta (AT-406) (http://clinicaltrials.gov), and Aegera (AEG40826). YM155 is a repressor of survivin transcription and has been evaluated in phase I studies [96]. A further phase II study on 60 patients with melanoma is planned in combination with Docetaxel. Further details of IAP targeted therapeutics are given in LaCasse et al. [92]. Common features of the drugs in vitro appear to be reduction primarily in cIAP1 and less so of cIAP2 and XIAP. They commonly have no direct apoptosis-inducing ability but enhance apoptosis induced by other agents such as TRAIL and chemotherapeutic agents.

Table 9.4 IAP-targeted therapeutics

Target	Compound	Class	Developmental stage	Company
XIAP	AEG35156/GEM640	Antisense	Phase 2	Aegera, Montreal, QC, Canada (Idera, Cambridge, MA, USA)
cIAP1, cIAP2, XIAP, livin	AEG40826/HGS1029	Smac mimetic	Phase 1	Aegera (Human Genome Sciences, Rockville, MD, USA)
	LCL161	Smac mimetic	Preclinical	Novartis, Cambridge, MA, USA
	Compound 11	Smac mimetic	Preclinical	Pfizer, New York, NY, USA (Idun, La Jolla, CA, USA/Abbot, Abbott Park, IL, USA)
	Compound C, compound 8	Smac mimetic	Phase 1	Genentech, San Francisco, CA, USA
	GT-T, compound A	Smac mimetic	Preclinical	Tetralogic, Malvern, PA, USA (Amgen, Thousand Oaks, CA, USA)
	AT-406	Smac mimetic	Preclinical	Asenta, Malvern, PA, USA
cIAP2	Ro106-9920	IKK ubiquitination inhibitor	Preclinical	Roche, Palo Alto, CA, USA
Survivin	LY218138/ISIS23722	Antisense	Phase 2	Eli Lilly, Indianapolis, IN, USA (Isis, Carlsbad, CA, USA)
	YM155	Transcriptional repressor	Phase 2	Astellas, Tokyo, Japan

Omi/HtrA2 is a serine protease also released from mitochondria. It regulates apoptosis by binding to XIAP and sensitizes cells to apoptosis [108]. Apoptosis-related protein in TGF-β signaling (*ARTS* – septin 4, isoform 2) [55] is another mitochondrial protein released during apoptosis which binds to BIR1 of XIAP and acts as a bridge to the E3 ligase, Siah, resulting in degradation of XIAP. It was reported to be deficient in some leukemias

XAF1 (XIAP-associated factor 1) is believed to bind to XIAP and to be inducible by IFN-β. It was considered crucial for induction of apoptosis by IFN-β in melanoma cells [129] and augmented TRAIL-induced apoptosis in melanoma but not normal cells [93]. It remains a potential anticancer agent

Apoptosis Induction by TRAIL

As reviewed elsewhere [6, 142, 169], a large number of clinical studies are in progress testing whether soluble TRAIL or agonistic antibodies against TRAIL receptors-R1 or R2 have antitumor effects. Very few of these studies have included melanoma patients because previous immunohistological studies have shown that progression of melanoma is associated with downregulation of TRAIL-R1 and -R2 on melanoma [186]. The reason for the receptor downregulation is not clear but appears to be posttranscriptional as mRNA levels show little variation despite loss or marked reduction in protein levels for TRAIL-R1 and -R2 [182].

As reported elsewhere, TRAIL-R2 can be upregulated in vitro by ER stress inducers such as Tunicamycin [76] and 2-Deoxyglucose (2DG) [101]. The transcription factor CHOP (Gadd153) was involved in ER stress receptor upregulation (36 h) but other factor(s) were involved at earlier periods [77]. In particular, the ATF6/IRE1/XBP-1 axis was involved in 2DG-mediated upregulation of TRAIL-R2. Tunicamycin is considered too toxic for clinical use but several other agents that are in clinical use, such as Cox-2 inhibitors [86] or Dipyridamole, may be useful for this purpose [53]. They and curcumin from curry powder appear to act on CHOP to upregulate TRAIL receptors [82].

One of the peculiarities of the TRAIL system is the concurrent delivery of opposing death and survival signals from its receptor [Yin (negative) and Yang (positive)]. It has been known for some time that TRAIL receptors may associate with other adaptor proteins rather than or in addition to FADD and result in different outcomes rather than cell death. Principal among these is activation of NF-κB and JNK, most likely through the RIP and TNF receptor-associating factor 2 (TRAF2) [35]. We and others have shown that activation of NF-κB in melanoma by TRAIL is strongly antiapoptotic [43]. One of the consequences of activation of NF-κB and Akt [122] is upregulation of Flice inhibitory protein (cFLIP), which can bind to DED of FADD and caspase 8 and inhibit apoptosis. cFLIP may also bind to TRAF1, 2 and RIP, resulting in activation of NF-κB and ERK1/2 [156, 174]. As discussed above, IAP1 and 2 were shown to be important in the activation of NF-κB via ubiquitin domains [61] by TNF-α [152]. Smac mimetics were shown to result in TNF-induced apoptosis by activation of caspase 8 either by inhibition of cFLIP production or formation of a RIP/FADD/caspase 8 complex [161].

In addition, the MEK pathway may be strongly activated by TRAIL. This is rapid but relatively transient, peaking at 1 h after exposure to TRAIL [179]. Activation of MEK is dependent on activation of protein kinase C (PKC), particularly PKC epsilon (ε), and the sensitivity of melanoma cells to TRAIL is inversely related to the activation of PKC-ε [51]. The activation of MEK by TRAIL occurs irrespective of whether BRAF is mutated or not [179].

These results therefore imply that within a polyclonal population of melanoma cells there is a range of activation signals in response to TRAIL. Sensitive cells have predominant activation of the FADD/caspase 8 pathway whereas resistant cells have dominant activation of NF-κB and MEK pathways. These results clearly have implications for selecting treatment combinations.

Table 9.5 Treatment combinations with TRAIL or agonistic antibodies to TRAIL

Agent	TRAIL/A. MAbs	Cancer	Mechanisms of action	References
Cox-2 inhibitors	TRAIL	Hepatocellular cancer	↑TRAIL-R1, R2, ↓Mcl-1	[86]
Dipyridamole	TRAIL	Colon and prostate cancer	CHOP mediated ↑TRAIL-R1, R2	[53]
Curcumin	TRAIL	Renal cancer	↑DR5	[82]
Bortezomib	A.MAbs	NSCLC	↓Mcl-1, ↓FLIP	[103]
Quercetin	TRAIL	Colon cancer	TRAIL-R1, R2 in lipid rafts	[127]
Sodium arsenite	TRAIL	Melanoma	↑TRAIL-R1, R2, ↓cFLIP	[71]
Resveratol	TRAIL	Melanoma	↓NF-κB, ↓Stat3, cFLIP, Bcl-XL	[72]
SBHA (HDAC)	TRAIL	Melanoma	↑Bim, ↓Mcl-1	[45]
Vorinostat (HDACi)	M.Ab MD5 (murine)	Mouse breast cancer	↓cFLIP	[51]
Triterpenoid CDOO-Me	TRAIL	Human lung cancer	↓cFLIP degradation	[187]

Table 9.5 summarizes some of the experimental studies on combinations with TRAIL that may increase apoptosis. In general, they can be viewed as agents which upregulate TRAIL death receptors or which downregulate antiapoptotic proteins. Bortezomib appears to mediate its effect by downregulation (directly or indirectly) of antiapoptotic proteins such as cFLIP, Mcl-1, and NF-κB and upregulation of Noxa [119]. Histone deacetylase inhibitors have had relatively little effects when used as single agents but may be most effective when used as sensitizing agents to induce apoptosis [104, 180].

MicroRNAs and Apoptosis

MicroRNAs (miRs) are small (~22 nucleotide) noncoding RNAs that regulate gene expression in a sequence-specific, imperfect-pairing manner. This is primarily accomplished through binding to the 3′ UTR of target mRNAs and either targeting the transcripts for degradation or blocking translation of the encoded protein. More than 70% of miR genes are located in either introns or exons of protein-coding genes and the remainder found to be present in intergenic regions. Like conventional protein-coding mRNA, miRs are transcribed by RNA polymerase II, spliced and polyadenylated (pri-miR). The pri-miRs are subsequently processed by Drosha, an RNAse III enzyme to become a ~70 nucleotide long stem-loop structure called precursor miR (pre-miR). Pre-miRs are then exported to cytoplasm by exportin 5

Table 9.6 Examples of regulation of apoptosis-related genes by miRNAs

Proapoptotic		Antiapoptotic	
miRNAs	Target genes	miRNAs	Target genes
Let-7 family	RAS, MYC	miR-17-92	E2F, Bim
miR-34a, b, c	Bcl-2, p53	miR-133	Caspase 9
miR-101	Mcl-1	miR-130	E2F1
miR-29a, b, c	E2F3, Mcl-1	miR-21	PTEN
miR-15/16	Bcl-2	miR-143	ERK5
		miR-221, 222	TRAIL

and cleaved by the cytoplasmic RNase III Dicer into a ~22-nucleotide miR duplex: one strand (miR*) of the usually nonfunctional short-lived duplex is degraded, whereas the other strand serves as a mature miR. The miRs are incorporated into the RNA-induced silencing complexes (RISCs) and target sequence-specific mRNAs through the RNA [70] interference pathway.

Many miRs have been found to play roles in regulating apoptosis by directly targeting putative apoptosis regulators. Some examples are listed in Table 9.6. While miRs that target proapoptotic genes are considered antiapoptotic, those that target antiapoptotic genes are proapoptotic (apoptomirs). Moreover, as expression patterns of miRs are highly tissue-specific, miRs that play roles in one tissue type may not have similar effects on regulating apoptosis in other tissues. In addition to direct regulation, many miRs may impinge on induction of apoptosis by indirectly acting on factors that regulate apoptosis-related proteins. For example, repression of FOXO3 by miR-182 may lead to downregulation of the BH3-only protein Bim that is known to be transcriptionally regulated by FOXO3. Given the increasing awareness of the significance of miRs in multiple biological processes, it is conceivable that the number of miRs that are involved, directly or indirectly, in regulation of apoptotic signaling will increase rapidly in the near future [170].

Relatively little has been published in melanoma in relation to apoptosis other than the association of miR-137 and miR-182 with MITF and MITF/FOXO3 expression [132]. miR-149* may also be involved in regulation of Mcl-1 [80]. It is evident from preclinical studies in leukemias that miR may be effective in treatment by either reintroduction of miRs lost in cancer or anti-miRs reduction in oncogenic miRs by anti-miRs, as reviewed elsewhere [70]. Delivery of siRNA via targeted nanoparticles appears a practical approach to such therapy [26].

Conclusions

Over the last 2 decades, there has been a considerable increase in information about the apoptotic pathways induced by oncogenes, ER stress and abnormal signal pathways, and how melanoma cells may adapt to and evade these pathways. It is highly likely that these adaptive antiapoptotic mechanisms are in large part responsible for resistance to treatment with chemotherapy, radiotherapy, and immunotherapy. As a result of this information, an impressive array of new drugs has been developed that may help to overcome tumor cell resistance to cell death due to the inherent apoptosis-inducing signal or in response to external agents such as chemotherapy. Several of these agents are being evaluated in early phase I/phase II trials as single agents and one (Genasense) has been the subject of a randomized trial in conjunction with chemotherapy.

Although some of the agents have activity as single agents, particularly in hematologic malignancies, it seems most likely that a strong external apoptotic signal supplied by chemotherapy, radiotherapy, or immunotherapy will be needed to show therapeutic effects, particularly in solid malignancies. Combinations may rationally involve not only agents targeting Bcl-2 family proteins but also those against IAP proteins. It may even be appropriate to combine agents that directly target the Bcl-2 and IAP families with signal pathway inhibitors.

Even with such combinations, it is likely that variation between different melanoma may limit responses and there is still a need to identify subgroups that may be more responsive than others. Studies in small cell lung carcinoma and leukemia/lymphoma suggest that expression of Bcl-2 and Noxa identified responders to ABT-263 whereas Mcl-1 was higher in resistant cells. Global gene expression patterns also helped to identify responders [138]. Mutation and copy number analysis of melanoma may further assist in patient selection [100]. BH3 profiling is another approach advocated to test whether cancer cells were dependent on particular antiapoptotic proteins and hence assist in selecting appropriate treatments [29]. The approach required viable cancer cells and was not considered robust enough for clinical studies.

References

1. Ackler S, Mitten MJ, Foster K, Oleksijew A, Refici M, Tahir SK, et al. The Bcl-2 inhibitor ABT-263 enhances the response of multiple chemotherapeutic regimens in hematologic tumors in vivo. Cancer Chemother Pharmacol. 2010;66(5):869–80.
2. Adams JM, Cory S. The Bcl-2 apoptotic switch in cancer development and therapy. Oncogene. 2007;26:1324–37.
3. Akiyama T, Dass CR, Choong PF. Bim-targeted cancer therapy: a link between drug action and underlying molecular changes. Mol Cancer Ther. 2009;8:3173–80.
4. Amaravadi RK, schuchter LM, MCDermott OF, Kramer A, Giles L, Gramlich K, et al. Phase II trial of temozolomide and sorafenib in advanced melanoma patients with or without brain metastases. Nlin Cancer Res. 2009;15(24):7711–18.
5. Amiri KI, Richmond A. Role of nuclear factor-kappa B in melanoma. Cancer Metastasis Rev. 2005;24:301–13.
6. Ashkenazi A. Directing cancer cells to self-destruct with pro-apoptotic receptor agonists. Nat Rev Drug Discov. 2008;7:1001–12.
7. Balmanno K, Cook SJ. Tumour cell survival signalling by the ERK1/2 pathway. Cell Death Differ. 2009;16:368–77.

8. Beadling C, Jacobson-Dunlop E, Hodi FS, Le C, Warrick A, Patterson J, et al. KIT gene mutations and copy number in melanoma subtypes. Clin Cancer Res. 2008;14:6821–8.

9. Becattini B, Kitada S, Leone M, Monosov E, Chandler S, Zhai D, et al. Rational design and real time, in-cell detection of the proapoptotic activity of a novel compound targeting Bcl-X(L). Chem Biol. 2004;11:389–95.

10. Bedikian AY, Millward M, Pehamberger H, Conry R, Gore M, Trefzer U, et al. Bcl-2 anti-sense (oblimersen sodium) plus dacarbazine in patients with advanced melanoma: the Oblimersen Melanoma Study Group. J Clin Oncol. 2006;24:4738–45.

11. Bennett DC. How to make a melanoma: what do we know of the primary clonal events? Pigment Cell Melanoma Res. 2008;21:27–38.

12. Berger AJ, Davis DW, Tellez C, Prieto VG, Gershenwald JE, Johnson MM, et al. Automated quantitative analysis of activator protein-2alpha subcellular expression in melanoma tissue microarrays correlates with survival prediction. Cancer Res. 2005;65:11185–92.

13. Cartlidge RA, Thomas GR, Cagnol S, Jong KA, Molton SA, Finch AJ, et al. Oncogenic BRAF(V600E) inhibits BIM expression to promote melanoma cell survival. Pigment Cell Melanoma Res. 2008;21:534–44.

14. Certo M, Del Gaizo Moore V, Nishino M, Wei G, Korsmeyer S, Armstrong SA, et al. Mitochondria primed by death signals determine cellular addiction to antiapoptotic BCL-2 family members. Cancer Cell. 2006;9:351–65.

15. Chen DJ, Huerta S. Smac mimetics as new cancer therapeutics. Anticancer drugs. 2009;20: 646–58.

16. Chen M, Osman I, Orlow SJ. Antifolate activity of pyrimethamine enhances temozolomide-induced cytotoxicity in melanoma cells. Mol Cancer Res. 2009;7:703–12.

17. Chen S, Dai Y, Harada H, Dent P, Grant S. Mcl-1 down-regulation potentiates ABT-737 lethality by cooperatively inducing Bak activation and Bax translocation. Cancer Res. 2007;67:782–91.

18. Chinnadurai G, Vijayalingam S, Rashmi R. BIK, the founding member of the BH3-only family proteins: mechanisms of cell death and role in cancer and pathogenic processes. Oncogene. 2008;27 Suppl 1:S20–9.

19. Chipuk JE, Moldoveanu T, Llambi F, Parsons MJ, Green DR. The BCL-2 family reunion. Mol Cell. 2010;37:299–310.

20. Chonghaile TN, Letai A. Mimicking the BH3 domain to kill cancer cells. Oncogene. 2008;27 Suppl 1:S149–57.

21. Coultas L, Terzano S, Thomas T, Voss A, Reid K, Stanley EG, et al. Hrk/DP5 contributes to the apoptosis of select neuronal populations but is dispensable for haematopoietic cell apoptosis. J Cell Sci. 2007;120:2044–52.

22. Cragg MS, Jansen ES, Cook M, Harris C, Strasser A, Scott CL. Treatment of B-RAF mutant human tumor cells with a MEK inhibitor requires Bim and is enhanced by a BH3 mimetic. J Clin Invest. 2008;118:3651–9.

23. Curtin JA, Fridlyand J, Kageshita T, Patel HN, Busam KJ, Kutzner H, et al. Distinct sets of genetic alterations in melanoma. N Engl J Med. 2005;353:2135–47.

24. Dankort D, Curley DP, Cartlidge RA, Nelson B, Karnezis AN, Damsky Jr WE, et al. Braf(V600E) cooperates with Pten loss to induce metastatic melanoma. Nat Genet. 2009;41:544–52.

25. Davies H, Bignell GR, Cox C, Stephens P, Edkins S, Clegg S, et al. Mutations of the BRAF gene in human cancer. Nature. 2002;417:949–54.

26. Davis ME, Zuckerman JE, Choi CH, Seligson D, Tolcher A, Alabi CA, et al. Evidence of RNAi in humans from systemically administered siRNA via targeted nanoparticles. Nature. 2010;464(7291):1067–70.

27. Dean E, Jodrell D, Connolly K, Danson S, Jolivet J, Durkin J, et al. Phase I trial of AEG35156 administered as a 7-day and 3-day continuous intravenous infusion in patients with advanced refractory cancer. J Clin Oncol. 2009;27:1660–6.

28. Degterev A, Lugovskoy A, Cardone M, Mulley B, Wagner G, Mitchison T, et al. Identification of small-molecule inhibitors of interaction between the BH3 domain and Bcl-xL. Nat Cell Biol. 2001;3:173–82.

29. Deng J, Carlson N, Takeyama K, Dal Cin P, Shipp M, Letai A. BH3 profiling identifies three distinct classes of apoptotic blocks to predict response to ABT-737 and conventional chemotherapeutic agents. Cancer Cell. 2007;12:171–85.

30. Dong L, Jiang CC, Thorne RF, croft A, yang F, Liu H, et al. Ets-1 mediates upregulation of Mcl-1 downstream of XBP-1 in human melanoma cells upon ER stress. Oncogene. 2011;30(34):3716–26. doi: 10.1038/onc.2011.87.

31. Dubrez-Daloz L, Dupoux A, Cartier J. IAPs: more than just inhibitors of apoptosis proteins. Cell Cycle. 2008;7:1036–46.

32. Dummer R, Robert C, Chapman PB, Sosman JA, Middleton M, Bastholt L, et al. AZD62444 (ARRy-142886) vs temozolomide (TMZ) in patients (pts) with advanced melanoma: an open-label, randomized, multicenter, phase II study. J Clin Oncol. 2008;26(May 20 Suppl):Abstract 9003.

33. Dry JR, Pavey S, pratilas CA, Harbron C, Runswick S, Hodgson D, et al. Transriptional pathway signatures predict MEK addiction and response to selunetinib A ZD6244. Cancer Res. 2010;70(6):2263–73.

34. Dynek JN, Chan SM, Liu J, Zha J, Fairbrother WJ, Vucic D. Microphthalmia-associated transcription factor is a critical transcriptional regulator of melanoma inhibitor of apoptosis in melanomas. Cancer Res. 2008;68:3124–32.

35. Ehrhardt H, Fulda S, Schmid I, Hiscott J, Debatin KM, Jeremias I. TRAIL induced survival and proliferation in cancer cells resistant towards TRAIL-induced apoptosis mediated by NF-kappaB. Oncogene. 2003;22:3842–52.

36. Emanuel PO, Phelps RG, Mudgil A, Shafir M, Burstein DE. Immunohistochemical detection of XIAP in melanoma. J Cutan Pathol. 2008;35:292–7.

37. Essner R, Kuo CT, Wang H, Wen DR, Turner RR, Nguyen T, et al. Prognostic implications of p53 overexpression in cutaneous melanoma from sun-exposed and nonexposed sites. Cancer. 1998;82:309–16.

38. Esteve-Puig R, Canals F, Colome N, Merlino G, Recio JA. Uncoupling of the LKB1-AMPKalpha energy sensor pathway by growth factors and oncogenic BRAF. PLoS One. 2009;4:e4771.

39. Fecher LA, Cummings SD, Keefe MJ, Alani RM. Toward a molecular classification of melanoma. J Clin Oncol. 2007;25:1606–20.

40. Flaherty KT. Chemotherapy and targeted therapy combinations in advanced melanoma. Clin Cancer Res. 2006;12:2366s–70.

41. Flaherty KT, Schiller J, Schuchter LM, Liu G, Tuveson DA, Redlinger M, et al. A phase I trial of the oral, multikinase inhibitor sorafenib in combination with carboplatin and paclitaxel. Clin Cancer Res. 2008;14:4836–42.

42. Fouladi M, Nicholson HS, Zhou T, Laningham F, Helton KJ, Holmes E, et al. A phase II study of the farnesyl transferase inhibitor, tipifarnib, in children with recurrent or progressive high-grade glioma, medulloblastoma/primitive neuroectodermal tumor, or brainstem glioma: a Children's Oncology Group study. Cancer. 2007;110:2535–41.

43. Franco AV, Zhang XD, Van Berkel E, Sanders JE, Zhang XY, Thomas WD, et al. The role of NF-kappa B in TNF-related apoptosis-inducing ligand (TRAIL)-induced apoptosis of melanoma cells. J Immunol. 2001;166:5337–45.

44. Franklin MC, Kadkhodayan S, Ackerly H, Alexandru D, Distefano MD, Elliott LO, et al. Structure and function analysis of peptide antagonists of melanoma inhibitor of apoptosis (ML-IAP). Biochemistry. 2003;42:8223–31.

45. Frew AJ, Lindemann RK, Martin BP, Clarke CJ, sharkey J, Anthony PA, Banks KM, Haynes NM, Gangatirkar P, stanley K, Bolden JE, Takeda K, Yagita H, secrist JP, smyth MJ, Johnstone RW. Combination therapy of established cancer using a histone deacetylase inhibitor and a TRAIL receptor agonist. Proc Natl Acad SCl USA. 2008;105(32):11317–22.

46. Fu Y, Li J, Lee AS. GRP78/BiP inhibits endoplasmic reticulum BIK and protects human breast cancer cells against estrogen starvation-induced apoptosis. Cancer Res. 2007;67:3734–40.

47. Fu Z, Tindall DJ. FOXOs, cancer and regulation of apoptosis. Oncogene. 2008;27:2312–9.

48. Gajewski TF, Niedzwiecki D, Johnson JC, Linette GP, Bucher C, Blaskovich MA, et al. Phase II tudy of farnesyltransferase inhibitor R115777 in advancd melanoma: CALGB 500104. J Clin Oncol. 2006;24:8014.
49. Gavathiotis E, Suzuki M, Davis ML, Pitter K, Bird GH, Katz SG, et al. BAX activation is initiated at a novel interaction site. Nature. 2008;455:1076–81.
50. Gillespie S, Borrow J, Zhang XD, Hersey P. Bim plays a crucial role in synergistic induction of apoptosis by the histone deacetylase inhibitor SBHA and TRAIL in melanoma cells. Apoptosis. 2006;11:2251–65.
51. Gillespie S, Zhang XD, Hersey P. Variable expression of protein kinase C epsilon in human melanoma cells regulates sensitivity to TRAIL-induced apoptosis. Mol Cancer Ther. 2005;4: 668–76.
52. Gilmartin AG, Bleam MR, Groy A, MOSS KG, Minthorn EA, Kulkarni SG, et al. GSK1120212 (JTP-74057) is an inhibitor of MEK activity and activation with favorable pharmacokinetic properties for sustained in vivo pathway inhibition. Clin Cancer Res. 2011;17(5):989–1000.
53. Goda AE, Yoshida T, Horinaka M, Yasuda T, Shiraishi T, Wakada M, et al. Mechanisms of enhancement of TRAIL tumoricidal activity against human cancer cells of different origin by dipyridamole. Oncogene. 2008;27:3435–45.
54. Goel VK, Ibrahim N, Jiang G, Singhal M, Fee S, Flotte T, et al. Melanocytic nevus-like hyperplasia and melanoma in transgenic BRAFV600E mice. Oncogene. 2009;28:2289–98.
55. Gottfried Y, Rotem A, Lotan R, Steller H, Larisch S. The mitochondrial ARTS protein promotes apoptosis through targeting XIAP. EMBO J. 2004;23:1627–35.
56. Gray-Schopfer VC, Cheong SC, Chong H, Chow J, Moss T, Abdel-Malek ZA, et al. Cellular senescence in naevi and immortalisation in melanoma: a role for p16? Br J Cancer. 2006;95: 496–505.
57. Gray-Schopfer VC, da Rocha Dias S, Marais R. The role of B-RAF in melanoma. Cancer Metastasis Rev. 2005;24:165–83.
58. Green DR, Chipuk JE. Apoptosis: stabbed in the BAX. Nature. 2008;455:1047–9.
59. Green DR, Evan GI. A matter of life and death. Cancer Cell. 2002;1:19–30.
60. Green DR, Kroemer G. Cytoplasmic functions of the tumour suppressor p53. Nature. 2009;458:1127–30.
61. Gyrd-Hansen M, Darding M, Miasari M, Santoro MM, Zender L, Xue W, et al. IAPs contain an evolutionarily conserved ubiquitin-binding domain that regulates NF-kappaB as well as cell survival and oncogenesis. Nat Cell Biol. 2008;10:1309–17.
62. Halaban R, Zhang W, Bacchiocchi A, Cheng E, Parisi F, Ariyan S, et al. PLX4032, a selective BRAF(V600E) kinase inhibitor, activates the ERK pathway and enhances cell migration and proliferation of BRAF(WT) melanoma cells. Pigment Cell Melanoma Res. 2010;23(2): 190–200.
63. Haluska P, Dy GK, Adjei AA. Farnesyl transferase inhibitors as anticancer agents. Eur J Cancer. 2002;38:1685–700.
64. Harris SL, Levine AJ. The p53 pathway: positive and negative feedback loops. Oncogene. 2005;24:2899–908.
65. Hauschild A, Agarwala SS, Trefzer U, Hogg D, Robert C, Hersey P, et al. Results of a phase III, randomized, placebo-controlled study of sorafenib in combination with carboplatin and paclitaxel as second-line treatment in patients with unresectable stage III or stage IV melanoma. J Clin Oncol. 2009;27:2823–30.
66. Heist RS, Fain J, Chinna-Sami B, Khan W, Molina J, Brainerd V, et al. A phase I/II (P1/P2) study of AT-101 in combination with topotecan (T) in patients with relapsed or refractory small cell lung cancer (SCLC) after prior platinum-containing first-line chemotherapy. In: ASCO Annual Meeting, Abstract No 8106; 2009.
67. Hersey P, Zhang XD. Adaptation to ER stress as a driver of malignancy and resistance to therapy in human melanoma. Pigment Cell Melanoma Res. 2008;21:358–67.
68. Hershko T, Ginsberg D. Up-regulation of Bcl-2 homology 3 (BH3)-only proteins by E2F1 mediates apoptosis. J Biol Chem. 2004;279:8627–34.

69. High LM, Szymanska B, Wilczynska-Kalak U, Barber N, O'Brien R, Khaw SL, et al. The Bcl-2 homology domain 3 mimetic ABT-737 targets the apoptotic machinery in acute lymphoblastic leukemia resulting in synergistic in vitro and in vivo interactions with established drugs. Mol Pharmacol. 2010;77:483–94.

70. Iorio MV, Croce CM. MicroRNAs in cancer: small molecules with a huge impact. J Clin Oncol. 2009;27:5848–56.

71. Ivanov VN, Hei TK. Sodium arsenite accelerates TRAIL-mediated apoptosis in melanoma cells through upregulation of TRAIL-R1/R2 surface levels and downregulation of CFLIP expression. Exp Cell Res. 2006;312(20):4120–38.

72. Ivanov VN, partridge MA, Johnson GE, Huang SX, Zhou H, Hei TK. Resveratrol sensitizes melanomas to TRAIL through modulation of antiapoptotic gene expression. Exp Cell Res. 2008;314(5): 1163–76.

73. Jane-Valbuena J, Widlund HR, Perner S, Johnson LA, Dibner AC, Lin WM, et al. An oncogenic role for ETV1 in melanoma. Cancer Res. 2010;70:2075–84.

74. Janku F, Novotny J, Julis I, Julisova I, Pecen L, Tomancova V, et al. KIT receptor is expressed in more than 50% of early-stage malignant melanoma: a retrospective study of 261 patients. Melanoma Res. 2005;15:251–6.

75. Jansen B, Wacheck V, Heere-Ress E, Schlagbauer-Wadl H, Hoeller C, Lucas T, et al. Chemosensitisation of malignant melanoma by BCL2 antisense therapy. Lancet. 2000;356: 1728–33.

76. Jiang CC, Chen LH, Gillespie S, Kiejda KA, Mhaidat N, Wang YF, et al. Tunicamycin sensitizes human melanoma cells to tumor necrosis factor-related apoptosis-inducing ligand-induced apoptosis by up-regulation of TRAIL-R2 via the unfolded protein response. Cancer Res. 2007;67:5880–8.

77. Jiang CC, Chen LH, Gillespie S, Wang YF, Kiejda KA, Zhang XD, et al. Inhibition of MEK sensitizes human melanoma cells to endoplasmic reticulum stress-induced apoptosis. Cancer Res. 2007;67:9750–61.

78. Jiang CC, Lucas K, Avery-Kiejda KA, Wade M, deBock CE, Thorne RF, et al. Up-regulation of Mcl-1 is critical for survival of human melanoma cells upon endoplasmic reticulum stress. Cancer Res. 2008;68:6708–17.

79. Jiang CC, Yang F, Thorne RF, Zhu BK, Hersey P, Zhang XD. Human melanoma cells under endoplasmic reticulum stress acquire resistance to microtubule-targeting drugs through XBP-1-mediated activation of Akt. Neoplasia. 2009;11:436–47.

80. Jin L, HU WL, Jiang CC, wang JX, Han CC, chu P, et al. MicroRNA-149*, a p53-responsive microRNA, functions as an oncogenic regulator in human melanoma. Proc Natl Acad sci USA. 2011;108(38):15840–5.

81. Jing N, Tweardy DJ. Targeting Stat3 in cancer therapy. Anticancer Drugs. 2005;16:601–7.

82. Jung EM, Park JW, Choi KS, Park JW, Lee HI, Lee KS, et al. Curcumin sensitizes tumor necrosis factor-related apoptosis-inducing ligand (TRAIL)-mediated apoptosis through CHOP-independent DR5 upregulation. Carcinogenesis. 2006;27:2008–17.

83. Kang MH, Kang YH, Szymanska B, Wilczynska-Kalak U, Sheard MA, Harned TM, et al. Activity of vincristine, L-ASP, and dexamethasone against acute lymphoblastic leukemia is enhanced by the BH3-mimetic ABT-737 in vitro and in vivo. Blood. 2007;110:2057–66.

84. Karjalainen JM, Kellokoski JK, Eskelinen MJ, Alhava EM, Kosma VM. Downregulation of transcription factor AP-2 predicts poor survival in stage I cutaneous malignant melanoma. J Clin Oncol. 1998;16:3584–91.

85. Kefford R, Millward M, Hersey P, Brady B, Graham M, Johnson RG, et al. Phase II trial of tanespimycin (KOS-953), a heat shock protein-90 (Hsp90) inhibitor in patients with metastatic melanoma. J Clin Oncol. 2007;25:8558.

86. Kern MA, Haugg AM, Koch AF, Schilling T, Breuhahn K, Walczak H, et al. Cyclooxygenase-2 inhibition induces apoptosis signaling via death receptors and mitochondria in hepatocellular carcinoma. Cancer Res. 2006;66:7059–66.

87. Kitevska T, Spencer DM, Hawkins CJ. Caspase-2: controversial killer or checkpoint controller? Apoptosis. 2009;14:829–48.

88. Kline MP, Rajkumar SV, Timm MM, Kimlinger TK, Haug JL, Lust JA, et al. R-(−)-gossypol (AT-101) activates programmed cell death in multiple myeloma cells. Exp Hematol. 2008;36:568–76.
89. Konopleva M, Contractor R, Tsao T, Samudio I, Ruvolo PP, Kitada S, et al. Mechanisms of apoptosis sensitivity and resistance to the BH3 mimetic ABT-737 in acute myeloid leukemia. Cancer Cell. 2006;10:375–88.
90. Konopleva M, Watt J, Contractor R, Tsao T, Harris D, Estrov Z, et al. Mechanisms of antileukemic activity of the novel Bcl-2 homology domain-3 mimetic GX15-070 (obatoclax). Cancer Res. 2008;68:3413–20.
91. Labi V, Grespi F, Baumgartner F, Villunger A. Targeting the Bcl-2-regulated apoptosis pathway by BH3 mimetics: a breakthrough in anticancer therapy? Cell Death Differ. 2008;15: 977–87.
92. LaCasse EC, Mahoney DJ, Cheung HH, Plenchette S, Baird S, Korneluk RG. IAP-targeted therapies for cancer. Oncogene. 2008;27:6252–75.
93. Leaman DW, Chawla-Sarkar M, Vyas K, Reheman M, Tamai K, Toji S, et al. Identification of X-linked inhibitor of apoptosis-associated factor-1 as an interferon-stimulated gene that augments TRAIL Apo2L-induced apoptosis. J Biol Chem. 2002;277:28504–11.
94. Lee EF, Fedorova A, Zobel K, Boyle MJ, Yang H, Perugini MA, et al. Novel Bcl-2 homology-3 domain-like sequences identified from screening randomized peptide libraries for inhibitors of the pro-survival Bcl-2 proteins. J Biol Chem. 2009;284:31315–26.
95. Leslie MC, Bar-Eli M. Regulation of gene expression in melanoma: new approaches for treatment. J Cell Biochem. 2005;94:25–38.
96. Lewis KD, Samlowski W, Ward J, Catlett J, Cranmer L, Kirkwood J, et al. A multi-center phase II evaluation of the small molecule survivin suppressor YM155 in patients with unresectable stage III or IV melanoma. Invest New Drugs. 2011;29(1):161–6.
97. Ley R, Ewings KE, Hadfield K, Cook SJ. Regulatory phosphorylation of Bim: sorting out the ERK from the JNK. Cell Death Differ. 2005;12:1008–14.
98. Liang S, Sharma A, Peng HH, Robertson G, Dong C. Targeting mutant (V600E) B-Raf in melanoma interrupts immunoediting of leukocyte functions and melanoma extravasation. Cancer Res. 2007;67:5814–20.
99. Lim JH, Lee ES, You HJ, Lee JW, Park JW, Chun YS. Ras-dependent induction of HIF-1alpha785 via the Raf/MEK/ERK pathway: a novel mechanism of Ras-mediated tumor promotion. Oncogene. 2004;23:9427–31.
100. Lin WM, Baker AC, Beroukhim R, Winckler W, Feng W, Marmion JM, et al. Modeling genomic diversity and tumor dependency in malignant melanoma. Cancer Res. 2008;68:664–73.
101. Liu H, Jiang CC, Lavis CJ, Croft A, Dong L, Tseng HY, et al. 2-Deoxy-D-glucose enhances TRAIL-induced apoptosis in human melanoma cells through XBP-1-mediated up-regulation of TRAIL-R2. Mol Cancer. 2009;8:122.
102. Lunghi P, Costanzo A, Mazzera L, Rizzoli V, Levrero M, Bonati A. The p53 family protein p73 provides new insights into cancer chemosensitivity and targeting. Clin Cancer Res. 2009;15:6495–502.
103. Luster TA, Carrell JA, McCormick K, Sun D, Humphreys R. Mapatumumab and lexatumumab induce apoptosis in TRAIL-R1 and TRAIL-R2 antibody-resistant NSCLC cell llnes when treated in combination with bortezomib. Mol Cancer Ther. 2009;(2):292–302.
104. Ma WW, Adjei AA. Novel agents on the horizon for cancer therapy. CA Cancer J Clin. 2009;59:111–37.
105. MacVicar GR, Greco A, Reeves J, Maleski J, Holmlund J, Leopold L. An open-label, multicenter, phase I/II study of AT-101 in combination with docetaxel (D) and prednisone (P) in men with castrate-resistant prostate cancer (CRPC). In: ASCO Annual Meeting, Abstract No 5062; 2009.
106. Maddodi N, Bhat KM, Devi S, Zhang SC, Setaluri V. Oncogenic BRAFV600E induces expression of neuronal differentiation marker MAP2 in melanoma cells by promoter demethylation and down-regulation of transcription repressor HES1. J Biol Chem. 2010;285:242–54.

107. Martin AP, Mitchell C, Rahmani M, Nephew KP, Grant S, Dent P. Inhibition of MCL-1 enhances lapatinib toxicity and overcomes lapatinib resistance via BAK-dependent autophagy. Cancer Biol Ther. 2009;8:2084–96.
108. Martins LM, Iaccarino I, Tenev T, Gschmeissner S, Totty NF, Lemoine NR, et al. The serine protease Omi/HtrA2 regulates apoptosis by binding XIAP through a reaper-like motif. J Biol Chem. 2002;277:439–44.
109. Maurer U, Charvet C, Wagman AS, Dejardin E, Green DR. Glycogen synthase kinase-3 regulates mitochondrial outer membrane permeabilization and apoptosis by destabilization of MCL-1. Mol Cell. 2006;21:749–60.
110. McDermott DF, Sosman JA, Gonzalez R, Hodi FS, Linette GP, Richards J, et al. Double-blind randomized phase II study of the combination of sorafenib and dacarbazine in patients with advanced melanoma: a report from the 11715 Study Group. J Clin Oncol. 2008;26:2178–85.
111. McDermott DF, Sosman JA, Hodi FS, Gonzalez R, Linette G, Richards J, et al. Randomized phase II study of dacarbazine with or without sorafenib in patients with advanced melanoma. J Clin Oncol. 2007;25:Abstract 8511.
112. McGill GG, Horstmann M, Widlund HR, Du J, Motyckova G, Nishimura EK, et al. Bcl2 regulation by the melanocyte master regulator Mitf modulates lineage survival and melanoma cell viability. Cell. 2002;109:707–18.
113. Michaloglou C, Vredeveld LC, Soengas MS, Denoyelle C, Kuilman T, van der Horst CM, et al. BRAFE600-associated senescence-like cell cycle arrest of human naevi. Nature. 2005;436:720–4.
114. Miller LA, Goldstein NB, Johannes WU, Walton CH, Fujita M, Norris DA, et al. BH3 mimetic ABT-737 and a proteasome inhibitor synergistically kill melanomas through Noxa-dependent apoptosis. J Invest Dermatol. 2009;129:964–71.
115. Mohammad RM, Goustin AS, Aboukameel A, Chen B, Banerjee S, Wang G, et al. Preclinical studies of TW-37, a new nonpeptidic small-molecule inhibitor of Bcl-2, in diffuse large cell lymphoma xenograft model reveal drug action on both Bcl-2 and Mcl-1. Clin Cancer Res. 2007;13:2226–35.
116. Moldoveanu T, Liu Q, Tocilj A, Watson M, Shore G, Gehring K. The X-ray structure of a BAK homodimer reveals an inhibitory zinc binding site. Mol Cell. 2006;24:677–88.
117. Montagut C, Settleman J. Targeting the RAF-MEK-ERK pathway in cancer therapy. Cancer Lett. 2009;283:125–34.
118. Nguyen M, Marcellus RC, Roulston A, Watson M, Serfass L, Murthy Madiraju SR, et al. Small molecule obatoclax (GX15-070) antagonizes MCL-1 and overcomes MCL-1-mediated resistance to apoptosis. Proc Natl Acad Sci USA. 2007;104:19512–7.
119. Nikiforov MA, Riblett M, Tang WH, Gratchouck V, Zhuang D, Fernandez Y, et al. Tumor cell-selective regulation of NOXA by c-MYC in response to proteasome inhibition. Proc Natl Acad Sci USA. 2007;104:19488–93.
120. Oltersdorf T, Elmore SW, Shoemaker AR, Armstrong RC, Augeri DJ, Belli BA, et al. An inhibitor of Bcl-2 family proteins induces regression of solid tumours. Nature. 2005;435:677–81.
121. Paik PK, Rudin CM, Brown A, Rizvi NA, Takebe N, Travis W, et al. A phase I study of obatoclax mesylate, a Bcl-2 antagonist, plus topotecan in solid tumor malignancies. Cancer Chemother Pharmacol. 2010;66(6):1079–85.
122. Panka DJ, Mano T, Suhara T, Walsh K, Mier JW. Phosphatidylinositol 3-kinase/Akt activity regulates c-FLIP expression in tumor cells. J Biol Chem. 2001;276:6893–6.
123. Patton EE, Widlund HR, Kutok JL, Kopani KR, Amatruda JF, Murphey RD, et al. BRAF mutations are sufficient to promote nevi formation and cooperate with p53 in the genesis of melanoma. Curr Biol. 2005;15:249–54.
124. Perez-Galan P, Roue G, Lopez-Guerra M, Nguyen M, Villamor N, Montserrat E, et al. BCL-2 phosphorylation modulates sensitivity to the BH3 mimetic GX15-070 (Obatoclax) and reduces its synergistic interaction with bortezomib in chronic lymphocytic leukemia cells. Leukemia. 2008;22:1712–20.
125. Polager S, Ginsberg D. p53 and E2f: partners in life and death. Nat Rev. 2009;9:738–48.

126. Prickett TD, Agrawal NS, Wei X, Yates KE, Lin JC, Wunderlich JR, et al. Analysis of the tyrosine kinome in melanoma reveals recurrent mutations in ERBB4. Nat Genet. 2009;41:1127–32.

127. psahoulia FH, Drosopoulos KG, Doubravska L, Andera L, pintzas A. Quercetin enhances TRAIL-mediated apoptosis in colon cancer cells by inducing the accumulation of death receptors in lipid rafts. Mol Cancer Ther. 2007;(9):2591–9.

128. Puthalakath H, O'Reilly LA, Gunn P, Lee L, Kelly PN, Huntington ND, et al. ER stress triggers apoptosis by activating BH3-only protein Bim. Cell. 2007;129:1337–49.

129. Reu FJ, Bae SI, Cherkassky L, Leaman DW, Lindner D, Beaulieu N, et al. Overcoming resistance to interferon-induced apoptosis of renal carcinoma and melanoma cells by DNA demethylation. J Clin Oncol. 2006;24:3771–9.

130. Schimmer AD, O'Brien S, Kantarjian H, Brandwein J, Cheson BD, Minden MD, et al. A phase I study of the pan bcl-2 family inhibitor obatoclax mesylate in patients with advanced hematologic malignancies. Clin Cancer Res. 2008;14:8295–301.

131. Schwickart M, Huang X, Lill JR, Liu J, Ferrando R, French DM, et al. Deubiquitinase USP9X stabilizes MCL1 and promotes tumour cell survival. Nature. 2010;463:103–7.

132. Segura MF, Hanniford D, Menendez S, Reavie L, Zou X, Alvarez-Diaz S, et al. Aberrant miR-182 expression promotes melanoma metastasis by repressing FOXO3 and microphthalmia-associated transcription factor. Proc Natl Acad Sci USA. 2009;106:1814–9.

133. Sheridan C, Brumatti G, Martin SJ. Oncogenic B-RafV600E inhibits apoptosis and promotes ERK-dependent inactivation of Bad and Bim. J Biol Chem. 2008;283:22128–35.

134. Simonin K, Brotin E, Dufort S, Dutoit S, Goux D, N'Diaye M, et al. Mcl-1 is an important determinant of the apoptotic response to the BH3-mimetic molecule HA14-1 in cisplatin-resistant ovarian carcinoma cells. Mol Cancer Ther. 2009;8:3162–70.

135. Smalley KS, Eisen TG. Farnesyl transferase inhibitor SCH66336 is cytostatic, pro-apoptotic and enhances chemosensitivity to cisplatin in melanoma cells. Int J Cancer. 2003;105:165–75.

136. Smoot RL, Blechacz BR, Werneburg NW, Bronk SF, Sinicrope FA, Sirica AE, et al. A bax-mediated mechanism for obatoclax-induced apoptosis of cholangiocarcinoma cells. Cancer Res. 2010;70:1960–9.

137. Strasser A, Harris AW, Bath ML, Cory S. Novel primitive lymphoid tumours in trangenic mice by cooperation between myc and bcl-2 Nature. 1990;(6299):331–3.

138. Tahir SK, Wass J, Joseph MK, Devanarayan V, Hessler P, Zhang H, et al. Identification of expression signatures predictive of sensitivity to the Bcl-2 family member inhibitor ABT-263 in small cell lung carcinoma and leukemia/lymphoma cell lines. Mol Cancer Ther. 2010;9(3):545–57.

139. Takimoto CH, Awada A. Safety and anti-tumor activity of sorafenib (Nexavar) in combination with other anti-cancer agents: a review of clinical trials. Cancer Chemother Pharmacol. 2008;61:535–48.

140. Tan J, Zhuang L, Jiang X, Yang KK, Karuturi KM, Yu Q. Apoptosis signal-regulating kinase 1 is a direct target of E2F1 and contributes to histone deacetylase inhibitor-induced apoptosis through positive feedback regulation of E2F1 apoptotic activity. J Biol Chem. 2006;281:10508–15.

141. Thallinger C, Wolschek MF, Wacheck V, Maierhofer H, Gunsberg P, Polterauer P, et al. Mcl-1 antisense therapy chemosensitizes human melanoma in a SCID mouse xenotransplantation model. J Invest Dermatol. 2003;120:1081–6.

142. Thorburn A, Behbakht K, Ford H. TRAIL receptor-targeted therapeutics: resistance mechanisms and strategies to avoid them. Drug Resist Updat. 2008;11:17–24.

143. Trudel S, Li ZH, Rauw J, Tiedemann RE, Wen XY, Stewart AK. Preclinical studies of the pan-Bcl inhibitor obatoclax (GX015-070) in multiple myeloma. Blood. 2007;109:5430–8.

144. Tsai J, Lee JT, Wang W, Zhang J, Cho H, Mamo S, et al. Discovery of a selective inhibitor of oncogenic B-Raf kinase with potent antimelanoma activity. Proc Natl Acad Sci USA. 2008;105:3041–6.

145. Tse C, Shoemaker AR, Adickes J, Anderson MG, Chen J, Jin S, et al. ABT-263: a potent and orally bioavailable Bcl-2 family inhibitor. Cancer Res. 2008;68:3421–8.
146. Tseng HY, Jiang CC, Croft A, Tay KH, Thorne RF, Yang F, et al. Contrasting effects of nutlin-3 on TRAIL- and docetaxel-induced apoptosis due to upregulation of TRAIL-R2 and Mcl-1 in human melanoma cells. Mol Cancer Ther. 2010; 9(12): 3363–74.
147. Tsujimoto Y, Cossman J, Jaffe E, Croce CM. Involvement of the bcl-2 gene in human follicular lymphoma. Science. 1985;228:1440–3.
148. Tzung SP, Kim KM, Basanez G, Giedt CD, Simon J, Zimmerberg J, et al. Antimycin A mimics a cell-death-inducing Bcl-2 homology domain 3. Nat Cell Biol. 2001;3:183–91.
149. van Delft MF, Wei AH, Mason KD, Vandenberg CJ, Chen L, Czabotar PE, et al. The BH3 mimetic ABT-737 targets selective Bcl-2 proteins and efficiently induces apoptosis via Bak/Bax if Mcl-1 is neutralized. Cancer Cell. 2006;10:389–99.
150. Van Raamsdonk CD, Bezrookove V, Green G, Bauer J, Gaugler L, O'Brien JM, et al. Frequent somatic mutations of GNAQ in uveal melanoma and blue naevi. Nature. 2009;457:599–602.
151. VanBrocklin MW, Verhaegen M, Soengas MS, Holmen SL. Mitogen-activated protein kinase inhibition induces translocation of Bmf to promote apoptosis in melanoma. Cancer Res. 2009;69:1985–94.
152. Varfolomeev E, Goncharov T, Fedorova AV, Dynek JN, Zobel K, Deshayes K, et al. c-IAP1 and c-IAP2 are critical mediators of tumor necrosis factor alpha (TNFalpha)-induced NF-kappaB activation. J Biol Chem. 2008;283:24295–9.
153. Varfolomeev E, Vucic D. (Un)expected roles of c-IAPs in apoptotic and NFkappaB signaling pathways. Cell Cycle. 2008;7:1511–21.
154. Vaux DL, Cory S, Adams JM. Bcl-2 gene promotes haemopoietic cell survival and cooperates with c-myc to immortalize pre-B cells. Nature. 1988;335:440–2.
155. Verhaegen M, Bauer JA, Martin de la Vega C, Wang G, Wolter KG, Brenner JC, et al. A novel BH3 mimetic reveals a mitogen-activated protein kinase-dependent mechanism of melanoma cell death controlled by p53 and reactive oxygen species. Cancer Res. 2006;66:11348–59.
156. Vilimanovich U, Bumbasirevic V. TRAIL induces proliferation of human glioma cells by c-FLIPL-mediated activation of ERK1/2. Cell Mol Life Sci. 2008;65:814–26.
157. Vogler M, Weber K, Dinsdale D, Schmitz I, Schulze-Osthoff K, Dyer MJ, et al. Different forms of cell death induced by putative BCL2 inhibitors. Cell Death Differ. 2009;16:1030–9.
158. Vucic D, Stennicke HR, Pisabarro MT, Salvesen GS, Dixit VM. ML-IAP, a novel inhibitor of apoptosis that is preferentially expressed in human melanomas. Curr Biol. 2000;10: 1359–66.
159. Walensky LD, Kung AL, Escher I, Malia TJ, Barbuto S, Wright RD, et al. Activation of apoptosis in vivo by a hydrocarbon-stapled BH3 helix. Science. 2004;305:1466–70.
160. Wang G, Nikolovska-Coleska Z, Yang CY, Wang R, Tang G, Guo J, et al. Structure-based design of potent small-molecule inhibitors of anti-apoptotic Bcl-2 proteins. J Med Chem. 2006;49:6139–42.
161. Wang L, Du F, Wang X. TNF-alpha induces two distinct caspase-8 activation pathways. Cell. 2008;133:693–703.
162. Wang YF, Jiang CC, Kiejda KA, Gillespie S, Zhang XD, Hersey P. Apoptosis induction in human melanoma cells by inhibition of MEK is caspase-independent and mediated by the Bcl-2 family members PUMA, Bim, and Mcl-1. Clin Cancer Res. 2007;13:4934–42.
163. Wang Z, Azmi AS, Ahmad A, Banerjee S, Wang S, Sarkar FH, et al. TW-37, a small-molecule inhibitor of Bcl-2, inhibits cell growth and induces apoptosis in pancreatic cancer: involvement of Notch-1 signaling pathway. Cancer Res. 2009;69:2757–65.
164. Weber A, Kirejczyk Z, Potthoff S, Ploner C, Hacker G. Endogenous Noxa determines the strong proapoptotic synergism of the BH3-mimetic ABT-737 with chemotherapeutic agents in human melanoma cells. Transl Oncol. 2009;2:73–83.
165. Weber A, Paschen SA, Heger K, Wilfling F, Frankenberg T, Bauerschmitt H, et al. BimS-induced apoptosis requires mitochondrial localization but not interaction with anti-apoptotic Bcl-2 proteins. J Cell Biol. 2007;177:625–36.
166. Wei J, Kitada S, Rega MF, Emdadi A, Yuan H, Cellitti J, et al. Apogossypol derivatives as antagonists of antiapoptotic Bcl-2 family proteins. Mol Cancer Ther. 2009;8:904–13.

167. Weiss J, Heine M, Korner B, Pilch H, Jung EG. Expression of p53 protein in malignant melanoma: clinicopathological and prognostic implications. Br J Dermatol. 1995;133:23–31.
168. Wellbrock C, Ogilvie L, Hedley D, Karasarides M, Martin J, Niculescu-Duvaz D, et al. V599EB-RAF is an oncogene in melanocytes. Cancer Res. 2004;64:2338–42.
169. Wiezorek J, Holland P, Graves J. Death receptor agonists as a targeted therapy for cancer. Clin Cancer Res. 2010;16(6):1701–8.
170. Wilmott JS, Zhang XD, Hersey P, Scolyer RA. The emerging important role of microRNAS in the pathogenesis, diagnosis and treatment of human cancers. Pathology. 2011;43(6):657–71.
171. Wu ZL, Zheng SS, Li ZM, Qiao YY, Aau MY, Yu Q. Polycomb protein EZH2 regulates E2F1-dependent apoptosis through epigenetically modulating Bim expression. Cell Death Differ. 2010;17(5):801–10.
172. Youle RJ, Strasser A. The BCL-2 protein family: opposing activities that mediate cell death. Nat Rev Mol Cell Biol. 2008;9:47–59.
173. Yu H, McDaid R, Lee J, Possik P, Li L, Kumar SM, et al. The role of BRAF mutation and p53 inactivation during transformation of a subpopulation of primary human melanocytes. Am J Pathol. 2009;174:2367–77.
174. Yu JW, Shi Y. FLIP and the death effector domain family. Oncogene. 2008;27:6216–27.
175. Zawacka-Pankau J, Kostecka A, Sznarkowska A, Hedstrom E, Kawiak A. p73 Tumor suppressor protein: a close relative of p53 not only in structure but also in anti-cancer approach? Cell Cycle. 2010;9(4):720–8.
176. Zerp SF, Stoter R, Kuipers G, Yang D, Lippman ME, van Blitterswijk WJ, et al. AT-101, a small molecule inhibitor of anti-apoptotic Bcl-2 family members, activates the SAPK/JNK pathway and enhances radiation-induced apoptosis. Radiat Oncol. 2009;4:47.
177. Zhang H, Nimmer PM, Tahir SK, Chen J, Fryer RM, Hahn KR, et al. Bcl-2 family proteins are essential for platelet survival. Cell Death Differ. 2007;14:943–51.
178. Zhang HJ, Li WJ, Gu YY, Li SY, An GS, Ni JH, et al. p14ARF interacts with E2F factors to form p14ARF-E2F/partner-DNA complexes repressing E2F-dependent transcription. J Cell Biochem. 2010;109(4):693–701.
179. Zhang XD, Borrow JM, Zhang XY, Nguyen T, Hersey P. Activation of ERK1/2 protects melanoma cells from TRAIL-induced apoptosis by inhibiting Smac/DIABLO release from mitochondria. Oncogene. 2003;22:2869–81.
180. Zhang XD, Gillespie SK, Borrow JM, Hersey P. The histone deacetylase inhibitor suberic bishydroxamate regulates the expression of multiple apoptotic mediators and induces mitochondria-dependent apoptosis of melanoma cells. Mol Cancer Ther. 2004;3:425–35.
181. Zhang XD, Zhang XY, Gray CP, Nguyen T, Hersey P. Tumor necrosis factor-related apoptosis-inducing ligand-induced apoptosis of human melanoma is regulated by smac/DIABLO release from mitochondria. Cancer Res. 2001;61:7339–48.
182. Zhang XY, Zhang XD, Borrow JM, Nguyen T, Hersey P. Translational control of tumor necrosis factor-related apoptosis-inducing ligand death receptor expression in melanoma cells. J Biol Chem. 2004;279:10606–14.
183. Zheng B, Jeong JH, Asara JM, Yuan YY, Granter SR, Chin L, et al. Oncogenic B-RAF negatively regulates the tumor suppressor LKB1 to promote melanoma cell proliferation. Mol Cell. 2009;33:237–47.
184. Zhong Q, Gao W, Du F, Wang X. Mule/ARF-BP1, a BH3-only E3 ubiquitin ligase, catalyzes the polyubiquitination of Mcl-1 and regulates apoptosis. Cell. 2005;121:1085–95.
185. Zhuang L, Lee CS, Scolyer RA, McCarthy SW, Zhang XD, Thompson JF, et al. Mcl-1, Bcl-XL and Stat3 expression are associated with progression of melanoma whereas Bcl-2, AP-2 and MITF levels decrease during progression of melanoma. Mod Pathol. 2007;20:416–26.
186. Zhuang L, Lee CS, Scolyer RA, McCarthy SW, Zhang XD, Thompson JF, et al. Progression in melanoma is associated with decreased expression of death receptors for tumor necrosis factor-related apoptosis-inducing ligand. Hum Pathol. 2006;37:1286–94.
187. zou w, Chen S, Liu x, yue P, Sporn MB, Khuri FR, Sun SY. C-FLIP downregulation contributes to apoptosis induction by the novel synthetic triterpenoid methyl-2-cyano-3, 12-dioxooleana-1, 9-dien-28-oate (CDDD-Me) in human lung cancer cells. Cancer Biol Ther. 2007 oct;6(10):1614–20. Epub 2007 Jul 19. PubMed PMID: 18253090.

Chapter 10
Anti-Angiogenesis Therapy in Melanoma

Daniel S. Chen

Abstract Malignant melanoma is a highly vascular tumor that tends to grow rapidly and metastasize aggressively. The formation of new tumor vasculature (angiogenesis) and lymphatics (lymphangiogenesis) are important steps in the development of melanoma and have been reported to be associated with a poor prognostic significance. Clinical studies of angiogenesis inhibitors suggest a role in the treatment of melanoma, while inhibitors of lymphangiogenesis have not yet been rigorously tested. Further studies of both of these classes of agents will be required to define whether combinations with chemotherapy, immune modulators, signaling inhibitors or other therapies will provide optimal clinical benefit. Together, angiogenesis and lymphangiogenesis are emerging as vital targets for the treatment of melanoma.

Keywords Angiogenesis • Melanoma • Anti-Angiogenic therapy • Combination therapy • Bevacizumab • Sorafenib • Axitinib • Novel therapies • VEGF • Clinical trials • Immunotherapy

Melanoma Is a Highly Vascular Malignancy

Malignant melanoma is a highly vascular tumor that tends to grow rapidly and metastasize aggressively. This vascular phenotype has been observed by both histologic and physiologic analysis [38, 121, 143, 157, 171, 172, 193]. In 1966, Warren and Shubik first observed that human melanoma explants placed into the cheek pouches of hamsters actively induced the formation of new vasculature, including capillary sprouts [187]. These observations have since been extended [90, 174, 187] and a tumor's ability to recruit a supportive vasculature is now clearly recognized as a critical step in

D.S. Chen, MD, PhD (✉)
Medical Oncology, Stanford University, Stanford, CA, USA

Oncology Clinical Development, Genentech Inc., South San Francisco, CA, USA
e-mail: dschen5@stanford.edu

T.F. Gajewski and F.S. Hodi (eds.), *Targeted Therapeutics in Melanoma*,
Current Clinical Oncology, DOI 10.1007/978-1-61779-407-0_10,
© Springer Science+Business Media, LLC 2012

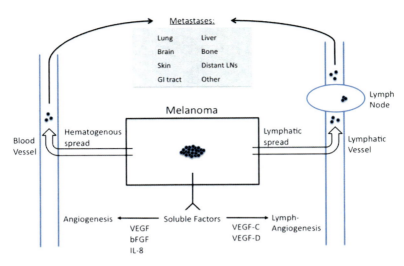

Fig. 10.1 Melanoma angiogenesis and lymphangiogenesis. Melanoma tumors can trigger angiogenesis and lymphangiogenesis. These processes can facilitate metastatic spread [2]

malignant transformation of tumors [76, 77]. Angiogenesis is the biologic process that leads to the formation of new blood vessels [77], and is necessary for expanded growth of tumors beyond 100–200 μm [59]. As the distance between a given melanoma cell and the nearest blood vessel grows, diffusion of nutrients and oxygen to the tumor and removal of carbon dioxide and waste products away from the tumor is diminished and can become inadequate to support further tumor growth [58]. The formation of new tumor vasculature and lymphatics (lymphangiogenesis) may also be important steps in the development of melanoma metastases (Fig. 10.1) [2, 4, 31]. Together, angiogenesis and lymphangiogenesis are emerging as vital targets for the treatment of melanoma.

Melanoma Angiogenesis During Disease Progression

Angiogenic factors can be released from melanoma cells, activated tumor stroma and tumor-infiltrating cells (myeloid cells, T cells, Mast cells), fibroblasts that together orchestrate the formation of a highly perfused tumor vascular bed (Figs. 10.2 and 10.3) [168]. The acquisition of the angiogenic phenotype [75] can be considered as a distinct stage in the evolution of melanoma, generally occurring between the transition from horizontal to vertical growth [8, 48, 116, 158]. Similarly, an analysis of melanoma perfusion using Doppler ultrasound showed blood flow in most melanomas greater than 0.9 mm in thickness, but rarely in thinner melanomas [171].

The vasculature that develops within malignant tumors tends to differ in anatomic structure, organization and function compared to the vessels that perfuse normal tissue [94]. Tumor blood vessels frequently exhibit a disorganized, tortuous

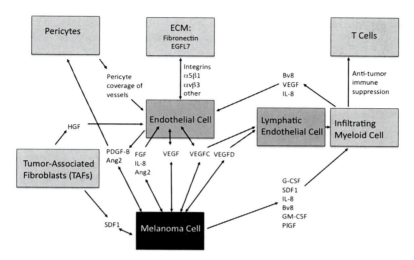

Fig. 10.2 Tumor angiogenesis. Angiogenesis (and lymphangiogenesis) in melanoma results from a complex interplay between different cell types and soluble factors

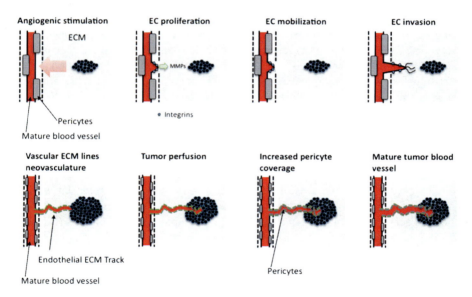

Fig. 10.3 Tumor neo-vascularization. 1. Angiogenic factors and chemokines from tumor act on nearby existing quiescent vessels and circulating endothelial cells; 2. endothelial cells respond to factors by dividing and expressing integrins; 3. secretion of MMPs and MT-MMPs break down ECM and open path for endothelial invasion from existing vessel; 4. endothelial integrins bind to ECM, enabling EC motility and invasion; 5. vessel sprouting led by a tip cell followed by stalk cells extends from existing vessel. Reiteration leads to branching. The new vessels are immature and highly permeable; 6. ECM tract forms around the new blood vessels; 7. pericytes are recruited to line the new blood vessel, decreasing its permeability; 8. further maturation of new blood vessel increases its stability and renders it less dependent on the presence of angiogenic factors

appearance with numerous branch-points and lack the regular pericyte coverage of normal mature vasculature [6]. Functionally, they exhibit an increased permeability, as has been observed through vascular imaging, such as Diffusion Contrast Enhanced MRI (DCE-MRI), that can lead to high interstitial fluid pressure [80]. These differences are likely driven by the dysregulated secretion of angiogenic factors in the tumor microenvironment. Additionally, some melanomas have been proposed to undergo vascular mimicry, where the malignant melanoma cells themselves form tubular structures that can carry blood without the presence of endothelial cells [84]. The similarity in these structures may be mediated by a common set of secreted and surface proteins found on both melanoma cells and endothelial cells, including Eph B4, N-cadherin, integrin $\alpha v \beta 3$ and vascular endothelial growth factor (VEGF) [83, 84, 180].

Mediators of Angiogenesis

Angiogenesis is mediated by a complex array of secreted factors, cell surface receptors, extracellular matrix (ECM) components, and cell types. However, the predominant angiogenic factor produced by melanoma cells is vascular endothelial growth factor (VEGF or VEGF-A) that along with its primary receptor, VEGF receptor-2 (VEGFR2 or KDR) serves as a potent pro-angiogenic and permeability factor. VEGF protein has several isoforms produced both by alternate splicing and post-translational processing. The major isoform is a soluble 45 kDa protein that induces endothelial cell proliferation, migration, permeability, and survival [54, 107]. It is expressed at high levels in human melanoma, as has been observed in all known melanoma lesions in nine patients studied by immunopet imaging using a radiolabelled anti-VEGF antibody tracer [130], and is central to the angiogenic process [40, 43, 53, 98, 130, 176]. Immunohistochemical analysis has also shown increased levels of VEGF in primary melanomas during the transition from horizontal to vertical growth phase [116]. These levels are further increased within metastases, as compared with primary tumors [158, 186]. VEGF family members bind and act through a family of related type III receptor tyrosine kinases (RTKs), VEGFR-1, VEGFR-2 and VEGFR-3, which are primarily expressed on blood and lymphatic endothelial cells (reviewed in [85, 101, 164]). Additionally, VEGF family members can also bind to the Neuropilin family of cell surface receptors, NRP-1 and NRP-2, which may act as co-receptors, modulating vascular biology [3, 46, 85, 105, 114].

Other soluble angiogenic factors likely to contribute to angiogenesis in human melanoma include VEGF-C, basic FGF (bFGF, FGF2), PDGFs, Ang2, IL-8, and uPA (Table 10.1 [113, 136]). VEGF-C can be secreted by melanoma cells, endothelial cells, tumor-associated macrophages (TAMs), and lymphocytes and promotes both angiogenesis and lymphangiogenesis through binding to VEGFR3 and VEGFR2 [16]. bFGF is associated with the ECM and basement membranes of melanoma neo-vasculature and can stimulate endothelial cell proliferation [182]. IL-8

Table 10.1 Mediators of angiogenesis in melanoma

Angiogenic factor	Receptor	Functions/associated with	References
VEGF	VEGFR2 (KDR), NRP1, NRP2, VEGFR1 (Flt-1)	Stimulates endothelial cell proliferation, survival, migration and permeability; central mediator of tumor angiogenesis	[19, 66, 106, 109, 113]
VEGF-C	VEGFR3, NRP2, VEGFR2	Stimulates lymphaendothelial and endothelial cell proliferation, survival and migration leading to lymphangiogenesis and angiogenesis	[19]
VEGF-D	VEGFR3, VEGFR2	Stimulates lymphangiogenesis and angiogenesis	[151, 179]
PIGF-1, PIGF-2	VEGFR1	Recruits bone marrow-derived hematopoietic precursors at site of angiogenesis	[106, 113]
bFGF, FGF family	FGFR family	Stimulates endothelial cell proliferation and vascular tube formation in melanoma	[113, 149, 177]
IL-8	CXCR1, CXCR2	Stimulates endothelial cell proliferation, survival and migration	[113, 119, 135]
HGF	c-met	Endothelial cell mitogen and survival factor	[96]
PDGF-BB, -AB	PDGFR-β	Pericyte mitogen and chemotactic	[9, 134]
Angiopoietin/ Ang1/Ang2/	Tie2	Involved in vascular remodeling and pericyte-mediated maturation	[33, 81, 127]
Bv8	PROKR1, PROKR2	Stimulates endothelial cell proliferation, hematopoietic mobilization	[165, 166]
SDF1 (CXCL12)	CXCR4, CXCR7	Recruits endothelial progenitors	[10]
MMPs	Targets ECM	MMP enzymic activity required for ECM remodeling and vascular invasion	[103]
EphrinB2	EphB4	Regulates tip cell dynamics and may function in vascular mimicry	[47, 89]
BMP9	ALK1	BMP9 (and BMP10) are specific ALK1 ligands that may physiologically trigger the effects of ALK1 on angiogenesis	[32, 124]
PEDF		Inhibits VEGF-VEGF-1/2 activity	[194]
PDGF-C	PDGFRα	Growth factor expressed by various cell types including vascular smooth muscle cells	[30]

(continued)

Table 10.1 (continued)

Endothelial integrins	Ligand	Vascular EC	Lymphatic EC	Endothelial-related function	References
αvβ3	Fibronectin, vitronectin, vWF, thrombospondin, tenascin, DEL1, osteopontin	⊙	⊙	Enables attachment to ECM, EC migration	[2, 113, 163]
α5β1	Fibronectin, L1-CAM	⊙	⊙	Enables attachment to ECM, EC migration. Increased EC expression following stimulation with IL-8, bFGF	[51, 113]
α6β4		⊙		Required for vascular maturation	[113, 133]
α2β1	Collagen, laminin, α3β1	⊙	⊙	Involved in angiogenesis and lymphangiogenesis	[2]
α4β1	CS1 fibronectin, VCAM-1	⊙	⊙	Involved in angiogenesis and lymphangiogenesis, infiltration of bone marrow derived cells	[15, 63]
α1β1	Collagen, laminin,	⊙	⊙	Involved in angiogenesis and lymphangiogenesis	[87]
α9β1	Fibronectin, VCAM, collagen, laminin, thrombospondin, tenascin	⊙	⊙	Involved in angiogenesis and lymphangiogenesis	[72]
αvβ5	Vitronectin, osteopontin, DEL1	⊙	⊙	Involved in angiogenesis, lymphangiogenesis and cell migration	[93, 128]
α6β1	Laminin, merosin, kalinin	⊙		Organization and maintenance of epithelial and endothelial cell layers	[175]
(αMβ2)	ICAM1, iC3b, fibrinogen			Enables leukocyte and myeloid infiltration	[155]

NRP-1	VEGF, Semaphorins	Regulatory role in VEGF-associated angiogenesis and vascular maturation	[106, 178]
NRP-2	VEGF, VEGF-C, Semaphorins	Modulating vascular and lymphatic biology	[46, 190]
uPA	uPAR	Increase tumor vasculature and migration	[113]
TSP-1	ECM, integrins	Associated with increased microvessel infiltration	[70]
Ephrin	Various	Ephrin/Eph signaling mechanisms associated with vasculogenesis, vascular remodeling, angiogenesis, cell migration	[37, 84]
PAR-1	Thrombin	Associated with tumor angiogenesis	[120]
DLL4	Notch1, Notch2	Regulation of VEGF signaling between tip and stalk cells	[13]
EGFL7		Vascular ECM component that forms tumor blood vessel tracts	[142]
MT1-MMP	ECM	Induces EC migration, invasion, differentiation, melanoma vascular mimicry	[65]
EC microtubules		EC structural component	

PlGF placental growth factor; *VEGFR-1* VEGF receptor-1; *uPA/uPAR* urokinase plasminogen activator/receptor; *bFGF* basic fibroblastic growth factor; *PAR-1* protease-activated receptor-1; *BMP* bone morphogenic protein; *TGF-B* transforming growth factor B; *TSP-1* thrombospondin-1 is expressed in malignant melanomas, but is not detectable in benign melanocytic lesions [135, 170] and can induce both endothelial and melanoma cell migration as well as vascular permeability [7]. uPA also mediates endothelial migration and organization [150]. Additional angiogenic factors, such as Bv8, have been shown to be associated with ancillary angiogenic pathways that can mediate active angiogenesis despite VEGF inhibition in pre-clinical melanoma models [165, 166].

The Prognostic Significance of Angiogenesis

The prognostic significance of angiogenesis in melanoma has remained controversial. Srivastava initially reported a correlation between higher vascular area at the base of melanomas and locoregional and systemic metastases [172]. However, some other studies have not corroborated these findings [21, 23]. One possibility is that tumor vascularity of primary melanoma may not be the strongest driver of metastases and disease-free survival in patients presenting with primary disease. In fact, the propensity for local and lymphatic spread of melanoma suggests that lymphangiogenesis may be a more common driver of early disease spread and would reasonably be a stronger prognostic factor for development of disseminated disease and ultimately survival. Indeed, recent reports have shown tumor lymphangiogenesis to be an important element of the metastatic process and a number of VEGF family members are implicated as key mediators of lymphangiogenesis in tumor biology [111, 162, 173]. Once melanoma presents as metastatic disease, metastases exhibiting higher vascularity (or other markers of angiogenesis) may prove to be strongly prognostic for poor overall survival [186]. This association has been recently reported for VEGF levels in patients with Stage IV melanoma [79].

Anti-Angiogenic Therapy in Melanoma

Anti-angiogenic therapy targets a genetically stable host compartment that is fundamental to cancer growth and survival. Its utility in treating cancer has been validated by the broad activity seen with the VEGF-targeted agents across many indications, either alone or in combination with other therapies. Clinical activity has been demonstrated through increased overall survival, improvements in progression-free survival and tumor response rates [20, 60, 91, 110, 122, 126, 159]. Early trials evaluated the effects of more modest anti-angiogenic therapies in melanoma patients. The past decade, however, has brought forward a number of VEGF-targeted agents for evaluation in patients with melanoma. These agents can be classified into those that are highly specific inhibitors of VEGF (or its receptor), the small molecule VEGFR tyrosine kinase inhibitors (VEGFR TKIs) and the indirect inhibitors of VEGF secretion. Additionally, therapies targeting other VEGF family members, angiogenic

Table 10.2 Completed trials of anti-angiogenic agents in melanoma

Anti-angiogenesis agent	Treatment	Study phase and size	Clinical setting	ORR (%)	mPFS (months)	mOS (months)	References
Axitinib	Axitinib (5 mg po bid)	Phase II, $N=32$	Stage IV	15.6	2.3	6.8	[61]
Bevacizumab	Bevacizumab (15 mg/kg IV q2 wk)	Phase II, $N=16$	Stage IV	0	3	8.5	[183]
	Carboplatin (AUC5 IV q3 wk) Paclitaxel (175 mg/m² IV q3 wk) Bevacizumab (15 mg/kg IV q3 wk) (CPB vs. CP)	Randomized Phase II (CP vs. CPB), $N=214$	Stage IV	25.5 (16.4% for CP)	5.6 (4.2 months for CP)	12.3 (8.6 for CP)	K.B. Kim, MD, unpublished data, (2011) [79]
	Carboplatin (AUC6 IV q2 wk) Paclitaxel (80 mg/m² IV q wk 3 of 4) Bevacizumab (10 mg/kg IV q2 wk)	Phase II, $N=53$	Stage IV	17	6	12	[144]
	Paclitaxel (70 mg/m² IV q wk) Bevacizumab (10 mg/kg IV q2 wk)	Phase II, $N=12$	Stage IV	16.6	3.7 (DFS)	7.8	[68]
	Nab-paclitaxel (150 mg/m² IV q wk 3 of 4) Bevacizumab (10 mg/kg IV q2 wk)	Phase II, $N=41$	FL Stage IV	29.7	5.8	NR	[14]
	DTIC (800 mg/m² IV q4 wk) Bevacizumab (10 mg/kg IV q2 wk)	Phase II, $N=40$	FL Stage IV	16.6	6 (TTP)	16.5	[41]
	Temozolomide (150 mg/m² po d 1–7 q2 wk) Bevacizumab (10 mg/kg IV q2 wk)	Phase II, $N=62$	FL Stage IV	16.1	4.2	9.3	[42]
	Oxaliplatin (85 mg/m² IV q2 wk) Sorafenib (200 mg po bid) Bevacizumab (5 mg/kg IV q2 wk)	Phase Ib, $N=6$	Stage IV	16.6	NR	NR	[117]
	Temozolomide (200 mg/m² po d 1–5 q28 d) Sorafenib 400 mg po bid Bevacizumab (5 mg/kg IV q2 wk)	Phase II, $N=35$	FL Stage IV acral melanoma	25.7	NR	NR	[167]
	Erlotinib (150 mg po qd) Bevacizumab (10 mg/kg IV q2 wk)	Phase II, $N=29$	Stage IV	9	3.2	NR	[189]

(continued)

Table 10.2 (continued)

Anti-angiogenesis agent	Treatment	Study phase and size	Clinical setting	ORR (%)	mPFS (months)	mOS (months)	References
	Everolimus (10 mg po qd) Bevacizumab (15 mg/kg IV q3 wk)	Phase II, N=57		12	4	8.6	[74]
	Everolimus (10 mg po qd) Bevacizumab (15 mg/kg IV q3 wk)	Phase II, N=31	Stage IV	4	3.5	NR	[147]
	Interferon 10 MU/m² sq MWF Bevacizumab (15 mg/kg IV q2 wk)	Phase II, N=25	Stage IV	24	4.8	17	[71]
	DTIC (200 mg/m² IV ×5 d q28 d) Interferon-α2a (3MIU sq qd d 15–28) Bevacizumab (5 mg/kg IV q2 wk)	Phase II, N=26	FL Stage IV	23	2.3	11.5	[185]
	DTIC (800 mg/m² IV q4 wk) Bevacizumab (10 mg/kg IV q2 wk)	Phase II, N=8	Stage IV	20	NR	NR	[129]
Cilengitide E7080	Cilengitide (2,000 mg IV twice weekly)	Phase II, N=29	Stage IV	NR	NR	NR	[104]
Etaracizumab	Etaracizumab (8.0 mg/kg IV q wk) ±DTIC (1,000 mg/m² IV q3 wk)	Phase II, N=112; E vs. ED	FL Stage IV	12.7 (0% in E)	2.6 (1.8 in E)	9.4 (12.6 in E)	[82]
MPC-6827 (4-arylamino-quinazoline)	Temozolomide (75 mg/m²/day po ×42 days) MPC-6827 (2.1 mg/m² IV q wk)	Phase I, N=6	Stage IV	17	4.5	NR	[92]
	Temozolomide (85 mg/m²/day po ×21 days) MPC-6827 (2.7 mg/m² IV q wk)	Phase I, N=4	Stage IV	25	4.9	NR	[92]
	Temozolomide (85 mg/m²/day po ×21 days) MPC-6827 (3.3 mg/m² IV q wk)	Phase I, N=12	Stage IV	0	1.5	NR	[92]

PI-88	PI-88 (250 mg/day, 4 consecutive days per week)	Phase II, $N=44$	Stage IV	2.4	NR	NR	[108]
Ramucimurab (IMC-1121B)	Ramucimurab (10 mg/kg q3 wk) ± DTIC (1,000 mg/m² q3 wk)	Phase II, $N=106$; D vs. DR	Stage IV	4 (10%+DTIC)	1.6 (2.7 months +DTIC)	NR	[24]
Semaxanib	Thalidomide (200 mg/day po qd) Semaxanib (145 mg/m² IV q wk) Semaxanib (145 mg/m² IV 2× week)	Phase II, $N=12$	Stage IV	20	NR	NR	[123] [146]
Sorafenib	Sorafenib 400 mg po bid	Phase I/II, $N=35$	Stage IV	31.4	NR	NR	[56]
	Sorafenib (400 mg po bid)	Phase II, $N=36$	FL Stage IIIc or IV	2.8	Median TTP of 63 days	NR	[140]
	Sorafenib (400 mg bid)	Phase II, $N=34$	Advanced melanoma	0	2.7	NR	[44]
	Carboplatin (AUC6 IV q3 wk) Paclitaxel (225 mg/m² IV q3 wk) Sorafenib (400 mg po bid)	Phase III, $N=823$	FL Stage IV	18 (16% for CP)	4.9 (4.1 months for CP)	11.1 (11.3 for CP)	[57]
	Carboplatin (AUC6 IV q3 wk) Paclitaxel (225 mg/m² IV q3 wk) Sorafenib (400 mg po bid)	Phase III, $N=270$	Stage IV	12 (11% for CP)	4.3 (4.4 months for CP)	NR	[78]
	Temozolomide (75 mg/m² po qd for 6 of every 8 weeks or 150 mg/m² daily po qd) Sorafenib (400 mg po qd)	Phase II, $N=167$	Stage IV	NR	5.9 (4.2 months with T)	NR	[1]
	DTIC (1,000 mg/m² q3 wk) Sorafenib (400 mg po bid)	Phase II, $N=101$	FL Stage IV	NR	5.2 (2.9 months with D)	11.8 (10.5 with D)	[118]
	DTIC (1,000 mg/m² IV q3 wk) Sorafenib (400 mg po bid)	Phase II, $N=24$	Advanced metastatic melanoma	NR	NR	NR	[69]

(continued)

Table 10.2 (continued)

Anti-angiogenesis agent	Treatment	Study phase and size	Clinical setting	ORR (%)	mPFS (months)	mOS (months)	References
Sunitinib	Sunitinib (37.5 mg/day po qd)	Pilot study, N=10	Stage IV uveal melanoma	NR	NR	NR	[26]
	Sunitinib (50 mg/day po qd for 4 of every 6 weeks)	Phase II, N=36	Stage IV	8.3	NR	NR	[36]
TKI258	TKI258 (100–175 mg/day)	Phase I, N=35	Stage IV	NR	NR	NR	[160]
Valatinib	Valatinib (dosing not specified)	Phase II, N=29	Stage IV	3.4	NR	NR	[29]
Volociximab	Volociximab (10 mg/kg IV q2 wk) DITC (1,000 mg/m² monthly)	Phase II, N=40	Stage IV	NR	NR	NR	[192]
	Volociximab (15 mg/kg weekly)	Phase II, N=19	Stage IV, relapsed	5.3	NR	NR	[11]
Vorinostat	Vorinostat (400 mg/day)	Phase II, N=32	Advanced melanoma	3.0	4	NR	[73]

factors, and combinations with other therapies have also entered into clinical studies in patients with melanoma (Table 10.2).

Specific Inhibitors of the VEGF Ligand

Specific inhibitors of VEGF signaling include monoclonal antibodies targeting VEGF or its receptor, VEGFR2, and the soluble VEGFR "traps." One example is bevacizumab, a fully humanized monoclonal IgG1 antibody that specifically neutralizes all isoforms of VEGF [55, 148]. The clinical efficacy of bevacizumab has been observed in multiple Phase III studies in metastatic colorectal cancer [91], breast cancer [122], lung cancer (Sandler et al. 2007), renal cell carcinoma [49, 153], and ovarian cancer [20, 145, 181], either in combination with chemotherapy or other biologic therapy. Published studies of bevacizumab in patients with metastatic melanoma have ranged from small single agent anecdotal observations to combination studies with targeted therapy, biologic therapy, and chemotherapy. Single agent bevacizumab therapy has resulted in only a handful of reported observed responses [95, 183] in melanoma patients. Larger studies of either single agent bevacizumab or combinations with interferon-α, erlotinib, and imatinib have also reported only a few responses, making the likelihood of clinical benefit from such regimens unclear. The largest single-agent bevacizumab study is currently being conducted in the adjuvant setting and efficacy results have not yet been reported [12]. In contrast, combinations of bevacizumab with various chemotherapy regimens have suggested potential clinical benefit, with observations of increased RECIST responses, prolonged progression-free survival, and overall survival when compared with historical controls or control arms lacking bevacizumab. Combinations of bevacizumab with DTIC or temozolomide have reported response rates of approximately 16% and median PFS of 4–6 months [42, 185] (Table 10.2). Combination with taxanes, such as paclitaxel or nanoparticle albumin-bound paclitaxel (nab-paclitaxel), has resulted in median PFS of 3–6 months, respectively [14, 68]. Bevacizumab combinations with carboplatin and paclitaxel have been tested in both a single arm multicenter Phase II study [144] and a large randomized placebo-controlled Phase II study (K.B. Kim, MD, unpublished data, 2011) [79]. This combination may be of particular interest, given the surprising activity recently observed with carboplatin and paclitaxel in large Phase III metastatic melanoma studies [57, 78] and the synergy observed between paclitaxel bevacizumab combinations in lung and breast cancer (Sandler et al. 2007) [122]. The single-arm multicenter treatment of 53 patients reported by Perez et al. showed a median overall survival of 12 months, a median progression free-survival of 6 months and an overall response rate of 17% [144]. In a Phase II study of 41 patients with chemotherapy-naive, unresectable stage III or IV melanoma, treatment with nab-paclitaxel and bevacizumab was associated with a median progression-free survival of 5.8 months and an objective response rate of 29.7% [14]. Similarly, the large randomized (214 patient) multicenter placebo-controlled Phase II study of carboplatin (AUC5) paclitaxel (175 mg/kg) and bevacizumab (15 mg/kg) or placebo IV every 21 days showed a median overall survival of 12.3 vs. 8.6 months (HR = 0.67, *p*-value 0.03), progression-free survival of 5.6 vs. 4.2 months (HR = 0.78, *p*-value 0.14), and an objective response rate of 25.5 vs. 16.4% (*p*-value 0.15) favoring the bevacizumab-containing arm at the protocol-defined analysis (K.B. Kim, MD, unpublished data, 2011) [79].

Interestingly, minimal benefit was seen for any of the three above endpoints in the approximately one third of patients that progressed prior to week 16 on study, with the remaining approximately two thirds of patients enrolled showing an even larger magnitude of benefit. Whether these observations reflect upon a less angiogenic-dependent mechanism for the rapidly progressing melanomas, or whether patients with tumors that are growing so quickly are poor candidates for a RECIST-based clinical study is unclear. Overall, the benefit for the addition of bevacizumab in this study was strongest in patients with Stage M1c disease or with an elevated LDH. While this might reflect a statistical anomaly, it seems plausible that the combination of a RECIST-based study and a combination with cytotoxic chemotherapy in melanoma may bias the observed benefit to patients that can stay on treatment long enough to provide adequate exposure to the bevacizumab and chemotherapy. While clinical studies of angiogenesis inhibitors have not adopted modified study approaches that tailor the study design to the expected activity of the therapy, this approach has been adopted by immune therapy modulators, such as anti-CTLA4, and the immune-related response criteria [112] (Wolchok et al. 2009). Alternatively, the rapidly progressing patients may have melanomas that are driven by multiple angiogenic and inflammatory factors, of which VEGF is only one component. The benefit seen in patients with elevated LDH may also reflect hypoxic conditions within the tumor, which may also be associated with VEGF up-regulation and tumor dependence on angiogenesis for further disease progression. Further validation of these findings and potential biomarkers for identifying patients that will receive the optimal clinical benefit will require a definitive Phase III study.

Small Molecule VEGFR TKIs

Small molecule tyrosine kinase inhibitors (TKIs) that inhibit VEGF receptor-mediated signaling have shown clear activity in a number of highly VEGF-responsive diseases, including renal cell carcinoma, hepatocellular carcinoma, neuroendocrine tumors, and thyroid-carcinoma [27, 34, 50, 126, 132, 152, 154]. While no truly VEGFR2-selective TKIs have been identified to date, the VEGFR2 TKIs currently in clinical development can be classified into those that are more VEGFR-specific (e.g. axitinib, Tivozanib), those which inhibit a broader spectrum of angiogenic targets, including those in the PDGFR family (e.g. sorafenib, semaxanib, ABT869), and those with a very broad spectrum of kinase targets (sunitinib). In contrast to the VEGF-targeted biologics, VEGFR TKIs are orally available and exhibit a range of half-lives and exposures. However, their utility can be complicated by off-target (non-VEGF) toxicities and pharmacokinetic variability, and thus have had limited success in tolerably combining with standard of care chemotherapies, given the potential for overlapping toxicities. Such toxicities can lead to dose reductions and sporadic VEGF inhibition, thereby limiting their therapeutic effects. Not surprisingly, the activity of these agents appears to be most evident in single agent treatment settings, rather than in combination with chemotherapy. In contrast to bevacizumab, sorafenib has failed to demonstrate efficacy in Phase III studies in combination with carboplatin and paclitaxel in lung cancer [64, 161] and in both first-line and second-line studies of melanoma patients [57, 78]. However, promising single agent results in melanoma have been reported with a number of VEGFR TKIs, including axitinib and sunitinib, where response rates have ranged from 8.3 to 15.6% [35, 61].

Agents with Indirect Effects on Angiogenesis

Agents that have an indirect effect on the angiogenic processes have been available for many years. These include thalidomide and its more potent derivative lenalidomide, as well as the cytokine interferon alpha (Interferon-α). Treatment with interferon-α, for example, has been shown to decrease levels of the pro-angiogenic factors bFGF and IL8 [137, 169, 184]. In clinical trials, thalidomide showed promising early results in combination with chemotherapy for the treatment of advanced melanoma [188]. More recently, however, Phase II clinical trials have shown that addition of thalidomide to dacarbazine [139] or temozolomide [28] was not associated with further benefits over chemotherapy alone. Lenalidomide monotherapy has been evaluated in patients with advanced refractory or relapsed melanoma, with limited evidence of efficacy [45, 67]. Phase I and II studies of lenalidomide in combination with chemotherapy are ongoing. Interferon-α has been evaluated in numerous studies in patients with melanoma, both as adjuvant therapy and for treatment of advanced disease. A recent meta-analysis of 14 randomized, controlled studies of adjuvant interferon-α found that treatment was associated with significant improvements in disease-free and overall survival [125]. High-dose interferon-α in patients with advanced melanoma has been evaluated in numerous studies, and appears to show benefits on disease-free progression without improving overall survival and with substantial toxicity [18]. However, it is unclear how much of the anti-melanoma activity of interferon is attributable to its modest anti-angiogenic properties compared to its immunomodulatory effects.

Other Anti-Angiogenic Therapies

The tumor-associated vasculature present in melanomas include several components that provide potential targets for emerging therapies. These components include (1) the small diameter, tortuous, immature blood vessels that are rapidly pruned by therapies that target VEGF, (2) larger, more mature (and less VEGF-dependent) blood vessels, (3) ECM components to which endothelial cells attach, (4) pericyte and other stromal cells that support endothelial cells, (5) lymphatic endothelial cells (6) infiltrating myeloid cells. The larger, less VEGF-dependent vessels are potentially a target of the class of vascular disrupting agents (VDAs) and recent studies suggest they may have activities complementary to VEGF inhibitors [92]. A number of monoclonal antibodies designed to inhibit ECM-endothelial cell interactions and thus prevent further angiogenesis are currently in testing, including anti-integrin $\alpha v\beta3$, anti-integrin $\alpha5\beta1$ and anti-EGFL7 [22, 39, 88, 156].

The integrins, specifically vascular-enriched integrins, contribute to tumor angiogenesis by supporting endothelial cell adhesion, migration, and modulation of growth factor signaling. $\alpha v\beta3$ is an integrin that binds vitronectin. Expressed on the surface of many melanomas and proliferating endothelial cells, inhibition of $\alpha v\beta3$ binding to vitronectin may interfere with angiogenesis. However, blockade of $\alpha v\beta3$ integrin binding by the monoclonal antibody etaracizumab when combined with dacarbazine in a phase II trial ($n=112$) has shown no significant improvement over dacarbazine alone [82]. In addition, a phase II trial ($n=26$) showed cilengitide, an antagonist of both $\alpha v\beta5$ and $\alpha v\beta3$ binding, to have minimal clinical efficacy as monotherapy for melanoma [104]. Similarly, $\alpha5\beta1$ is an integrin that binds fibronectin and is reported to support embryonic and tumor vascular growth. Volocizumab, an antibody directed against $\alpha5\beta1$ showed only a 5.3% response rate as monotherapy in a phase II study in melanoma.

EGFL7 is another ECM component that forms peri-vascular tracks along which blood vessels grow and provide both adhesive function and pro-survival signals to endothelial cells. Anti-angiogenic therapy that leads to pruning of tumor-associated blood vessels leave behind these EGFL7 "ghost" tracks. Cessation of therapy has been observed to result in rapid re-growth of the tumor blood vessels along the existing tracks [115]. Clinical trials examining monoclonal antibodies directed against each of these ECM components are currently on-going. However, the optimal approach to using such therapies may require further investigation. Pericyte biology can also be affected by inhibitors of PDGFR-β, endoglin, angiopoeitin-2 (Ang2) or neuropilin-1 (NRP1) [46, 136]. This inhibition may prevent the further maturation of VEGF-dependent tumor blood vessels to a VEGF-independent state, and the clinical impact of this inhibition is currently being investigated [141]. Inhibitors of lymphangiogenesis and tumor-infiltrating inflammatory myeloid cells have shown anti-tumor activity in pre-clinical models and represent further approaches to blocking tumor perfusion, spread and immune evasion [4, 97, 165].

Several different subtypes of tumor-infiltrating myeloid cells have been recently identified. These include immature myeloid cells (which include myeloid-derived suppressor cells, or MDSCs), Tie2-expressing monocytes (TEMs) and M2 TAMs; collectively, their described functions support the interaction between angiogenesis and inflammation. Each of these populations of myeloid cells can infiltrate tumors, promote tumor angiogenesis through the secretion of pro-angiogenic factors, such as VEGF, IL-8 and Bv8, and play a role in the progression of tumors. Additionally, tumor-infiltrating immature myeloid cells and MDSCs can increase in response to treatment, such as with chemotherapy [102, 138, 165, 191] and suppress anti-tumor immune responses through numerous immune regulatory factors, including IL-10 and arginase. Targeting these cells directly, or the factors that stimulate their increase in tumors, may result in blocking a potential tumor angiogenesis-escape pathway as well as improve anti-tumor immune responses.

Inhibition of lymphangiogenesis has recently been shown to reduce the formation of lymph node and distant organ metastasis in a number of pre-clinical studies [25, 190]. The mediators of lymphangiogenesis are not yet comprehensively understood, but is rapidly increasing. The most compelling evidence comes from the VEGF-C/D signaling axis, where overexpression in cell lines with limited metastatic capacity or inhibition of endogenous or over-expressed factors have led to observations that include changes in metastatic spread to regional lymph nodes and distant organs. Further clinical studies that elucidate the impact of lymphangiogenic inhibition on adjuvant treatment of stage II or stage III melanoma, and perhaps specifically, in transit disease, will likely determine the potential value of targeting this pathway in the treatment of melanoma.

Anti-Angiogenic Combinations

Numerous studies are investigating the potential for combining anti-angiogenic agents with other biologic or cytotoxic agents (Table 10.3). Highly specific anti-angiogenic inhibitors can be used in combination with many other therapeutic agents, due to non-overlapping adverse effects. The most common anti-VEGF class effects include hypertension and proteinuria, which are uncommon toxicities of other therapies. More severe toxicities, such as gastrointestinal perforations, have occurred rarely with anti-angiogenic therapy in melanoma, despite initial concerns given frequent metastasis to the intestinal tract. No new adverse events specific to melanoma treatment with anti-angiogenic agents have been observed in clinical studies. In addition to having a favorable toxicity profile for combination treatment, synergy with other therapies has been best defined with chemotherapy combinations thus far. Theories for why chemotherapy may combine well with anti-angiogenesis agents include: (1) "vascular normalization," where anti-angiogenic treatment leads to rapid pruning of the abnormal tumor vasculature, leading to decreased interstitial tumor pressure and increased delivery of chemotherapy to tumor cells, (2) synergistic anti-angiogenic activity of chemotherapy agents and anti-angiogenic therapy, particularly in the setting of metronomic taxanes, and (3) blunting of post-chemotherapy re-growth (such as increased VEGF production [100, 102, 144]), (4) direct effects of chemotherapy on endothelial cells [5]. Regardless of the mechanism, the combination of chemotherapy and anti-angiogenesis inhibitors has proven highly successful in colon, breast, lung cancers, and thus far, the combination of carboplatin, paclitaxel, and bevacizumab also appears to be active in melanoma.

Beyond chemotherapy, anti-angiogenesis agents have been combined with a number of other targeted therapies. These combinations can be separated into combinations of multiple angiogenesis inhibitors vs. combinations with other non-angiogenesis targeted therapies. In renal cell carcinoma, high dose IL-2, Interferon and mTOR inhibitors have been combined with bevacizumab and various VEGFR TKIs. In melanoma, small signal-seeking studies of bevacizumab and erlotinib (EGFRi) or imatinib (PDGF/cKITi) combinations have not shown

Table 10.3 On-going/unpublished trials of anti-angiogenic agents in melanoma

Primary molecular target	Agent	Clinical setting	Treatment	PI/cooperative group	Clinicaltrials. gov reference
VEGF	Bevacizumab	Neoadjuvant uveal	Monotherapy	David Abramson, MD	NCT00596362
		Adjuvant	Monotherapy	Pippa Corrie, PhD, FRCP	N/A (AVAST-M study)
		Stage IV	+Ipilimumab (Phase I)	F. Stephen Hodi, MD	NCT00790010
		Stage IV	+Fotemustine	Not stated	NCT01069627
		Stage IV	+Carboplatin+paclitaxel ± everolimus	Robert McWilliams, MD/NCCTG	NCT00976573
		CNS+	+Temozolomide	Jose Lutzky, MD	NCT01048554
		Stage IV	+Temozolomide vs. +carboplatin+paclitaxel	Svetomir Markovic, MD, PhD/NCCTG	NCT00626405
		Stage IV	+Rad001	John D. Hainsworth, MD/SCRI	NCT00591734
		Stage IV	+Sorafenib+oxaliplatin	Edward F. McClay, MD	NCT00538005
		Stage IV	Monotherapy vs. +IFN-α2b	William E. Carson, MD/NCI	NCT00026221
		Stage IV	+Temsirolimus	Craig L. Slingluff, MD/NCI	NCT00397982
		Stage IV	+Carboplatin+paclitaxel	Not stated	NCT00434252
	Aflibercept	Stage IV	Monotherapy	Ahmad A. Tarhini, MD, MS/ California Cancer Consortium	NCT00450255
	Sorafenib	Stage IV	+Bortezomib (Phase I)	Ryan J. Sullivan, MD	NCT01078961
		Stage III extremity	+Melphalan (Phase I)	Douglas S. Tyler, MD	NCT00565968
		Stage IV	+Temsirolimus (Phase I)	Kevin Kim, MD	NCT00349206
		Stage IV	+Biochemo (temozolomide +vinblastine+cisplatin+IL-2+IFN-α)	Michael A. Morse, MD	NCT00673361

Class	Drug	Regimen	Stage	Investigator	NCT number
		+Tamoxifen+Cisplatin	Adjuvant	Edward F. McClay, MD	NCT00492505
		+CP-4055	Stage IV	Svein Dueland, MD	NCT00498836
		+Pegylated IFN-α2b		Axel Hauschild, MD	NCT00623402
		+Carboplatin+paclitaxel	Uveal	Jeffrey S. Weber, MD, PhD/SWOG	NCT00329641
		+Temsirolimus vs. +tipifarnib	Stage IV	Vernon K. Sondak, MD/SWOG	NCT00281957
		+Bevacizumab+oxaliplatin	Stage IV	Edward F McClay, MD	NCT00538005
	Cediranib	Monotherapy	Stage IV	Elaine McWhirter, MD, MSC, FRCPC	NCT00243061
	Pazopanib	Monotherapy	Stage IV	Amy Weise, DO	NCT00861913
		+Paclitaxel	Stage IV	John Fruehauf, MD, PhD	NCT01107665
	Vatalanib	Monotherapy	Stage IV	Pippa Corrie, PhD, FRCP	NCT00563823
		+Everolimus	Stage IV	Julian Molina, MD, PhD	NCT00655655
	TKI258	Monotherapy	Stage IV	Not stated	NCT00303251
BRAF/VEGF	RAF265	Monotherapy	Stage III or IV	Amanda May, MD, William	NCT00304525
Multitarget TKI	Sunitinib	+Temozolomide	Stage IV	Bartosz Chmielowski, MD	NCT01005472
		+Temozolomide	Stage IV	Bartosz Chmielowski, MD, PhD	NCT00859326
		+Tamoxifen+cisplatin	Adjuvant uveal	Edward F. McClay, MD	NCT00489944
		+Lenalidomide+cyclophosphamide	Stage IV uveal	Steven K. Libutti, MD	NCT00482911

(continued)

Table 10.3 (continued)

Primary molecular target	Agent	Clinical setting	Treatment	PI/cooperative group	Clinicaltrials. gov reference
Heparanase	PI-88	Stage IV	Monotherapy	Not stated	NCT00068172
		Stage IV	Monotherapy	S.G. Eckhardt, MD	NCT00073892
		Stage IV	+Dacarbazine	Damien Thomson, MD	NCT00130442
Integrin avb3	Cilengitide	Stage IV	Monotherapy	Kevin B. Kim, MD	NCT00082875
	CNTO95	Stage IV	Monotherapy vs. +DITC vs. DITC	Centocor, Inc.	NCT00246012
Integrin a5b1	Volociximab	Stage IV	+DITC	Steven J. O'Day, MD	NCT00099970
MMPs	COL-3 (NSC-683551)	Stage IV	Monotherapy	National Cancer Institute	NCT00001683
Vascular disrupting agent	Vorinostat	Metastatic or unresectable	MONOTHERAPY	Naomi S. Balzer-Haas, MD	NCT00121225
		N/A	+NPI-0052	Christopher Sweeney, MD	NCT00667082

clearly appreciable activity. However, recent results from a study of bevacizumab with everolimus (mTOR inhibitor) suggest activity for the combination of two targeted therapies in melanoma without the addition of chemotherapy [74]. Combinations between anti-angiogenic therapies and B-RAF inhibitors have not been initiated, but may well be warranted, particularly if the possibility that anti-angiogenic therapy might prevent or slow the development of resistance to B-RAF inhibition in melanoma.

There is strong interest in combinations of anti-angiogenic therapies and immune modulatory agents, such as CTLA-4 inhibitors. As reported by Gabrilovich et al., VEGF may affect monocyte maturation and activation and has been proposed to affect certain subsets of dendritic cells [62]. VEGF blockade can also decrease tumor interstitial fluid pressure and tumor hypoxia and may improve lymphocyte-vessel wall interactions, which could improve trafficking and activity of tumor-infiltrating lymphocytes, NK or other hematopoietic cells [17, 99, 131]. Additionally, this inhibition may also decrease the infiltration of pro-angiogenic myeloid cells as previously described. The combination of bevacizumab and interferon in 25 patients with Stage IV melanoma was recently reported by Grignol et al. and found to be tolerable and associated with a response rate of 24% and a median survival of 17 months [71]. While the study was small, it clearly contrasts with the limited activity reported by the same group for a combination of bevacizumab and a low, non-immunomodulatory dose of interferon [183]. A study of bevacizumab and ipilimumab (anti-CTLA4) is currently examining a more active immune-modulatory agent combined with anti-angiogenic therapy, and will hopefully provide results for both the tolerability and efficacy of the combination soon [86].

Conclusions

Malignant melanoma is a highly vascular tumor associated with limited treatment options and short survival. However, therapy for this disease is rapidly changing. Advances in our understanding of the molecular alterations that drive its behavior are leading to encouraging results from clinical studies. Therapies that target critical mutations that lead to uncontrolled growth and escape from immune surveillance are now well established for the treatment of metastatic melanoma. Completed clinical studies already have demonstrated the potential benefit of anti-angiogenic treatment. Monoclonal antibodies targeting VEGF, in combination with chemotherapy have shown activity leading to improvements in response rates and survival in metastatic melanoma, whereas small molecule TKIs that inhibit signaling through multiple angiogenic receptors have shown responses as monotherapy. Given the number of genetic alterations present in melanoma cells [52] it is most likely that patients will benefit most from combination therapies that inhibit multiple pathways in a highly selective manner. Anti-angiogenic and anti-lymphangiogenic therapy will likely represent one such approach, and benefit from targeting a genetically stable pathway associated with both melanoma disease progression and prognosis. Its limited overlapping treatment toxicity with other therapies and synergistic potential, observed thus far with immunotherapy and cytotoxic therapy, make it an important approach to further investigate in on-going and future clinical studies. Increasing our understanding of these therapies in melanoma, whether they should be used in combination with other therapies or sequentially, and in which patient subsets should be key objectives in melanoma treatment for years to come.

References

1. Amaravadi RK, Schuchter LM, McDermott DF, et al. Phase II trial of temozolomide and sorafenib in advanced melanoma patients with or without brain metastases. Clin Cancer Res. 2009;15:7711–8.
2. Avraamides CJ, Garmy-Susini B, Varner JA. Integrins in angiogenesis and lymphangiogenesis. Nat Rev Cancer. 2008;8:604–17.
3. Bagri A, Tessier-Lavigne M, Watts RJ. Neuropilins in tumor biology. Clin Cancer Res. 2009;15:1860–4.
4. Bagri A, Kouros-Mehr H, Leong KG, Plowman GD. Use of anti-VEGF adjuvant therapy in cancer: challenges and rationale. Trends Mol Med. 2010;16:122–32.
5. Bagri A, Berry L, Gunter B, et al. Effects of anti-VEGF treatment duration on tumor growth, tumor regrowth, and treatment efficacy. Clin Cancer Res. 2010;16:3887–900.
6. Baluk P, Hashizume H, McDonald DM. Cellular abnormalities of blood vessels as targets in cancer. Curr Opin Genet Dev. 2005;15:102–11.
7. Bar-Eli M. Role of interleukin-8 in tumor growth and metastasis of human melanoma. Pathobiology. 1999;67:12–8.
8. Barnhill RL. Melanocytic nevi and tumor progression: perspectives concerning histomorphology, melanoma risk and molecular genetics. Dermatology. 1993;187:86–90.
9. Barnhill RL, Xiao M, Graves D, et al. Expression of platelet-derived growth factor (PDGF)-A, PDGF-B and the PDGF-alpha receptor, but not the PDGF-beta receptor, in human malignant melanoma in vivo. Br J Dermatol. 1996;135:898–904.
10. Bartolomé RA, Gálvez BG, Longo N, et al. Stromal cell-derived factor-1alpha promotes melanoma cell invasion across basement membranes involving stimulation of membrane-type 1 matrix metalloproteinase and Rho GTPase activities. Cancer Res. 2004;64:2534–43.
11. Barton J. A multicenter phase II study of volociximab in patients with relapsed metastatic melanoma. J Clin Oncol. 2008;26(Suppl):495s (Abstract 9051).
12. Basu B, Biswas S, Wrigley J, Sirohi B, Corrie P. Angiogenesis in cutaneous malignant melanoma and potential therapeutic strategies. Expert Rev Anticancer Ther. 2009;9:1583–98.
13. Bentley K, Mariggi G, Gerhardt H, Bates PA. Tipping the balance: robustness of tip cell selection, migration and fusion in angiogenesis. PLoS Comput Biol. 2009;5:e1000549.
14. Boasberg P, Cruickshank S, Hamid O, O'Day S, Weber R, Spitler L. Nab-paclitaxel and bevacizumab as first-line therapy in patients with unresectable stage III and IV melanoma. J Clin Oncol. 2009;27(15s Suppl):476s (Abstract 9061).
15. Boehmler AM, Drost A, Jaggy L, et al. The CysLT1 ligand leukotriene D4 supports alpha-4beta1- and alpha5beta1-mediated adhesion and proliferation of CD34+ hematopoietic progenitor cells. J Immunol. 2009;182:6789–98.
16. Boone B, Blokx W, De Bacquer D, et al. The role of VEGF-C staining in predicting regional metastasis in melanoma. Virchows Arch. 2008;453:257–65.
17. Bouzin C, Brouet A, De Vriese J, et al. Effects of vascular endothelial growth factor on the lymphocyte-endothelium interactions: identification of caveolin-1 and nitric oxide as control points of endothelial cell anergy. J Immunol. 2007;178:1505–11.
18. Bracarda S, Eggermont AM, Samuelsson J. Redefining the role of interferon in the treatment of malignant diseases. Eur J Cancer. 2010;46:284–397.

19. Brychtova S, Bezdekova M, Brychta T, Tichy M. The role of vascular endothelial growth factors and their receptors in malignant melanomas. Neoplasma. 2008;55:273–9.
20. Burger RA, Brady MF, Bookman MA, et al. Phase III trial of bevacizumab (BEV) in the primary treatment of advanced epithelial ovarian cancer (EOC), primary peritoneal cancer (PPC), or fallopian tube cancer (FTC): A Gynecologic Oncology Group study. J Clin Oncol. 2010;28(15s Suppl):946s (Abstract LBA1).
21. Busam KJ, Berwick M, Blessing K, et al. Tumor vascularity is not a prognostic factor for malignant melanoma of the skin. Am J Pathol. 1995;147:1049–56.
22. Campagnolo L, Leahy A, Chitnis S, et al. EGFL7 is a chemoattractant for endothelial cells and is up-regulated in angiogenesis and arterial injury. Am J Pathol. 2005;167:275–84.
23. Carnochan P, Briggs JC, Westbury G, Davies AJ. The vascularity of cutaneous melanoma: a quantitative histological study of lesions 0.85-1.25 mm in thickness. Br J Cancer. 1991;64:102–7.
24. Carvajal RD, Wong MK, Thompson JA, et al. A phase II randomized study of ramucirumab (IMC-1121B) with or without dacarbazine (DTIC) in patients (pts) with metastatic melanoma (MM). J Clin Oncol. 2010;28(15s Suppl):615s (Abstract 8519).
25. Caunt M, Mak J, Liang WC, et al. Blocking neuropilin-2 function inhibits tumor cell metastasis. Cancer Cell. 2008;13:331–42.
26. Chan KR, Gundala S, Laudadio M, Mastrangelo M, Yamamoto A, Sato T. A pilot study using sunitinib malate as therapy in patients with stage IV uveal melanoma. J Clin Oncol. 2008;26(Suppl):494s (Abstract 9047).
27. Cheng AL, Kang YK, Chen Z, et al. Efficacy and safety of sorafenib in patients in the Asia-Pacific region with advanced hepatocellular carcinoma: a phase III randomised, double-blind, placebo-controlled trial. Lancet Oncol. 2009;10:25–34.
28. Clark JI, Moon J, Hutchins LF, et al. Phase 2 trial of combination thalidomide plus temozolomide in patients with metastatic malignant melanoma: Southwest Oncology Group S0508. Cancer. 2010;116:424–31.
29. Cook N, Kareclas P, Mann C, et al. A phase II study of PTK787 in patients with metastatic melanoma (CAMEL02). National Cancer Research Institute Cancer Conference 2008 (Abstract BOA20).
30. Crawford Y, Kasman I, Yu L, et al. PDGF-C mediates the angiogenic and tumorigenic properties of fibroblasts associated with tumors refractory to anti-VEGF treatment. Cancer Cell. 2009;15:21–34.
31. Dadras SS, Paul T, Bertoncini J, et al. Tumor lymphangiogenesis: a novel prognostic indicator for cutaneous melanoma metastasis and survival. Am J Pathol. 2003;162:1951–60.
32. David L, Mallet C, Mazerbourg S, Feige JJ, Bailly S. Identification of BMP9 and BMP10 as functional activators of the orphan activin receptor-like kinase 1 (ALK1) in endothelial cells. Blood. 2007;109:1953–61.
33. De Palma M, Venneri MA, Rossella Galli R, et al. Tie2 identifies a hematopoietic lineage of proangiogenic monocytes required for tumor vessel formation and a mesenchymal population of pericyte progenitors. Cancer Cell. 2005;8:211–26.
34. De Souza JA, Busaidy N, Zimrin A, et al. Phase II trial of sunitinib in medullary thyroid cancer (MTC). J Clin Oncol. 2010;28(15s Suppl):422s (Abstract 5504).
35. Decoster L, Vande Broek I, Declerq D, et al. Activity of sunitinib in advanced malignant melanoma and its correlation with potential predictive biomarkers. Eur J Cancer Suppl. 2009;7:577–8 (Abstract 9305).
36. Decoster L, Neyns B, Vande Broek I, et al. Activity of sunitinib in advanced malignant melanoma and its correlation with potential predictive biomarkers. J Clin Oncol. 2010;28(15s Suppl):615s (Abstract 8518).
37. Demou ZN, Hendrix MJ. Microgenomics profile the endogenous angiogenic phenotype in subpopulations of aggressive melanoma. J Cell Biochem. 2008;105:562–73.
38. Denijn M, Ruiter DJ. The possible role of angiogenesis in the metastatic potential of human melanoma. Clinicopathological aspects. Melanoma Res. 1993;3:5–14.
39. Desgrosellier JS, Cheresh DA. Integrins in cancer: biological implications and therapeutic opportunities. Nat Rev Cancer. 2010;10:9–22.

40. Detmar M. Molecular regulation of angiogenesis in the skin. J Invest Dermatol. 1996;106:207–8.
41. Di Pietro A, Ferrucci P, Munzone E, et al. Dacarbazine (DTIC) plus bevacizumab (B) combination therapy in chemotherapy (CTh)-naïve advanced melanoma (MM) patients (pts): a phase II study. J Clin Oncol. 2010;28(15s Suppl):620s (Abstract 8536).
42. Dummer R, Michielin O, Seifert B, et al. First-line temozolomide (TEM) combined with bevacizumab (BEV) in metastatic melanoma (MM): a multicenter phase II trial (SAKK 50/07). J Clin Oncol. 2010;28(15s Suppl):616s (Abstract 8521).
43. Dvorak HF, Detmar M, Claffey KP, Nagy JA, van de Water L, Senger DR. Vascular permeability factor/vascular endothelial growth factor: an important mediator of angiogenesis in malignancy and inflammation. Int Arch Allergy Immunol. 1995;107:233–5.
44. Eisen T, Ahmad T, Flaherty KT, et al. Sorafenib in advanced melanoma: a Phase II randomised discontinuation trial analysis. Br J Cancer. 2006;95:581–6.
45. Eisen T, Trefzer U, Hamilton A, et al. Results of a multicenter, randomized, double-blind phase 2/3 study of lenalidomide in the treatment of pretreated relapsed or refractory metastatic malignant melanoma. Cancer. 2010;116:146–54.
46. Ellis LM. The role of neuropilins in cancer. Mol Cancer Ther. 2006;5:1099–107.
47. Erber R, Eichelsbacher U, Powajbo V, et al. EphB4 controls blood vascular morphogenesis during postnatal angiogenesis. EMBO J. 2006;25:628–41.
48. Erhard H, Rietveld FJ, van Altena MC, Bröcker EB, Ruiter DJ, de Waal RM. Transition of horizontal to vertical growth phase melanoma is accompanied by induction of vascular endothelial growth factor expression and angiogenesis. Melanoma Res. 1997;7 Suppl 2:S19–26.
49. Escudier B, Pluzanska A, Koralewski P, et al., for the AVOREN Trial investigators. Bevacizumab plus interferon alfa-2a for treatment of metastatic renal cell carcinoma: a randomised, double-blind phase III trial. Lancet. 2007;370:2103–11.
50. Escudier B, Eisen T, Stadler WM, et al. Sorafenib for treatment of renal cell carcinoma: final efficacy and safety results of the phase III treatment approaches in renal cancer global evaluation trial. J Clin Oncol. 2009;27:3312–8.
51. Eskens FA, Dumez H, Hoekstra R, et al. Phase I and pharmacokinetic study of continuous twice weekly intravenous administration of Cilengitide (EMD 121974), a novel inhibitor of the integrins alphavbeta3 and alphavbeta5 in patients with advanced solid tumours. Eur J Cancer. 2003;39:917–26.
52. Fecher LA, Cummings SD, Keefe MJ, et al. Toward a molecular classification of melanoma. J Clin Oncol. 2007;25:1606–20.
53. Ferrara N. Molecular and biological properties of vascular endothelial growth factor. J Mol Med. 1999;77:527–43.
54. Ferrara N, Gerber HP, LeCouter J. The biology of VEGF and its receptors. Nat Med. 2003;9(6):669–76.
55. Ferrara N, Hillan KJ, Gerber HP, Novotny W. Discovery and development of bevacizumab, an anti-VEGF antibody for treating cancer. Nat Rev Drug Discov. 2004;3:391–400.
56. Flaherty K, Brose M, Schuchter L, et al. Phase I/II trial of BAY 43-9006, carboplatin (C) and paclitaxel (P) demonstrates preliminary antitumor activity in the expansion cohort of patients with metastatic melanoma. Proc Am Soc. 2004;23:708 (Abstract 7507).
57. Flaherty KT, Lee SJ, Schuchter LM, et al. Final results of E2603: A double-blind, randomized phase III trial comparing carboplatin (C)/paclitaxel (P) with or without sorafenib (S) in metastatic melanoma. J Clin Oncol. 2010;28(15s Suppl):613s (Abstract 8511).
58. Folkman J. Tumor angiogenesis: therapeutic implications. N Engl J Med. 1971;285:1182–6.
59. Folkman J. Angiogenesis and apoptosis. Semin Cancer Biol. 2003;13:159–67.
60. Friedman HS, Prados MD, Wen PY, et al. Bevacizumab alone and in combination with irinotecan in recurrent glioblastoma. J Clin Oncol. 2009;27:4733–40.
61. Fruehauf JP, Lutzky J, McDermott DF, et al. Axitinib (AG-013736) in patients with metastatic melanoma: a phase II study. J Clin Oncol. 2008;26(20 Suppl):484s (Abstract 9006).
62. Gabrilovich DI, Chen HL, Girgis KR, et al. Production of vascular endothelial growth factor by human tumors inhibits the functional maturation of dendritic cells. Nat Med. 1996;2:1096–103.

63. Garmy-Susini B, Avraamides CJ, Schmid MC. Integrin alpha4beta1 signaling is required for lymphangiogenesis and tumor metastasis. Cancer Res. 2010;70:3042–51.
64. Gatzemeier U, Eisen T, Santoro A, et al. Sorafenib (S) + gemcitabine/cisplatin (GC) vs GC alone in the first-line treatment of advanced non-small cell lung cancer (NSCLC): phase III NSCLC Research Experience Utilizing Sorafenib (NEXUS) trial. Ann Oncol. 2010;21(Suppl 8):viii7 (Abstract LBA16).
65. Gingras D, Béliveau R. Emerging concepts in the regulation of membrane-type 1 matrix metalloproteinase activity. Biochim Biophys Acta. 2010;1803:142–50.
66. Gitay-Goren H, Halaban R, Neufeld G. Human melanoma cells but not normal melanocytes express vascular endothelial growth factor receptors. Biochem Biophys Res Commun. 1993;190:702–8.
67. Glaspy J, Atkins MB, Richards JM, et al. Results of a multicenter, randomized, double-blind, dose-evaluating phase 2/3 study of lenalidomide in the treatment of metastatic malignant melanoma. Cancer. 2009;115:5228–36.
68. González-Cao M, Viteri S, Díaz-Lagares A, et al. Preliminary results of the combination of bevacizumab and weekly Paclitaxel in advanced melanoma. Oncology. 2008;74:12–6.
69. Gonzalez-Larriba JL, Guillem V, Mármol M, et al. Open-label phase II study of sorafenib + dacarbazine in patients with advanced metastatic melanoma. Ann Oncol. 2008;19(Suppl 8):viii246 (Abstract 791P).
70. Grant SW, Kyshtoobayeva AS, Kurosaki T, et al. Mutant p53 correlates with reduced expression of thrombospondin-1, increased angiogenesis, and metastatic progression in melanoma. Cancer Detect Prev. 1998;22:185–94.
71. Grignol VP, Olencki T, Taylor C, et al. Phase II trial of bevacizumab and high-dose interferon alpha-2b in metastatic melanoma. J Clin Oncol. 2010:28(15s Suppl):616s (Abstract 8520).
72. Gupta SK, Vlahakis NE. Integrin alpha9beta1: unique signaling pathways reveal diverse biological roles. Cell Adh Migr. 2010;4:194–8.
73. Haas NB, McWhirter E, Hogg D, et al. Phase II study of vorinostat in patients with advanced melanoma. J Clin Oncol. 2010;28(15s Suppl):618s (Abstract 8530).
74. Hainsworth JD, Infante JR, Spigel DR, et al. Bevacizumab and everolimus in the treatment of patients with metastatic melanoma: a phase 2 trial of the Sarah Cannon Oncology Research Consortium. Cancer. 2010;116:4122–9.
75. Hanahan D, Folkman J. Patterns and emerging mechanisms of the angiogenic switch during tumorigenesis. Cell. 1996;86:353–64.
76. Hanahan D, Weinberg RA. The hallmarks of cancer. Cell. 2000;100:57–70.
77. Hanahan D, Weinberg RA. Hallmarks of cancer: the next generation. Cell. 2011;144: 646–74.
78. Hauschild A, Agarwala SS, Trefzer U, et al. Results of a phase III, randomized, placebo-controlled study of sorafenib in combination with carboplatin and paclitaxel as second-line treatment in patients with unresectable stage III or stage IV melanoma. J Clin Oncol. 2009;27:2823–30.
79. Hegde P, Xing B, O'Day S, et al. Biomarkers of treatment benefit in a randomized phase II study of bevacizumab in combination with carboplatin and paclitaxel in metastatic melanoma patients (BEAM). J Clin Oncol. 2010;28(15s Suppl):738s (Abstract 10563).
80. Heldin CH, Rubin K, Pietras K, Ostman A. High interstitial fluid pressure – an obstacle in cancer therapy. Nat Rev Cancer. 2004;4:806–13.
81. Helfrich I, Edler L, Sucker A, et al. Angiopoietin-2 levels are associated with disease progression in metastatic malignant melanoma. Clin Cancer Res. 2009;15:1384–92.
82. Hersey P, Sosman J, O'Day S, et al. Etaracizumab Melanoma Study Group. A randomized phase 2 study of etaracizumab, a monoclonal antibody against integrin alpha(v) beta(3), + or - dacarbazine in patients with stage IV metastatic melanoma. Cancer. 2010;116:1526–34.
83. Hess AR, Seftor EA, Gruman LM, et al. VE-cadherin regulates EphA2 in aggressive melanoma cells through a novel signaling pathway: implications for vasculogenic mimicry. Cancer Biol Ther. 2006;5:228–33.

84. Hess AR, Margaryan NV, Seftor EA, et al. Deciphering the signaling events that promote melanoma tumor cell vasculogenic mimicry and their link to embryonic vasculogenesis: role of the Eph receptors. Dev Dyn. 2007;236:3283–96.
85. Hicklin DJ, Ellis LM. Role of the vascular endothelial growth factor pathway in tumor growth and angiogenesis. J Clin Oncol. 2005;23:1011–27.
86. Hodi FS, Friedlander P, Atkins M, et al. A phase I trial of ipilimumab plus bevacizumab in patients with unresectable stage III or stage IV melanoma. In: Presented at 47th annual meeting of the American Society of Clinical Oncology, 3–7 June 2011, Chicago. http://www.asco.org. Accessed 18 April 2011.
87. Hong YK, Lange-Asschenfeldt B, Velasco P, et al. VEGF-A promotes tissue repair-associated lymphatic vessel formation via VEGFR-2 and the alpha1beta1 and alpha2beta1 integrins. FASEB J. 2004;18:1111–3.
88. Hong JY, Kim G-Y, Kim J-H. Role of the low-affinity leukotriene B4 receptor BLT2 in VEGF-induced angiogenesis. In: Proceedings of the 101st annual meeting of the American Association for Cancer Research, 17–21 April 2010. Washington: AACR (Abstract 1302).
89. Huang X, Yamada Y, Kidoya H, et al. EphB4 overexpression in B16 melanoma cells affects arterial-venous patterning in tumor angiogenesis. Cancer Res. 2007;67:9800–8.
90. Hubler Jr WR, Wolf Jr JE. Melanoma. Tumor angiogenesis and human neoplasia. Cancer. 1976;38:187–92.
91. Hurwitz H, Fehrenbacher L, Novotny W, et al. Bevacizumab plus irinotecan, fluorouracil, and leucovorin for metastatic colorectal cancer. N Engl J Med. 2004;350:2335–42.
92. Hwu W, Akerley WL, Stephenson J, et al. Final report: combination of MPC-6827 with temozolomide for the treatment of patients with metastatic melanoma. J Clin Oncol. 2010:28(15s Suppl):618s (Abstract 8531).
93. Hynes RO. A reevaluation of integrins as regulators of angiogenesis. Nat Med. 2002;8: 918–21.
94. Jain RK. Normalization of tumor vasculature: an emerging concept in antiangiogenic therapy. Science. 2005;307:58–62.
95. Jaissle GB, Ulmer A, Henke-Fahle S, et al. Suppression of melanoma-associated neoangiogenesis by bevacizumab. Arch Dermatol. 2008;144:525–7.
96. Jiang WG, Martin TA, Parr C, et al. Hepatocyte growth factor, its receptor, and their potential value in cancer therapies. Crit Rev Oncol Hematol. 2005;53:35–69.
97. Jimenez X, Lu D, Brennan L, et al. A recombinant, fully human, bispecific antibody neutralizes the biological activities mediated by both vascular endothelial growth factor receptors 2 and 3. Mol Cancer Ther. 2005;4:427–34.
98. Jubb AM, Pham TQ, Hanby AM, et al. Expression of vascular endothelial growth factor, hypoxia inducible factor 1alpha, and carbonic anhydrase IX in human tumours. J Clin Pathol. 2004;57:504–12.
99. Kamrava M, Bernstein MB, Camphausen K, et al. Combining radiation, immunotherapy, and antiangiogenesis agents in the management of cancer: the Three Musketeers or just another quixotic combination? Mol Biosyst. 2009;5:1262–70.
100. Kerbel RS. Antiangiogenic therapy: a universal chemosensitization strategy for cancer? Science. 2006;312:1171–5.
101. Kerbel RS. Tumor angiogenesis. N Engl J Med. 2008;358:2039–49.
102. Kerbel RS. Issues regarding improving the impact of antiangiogenic drugs for the treatment of breast cancer. Breast. 2009;18 Suppl 3:S41–7.
103. Kessenbrock K, Plaks V, Werb Z. Matrix metalloproteinases: regulators of the tumor microenvironment. Cell. 2010;141:52–67.
104. Kim KB, Diwan AH, Papadopoulos NE, et al. A randomized phase II study of EMD 121974 in patients (pts) with metastatic melanoma (MM). J Clin Oncol. 2007;25(18s Suppl):484s (Abstract 8548).
105. Klagsbrun M, Takashima S, Mamluk R. The role of neuropilin in vascular and tumor biology. Adv Exp Med Biol. 2002;515:33–48.

106. Lacal PM, Failla CM, Pagani E, et al. Human melanoma cells secrete and respond to placenta growth factor and vascular endothelial growth factor. J Invest Dermatol. 2000;115:1000–7.
107. Leung et al. VEGF is a secreted angiogenic mitogen; 1989.
108. Lewis KD, Robinson WA, Millward MJ, et al. A phase II study of the heparanase inhibitor PI-88 in patients with advanced melanoma. Invest New Drugs. 2008;26:89–94.
109. Liu B, Earl HM, Baban D, et al. Melanoma cell lines express VEGF receptor KDR and respond to exogenously added VEGF. Biochem Biophys Res Commun. 1995;217:721–7.
110. Llovet JM, Ricci S, Mazzaferro V, et al., for the SHARP Investigators Study Group. Sorafenib in advanced hepatocellular carcinoma. N Engl J Med. 2008;359:378–90.
111. Lohela M, Bry M, Tammela T, Alitalo K. VEGFs and receptors involved in angiogenesis versus lymphangiogenesis. Curr Opin Cell Biol. 2009;21:154–65.
112. Lynch TJ, Bondarenko IN, Luft A, et al. Phase II trial of ipilimumab and paclitaxel/carboplatin (P/C) in first-line stage IIIb/IV non-small cell lung cancer (NSCLC). J Clin Oncol. 2010;28(15s Suppl):545s (Abstract 7531).
113. Mahabeleshwar GH, Byzova TV. Angiogenesis in melanoma. Semin Oncol. 2007;34:555–65.
114. Mak J, Tong R, Koch A, et al. Broad vascular distribution of Neuropilin-1 and its ligands in human tumors. In: Proceedings of the 101st annual meeting of the American Association for Cancer Research, 17–21 April 2010. Washington: AACR (Abstract 1292).
115. Mancuso MR, Davis R, Norberg SM, et al. Rapid vascular regrowth in tumors after reversal of VEGF inhibition. J Clin Invest. 2006;116:2610–21.
116. Marcoval J, Moreno A, Graells J, et al. Angiogenesis and malignant melanoma. Angiogenesis is related to the development of vertical (tumorigenic) growth phase. J Cutan Pathol. 1997;24:212–8.
117. McClay EF, Bessudo A, Frakes L, et al. phase I/II trial of the combination of bevacizumab, oxaliplatin, and sorafenib in patients with metastatic melanoma. J Clin Oncol. 2008;26(Suppl):723s (Abstract 20020).
118. McDermott DF, Sosman JA, Gonzalez R, et al. Double-blind randomized phase II study of the combination of sorafenib and dacarbazine in patients with advanced melanoma: a report from the 11715 Study Group. J Clin Oncol. 2008;26:2178–85.
119. Melnikova VO, Bar-Eli M. Bioimmunotherapy for melanoma using fully human antibodies targeting MCAM/MUC18 and IL-8. Pigment Cell Res. 2006;19:395–405.
120. Melnikova VO, Villares GJ, Bar-Eli M. Emerging roles of PAR-1 and PAFR in melanoma metastasis. Cancer Microenviron. 2008;1:103–11.
121. Mihm Jr MC, Clark Jr WH, Reed RJ. The clinical diagnosis of malignant melanoma. Semin Oncol. 1975;2:105–18.
122. Miller K, Wang M, Gralow J, et al. Paclitaxel plus bevacizumab versus paclitaxel alone for metastatic breast cancer. N Engl J Med. 2007;357:2666–76.
123. Mita MM, Rowinsky EK, Forero L, et al. A phase II, pharmacokinetic, and biologic study of semaxanib and thalidomide in patients with metastatic melanoma. Cancer Chemother Pharmacol. 2007;59:165–74.
124. Mitchell D, Pobre EG, Mulivor AW, et al. ALK1-Fc inhibits multiple mediators of angiogenesis and suppresses tumor growth. Mol Cancer Ther. 2010;9:379–88.
125. Mocellin S, Pasquali S, Rossi CR, Nitti D. Interferon alpha adjuvant therapy in patients with high-risk melanoma: a systematic review and meta-analysis. J Natl Cancer Inst. 2010;102:493–501.
126. Motzer RJ, Hutson TE, Tomczak P, et al. Overall survival and updated results for sunitinib compared with interferon alfa in patients with metastatic renal cell carcinoma. J Clin Oncol. 2009;27:3584–90.
127. Mouawad R, Spano J, Conforti R, et al. Evaluation of circulating angiopoietin levels with prognosis and disease progression in metastatic malignant melanoma. J Clin Oncol. 2010;28(15s Suppl):616s (Abstract 8522).
128. Mousa SA. alphav Vitronectin receptors in vascular-mediated disorders. Med Res Rev. 2003;23:190–9.
129. Munzone E, Testori A, Minchella I, et al. A phase II trial of dacarbazine (DTIC) and bevacizumab in patients with metastatic melanoma. J Clin Oncol. 2007;25(18s Suppl):491s (Abstract 8579).

130. Nagengast WB, Hooge MN, van Straten EM, et al. VEGF-SPECT with (111)In-bevacizumab in stage III/IV melanoma patients. Eur J Cancer. 2011;47(10):1595–602.

131. Nair S, Boczkowski D, Moeller B, et al. Synergy between tumor immunotherapy and antiangiogenic therapy. Blood. 2003;102:964–71.

132. Niccoli P, Raoul J, Bang Y, et al. Updated safety and efficacy results of the phase III trial of sunitinib (SU) versus placebo (PBO) for treatment of pancreatic neuroendocrine tumors (NET). J Clin Oncol. 2010;28(15s Suppl):301s (Abstract 4000).

133. Nikolopoulos SN, Blaikie P, Yoshioka T, et al. Integrin beta4 signaling promotes tumor angiogenesis. Cancer Cell. 2004;6:471–83.

134. Nissen LJ, Cao R, Hedlund EM, et al. Angiogenic factors FGF2 and PDGF-BB synergistically promote murine tumor neovascularization and metastasis. J Clin Invest. 2007;117:2766–77.

135. Nürnberg W, Tobias D, Otto F, Henz BM, Schadendorf D. Expression of interleukin-8 detected by in situ hybridization correlates with worse prognosis in primary cutaneous melanoma. J Pathol. 1999;189:546–51.

136. Oliner J, Min H, Leal J, et al. Suppression of angiogenesis and tumor growth by selective inhibition of angiopoietin-2. Cancer Cell. 2004;6:507–16.

137. Oliveira IC, Sciavolino PJ, Lee TH, Vilcek J. Downregulation of interleukin 8 gene expression in human fibroblasts: unique mechanism of transcriptional inhibition by interferon. Proc Natl Acad Sci USA. 1992;89:9049–53.

138. Ostrand-Rosenberg S, Sinha P. Myeloid-derived suppressor cells: linking inflammation and cancer. J Immunol. 2009;182:4499–506.

139. Ott PA, Chang JL, Oratz R, et al. Phase II trial of dacarbazine and thalidomide for the treatment of metastatic melanoma. Chemotherapy. 2009;55:221–7.

140. Ott PA, Hamilton A, Min C, et al. A phase II trial of sorafenib in metastatic melanoma with tissue correlates. PLoS One. 2010;5:e15588.

141. Pan Q, Chanthery Y, Liang WC, et al. Blocking neuropilin-1 function has an additive effect with anti-VEGF to inhibit tumor growth. Cancer Cell. 2007;11:53–67.

142. Parker LH, Schmidt M, Jin SW, et al. The endothelial-cell-derived secreted factor Egfl7 regulates vascular tube formation. Nature. 2004;428:754–8.

143. Pawlak WZ, Legha SS. Phase II study of thalidomide in patients with metastatic melanoma. Melanoma Res. 2004;14:57–62.

144. Perez DG, Suman VJ, Fitch TR, et al. Phase 2 trial of carboplatin, weekly paclitaxel, and biweekly bevacizumab in patients with unresectable stage IV melanoma: a North Central Cancer Treatment Group study, N047A. Cancer. 2009;115:119–27.

145. Perren T, Swart AM, Pfisterer J, et al. ICON7: a phase III Gynecologic Cancer InterGroup (GCIG) trial of adding bevacizumab to standard chemotherapy in women with newly diagnosed epithelial ovarian, primary peritoneal or fallopian tube cancer. Ann Oncol. 2010;21(Suppl 8):viii2–3 (Abstract LBA4).

146. Peterson AC, Swiger S, Stadler WM, Medved M, Karczmar G, Gajewski TF. Phase II study of the Flk-1 tyrosine kinase inhibitor SU5416 in advanced melanoma. Clin Cancer Res. 2004;10:4048–54.

147. Peyton JD, Spigel DR, Burris HA, et al. Phase II trial of bevacizumab and everolimus in the treatment of patients with metastatic melanoma: preliminary results. J Clin Oncol. 2009;27(15s Suppl):467s (Abstract 9027).

148. Presta LG, Chen H, O'Connor SJ, et al. Humanization of an anti-vascular endothelial growth factor monoclonal antibody for the therapy of solid tumors and other disorders. Cancer Res. 1997;57:4593–9.

149. Reed JA, McNutt NS, Albino AP. Differential expression of basic fibroblast growth factor (bFGF) in melanocytic lesions demonstrated by in situ hybridization. Implications for tumor progression. Am J Pathol. 1994;144:329–36.

150. Reuning U, Sperl S, Kopitz C, et al. Urokinase-type plasminogen activator (uPA) and its receptor (uPAR): development of antagonists of uPA/uPAR interaction and their effects in vitro and in vivo. Curr Pharm Des. 2003;9:1529–43.

151. Ribatti D, Annese T, Longo V. Angiogenesis and melanoma. Cancer. 2010;2:114–32.
152. Rini BI, Wilding GT, Hudes G, et al. Axitinib (AG-013736; AG) in patients (pts) with metastatic renal cell cancer (RCC) refractory to sorafenib. J Clin Oncol. 2007;25(18s Suppl):242s (Abstract 5032).
153. Rini BI, Halabi S, Rosenberg JE, et al. Bevacizumab plus interferon alfa compared with interferon alfa monotherapy in patients with metastatic renal cell carcinoma: CALGB 90206. J Clin Oncol. 2008;26:5422–8.
154. Rixe O, Bukowski RM, Michaelson MD, et al. Axitinib treatment in patients with cytokine-refractory metastatic renal-cell cancer: a phase II study. Lancet Oncol. 2007;8:975–84.
155. Ross GD. Regulation of the adhesion versus cytotoxic functions of the Mac-1/CR3/alphaM-beta2-integrin glycoprotein. Crit Rev Immunol. 2000;20:197–222.
156. Rüegg C, Alghisi GC. Vascular integrins: therapeutic and imaging targets of tumor angiogenesis. Recent Results Cancer Res. 2010;180:83–101.
157. Ruiter DJ, Bröcker EB. Immunohistochemistry in the evaluation of melanocytic tumors. Semin Diagn Pathol. 1993;10:76–91.
158. Salven P, Heikkilä P, Joensuu H. Enhanced expression of vascular endothelial growth factor in metastatic melanoma. Br J Cancer. 1997;76:930–4.
159. Sandler A, Gray R, Perry MC, et al. Paclitaxel-carboplatin alone or with bevacizumab for non-small-cell lung cancer. N Engl J Med. 2006;355:2542–50.
160. Sarker D, Molife R, Evans TR, et al. A phase I pharmacokinetic and pharmacodynamic study of TKI258, an oral, multitargeted receptor tyrosine kinase inhibitor in patients with advanced solid tumors. Clin Cancer Res. 2008;14:2075–81.
161. Scagliotti G, Novello S, von Pawel J, et al. Phase III study of carboplatin and paclitaxel alone or with sorafenib in advanced non-small-cell lung cancer. J Clin Oncol. 2010;28:1835–42.
162. Schietroma C, Cianfarani F, Lacal PM, et al. Vascular endothelial growth factor-C expression correlates with lymph node localization of human melanoma metastases. Cancer. 2003;98:789–97.
163. Seftor RE. Role of the beta3 integrin subunit in human primary melanoma progression: multifunctional activities associated with alpha(v)beta3 integrin expression. Am J Pathol. 1998;153:1347–51.
164. Shibuya M, Claesson-Welsh L. Signal transduction by VEGF receptors in regulation of angiogenesis and lymphangiogenesis. Exp Cell Res. 2006;312:549–60.
165. Shojaei F, Wu X, Zhong C, et al. Bv8 regulates myeloid-cell-dependent tumour angiogenesis. Nature. 2007;450:825–31.
166. Shojaei F, Wu X, Qu X, et al. G-CSF-initiated myeloid cell mobilization and angiogenesis mediate tumor refractoriness to anti-VEGF therapy in mouse models. Proc Natl Acad Sci USA. 2009;106:6742–7.
167. Si L, Han M, Chi ZH, et al. Durable response of the triple combination of temozolomide, sorafenib, and bevacizumab to treat refractory stage IV acral melanoma. J Clin Oncol. 2010;28(15s Suppl):627s (Abstract 8564).
168. Sidky YA, Auerbach R. Lymphocyte-induced angiogenesis in tumor-bearing mice. Science. 1976;192:1237–8.
169. Singh RK, Gutman M, Llansa N, Fidler IJ. Interferon-beta prevents the upregulation of interleukin-8 expression in human melanoma cells. J Interferon Cytokine Res. 1996;16:577–84.
170. Singh RK, Varney ML, Bucana CD, Johansson SL. Expression of interleukin-8 in primary and metastatic malignant melanoma of the skin. Melanoma Res. 1999;9:383–7.
171. Srivastava A, Laidler P, Hughes LE, Woodcock J, Shedden EJ. Neovascularization in human cutaneous melanoma: a quantitative morphological and Doppler ultrasound study. Eur J Cancer Clin Oncol. 1986;22:1205–9.
172. Srivastava A, Laidler P, Davies RP, Horgan K, Hughes LE. The prognostic significance of tumor vascularity in intermediate-thickness (0.76-4.0 mm thick) skin melanoma. A quantitative histologic study. Am J Pathol. 1988;133:419–23.
173. Stacker SA, Achen MG, Jussila L, Baldwin ME, Alitalo K. Lymphangiogenesis and cancer metastasis. Nat Rev Cancer. 2002;2:573–83.

174. Stenzinger W, Brüggen J, Macher E, Sorg C. Tumor angiogenic activity (TAA) production in vitro and growth in the nude mouse by human malignant melanoma. Eur J Cancer Clin Oncol. 1983;19:649–56.
175. Stipp CS. Laminin-binding integrins and their tetraspanin partners as potential antimetastatic targets. Expert Rev Mol Med. 2010;12:e3.
176. Stollman TH, Scheer MG, Franssen GM, et al. Tumor accumulation of radiolabeled bevacizumab due to targeting of cell- and matrix-associated VEGF-A isoforms. Cancer Biother Radiopharm. 2009;24:195–200.
177. Straume O, Akslen LA. Importance of vascular phenotype by basic fibroblast growth factor, and influence of the angiogenic factors basic fibroblast growth factor/fibroblast growth factor receptor-1 and ephrin-A1/EphA2 on melanoma progression. Am J Pathol. 2002;160:1009–19.
178. Straume O, Akslen LA. Increased expression of VEGF-receptors (FLT-1, KDR, NRP-1) and thrombospondin-1 is associated with glomeruloid microvascular proliferation, an aggressive angiogenic phenotype, in malignant melanoma. Angiogenesis. 2003;6:295–301.
179. Streit M, Detmar M. Angiogenesis, lymphangiogenesis, and melanoma metastasis. Oncogene. 2003;22:3172–9.
180. Sun B, Zhang D, Zhang S, et al. Hypoxia influences vasculogenic mimicry channel formation and tumor invasion-related protein expression in melanoma. Cancer Lett. 2007;249:188–97.
181. Third phase III study of Avastin-based regimen met primary endpoint in ovarian cancer [press release]. Basel, Switzerland: F. Hoffmann-La Roche Ltd.; 8 Feb 8 2011.
182. Vacca A, Ria R, Ribatti D, et al. Angiogenesis and tumor progression in melanoma. Recenti Prog Med. 2000;91:581–7.
183. Varker KA, Biber JE, Kefauver C, et al. A randomized phase 2 trial of bevacizumab with or without daily low-dose interferon alfa-2b in metastatic malignant melanoma. Ann Surg Oncol. 2007;14:2367–76.
184. Vermeulen PB, Dirix LY, Martin M, et al. Serum basic fibroblast growth factor and vascular endothelial growth factor in metastatic renal cell carcinoma treated with interferon alfa-2b. J Natl Cancer Inst. 1997;89:1316–7.
185. Vihinen PP, Hernberg M, Vuoristo MS, et al. A phase II trial of bevacizumab with dacarbazine and daily low-dose interferon-alpha2a as first line treatment in metastatic melanoma. Melanoma Res. 2010;20 318–25.
186. Vlaykova T, Laurila P, Muhonen T, et al. Prognostic value of tumour vascularity in metastatic melanoma and association of blood vessel density with vascular endothelial growth factor expression. Melanoma Res. 1999;9:59–68.
187. Warren BA, Shubik P. The growth of the blood supply to melanoma transplants in the hamster cheek pouch. Lab Invest. 1966;15:464–78.
188. Wu JJ, Huang DB, Pang KR, Hsu S, Tyring SK. Thalidomide: dermatological indications, mechanisms of action and side-effects. Br J Dermatol. 2005;153:254–73.
189. Wyman K, Spigel D, Puzanov I, et al. A multicenter phase II study of erlotinib and bevacizumab in patients with metastatic melanoma. J Clin Oncol. 2007;25(18s Suppl):481s (Abstract 8539).
190. Xu Y, Yuan L, Mak J, et al. Neuropilin-2 mediates VEGF-C-induced lymphatic sprouting together with VEGFR3. J Cell Biol. 2010;188:115–30.
191. Yang L, DeBusk LM, Fukuda K, et al. Expansion of myeloid immune suppressor Gr+CD11b+ cells in tumor-bearing host directly promotes tumor angiogenesis. Cancer Cell. 2004;6:409–21.
192. Yazji S, Figlin RA, Kirkwood JM, et al. Safety of Volociximab as a monotherapy and in combination with chemotherapy the result of three phase II studies. Eur J Cancer Suppl. 2006;4(12):24 (Abstract 65).
193. Yu JL, Rak JW, Klement G, Kerbel RS. Vascular endothelial growth factor isoform expression as a determinant of blood vessel patterning in human melanoma xenografts. Cancer Res. 2002;62:1838–46.
194. Zhang SX, Wang JJ, Gao G, et al. Pigment epithelium-derived factor downregulates vascular endothelial growth factor (VEGF) expression and inhibits VEGF-VEGF receptor 2 binding in diabetic retinopathy. J Mol Endocrinol. 2006;37:1–12.

Part III
Rational Immunotherapy Approaches in Melanoma

Chapter 11
Melanoma Antigens Recognized by T Lymphocytes

Nicolas van Baren, Jean-François Baurain, Francis Brasseur, and Pierre G. Coulie

Abstract The antigenicity of melanomas is known better than that of all other human tumors. Melanoma antigens recognized by T lymphocytes fall into four groups. They can be encoded by genes that are mutated in the tumor cells, by the cancer-germline genes which are not expressed in non-tumor cells that bear HLA molecules, by melanocyte differentiation genes, and by genes that are overexpressed in tumor cells. Only the antigens of the first two groups can be considered as melanoma-specific and therefore can be used safely in active or passive immunizations.

Keywords Melanoma • Antigen • Immunotherapy • Vaccination

N. van Baren, MD, PhD
de Duve Institute and Université catholique de Louvain 74, B1.74.04, Brussels 1200, Belgium

Ludwig Institute for Cancer Research, Brussels Branch, Belgium

Centre du Cancer, Unité d'Oncologie Médicale, Cliniques universitaires, Saint-Luc, Université catholique de Louvain, Brussels 1200, Belgium

J.-F. Baurain, MD, PhD
Centre du Cancer, Cliniques universitaires Saint-Luc, Université catholique de Louvain, Brussels 1200, Belgium

F. Brasseur, PhD
de Duve Institute and Université catholique de Louvain 74, B1.74.04, Brussels 1200, Belgium

Ludwig Institute for Cancer Research, Brussels Branch, Belgium

P.G. Coulie, MD, PhD (⊠)
de Duve Institute and Université catholique de Louvain, Avenue Hippocrate 74, B1.74.04, Brussels 1200, Belgium
e-mail: pierre.coulie@uclouvain.be

T.F. Gajewski and F.S. Hodi (eds.), *Targeted Therapeutics in Melanoma*,
Current Clinical Oncology, DOI 10.1007/978-1-61779-407-0_11,
© Springer Science+Business Media, LLC 2012

Abbreviations

CTL   Cytolytic T lymphocyte
MLTC   Mixed lymphocyte-tumor cell cultures
TILs   Tumor-infiltrating lymphocytes

Introduction

Most if not all human tumors bear antigens that can be recognized by T lymphocytes. These antigens are small peptides, derived mostly from endogenous proteins, and presented at the cell surface by HLA molecules. The antigenicity of melanoma is better known than that of all other human tumors, for several reasons. Firstly, from a historical perspective, melanomas have always been considered as privileged "immunogenic" tumors. There are histological and clinical suggestions that melanomas, during their development and progression, are the target of immune reactions mediated by T lymphocytes, and that these reactions influence the clinical course of the disease. About 10–20% of primary melanomas show signs of partial tumor regression, often associated with infiltrates of inflammatory cells including T lymphocytes. In 10% of new melanoma cases, the diagnosis is made on a metastatic lesion, without any detectable primary tumor, suggesting that the latter regressed spontaneously. Primary melanomas often contain tumor-infiltrating lymphocytes (TILs), whose extent and pattern of infiltration has a clear impact on metastatic spread and prognosis [1]. Clinical observations that a fraction of melanoma patients benefit from various forms of immunotherapy, including BCG [2], IL-2 [3–5], IFN-α [6], and adoptive transfer of blood or tumor-derived lymphocytes activated by IL-2 [7, 8], further drew the attention of immunologists to melanoma. The high rate of success of melanoma cell line establishment, about 40% from metastatic melanoma as compared to 1–10% for other tumors, provided researchers with a stable and renewable source of tumor antigens for the stimulation of autologous lymphocytes, which proved to be a key step toward the molecular identification of these antigens.

This review deals with antigens recognized on human melanoma cells by T lymphocytes. Today more than 200 such antigens have been identified, about two thirds of which are being presented by HLA class I molecules to CD8+ cytolytic T cells (CTLs) and one third by HLA class II molecules to CD4+ T cells. An updated list of T cell-recognized tumor antigens is available at [9].

Antigen Discovery Process

The molecular identification of melanoma antigens has followed three approaches. In the first, the starting material is a population of tumor-specific T cells, and preferably a T cell clone. They can be derived from autologous mixed lymphocyte-tumor cell cultures (MLTC), in which T lymphocytes from the patient's blood or melanoma are restimulated in vitro with the autologous tumor cells. From the beginning of the identification work, one knows that the examined antigen is naturally processed in the melanoma cells and expressed at their surface at a sufficient level for recognition by T cells. The antigenic peptide itself can be identified either by eluting HLA-bound peptides from the tumor cells, fractionating and testing them for recognition by the T cells, or by cloning the gene encoding the peptide by transfecting a cDNA library derived from the autologous melanoma line [10].

In the second approach, often referred to as "reverse immunology" [10], one starts with the sequence of a gene of particular interest such as an oncogene frequently mutated in melanoma, a gene selectively expressed or overexpressed in melanomas, or in the SEREX methodology the gene coding for a protein against which melanoma patients have mounted an antibody response [11]. The work then consists in finding a candidate antigenic peptide encoded by this gene, verify its binding to HLA molecules, use it to prime T cells in vitro, derive a T cell line or clone that specifically recognizes the peptide and, last but not least, verify that these lymphocytes do recognize melanoma cells that naturally express the gene of interest and the appropriate HLA. Compared to the MLTC approach, there is a fairly high dropout rate over this difficult course, mainly at the final step of melanoma cell recognition.

Finally, a direct biochemical approach consists in immunoaffinity purification of detergent-solubilized MHC-peptide complexes from melanoma cells, followed by acid elution of peptides and their identification with liquid chromatography and mass spectrometry [12]. The resulting "MHC-ligandome" contains mostly non-antigenic normal self peptides, and the tumor-specific antigenic peptides.

These methods have led to the identification of four main categories of melanoma antigens, classified according to the genetic mechanisms leading to their expression.

Melanoma Antigens Resulting from Mutations

These antigenic peptides are encoded by genes that bear somatic mutations in melanoma cells. About 25 antigenic peptides resulting from a mutation have been described in melanoma, 18 presented on HLA class I and 9 on HLA class II molecules [9]. Without a doubt, there is a multitude of other such peptides. In most cases, the mutation changes one amino acid in the antigenic peptide recognized by the T cells. Either this change enables peptide binding to a presenting HLA molecule, to which the wild type peptide does not bind [13], or both the wild type and mutated peptides bind to an HLA molecule but the mutation creates a new antigenic determinant that is recognized by the T cell receptor [14]. In this case, the wild type peptide is not recognized because the specific T cells have been deleted or anergized during the establishment of natural tolerance. Sometimes the mutation is not in a codon of the antigenic peptide, but either creates a new start codon that opens an alternative open reading frame encoding the peptide [15], or generates a frameshift

[16], or is thought to modify the intracellular localization of the protein and its processing into antigenic peptides [17]. In all cases, the resulting antigens are strictly tumor-specific.

As expected, several point mutations resulting in antigenic peptides are oncogenic such as in CDK4 [18], B-raf [19, 20], N-ras [21], or CDKN2A [16]. The corresponding peptides are attractive candidates for immunotherapy because the mutations are shared between several melanomas, and because antigen loss is unlikely since the mutated gene product drives the tumor. However, the prevalence of such antigens in melanoma is often low, as it equals the prevalence of the specific mutation in melanoma multiplied by the prevalence of the presenting HLA molecule in the target population.

The vast majority of antigen-producing melanoma mutations could not be associated with tumoral transformation, and were individual to single tumors. These results led to the inference that in any given tumor the number of "antigenic" mutations could be high, with only a small proportion corresponding to common mutated oncogenes. Thus far, this notion seems to have been confirmed. The first complete catalogue of somatic mutations in a melanoma was recently obtained by comparing the full genome of a melanoma cell line with that of autologous EBV-transformed B cells and with a reference genome [22]. The melanoma cells contained about 33,000 somatic base substitutions, of which approximately 300 were in protein-coding sequences with around 200 that caused amino acid changes [22]. Assuming that about 40% of the protein-coding sequences are indeed expressed in the melanoma cells, we are left with 80 amino acid changes. Of these, less than 10 are estimated to be "driver" mutations, i.e., causing the neoplastic process and probably selected for during tumorigenesis and metastasis, the remainder being "passenger" mutations that do not contribute to oncogenesis [23]. How many of these 80 amino acid changes produce an antigen is not known. It will depend on the amount of protein present, or on the amount of the so-called defective ribosomal products which seem to be a good source of antigenic peptides presented by HLA class I molecules [24], on the capacity of the antigen processing pathways to generate the appropriate peptide, and on the ability of the latter to be presented by HLA molecules present in the melanoma cells. A conservative estimation of 10–15% leads to ±10 different mutated peptides available to T cell recognition at the surface of melanoma cells, always with a driver to passenger mutated peptides ratio of only 1:10. It is therefore not surprising that most of the mutated peptides identified with anti-melanoma CTL clones did not derive from oncoproteins.

Shared Tumor-Specific Antigens on Melanoma

The other genetic mechanism responsible for the tumor specificity of antigens is the expression in tumor cells of genes that are silent in normal cells. These antigens can be shared if encoded by genes that are expressed in many melanomas or in other tumors. Most of such tumor-specific shared antigens are encoded by the "cancer-germline" genes [25] that are expressed in various proportions of tumors of different histological types, and also in male germline cells. But male germline cells do not present antigenic peptides to T lymphocytes because they do not express HLA molecules [26, 27]. Thus, these tumor antigens recognized by T cells are not present in testis, and the widely used designation "cancer testis (CT) antigens" is not only unfortunate, but also misleading as it suggests that autoimmunity to testis is a concern. Some cancer-germline genes such as *MAGE-A3* and *-A4* are expressed in placenta [28], with proteins detected in the cytotrophoblast, which does not express the classical polymorphic HLA molecules [29]. As with antigens encoded by mutated genes, the tumor specificity of antigens encoded by cancer-germline genes and recognized by T cells appears to be strict.

The cancer-germline genes are categorized in gene families including *MAGE-A*, *-B*, and *-C* [28, 30], *BAGE* [31], *GAGE* [32], *LAGE* with *LAGE-1* and *LAGE-2/ NY-ESO-1* [33, 34], *SSX* [35], or *TAG* [36]. In melanoma, expression of cancer-germline genes is more frequent in metastases than in primary tumors (Table 11.1, Fig. 11.1), suggesting that activation of these genes occurs during tumor progression. It is worth noting that contrary to cutaneous melanomas, most ocular melanomas do not express *MAGE* genes [37] (Table 11.1, Fig. 11.1). The reason for the expression of cancer-germline genes in tumors has been examined in detail for gene *MAGE-A1*. The triggering event is demethylation of its promoter, which has a high CpG content, while the transcription factors that activate the promoter are ubiquitous [38, 39]. Accordingly, *MAGE-A1* expression can be induced in vitro in non-tumoral dividing cells treated with the demethylating agent deoxy-azacytidine [38]. Similar results were obtained for *LAGE-1* and other cancer-germline genes [40]. In tumor cells, after an initial and transient demethylation of cancer-germline genes' promoters, hypomethylation is locally maintained due to the presence of ubiquitous transcription factors [41, 42]. Melanoma samples often co-express several cancer-germline genes, as shown in Fig. 11.1 for genes *MAGE-A1*, *-A2*, *-A3*, *-A4*, *-A6*, *-A10*, and *-A12*. About 50% of primary tumors and 70–75% of cutaneous or lymph node metastases express at least one of these seven genes (Fig. 11.1). When several melanoma metastases of the same patient are tested, one usually observes a conserved pattern of cancer-germline genes expression across the different samples [43] (Fig. 11.2).

Beside the members of the cancer-germline gene families reported above, other genes such as *TRAG-3* [44], *HAGE* [45], *KM-HN-1* (*CCDC110*) [46], or the *CT45* gene family [47], are also expressed in testis and in some tumors, including melanomas. So far only a few antigenic peptides encoded by these genes have been identified.

A few transcripts that code for antigens recognized by T cells are expressed in a sizeable proportion of melanomas but are silent or expressed at very low levels in other tumors and in normal tissues including testis and melanocytes. In the gene coding for N-acetylglucosaminyltransferase V, a cryptic promoter active in most cutaneous and ocular melanomas controls transcript NA17, which encodes a polypeptide of 74 amino acids [48]. An antigenic peptide presented by HLA-A2 corresponds to residues 1–9 of this polypeptide. A pseudogene very similar to gene

Table 11.1 Expression of the main genes that encode tumor antigens, assessed by conventional RT-PCR, in a large panel of melanoma samples

| Gene | Cutaneous melanomas | | | | Ocular melanomas | | | |
| | Primary tumors | | Metastases | | Primary tumors | | Metastases | |
	%	n	%	n	%	n	%	n
MAGEA1	22	76	40	551	0	23	9	33
MAGEA2	46	68	68	364			0	12
MAGEA3	49	82	63	643	0	23	3	33
MAGEA4	19	70	32	429			17	12
MAGEA5			25	20				
MAGEA6	46	68	67	359			0	12
MAGEA8			10	52				
MAGEA9			12	50				
MAGEA10	28	18	45	349				
MAGEA11			54	56				
MAGEA12	27	67	50	372			0	11
MAGEB1			18	33				
MAGEB2			22	58				
MAGEC1	33	33	39	38				
MAGEC2	39	31	60	92				
BAGE	14	28	38	128				
GAGE-1,2,8	39	41	41	186				
GAGE-3-7	36	59	46	197				
CTAG1/LAGE-2			33	171	0	16		
CTAG2/LAGE-1			29	171				
SSX1			15	20				
SSX2			30	33				
SSX4			5	20				
HAGE			16	19				
SAGE			5	19				
NXF2			11	19				
PRAME	97	30	96	71				
NA17	35	20	74	238	100	12	91	34
TYR	91	64	79	509	87	23	89	35
MLANA	95	64	80	496	91	23	100	35
SILV/gp100	75	52	65	399	86	21	94	33

The table shows, for each gene, the proportion of positive samples and the number of samples tested. Results obtained with less than 10 samples are not included. Quantity of the amplified product was estimated visually on an ethidium bromide-stained agarose gel by comparing the intensity of the band to that resulting from RT-PCR performed on serial dilutions (1:1, 1:3, 1:9, 1:27) of the RNA of reference melanoma cell lines. Samples were scored positive if the amount of the amplified product was equal to or greater than that obtained with the 1:9 dilution of the reference RNA. Lower levels of expression were scored negative. All samples expressed gene β-ACTIN at levels comparable to those of the reference lines

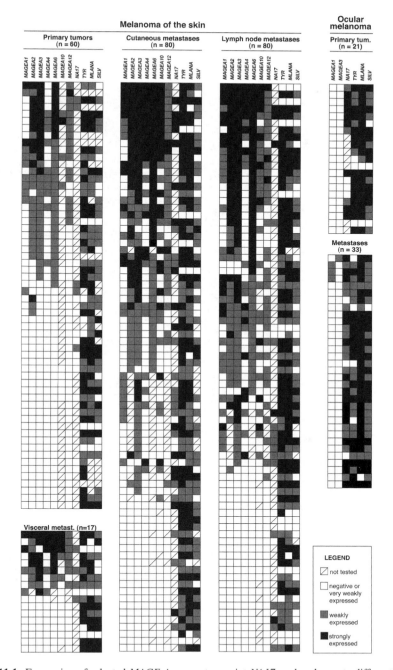

Fig. 11.1 Expression of selected *MAGE-A* genes, transcript *NA17*, and melanocyte differentiation genes, assessed by conventional RT-PCR, in unique tumor samples from melanoma patients. Assessment of the PCR product was performed visually on an ethidium bromide-stained agarose gel by comparing the intensity of the band to that resulting from RT-PCR performed on serial dilutions (1:1, 1:3, 1:9, 1:27) of the RNA reference melanoma cell line. Samples were scored *filled squares* or *gray boxes* if the amount of the amplified product was equal to or greater than that obtained with the 1:1 or 1:9 dilutions of the reference RNA, respectively. Lower levels of expression were scored *open squares*. All samples expressed gene *β-ACTIN* at a level comparable to that of the positive control

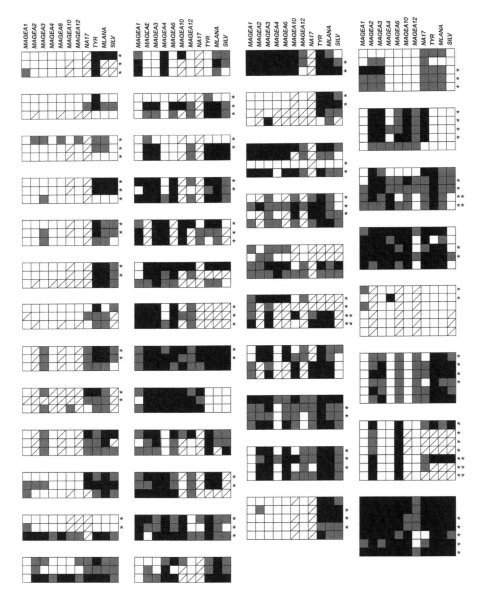

Fig. 11.2 Expression of selected *MAGE-A* genes, transcript NA17, and melanocyte differentiation genes in multiple melanoma samples from individual patients. Each group of 2–7 samples corresponds to a single patient. *Asterisks* and *double asterisks* indicate metastases that were resected simultaneously. Gene expression levels are represented as in Fig. 11.1

HPX42B contains a very short open reading frame that codes for an antigenic peptide presented by HLA-A2 [49]. This pseudogene is expressed in about 10% of melanomas. Finally, an endogenous retroviral sequence expressed in more than 80% of melanomas was found to code for an antigenic peptide recognized by CTL [50].

Is there some level of natural tolerance to antigens encoded by cancer-germline genes, considering their strict tumor-specific expression? A degree of central tolerance is possible since human medullary thymic epithelial cells express several cancer-germline genes, albeit at low and varying levels [51]. The same is true in mice for cancer-germline gene *P1A* [52], which is expressed on the mastocytoma cells P815. In *P1A*$^{-/-}$ mice, the tumor rejection responses obtained after inoculation of P815 cells are stronger than in wild type animals, while anti-P1A CTL responses obtained after immunization with peptide are only slightly increased [100]. These results are compatible with a partial T cell tolerance toward antigen P1A in DBA/2 mice. The situation might be similar for human tumor antigens encoded by cancer-germline genes. We have observed low functional avidity of all the anti-MAGE-3. A1 (peptide MAGE-A3$_{168-176}$ presented by HLA-A1) CTL clones that we have analyzed [53–56]. Thus, high-affinity anti-MAGE-3.A1 CTL may be either deleted from the repertoire or anergized. However, the situation is different for several other MAGE-encoded antigens against which we obtained high-affinity CTL clones from melanoma patients [54].

Melanocyte Differentiation Antigens

A significant proportion of the tumor-specific CTL clones derived from melanoma patients were found also to recognize normal melanocytes [57]. Their target antigens are encoded by the melanocyte-specific genes *tyrosinase* (*TYR*) [58], *Melan-A/MART-1 (MLANA)* [59, 60], *Pmel17/gp100 (SILV)* [61, 62], *tyrosinase-related protein-1 (TRP1)* [63], and *dopachrome tautomerase (DCT or TRP2)* [9, 64]. These genes are expressed in normal melanocytes and in melanoma cells, and are silent in other cancerous and non-cancerous cells. The corresponding proteins participate either in melanin synthesis or in the biogenesis of melanosomes, the pigment-rich organelles that, in the epidermis, are transferred from melanocytes to adjacent keratinocytes. Expression of these five melanocyte differentiation genes is induced by MITF-M, the melanocyte-specific isoform of transcription factor MITF (MIcrophtalmia associated Transcription Factor) [65]. Beside the skin, melanocytes are also present in the uvea, the retina, the membranous labyrinth of the inner ear, and the leptomeninges.

To date, about 60 different associations of HLA and peptides encoded by these melanocyte differentiation genes have been identified. Almost one third are antigens presented by HLA class II molecules: either an HLA-DR allele, or HLA-DQ6. Among all these combinations, one deserves a comment: peptide Melan-A/MART-1$_{26-35}$ presented by HLA-A2 molecules [66]. Initial results indicated that anti-melanoma CTL lines, and one CTL clone, recognized both the Melan-A/MART-1 nonamer AAGIGILTV and decamer EAAGIGILTV [66]. The decamer was shown to bind to HLA-A2 better than the nonamer, and the binding was even stronger for a modified decamer with leucine instead of alanine in position 2 [67]. In vitro, this ELAGIGILTV or Melan-A$_{26-35(A27L)}$ peptide stimulated CD8$^+$ T cells better than the natural peptides, and the responding cells recognized HLA-A2$^+$ melanoma cells [68]. On this basis, Melan-A$_{26-35(A27L)}$ has been used in many clinical studies of anti-melanoma vaccination. Another reason for the attractiveness of this peptide was that, when injected into patients, it stimulated T cell responses that could be detected easily. CTL responses could even be found in non-vaccinated HLA-A2$^+$ melanoma patients. Part of the explanation lies in a remarkable property of this antigen: it is recognized by a frequency of naive T lymphocytes that is between 10^{-4} and 10^{-3} of the CD8$^+$ cells, considerably higher than the frequency of naive T cells to other HLA/peptide combinations, estimated to be between 10^{-6} and 10^{-7} [53, 69]. Recently, the unmodified decamer administered with CpG was found to stimulate T cells that recognized melanoma cells better than did T cells induced by vaccination with the modified decamer [70]. The best can be the enemy of the good, and it is an interesting illustration of what can be obtained with peptides modified to increase their stability or binding to HLA: the fine specificity of all or some of the responding T cells may be such that the natural tumor antigen is not efficiently targeted. Other modified peptides that are often used in vaccination studies include gp100$_{209-217(T210M)}$ [71], or LAGE-2/NY-ESO-1$_{157-165(C165V \text{ or L or I})}$.

In addition to the five genes mentioned above, two others were found to code for melanocyte differentiation antigens, *RAB38* [72] and *OA1/GPR143* (Ocular albinism 1) [73]. Gene *OA1* is present on chromosome X and, interestingly, a male patient deleted for this gene produced anti-OA1 T cells that had a higher functional avidity than that of anti-OA1 T cells from normal controls, suggesting that there is some natural tolerance to melanocytic differentiation antigens [73].

Overexpressed Antigens on Melanoma Cells

The last group of melanoma antigens contains those that are considered to be overexpressed in tumors. That a gene is overexpressed is an ambiguous statement. A gene can be expressed in tumor cells at much higher levels than in normal cells, leading to more antigenic peptides displayed on HLA at the surface of tumor cells than on that of normal cells, thus explaining tumor-specificity of the T lymphocytes. Demonstration of this overexpression requires quantitative RT-PCR analysis of pure populations of each cell type tested. Overexpression may also mean that a gene is expressed at higher levels in tumor samples than in normal tissues because of higher proportions of cells expressing the gene, without real tumor specificity. Moreover, overexpression is often claimed on the basis of immunohistochemical analyses, not easy to quantify. From a long list [9], a few "overexpressed" melanoma antigens are described below.

Gene *PRAME* is expressed in almost all melanomas, and in many other tumors [74–77]. Protein PRAME binds to retinoic acid receptor alpha, inhibiting its effects on gene transcription [78]. Thus, PRAME could suppress the proliferation arrest and differentiation normally induced by retinoic acid [79]. Gene *PRAME* is expressed in some normal tissues such as testis, endometrium, adrenals or ovary, at levels that are about 100-fold lower than in melanomas [74]. So far, the distribution of PRAME-positive cells in these tissues is, however, unknown, and it is possible that a few normal cells express *PRAME* at levels comparable to those observed in tumors. Even though the presence of anti-PRAME T cells has been reported in cancer patients and in some normal individuals [74, 80, 81], these lymphocytes are rare ($\leq 10^{-5}$ of circulating T cells) and the consequences of anti-PRAME immunization remain uncertain.

Telomerase reverse transcriptase is often mentioned as an attractive source of tumor antigens. Antigenic peptides recognized by CTLs or CD4+ T cells have been identified [82–84]. But telomerase is also expressed in stem cells and mature hematopoietic cells, probably at the same level as in tumors. In vitro experiments showed that hematopoietic cells were not lysed by anti-telomerase$_{865-873}$ CTL that lysed tumor cells, leaving open the possibility to use this epitope for vaccination [84].

MELOE-1 is a gene product transcribed from an intron of the gene coding for histone deacetylase 4 [85]. An antigenic peptide presented by HLA-A2 is encoded by one of several short open reading frames. T cells recognizing this peptide were found in TILs, and their presence was correlated with good prognosis after TIL adoptive transfer [85].

About Tumor Specificity

Every physician or laboratory scientist agrees with the obvious notion that vaccination or adoptive transfer for cancer immunotherapy requires target antigens that are not present on normal cells, to avoid their destruction. Finding such antigens was the Holy Grail of many tumor immunologists. Today, many such antigens have been identified. And it is interesting to observe the consequences of a drift from the tumor specificity rule. The identification of the melanocytic antigens, recognized by T cell clones derived from blood or TILs of melanoma patients, was a surprise and an indication, or rather a confirmation, of incomplete tolerance. The absence of overt autoimmunity in the corresponding patients eroded the notion that tumor specificity was required. With Pandora's box opened, misleading terminology such as "tumor self antigens," "tumor-associated antigens," or "cancer-testis" antigens added to the confusion, and many antigens that were not at all tumor-specific were reported to be recognized by anti-tumor T cells. As a result, in many clinical studies, cancer patients receive immunotherapy with antigens that are not truly tumor-specific.

Is this a problem? For active immunization, probably no, at least not with today's techniques and adjuvants which are not yet very good at inducing high magnitude CTL responses. For the adoptive transfer of anti-tumor T cells, and its remarkable progresses over the last 10 years, obviously yes. Melanoma patients, who can display vitiligo in the absence of immunotherapy [86], also can develop vitiligo after administration of IL-2 and of T cells recognizing melanocytic differentiation antigens [87, 88]. In one such patient, the T cells infiltrating the depigmented skin were identical to the infused anti-Melan-A CTL clones, confirming that normal tissues could be destroyed by anti-Melan-A T cells [87]. Anterior uveitis was reported in a few patients who received melanocyte-specific T cells and IL-2 [87, 89]. In one patient, it was more severe [90]. Destruction of melanocytes in skin, eye, and inner ear were observed in up to 50% of patients after infusion of T cells transduced with high affinity T cell receptors to Melan-A/MART-1 or gp100 peptides [90]. Beyond melanoma, liver toxicity was observed after transfer of T cells engineered to express a chimeric receptor targeting carbonic anhydrase IX, present on renal carcinoma cells but also on normal bile duct epithelial cells [91]. Lethal toxicity occurred after transfer of T cells carrying a chimeric anti-ERBB2 receptor, probably because the infused cells localized immediately to the lungs and recognized ERBB2 on epithelial cells [92]. While these reports confirm the efficiency of the transferred cells, they also demonstrate the importance of a strict tumor specificity of the targeted antigens.

In vaccination, we believe that if the use of non-specific tumor antigens has not been associated with overt autoimmunity, it is because the induced T cell responses have usually been weak. However, progress is being made toward more immunogenic vaccine modalities, and with non-specific tumor antigens, vaccination inocuity may fade away as immunogenicity increases. Moreover, vaccination aims at inducing long-term T cell responses, even more so if there is a chronic stimulation by residual tumor cells. And if autoimmunity occurs, it might be considerably more difficult to control than after adoptive transfer.

Multiplicity of Antigens on Melanomas

It is obvious that melanoma cells carry multiple HLA/peptide associations that can be recognized by autologous T cells. Many of these antigens are immunogenic in vivo, i.e. induce spontaneous anti-tumor T cell responses. Figure 11.3 illustrates this point, with four melanoma lines and their sets of antigens recognized by autologous CTL clones. We believe that these sets correspond to antigens recognized by spontaneous anti-melanoma CTL responses of the patients because the CTL clones were obtained simply through stimulation of blood mononuclear cells with autologous melanoma cells and T cell growth factors, which in our hands is insufficient for de novo CTL priming. Thus, we think that all these melanoma-specific CTL were primed in vivo, and restimulated in vitro. Comparing the four melanomas, it appears that immunogenicity can result mostly from either mutated antigens (MZ7-MEL [93] or LB33-MEL), or antigens encoded by cancer-germline genes (MZ2-MEL). It is perhaps not coincidental that only one of the 28 identified antigens presented in Fig. 11.3 is coded by a gene (*PRAME*) that is expressed by normal cells other than male germline cells or melanocytes. Spontaneous T cell responses

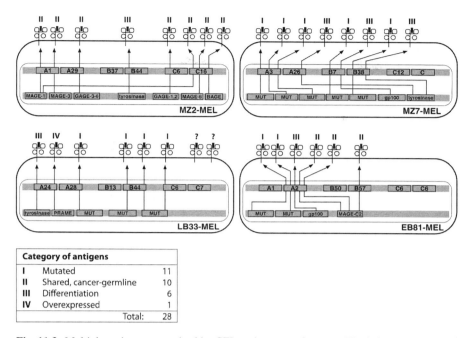

Category of antigens		
I	Mutated	11
II	Shared, cancer-germline	10
III	Differentiation	6
IV	Overexpressed	1
	Total:	28

Fig. 11.3 Multiple antigens recognized by CTL on human melanomas. The indicated HLA/peptide combinations were identified with autologous CTL clones obtained from MLTC experiments. On LB33-MEL at least two different antigens were not identified, they are indicated with question marks. MUT stands for various ubiquitously expressed, mutated genes

against the "overexpressed" tumor antigens are probably prevented by natural immunological tolerance.

One interesting question is whether all the cells of a melanoma, or all the metastases, bear the same set of antigens. When several metastases of a patient could be tested for the expression of genes coding for tumor antigens, the expression profiles were found to be similar [43]. We made similar observations, summarized in Fig. 11.2. Many reports mention the intratumoral heterogeneity of staining with antibodies recognizing MAGE or LAGE-2/NY-ESO1 [94, 95]. The reasons for this heterogeneity are not known.

The multiplicity of antigens recognized by T lymphocytes on melanoma cells is an important point for immunotherapy. Melanoma cells can escape recognition by CTL to a given antigen by losing expression of the presenting HLA molecule, which appears to be frequent [96]. But complete CTL evasion can only result from loss of β2-microglobulin or of a component of the antigen processing machinery, requiring invalidation of the two copies of the corresponding gene. Moreover, HLA-loss melanoma cells would then have to select additional mechanisms to resist NK cell lysis. Another consequence of antigen multiplicity is antigen spreading, which we found to be important if not decisive in melanoma patients displaying tumor regression following vaccination with one or two tumor-specific antigens [97, 98]. Antigen spreading is also observed after adoptive transfer [99], and it is probably one of the major mechanisms behind the rare complete and durable melanoma regressions observed after immunotherapy. Another mechanism underlying success is likely the absence or minimal contribution of local immunosuppressive mechanisms.

Conclusions

The rules governing melanoma antigenicity toward autologous T cells are now well established. They apply to most other tumor types. It is likely that the important immunogenicity of melanomas, illustrated by the spontaneous anti-tumor T cell responses in melanoma patients, owes much to the melanocyte differentiation antigens and to the low level of natural T cell tolerance to them. Published data on immunotherapy in melanoma patients do not yet allow to conclude that particular antigens will provide more clinical benefit than others. However, there are already confirmations that using not strictly tumor-specific antigens can lead to clinical autoimmunity.

Acknowledgments We thank Jerôme Degueldre for data processing, Suzanne Depelchin for editorial assistance, and Thomas Wölfel (Mainz, Germany) for critical reading of the manuscript and inclusion in Fig. 11.3 of results from patient MZ7-MEL.

References

1. Oble DA, Loewe R, Yu P, Mihm Jr MC. Focus on TILs: prognostic significance of tumor infiltrating lymphocytes in human melanoma. Cancer Immun. 2009;9:3.
2. Morton DL, Eilber FR, Holmes EC, et al. BCG immunotherapy of malignant melanoma: summary of a seven-year experience. Ann Surg. 1971;180:635–43.
3. Rosenberg SA, Lotze MT, Yang JC, et al. Prospective randomized trial of high-dose interleukin-2 alone or in conjunction with lymphokine-activated killer cells for the treatment of patients with advanced cancer. J Natl Cancer Inst. 1993;85:622–32.
4. Atkins MB, Lotze MT, Dutcher JP, et al. High-dose recombinant interleukin 2 therapy for patients with metastatic melanoma: analysis of 270 patients treated between 1985 and 1993. J Clin Oncol. 1999;17:2105–16.
5. Petrella T, Quirt I, Verma S. Haynes AE, Charette M, Bak K. Single-agent interleukin-2 in the treatment of metastatic melanoma: a systematic review. Cancer Treat Rev. 2007;33:484–96.
6. Kirkwood JM, Strawderman MH, Ernstoff MS, Smith TJ, Borden EC, Blum RH. Interferon alfa-2b adjuvant therapy of high-risk resected cutaneous melanoma: the Eastern Cooperative Oncology Group Trial EST 1684. J Clin Oncol. 1996;14:7–17.
7. Rosenberg SA, Lotze MT, Muul LM, et al. Observations on the systemic administration of autologous lymphokine-activated killer cells and recombinant interleukin-2 to patients with metastatic cancer. New Engl J Med. 1985;313:1485–92.
8. Topalian SL, Solomon D, Davis FP, et al. Immunotherapy of patients with advanced cancer using tumor-infiltrating lymphocytes and recombinant interleukin-2: a pilot study. J Clin Oncol. 1988;6:839–53.
9. van der Bruggen P, Stroobant V, Van Pel A, Van den Eynde B. Peptide database of T-cell defined tumor antigens; 2009. URL: http://www.cancerimmunity.org/peptidedatabase/Tcellepitopes.htm.

10. Boon T, van der Bruggen P. Human tumor antigens recognized by T lymphocytes. J Exp Med. 1996;183:725–9.
11. Tureci O, Sahin U, Schobert I, et al. The SSX-2 gene, which is involved in the t(X;18) translocation of synovial sarcomas, codes for the human tumor antigen HOM-MEL-40. Cancer Res. 1996;56:4766–72.
12. Falk K, Rötzschke O, Rammensee H-G. Cellular peptide composition governed by major histocompatibility complex class I molecules. Nature. 1990;348:248–51.
13. Lurquin C, Van Pel A, Mariamé B, et al. Structure of the gene of tum- transplantation antigen P91A: the mutated exon encodes a peptide recognized with Ld by cytolytic T cells. Cell. 1989;58:293–303.
14. Sibille C, Chomez P, Wildmann C, et al. Structure of the gene of tum- transplantation antigen P198: a point mutation generates a new antigenic peptide. J Exp Med. 1990;172:35–45.
15. Wang HY, Peng G, Guo Z, Shevach EM, Wang RF. Recognition of a new ARTC1 peptide ligand uniquely expressed in tumor cells by antigen-specific CD4+ regulatory T cells. J Immunol. 2005;174:2661–70.
16. Huang J, El-Gamil M, Dudley ME, Li YF, Rosenberg SA, Robbins PF. T cells associated with tumor regression recognize frameshifted products of the CDKN2A tumor suppressor gene locus and a mutated HLA class I gene product. J Immunol. 2004;172:6057–64.
17. Wang R-F, Wang X, Atwood AC, Topalian SL, Rosenberg SA. Cloning genes encoding MHC class II-restricted antigens: mutated CDC27 as a tumor antigen. Science. 1999;284:1351–4.
18. Wölfel T, Hauer M, Schneider J, et al. A p16[INK4a]-insensitive CDK4 mutant targeted by cytolytic T lymphocytes in a human melanoma. Science. 1995;269:1281–4.
19. Sharkey MS, Lizee G, Gonzales MI, Patel S, Topalian SL. CD4[(+)] T-cell recognition of mutated B-RAF in melanoma patients harboring the V599E mutation. Cancer Res. 2004;64:1595–9.
20. Andersen MH, Fensterle J, Ugurel S, et al. Immunogenicity of constitutively active [V599E]BRaf. Cancer Res. 2004;64:5456–60.
21. Linard B, Bézieau S, Benlalam H, et al. A ras-mutated peptide targeted by CTL infiltrating a human melanoma lesion. J Immunol. 2002;168:4802–8.
22. Pleasance ED, Cheetham RK, Stephens PJ, et al. A comprehensive catalogue of somatic mutations from a human cancer genome. Nature. 2010;463:191–6.
23. Wood LD, Parsons DW, Jones S, et al. The genomic landscapes of human breast and colorectal cancers. Science. 2007;318:1108–13.
24. Yewdell JW, Nicchitta CV. The DRiP hypothesis decennial: support, controversy, refinement and extension. Trends Immunol. 2006;27:368–73.
25. van der Bruggen P, Traversari C, Chomez P, et al. A gene encoding an antigen recognized by cytolytic T lymphocytes on a human melanoma. Science. 1991;254:1643–7.
26. Haas GGJ, D'Cruz OJ, De Bault LE. Distribution of human leukocyte antigen-ABC and -D/DR antigens in the unfixed human testis. Am J Reprod Immunol Microbiol. 1988;18:47–51.
27. Fiszer D, Kurpisz M. Major histocompatibility complex expression on human, male germ cells: a review. Am J Reprod Immunol. 1998;40:172–6.
28. De Plaen E, Arden K, Traversari C, et al. Structure, chromosomal localization and expression of twelve genes of the MAGE family. Immunogenetics. 1994;40:360–9.
29. Jungbluth AA, Silva Jr WA, Iversen K, et al. Expression of cancer-testis (CT) antigens in placenta. Cancer Immun. 2007;7:15.
30. Chomez P, De Backer O, Bertrand M, De Plaen E, Boon T, Lucas S. An overview of the MAGE gene family with the identification of all human members of the family. Cancer Res. 2001;61:5544–51.
31. Boël P, Wildmann C, Sensi M-L, et al. BAGE, a new gene encoding an antigen recognized on human melanomas by cytolytic T lymphocytes. Immunity. 1995;2:167–75.
32. Van den Eynde B, Peeters O, De Backer O, Gaugler B, Lucas S, Boon T. A new family of genes coding for an antigen recognized by autologous cytolytic T lymphocytes on a human melanoma. J Exp Med. 1995;182:689–98.
33. Chen Y-T, Scanlan MJ, Sahin U, et al. A testicular antigen aberrantly expressed in human cancers detected by autologous antibody screening. Proc Natl Acad Sci USA. 1997;94:1914–8.

34. Lethé B, Lucas S, Michaux L, et al. LAGE-1, a new gene with tumor specificity. Int J Cancer. 1998;76:903–8.
35. Gure AO, Wei IJ, Old LJ, Chen YT. The SSX gene family: characterization of 9 complete genes. Int J Cancer. 2002;101:448–53.
36. Hogan KT, Coppola MA, Gatlin CL, et al. Identification of novel and widely expressed cancer/testis gene isoforms that elicit spontaneous cytotoxic T-lymphocyte reactivity to melanoma. Cancer Res. 2004;64:1157–63.
37. Mulcahy KA, Rimoldi D, Brasseur F, et al. Infrequent expression of the MAGE gene family in uveal melanomas. Int J Cancer. 1996;66:738–42.
38. De Smet C, Lurquin C, Lethé B, Martelange V, Boon T. DNA methylation is the primary silencing mechanism for a set of germ line- and tumor-specific genes with a CpG-rich promoter. Mol Cell Biol. 1999;19:7327–35.
39. De Smet C, De Backer O, Faraoni I, Lurquin C, Brasseur F, Boon T. The activation of human gene MAGE-1 in tumor cells is correlated with genome-wide demethylation. Proc Natl Acad Sci USA. 1996;93:7149–53.
40. Sigalotti L, Fratta E, Coral S, et al. Intratumor heterogeneity of cancer/testis antigens expression in human cutaneous melanoma is methylation-regulated and functionally reverted by 5-aza-2'-deoxycytidine. Cancer Res. 2004;64:9167–71.
41. De Smet C, Loriot A, Boon T. A promoter-dependent mechanism leading to selective hypomethylation within the 5' region of gene MAGE-A1 in tumor cells. Mol Cell Biol. 2004;24: 4781–90.
42. Loriot A, De Plaen E, Boon T, De Smet C. Transient down-regulation of DNMT1 methyltransferase leads to activation and stable hypomethylation of MAGE-A1 in melanoma cells. J Biol Chem. 2006;281:10118–25.
43. Dalerba P, Ricci A, Russo V, et al. High homogeneity of MAGE, BAGE, GAGE, tyrosinase and Melan-A/MART-1 gene expression in clusters of multiple simultaneous metastases of human melanoma: implications for protocol design of therapeutic antigen-specific vaccination strategies. Int J Cancer. 1998;77:200–4.
44. Feller AJ, Duan Z, Penson R, Toh HC, Seiden MV. TRAG-3, a novel cancer/testis antigen, is overexpressed in the majority of melanoma cell lines and malignant melanoma. Anticancer Res. 2000;20:4147–51.
45. Martelange V, De Smet C, De Plaen E, Lurquin C, Boon T. Identification on a human sarcoma of two new genes with tumor-specific expression. Cancer Res. 2000;60:3848–55.
46. Monji M, Nakatsura T, Senju S, et al. Identification of a novel human cancer/testis antigen, KM-HN-1, recognized by cellular and humoral immune responses. Clin Cancer Res. 2004;10:6047–57.
47. Chen YT, Scanlan MJ, Venditti CA, et al. Identification of cancer/testis-antigen genes by massively parallel signature sequencing. Proc Natl Acad Sci USA. 2005;102:7940–5.
48. Guilloux Y, Lucas S, Brichard VG, et al. A peptide recognized by human cytolytic T lymphocytes on HLA-A2 melanomas is encoded by an intron sequence of the N-acetylglucosaminyltransferase V gene. J Exp Med. 1996;183:1173–83.
49. Moreau-Aubry A, Le Guiner S, Labarrière N, Gesnel MC, Jotereau F, Breathnach R. A processed pseudogene codes for a new antigen recognized by a CD8(+) T cell clone on melanoma. J Exp Med. 2000;191:1617–24.
50. Schiavetti F, Thonnard J, Colau D, Boon T, Coulie PG. A human endogenous retroviral sequence encoding an antigen recognized on melanoma by cytolytic T lymphocytes. Cancer Res. 2002;62:5510–6.
51. Gotter J, Brors B, Hergenhahn M, Kyewski B. Medullary epithelial cells of the human thymus express a highly diverse selection of tissue-specific genes colocalized in chromosomal clusters. J Exp Med. 2004;199:155–66.
52. Derbinski J, Schulte A, Kyewski B, Klein L. Promiscuous gene expression in medullary thymic epithelial cells mirrors the peripheral self. Nat Immunol. 2001;2:1032–9.
53. Lonchay C, van der Bruggen P, Connerotte T, et al. Correlation between tumor regression and T cell responses in melanoma patients vaccinated with a MAGE antigen. Proc Natl Acad Sci USA. 2004;101:14631–8.

54. Hanagiri T, van Baren N, Neyns B, Boon T, Coulie PG. Analysis of a rare melanoma patient with a spontaneous CTL response to a MAGE-A3 peptide presented by HLA-A1. Cancer Immunol Immunother. 2006;55:178–84.

55. Godelaine D, Carrasco J, Lucas S, et al. Polyclonal CTL responses observed in melanoma patients vaccinated with dendritic cells pulsed with a MAGE-3.A1 peptide. J Immunol. 2003;171:4893–7.

56. Karanikas V, Lurquin C, Colau D, et al. Monoclonal anti-MAGE-3 CTL responses in melanoma patients displaying tumor regression after vaccination with a recombinant canarypox virus. J Immunol. 2003;171:4898–904.

57. Anichini A, Maccalli C, Mortarini R, et al. Melanoma cells and normal melanocytes share antigens recognized by HLA-A2-restricted cytotoxic T cell clones from melanoma patients. J Exp Med. 1993;177:989–98.

58. Brichard V, Van Pel A, Wölfel T, et al. The tyrosinase gene codes for an antigen recognized by autologous cytolytic T lymphocytes on HLA-A2 melanomas. J Exp Med. 1993;178:489–95.

59. Kawakami Y, Eliyahu S, Delgado CH, et al. Cloning of the gene coding for a shared human melanoma antigen recognized by autologous T cells infiltrating into tumor. Proc Natl Acad Sci USA. 1994;91:3515–9.

60. Coulie PG, Brichard V, Van Pel A, et al. A new gene coding for a differentiation antigen recognized by autologous cytolytic T lymphocytes on HLA-A2 melanomas. J Exp Med. 1994;180:35–42.

61. Kawakami Y, Eliyahu S, Delgado CH, et al. Identification of a human melanoma antigen recognized by tumor-infiltrating lymphocytes associated with in vivo tumor rejection. Proc Natl Acad Sci USA. 1994;91:6458–62.

62. Cox AL, Skipper J, Chen Y, et al. Identification of a peptide recognized by five melanoma-specific human cytotoxic T cell lines. Science. 1994;264:716–9.

63. Wang R-F, Parkhurst MR, Kawakami Y, Robbins PF, Rosenberg SA. Utilization of an alternative open reading frame of a normal gene in generating a novel human cancer antigen. J Exp Med. 1996;183:1131–40.

64. Wang R-F, Appella E, Kawakami Y, Kang X, Rosenberg SA. Identification of TRP-2 as a human tumor antigen recognized by cytotoxic T lymphocytes. J Exp Med. 1996;184:2207–16.

65. Hoek KS, Schlegel NC, Eichhoff OM, et al. Novel MITF targets identified using a two-step DNA microarray strategy. Pigment Cell Melanoma Res. 2008;21:665–76.

66. Kawakami Y, Eliyahu S, Sakaguchi K, et al. Identification of the immunodominant peptides of the MART-1 human melanoma antigen recognized by the majority of HLA-A2-restricted tumor infiltrating lymphocytes. J Exp Med. 1994;180:347–52.

67. Romero P, Gervois N, Schneider J, et al. Cytolytic T lymphocyte recognition of the immunodominant HLA-A*0201-restricted Melan-A/MART-1 antigenic peptide in melanoma. J Immunol. 1997;159:2366–74.

68. Valmori D, Fonteneau J-F, Lizana CM, et al. Enhanced generation of specific tumor-reactive CTL in vitro by selected Melan-A/MART-1 immunodominant peptide analogues. J Immunol. 1998;160:1750–8.

69. Chaux P, Vantomme V, Coulie P, Boon T, van der Bruggen P. Estimation of the frequencies of anti-MAGE-3 cytolytic T lymphocyte precursors in blood from individuals without cancer. Int J Cancer. 1998;77:538–42.

70. Speiser DE, Baumgaertner P, Voelter V, et al. Unmodified self antigen triggers human CD8 T cells with stronger tumor reactivity than altered antigen. Proc Natl Acad Sci USA. 2008;105:3849–54.

71. Parkhurst MR, Salgaller ML, Southwood S, et al. Improved induction of melanoma-reactive CTL with peptides from the melanoma antigen gp100 modified at HLA-A*0201-binding residues. J Immunol. 1996;157:2539–48.

72. Walton SM, Gerlinger M, de la Rosa O, et al. Spontaneous CD8 T cell responses against the melanocyte differentiation antigen RAB38/NY-MEL-1 in melanoma patients. J Immunol. 2006;177:8212–8.

73. Touloukian CE, Leitner WW, Schnur RE, et al. Normal tissue depresses while tumor tissue enhances human T cell responses in vivo to a novel self/tumor melanoma antigen, OA1. J Immunol. 2003;170:1579–85.
74. Ikeda H, Lethé B, Lehmann F, et al. Characterization of an antigen that is recognized on a melanoma showing partial HLA loss by CTL expressing an NK inhibitory receptor. Immunity. 1997;6:199–208.
75. Oberthuer A, Hero B, Spitz R, Berthold F, Fischer M. The tumor-associated antigen PRAME is universally expressed in high-stage neuroblastoma and associated with poor outcome. Clin Cancer Res. 2004;10:4307–13.
76. van Baren N, Chambost H, Ferrant A, et al. PRAME, a gene encoding an antigen recognized on a human melanoma by cytolytic T cells, is expressed in acute leukaemia cells. Br J Haematol. 1998;102:1376–9.
77. Pellat-Deceunynck C, Mellerin MP, Labarriere N, et al. The cancer germ-line genes MAGE-1, MAGE-3 and PRAME are commonly expressed by human myeloma cells. Eur J Immunol. 2000;30:803–9.
78. Epping MT, Wang L, Edel MJ, Carlee L, Hernandez M, Bernards R. The human tumor antigen PRAME is a dominant repressor of retinoic acid receptor signaling. Cell. 2005;122:835–47.
79. Epping MT, Bernards R. A causal role for the human tumor antigen preferentially expressed antigen of melanoma in cancer. Cancer Res. 2006;66:10639–42.
80. Greiner J, Schmitt M, Li L, et al. Expression of tumor-associated antigens in acute myeloid leukemia: Implications for specific immunotherapeutic approaches. Blood. 2006;108: 4109–17.
81. Griffioen M, Kessler JH, Borghi M, et al. Detection and functional analysis of CD8+ T cells specific for PRAME: a target for T-cell therapy. Clin Cancer Res. 2006;12:3130–6.
82. Schroers R, Huang XF, Hammer J, Zhang J, Chen SY. Identification of HLA DR7-restricted epitopes from human telomerase reverse transcriptase recognized by CD4+ T-helper cells. Cancer Res. 2002;62:2600–5.
83. Vonderheide RH, Hahn WC, Schultze JL, Nadler LM. The telomerase catalytic subunit is a widely expressed tumor-associated antigen recognized by cytolytic T lymphocytes. Immunity. 1999;10:673–9.
84. Minev B, Hipp J, Firat H, Schmidt JD, Langlade-Demoyen P, Zanetti M. Cytotoxic T cell immunity against telomerase reverse transcriptase in humans. Proc Natl Acad Sci USA. 2000;97:4796–801.
85. Godet Y, Moreau-Aubry A, Guilloux Y, et al. MELOE-1 is a new antigen overexpressed in melanomas and involved in adoptive T cell transfer efficiency. J Exp Med. 2008;205:2673–82.
86. Le Gal FA, Avril MF, Bosq J, et al. Direct evidence to support the role of antigen-specific CD8(+) T cells in melanoma-associated vitiligo. J Invest Dermatol. 2001;117:1464–70.
87. Yee C, Thompson JA, Roche P, et al. Melanocyte-destruction after antigen-specific immunotherapy of melanoma: direct evidence of T-cell mediated vitiligo. J Exp Med. 2000;192:1637–43.
88. Powell Jr DJ, Dudley ME, Hogan KA, Wunderlich JR, Rosenberg SA. Adoptive transfer of vaccine-induced peripheral blood mononuclear cells to patients with metastatic melanoma following lymphodepletion. J Immunol. 2006;177:6527–39.
89. Dudley ME, Wunderlich JR, Robbins PF, et al. Cancer regression and autoimmunity in patients after clonal repopulation with antitumor lymphocytes. Science. 2002;298:850–4.
90. Johnson LA, Morgan RA, Dudley ME, et al. Gene therapy with human and mouse T-cell receptors mediates cancer regression and targets normal tissues expressing cognate antigen. Blood. 2009;114:535–46.
91. Lamers CH, Sleijfer S, Vulto AG, et al. Treatment of metastatic renal cell carcinoma with autologous T-lymphocytes genetically retargeted against carbonic anhydrase IX: first clinical experience. J Clin Oncol. 2006;24 (13):e20–2.
92. Morgan RA, Yang JC, Kitano M, Dudley ME, Laurencot CM, Rosenberg SA. Case report of a serious adverse event following the administration of T cells transduced with a chimeric antigen receptor recognizing ERBB2. Mol Ther. 2010;18:843–51.

93. Lennerz V, Fatho M, Gentilini C, et al. The response of autologous T cells to a human melanoma is dominated by mutated neoantigens. Proc Natl Acad Sci USA. 2005;102:16013–8.
94. Barrow C, Browning J, MacGregor D, et al. Tumor antigen expression in melanoma varies according to antigen and stage. Clin Cancer Res. 2006;12:764–71.
95. Jungbluth AA, Chen YT, Stockert E, et al. Immunohistochemical analysis of NY-ESO-1 antigen expression in normal and malignant human tissues. Int J Cancer. 2001;92:856–60.
96. Rodriguez T, Mendez R, Roberts CH, et al. High frequency of homozygosity of the HLA region in melanoma cell lines reveals a pattern compatible with extensive loss of heterozygosity. Cancer Immunol Immunother. 2005;54:141–8.
97. Germeau C, Ma W, Schiavetti F, et al. High frequency of anti-tumor T cells in the blood of melanoma patients before and after vaccination with tumor antigens. J Exp Med. 2005; 201:241–8.
98. Carrasco J, Van Pel A, Neyns B, et al. Vaccination of a melanoma patient with mature dendritic cells pulsed with MAGE-3 peptides triggers the activity of nonvaccine anti-tumor cells. J Immunol. 2008;180:3585–93.
99. Hunder NN, Wallen H, Cao J, et al. Treatment of metastatic melanoma with autologous CD4+ T cells against NY-ESO-1. N Engl J Med. 2008;358:2698–703.
100. Huijbers IJ, Soudja SM, Uyttenhove C, et al. Minimal tolerance to a tumor antigen encoded by a cancer-germline gene. Journal of J Immunol. in press.

Chapter 12
Melanoma Vaccines

Pedro Romero and Daniel E. Speiser

Abstract Many vaccines have been very successful. They can protect from many different infectious diseases, and thus contribute enormously to public health. The majority of successful vaccines induce neutralizing antibodies, which are essential for protection from disease, by the inhibition of microbe invasion and spread through the body, via extracellular compartments, or by neutralization of toxins. In contrast to infectious diseases, the pathological process in cancer is primarily intracellular. Immunity to cancer depends mainly on T cells which are capable of identifying and eliminating abnormal cells, via recognition of peptide antigens presented by major histocompatibility complex molecules at the cell surface. In some instances, tumor-specific antibodies can contribute to immune defense against cancer. Unfortunately, for many solid tumors (including melanoma), this mechanism is insufficient. Nevertheless, the search for cancer-neutralizing antibodies continues, similar to, e.g., HIV neutralizing antibodies. In this chapter, we focus on the development of T cell vaccines, a great challenge but also a promising approach as a new therapy for melanoma, other cancers, and intracellular pathogens.

Keywords Antigen • Adjuvant • Vaccine • T cell • Dendritic cell • TLR • Viral vectors

P. Romero, MD (✉)
Therapeutic cancer vaccines, Ludwig Center for Cancer Research
of the University of Lausanne, Lausanne, Switzerland
e-mail: Pedro.Romero@inst.hospvd.ch

D.E. Speiser, MD
Ludwig Center for Cancer Research of the University of Lausanne, Lausanne, Switzerland

T.F. Gajewski and F.S. Hodi (eds.), *Targeted Therapeutics in Melanoma*,
Current Clinical Oncology, DOI 10.1007/978-1-61779-407-0_12,
© Springer Science+Business Media, LLC 2012

Introduction: Development of T Cell Vaccines

Synthetic vaccines are composed of at least two basic components: Antigen and adjuvant. A detailed discussion of specific antigens has been presented in Chap. 11. There is a relatively large consensus that immune protection against malignant disease requires antigen-specific (adaptive) immune responses including T cells. Some experts argue that stimulation of the innate immune system alone may be sufficient to generate tumor-specific immunity, since cancer tissue often produces tumor antigen allowing some activation of antigen-specific immune responses. Therefore, an increasing number of novel immune therapies are developed without taking advantage of (synthetic or recombinant) tumor antigens, essentially also because this approach simplifies drug production and application. However, tumor cells often produce only low amounts of antigen, which often are not present at the optimal location and/or time. Therefore, immune responses triggered by naturally expressed antigen may not be sufficiently timed, strong and/or anatomically focused to protect from tumor progression. In addition, immunotherapy without antigen often requires high and in part toxic drug doses in contrast to vaccines containing synthetic antigens that can have powerful effects already at low doses. For these reasons, we propose that synthetic cancer vaccines should include tumor antigens.

The second essential vaccine component is the so-called immunological "adjuvant". Adjuvants are immune stimulating agents which typically provide innate immune activation. They are important because immune responses remain poor when antigens are administered alone. For many years, adjuvants have been developed empirically, without significant progress in the understanding of their molecular nature and mechanisms of action. The discovery of dendritic cells (DC), and of their central role to link innate with adaptive immune responses, was key for progress. Besides regulating central mechanisms of the innate immune system, DCs are the most effective antigen-presenting cells for enabling antigen-specific T and B cell responses. But how are they put into action? Only about 15 years ago it was discovered that DCs become activated due to triggering of their pathogen recognition receptors (PRR). These receptors typically enable the innate immune system to sense microbes, but host-derived "stress" ligands also can be recognized. The best-characterized family of PRRs is the Toll-like receptors (TLRs) that bind microbial products [15, 48, 60, 144].

Four major criteria that adjuvants may need to fulfill for optimal promotion of T cell responses are:

- To promote vaccine depot formation at the site of injection
- To promote antigen uptake by DCs
- To promote DC migration to lymph nodes
- To induce DC activation, such that they upregulate major histocompatibility complex (MHC) and present antigens, express costimulatory and adhesion molecules, and produce cytokines.

Through these mechanisms, DCs produce Th1-type immune activators (e.g., IL-12 and type I IFNs), resulting in CD4+ and CD8+ T cell responses.

Based on these theoretical considerations, vaccine development is performed in preclinical studies, followed by clinical trials. Preclinical experiments include animal studies, because immune responses and tumor immune defense can only partially be simulated in vitro. The complex nature of the whole organism can generate surprises; predictions based on preclinical studies remain imprecise. After careful consideration, novel vaccine components are introduced in the clinic, whereby first-in-human applications are done in the context of clinical phase I trials. These trials have the purpose to evaluate toxicity and biological/immunological activity. The essential principles guiding the current and future development of T cell vaccination are summarized as follows:

- For enhanced efficacy of immunological therapies against cancer and infectious diseases, it is necessary to improve T cell vaccines, such that they activate T cells as profoundly as observed in natural immune responses against some viruses.
- Results from basic research have identified key molecules implied in T cell activation, which progressively become available and can be used as vaccine components. However, the number of candidate molecules is rapidly increasing, emphasizing the need for selection of the most promising ones for clinical testing.
- A suitable vaccine component is capable to promote human immune responses. This can be tested in small-scale phase I/II clinical studies, involving small numbers of patients and reasonably low costs, providing results rapidly.
- Clinical research and advanced laboratory techniques are required to precisely determine biological responses to vaccines. Cellular and molecular features can be assessed quantitatively and qualitatively.
- Results from such studies are used to eliminate useless approaches, and to select optimal vaccine components for testing in large phase III clinical studies (with 100s–1,000s of patients) assessing therapeutic efficacy.

The goal of therapeutic vaccination aimed at inducing specific T cell mediated immunity is to induce high frequencies of T cells, mainly CD8+ T cells, a good proportion of which should possess the ability to lyse tumor cells and to secrete at least IL-2, TNF-α, and IFN-γ. In addition, vaccination should also induce a tissue homing program in specific effector T cells that leads to efficient migration of T cells from the secondary lymphoid organs, where they were primed, to the tumor sites via the blood vessel network. Last, but not least, a definite proportion of vaccine induced T cells should possess memory qualities such as long-term persistence, poised to undergo expansion and proliferation upon reexposure to tumor antigen and a migratory program similar to that exhibited by naïve T cell precursors and the so-called central memory T cells. These ideal attributes of the response are some of the hallmarks of protective CD8 T cell responses in the case of intracellular pathogens, mainly viruses (Fig. 12.1). Clearly, while modern vaccines meet some of these criteria, much work remains to accomplish a detailed understanding of the molecular and cellular interactions required to mount such protective T cell immunity.

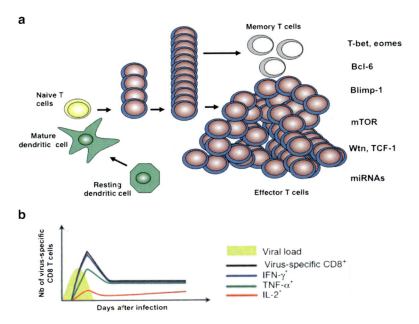

Fig. 12.1 Robust lymphocyte expansion and differentiation during a primary CD8+ T cell response to an acute viral infection, a paradigm of a protective MHC-I-restricted T cell response. (**a**) Naive CD8+ precursor cells exist in the peripheral mature immune system at very low frequencies. During priming, activated dendritic cells carry viral antigen to draining lymph nodes and interact with naïve antigen-specific CD8+ T cell precursors. Upon a productive interaction, T cells are activated and undergo rapid expansion involving one to two cell divisions per day, during the first week post infection. Coupled to cell division, CD8+ T cells acquire effector functions including lytic granules filled with perforin and granzymes and the ability to secrete several effector cytokines. A large number of effector cells is thus rapidly generated. At some point, a relatively small fraction of responding CD8+ T cells differentiate into memory cells. These processes are regulated by signaling pathways such as mTOR and Wnt/TCF-1 downstream of TCR and costimulatory receptors and by several transcription factors and microRNAs (for review cfr [30]). (**b**) Schematic representation of the kinetics of viral antigen load during an acute viral infection in a mouse model and the expansion of viral antigen-specific CD8 T cells. Antigen increases as a result of rapid viral replication; in parallel, viral antigen-specific CD8+ T cell numbers increase with a lag time of a few days. As the latter reach the peak expansion, viral antigen load decreases sharply. As viral infection subsides due to massive elimination of viral infected cells by specific CD8 effector T cells, the latter undergo massive attrition by activation induced cell death. A relatively small population of viral antigen-specific CD8+ T cells persists for long periods of time, which represents the memory pool. Please note that protective effector T cells typically secrete one or more cytokines, mainly IFN-γ, TNF-α, and IL-2. Double and triple cytokine producers are deemed multifunctional T cells and their presence often correlates with protection (adapted from Yi et al. [166])

Past and Present Melanoma Vaccine Development

The first vaccines to be considered for melanoma were based on tumor cells. The rationale for these came from animal model experimentation showing that repeated vaccination with irradiated tumor cells could elicit solid protective immunity. Large phase III clinical trials were conducted over the last three decades, which involved several thousand metastatic melanoma patients worldwide. Subsequently, progress in the understanding of T cell recognition of antigen led to the design of a whole new generation of vaccines based on the use of defined antigens. Since then, the field has focused on the testing of a large variety of antigen delivery systems for vaccination. Some lead candidates are today undergoing advanced phase clinical trial testing.

Cell Based Vaccines

An allogeneic cancer vaccine (Canvaxin™) developed from three melanoma cell lines, expressing at least 20 T cell defined tumor antigens, has been extensively tested in melanoma patients. In large trials involving 1,166 patients with stage III melanoma and 496 patients with resected stage IV melanoma, patients were randomized to Canvaxin™ plus BCG or placebo plus BCG after surgery. Matched pair analyses on patients who had received this vaccine after melanoma metastasis resection suggested efficacy and important survival benefit [57]. However, the two trials were prematurely terminated after the interim analysis suggested lack of clinical benefit [92]. Follow up in fact suggested a median survival in the vaccine arm shorter than in the placebo control group [38].

Another allogeneic melanoma vaccine reached the phase III testing in adjuvant high risk for recurrence melanoma. The vaccine consists of cell lysates (Melacine®) of two cell lines derived from metastases from two different patients. It is coadministered with an immunologic adjuvant, DETOX composed of monophosphoryl lipid A and mycobacterial (BCG) cell wall skeleton in an oil-in-water emulsion. The peptidoglycan in this adjuvant contains the NOD-2 agonist muramyl dipeptide. A phase II trial in 22 patients with metastatic melanoma suggested a 6% objective tumor response rate with some durable complete responses [90]. On the basis of these results, the Canadian authorities approved its use. Induction of tumor lysate specific cell mediated immunity was observed in a significant proportion of patients that correlated with clinical efficacy. Similar results were reported using autologous tumor cell lysates as vaccines in combination with the same DETOX adjuvant [42].

Melacine® vaccination in conjunction with IFN-α showed encouraging results which led to the initiation of a phase III trial to measure the clinical efficacy of this combined immunotherapy. The adjuvant trial of the Melacine® vaccine in stage II patients showed no benefit for the total study population [133]. Of interest, however, a significant clinical benefit was measured in the subset of patients expressing HLA-A2 and/or Cw3 [134]. These results remain to be confirmed in prospective studies with appropriately selected patients.

Gangliosides

The ganglioside GM2 is a serologically defined melanoma antigen which possesses strong immunogenicity. Administration of GM2 in combination with BCG induced specific IgM antibodies in the majority of patients which reportedly were correlated with improved recurrence-free survival and overall survival in stage III melanoma patients [82]. Multiple GM2 vaccine formulations were screened and a commercial preparation consisting of GM2 coupled to the multimeric protein keyhole limpet hemocyanin (KLH), a potent primary antigen, combined with QS-21 a saponin based adjuvant (GMK vaccine, Progenic Pharmaceuticals) was chosen for testing of clinical efficacy. Such vaccine formulation induced GM2-specific antibody responses in the majority of patients, even of the IgG type [25]. A large phase III study in stage II melanoma was performed in Europe to determine the efficacy of subcutaneous administration of GM2 conjugated to KLH compared to an observation group. Upon a median follow up of 1.8 years it was concluded that the adjuvant vaccination was ineffective and could even be detrimental in stage II melanoma patients [39]. Similar results were obtained in a trial including 880 patients with stage IIb-III melanoma randomized to high dose interferon therapy and the GM2-KLH conjugate vaccine [66]. Indeed, the trial was closed after the interim analysis indicated inferiority of GMK compared to high dose IFN in terms of both relapse-free survival and overall survival. Another phase III trial including 1,300 patients at immediate risk of recurrence randomized after surgery to vaccine or standard of care was also closed after the interim analysis revealed that the GMK vaccine failed to show effectiveness in terms of relapse-free survival over observation. Thus, the negative results impeded to measure in both of these large trials the impact of the vaccine on survival.

Peptide and Recombinant Protein Vaccines

Numerous vaccines based on synthetic peptides representing exact MHC class I molecule restricted epitopes have been tested in early phase clinical trials in patients with metastatic melanoma. Peptides have enormous advantages such as the possibility to rigorously define them as highly purified compounds at relatively low cost and to perform in depth monitoring of the specific T cell response. However, significant disadvantages are their intrinsic poor immunogenicity, the restricted population of melanoma patients eligible for vaccination and the narrow targeting which may cause selection of tumor escape variants. Defined peptide vaccines tried in melanoma have been exhaustively reviewed in the recent past [118, 120]. In general, peptides derived from both melanoma differentiation and cancer testis antigens have been extensively tested in conjunction with various defined adjuvants or loaded onto autologous dendritic cells. Peptide vaccine-specific T cell responses have been detected in most vaccinated patients albeit it generally required a step of short expansion in in vitro culture. A prominent exception is the response to the HLA-A2 restricted Melan-A/MART-1$_{26-35\ A27L}$ peptide analog when administered as an emulsion in mineral oil (Montanide ISA51) [79]. Remarkably, we could show that addition of a TLR-9 agonist to the emulsion containing the vaccinating peptide converted the vaccine into the most potent peptide vaccine formulation known to date [140]. Indeed, specific ex vivo detectable T cell responses were apparent in all vaccinated patients after two or more immunizations. The mean frequency of HLA-A2/Melan-A/MART-$1_{26\text{-}35\ A27L}$ tetramer$^+$ CD8$^+$ T cells was around 0.5% which progressively differentiated to effector memory T cells with enhanced lytic capacity upon repeated vaccination. It was interesting to find that the use of such potent adjuvant formulation conferred strong immunogenicity to the wild type Melan-A/MART-1 peptide [138]. In this case, the frequencies of peptide specific CD8$^+$ T cells were two folds lower than those induced by the enhanced peptide analog. However, on a per cell basis, specific CD8$^+$ T cells induced by vaccination with the wild type peptide were of a higher quality. They produced more IFN-γ in response to antigen and practically all cells recruited to the response had strong tumor reactivity and lytic activity. In contrast, close to 40% of those induced by enhanced peptide analog were poorly tumor reactive [138].

Another extensively tested peptide in vaccination trials has been the gp100$_{209\text{-}217\ 210M}$. This is also an enhanced peptide analog. Large trials have used this peptide emulsified in mineral oil based adjuvant ISA51. It has been found that repeated immunization can result in the induction of large specific T cell responses which nevertheless do not seem to translate into clinical benefit [119]. As with the Melan-A/MART-1 peptide vaccination studies mentioned above, the cross-reactivity of peptide analog-induced CD8 T cells with the naturally processed and presented gp100 tumor antigen in tumor cells is limited and only a fraction of tetramer$^+$ cells are able to recognize and lyse gp100$^+$ HLA-A2$^+$ tumor cells. A randomized phase II trial showed that immunization with the peptide emulsion every 3 weeks induced frequencies of specific T cells that were no different from those induced on a biweekly vaccination schedule [132]. In this case, robust memory specific CD8$^+$ T cell responses were recorded [153]. This peptide vaccine has also been tested for clinical efficacy in large randomized phase III trials. In one case, it was part of the pivotal study testing the antihuman CTLA-4 mAb ipilimumab. It was shown that the vaccine arm alone conferred no overall survival benefit while the anti-CTLA-4 alone or in combination with the gp100 peptide vaccine did double the median overall survival time in metastatic melanoma [56]. On the basis of these results, anti-CTLA-4 (ipilimumab, Yervoy$^®$) treatment was approved by the FDA on March 25th 2011 for the indication of advanced metastatic melanoma. In the other case, statistically significant extension of progression free survival and response rate were reported for the gp100 vaccine when combined with high dose IL-2 administration following vaccination [125]. It is intriguing that high dose IL-2 but not CTLA-4 blockade appears to confer some measure of clinical efficacy to the peptide vaccine. Future studies will address the many issues raised by these observations.

A way to overcome the narrow target population imposed by MHC restriction would be to combine various peptides, derived from various tumor antigens and restricted by various MHC class I and class II alleles, in the same vaccine formulation. This has been demonstrated to be feasible in multiple independent studies [28, 54, 112, 149]. In vivo competition for binding to the same MHC allelic product does not seem to be a limiting factor [9], even when a relatively large number of peptides is put together in the same emulsion for subcutaneous injections [128].

Heat shock proteins (hsp), particularly the hsp gp96 one, may possess intrinsic immunogenicity and carry tumor petides even after the purification procedure. The concept that these proteins may represent tumor vaccines has been tested in melanoma and the phase I/II clinical study could demonstrate elicitation of melanoma antigen-specific CD8 T cell responses in about half of immunized patients [10]. While there have been encouraging tumor responses, pursuing this approach is labor intensive and difficult to standardize as it involves the biochemical isolation of autologous tumor hsp gp96.

Two recombinant full-length proteins, MAGE-A3 and NY-ESO-1, have been successfully tested in the clinic. The recombinant MAGE-A3 protein is produced as a fusion with the lipoprotein D derived from *Haemophilus influenza* at its N-terminus and a polyhistidine tag on the C-terminus. The initial clinical study with this protein in patients with metastatic melanoma showed induction of specific immune responses in some patients and, importantly, encouraging clinical activity [73]. More recently, a randomized phase II clinical trial was performed to establish the relative efficacy of the adjuvant in which the recombinant MAGE-A3 fusion protein was formulated. Patients in one arm received an adjuvant containing the TLR-4 agonist morophosphoryl lipid A, the saponin QS21 and oil-in-water emulsion. Patients in the second arm received the same adjuvant components supplemented with liposomes containing CpG-ODNs that are TLR-9 agonists. The latter adjuvant mixture proved to be more potent both in terms of elicited immune responses and of clinical benefit [72]. A pivotal phase III trial is now underway (DERMA) sponsored by GlaxoSmithKline Bio to measure the clinical efficacy of recombinant MAGE-A3 with the complex adjuvant formulation (AS15™). This trial is recruiting in parallel with another pivotal phase III trial in patients with locally advanced non-small cell lung carcinoma patients bearing tumors that express the targeted tumor antigen. It should possible to have these decisive results available by approximately 2013.

The second recombinant protein is NY-ESO-1 produced in bacteria and sponsored jointly by the Ludwig Institute for Cancer Research and the Cancer Research Institute. This is a 180 amino acid long polypeptide which has turned out to be one of the most immunogenic of all the tumor antigens characterized thus far, and certainly, of those in the category of cancer testis antigens [50]. Melanoma patients have been vaccinated with this protein in conjunction with various adjuvants including adjuvanted nanoparticles (ISCOMatrix® [34, 98]), emulsified in the mineral oil based adjuvant ISA51 together with CpG-ODNs [150], covalently linked to cholesteryl-pullulan [62, 148], or injected intradermally at sites preconditioned by topical application of imiquimod [3].

Full-length proteins have the potential to provide multiple epitopes for T cell recognition, thus alleviating the MHC restriction of antigen recognition. One drawback, however, is the bias towards MHC class II antigen presentation and, conversely, poor presentation of MHC class I restricted antigens, due to the default delivery of proteins to the endocytic compartment. In this regard, long synthetic peptides (LSPs) may offer a more balanced presentation of antigens for both CD8 and CD4 T cells. Consensus is building that the optimal length of LSPs may be around 25–30 amino acids. The approach to cancer vaccination with LSPs has been tested in the clinics in women with HPV-16 vulvar intraepithelial neoplasia. In this trial, a tumor response rate of 50% was observed that correlated with the elicitation of broad systemic peptide specific T cell immunity [65]. Immunization with a 14 amino acid long peptide from the NY-ESO-1 antigen, emulsified in mineral oil, elicited both CD4+ and CD8+ T cell responses in the majority of ovarian carcinoma patients included in the study [102]. Similar studies are being conducted in patients with metastatic melanoma in the context of the Cancer Vaccine Collaborative consortium.

Dendritic Cell-Based Vaccines

Many of the concepts of therapeutic vaccines based on dendritic cells have been tested in patients with advanced metastatic melanoma. One of the first trials to be published included 16 melanoma patients vaccinated with monocyte-derived dendritic cells loaded with peptides and KLH [96]. The reported clinical benefit was encouraging and prompted a randomized phase III clinical study that compared this vaccine to chemotherapy with dacarbazine (DTIC) in a total of 108 melanoma patients. Despite the initial promise, the autologous peptide pulsed DC vaccination did not show superiority to the DTIC treatment [123].

DC can be loaded ex vivo with either peptides [124], as in these prototypic trials, recombinant proteins [44], or transduced with recombinant viruses, such as adenovirus [21], or even with mRNA by electroporation [17]. In one interesting phase I study, the Melan-A/MART-1 antigenic peptide was pulsed onto autologous peripheral blood mononuclear cells (PBMCs) and administered together with IL-12. Encouraging immunological and clinical results were reported [107]. It might be speculated that the low frequency circulating dendritic cells present in the PBLs were the active antigen presenting cells in the cell mixture. One of the parameters that are thought to be central to the success of DC-based vaccines is the type of DCs, as well as their state of differentiation [2]. In this regard, while CD34-derived DCs supplemented with IFN-α and loaded with melanoma antigenic peptides were deemed to be superior to the monocyte-derived DCs, the results of a carefully analyzed phase I trial including 22 advanced melanoma patients led to the conclusion that more knowledge is required about the appropriate DC to be used in the clinic [8]. A more recent study compared the immunogenicity of peptide loaded monocyte-derived DCs to that of Langerhans DC (LC), and again could not conclude on the superiority of either cell type [117].

Other studies have compared the immunological efficacy of monocyte-derived DCs (moDC) loaded with peptides to that of the same peptides administered in water-in-oil emulsions. The results showed that multiple peptides administered in the emulsion together with GM-CSF appeared superior to the same peptides loaded onto autologous moDCs [129]. A major issue when using DCs as vaccines is their relatively poor migration to the draining lymph nodes as well as their limited survival at the injection sites [152]. A mechanistic study conducted in a mouse model casts doubt on the ability of ex vivo prepared DCs to directly present antigen when used as vaccine and indicates that transfer of antigen to an endogenous antigen presenting cell is required [165]. Thus, alternative approaches to ex vivo generation of DCs may be advantageous. One possibility that is gaining favor is the use of antibodies directed against molecules selectively expressed on the surface of DCs to target antigens directly in vivo [16, 143].

Recombinant Vector-Based Vaccines

Numerous recombinant viral vectors have been tried in patients with advanced metastatic melanoma. The antigens delivered have included single minigenes encoding exact MHC-I restricted T cell epitopes, strings of epitopes, or full-length tumor antigens. Induction of specific T cell immunity has been documented and even, in some cases, favorable clinical outcomes after vaccination with viral vectors such as modified vaccinia Ankara (MVA), canary pox, fowl pox, and adenovirus [1, 59, 83, 109, 130, 135, 151].

Generally, viral vectors, in contrast to proteins, are efficient inducers of MHC-I restricted CD8 T cell immunity because they can infect cells and replicate to various extents depending upon the degree of attenuation. In this regard, such vectors are desired for the purpose of therapeutic vaccination against cancer. However, safety considerations usually require that vectors cannot be replicative or are highly attenuated. This is detrimental to their capacity to induce robust CD8 T cell immunity, although attenuation does not completely abrogate this property. Another, perhaps more important, drawback of most viral vectors is the immunodominance of viral antigens that may outcompete the recruitment and expansion of T cells specific for the insert encoding the tumor-associated antigen. This has been clearly shown to be the case of the STEP trial using recombinant adenovirus to induce anti-HIV therapeutic immunity and it has been clearly documented in the case of recombinant vaccinia carrying a string of MHC-I restricted melanoma associated epitopes [87, 131]. Thus, the choice of appropriate recombinant viral vector is a tradeoff between attenuation, intrinsic vector backbone immunogenicity, and antigen to be delivered. Moreover, prime and boost regimens with two different vectors may minimize neutralization by specific antiviral antibodies and therefore contribute to efficient antitumor vaccination [59, 80, 105, 115].

A few bacterial vectors are also at different stages of preclinical or even clinical development for the immunotherapy of cancer, particularly of melanoma. *Listeria monocytogenes* is one that has been extensively characterized as a vector capable of inducing strong antigen-specific CD8 T cell responses in mouse models and is under development for use in humans [163]. The type III secretion system in various gram negative bacteria such as *Salmonella* [122, 169] or *Pseudomonas aeruginosa* [40] are also being used successfully to deliver recombinant antigens to antigen presenting cells.

Nucleic Acid-Based Vaccines

Naked DNA has been extensively used for vaccination. Major advantages are the possibility to isolate and produce relatively large quantities of cDNA in expression plasmids, the feasibility to produce this material in GMP grade and the good safety record in preclinical settings as well as in humans. However, the results obtained so far in many different vaccine contexts show that DNA vaccines are weakly immunogenic. Repeated immunization with DNA plasmid leads to only weak specific antibody and T cell responses, although these can be efficiently boosted by other antigen delivery systems. This has been the case for the DNA vaccines tested thus far in early phase clinical trials of patients with metastatic melanoma. They have included plasmids encoding melanoma associated antigens such as tyrosinase [161], human gp100 [24], xenogeneic gp100 [49], or strings of DNA encoding defined epitopes recognized by tumor reactive CD8 T cells [32, 113].

It is also interesting that mRNAs stabilized with protamine and encoding several melanoma associated antigens have been injected directly via the intradermal route to 21 metastatic melanoma patients. Induction of specific T cell responses and even some evidence of clinical efficacy were reported for some of the patients included in that study [155]. Several other trials have tested the approach of ex vivo transduction of autologous monocyte-derived dendritic cells with either total tumor mRNA [75, 84] or mRNAs encoding defined tumor antigens [51, 88]. In both approaches, mRNAs ensure transient expression of the desired antigens, approximately 2–4 days. A great deal of effort has gone into their optimization for enhanced in vitro and in vivo stability as well as their ability to direct expression of antigen in the appropriate antigen processing and presentation compartments [71, 74].

Immunological Tolerance

Some tumor antigens are derived from mutated genes. Antigen-specific T cells often respond efficiently to such antigens, since these are neoantigens to which immunological tolerance is not readily established. However, these antigens are patient-specific, meaning that vaccines would need to be produced individually for each patient, which is rarely possible. In contrast, tumors from different patients and different histotypes often share antigens. These antigens are usually "self," with the consequence of some degree of immune tolerance. Thymic selection results in T cell repertoires that are partially deficient of TCRs with high affinity to self-molecules. Consequently, T cells to self-antigens are less reactive and relatively rare. Moreover, mechanisms of peripheral tolerance further compromise T cell function [43, 76, 101, 157, 159, 160]. There are profound deficits in functions of tumor antigen-specific T cells in metastatic lesions [170]. The reasons for this are probably numerous, and are only briefly mentioned here. We distinguish cell intrinsic and cell extrinsic mechanisms of T cell tolerance or anergy. T cell intrinsic anergy is due to various mechanisms, associated with expression of Egr-2, Egr-3, and Grail [157], but the regulation of T cell anergy still requires further elucidation. Multiple T cell extrinsic mechanisms are also involved. Most cells of the body, including tumor cells, are deficient in costimulatory molecules, with the result of insufficient T cell stimulation. In turn, ligands for inhibitory T cell receptors (TCRs) are frequently expressed in tumor tissue, with functional impact on T cell mediated immune defense [35, 37, 45, 108, 147]. Furthermore, the microenvironment of malignant tissue is immune suppressive, due to tumor-associated macrophages [94], myeloid-derived suppressor cells [19, 46, 103], plasmacytoid DCs [85], and immature myeloid-derived dendritic cells [11]. In animal models, it has been found that T cell function is reduced already early during disease development [142]. Thus, although self-tolerance and suppressive mechanisms are mostly evident in individuals with large tumor burden, they may be functional already much earlier.

Deficient T cell function in malignant disease may have similarities to T cells in chronic infection. Therefore, animal models of infectious diseases are investigated to study T cell mediated immunity. Microbes causing acute infections are often eliminated by T cells. However, when viruses persist at high copy numbers and for several months, T cells are exhausted and eventually deleted. Thus, prolonged infection is associated with functional T cell deficits. The underlying mechanisms have been carefully studied in the murine model of infection with lymphocytic choriomeningitis virus (LCMV). During prolonged infection, T cells progressively lose the capacity to produce IL-2, TNF-α, IFN-γ, and finally cytotoxicity [156, 157]. Thus, T cells become progressively exhausted, and may eventually even undergo apoptosis. However, in malignant disease, T cell exhaustion is often not evident. Although it may occur in some instances [68], circulating T cells in cancer patients are often functionally competent [141, 170]. Deficits in cytokine production are observed among T cells from metastases, but the reasons remain poorly understood. Therefore, it is necessary to further elucidate whether cellular and molecular features of T cell exhaustion are frequent in cancer, or whether low T cell activity in malignant disease is more prominently explained by mechanisms of T cell anergy and self-tolerance.

There exist several strategies to improve T cell function against cancer. One approach is to combine vaccination with agents that modulate T cell responses. The elucidation of questions on T cell exhaustion, anergy, and self-tolerance is important, in order to find the most promising molecular pathways that can be targeted for cancer therapy. Various approaches, such as CTLA-4 blockade or PD-1 blockade, neutralization of IL-10 [20], or of STAT3, are described elsewhere in this book.

Analysis of Cancer Specific T Cell Responses, and Correlates of T Cell Mediated Protection from Disease

T cells are highly "sensitive detectors" of immune stimulation. Upon natural infection with a virus, antigen-specific naïve T cells proliferate during the first 1–2 weeks to reach high T cell frequencies, with up to 10^5-fold expansion [22, 93] thus, exceeding the proliferative potential of most other cells in the body. In contrast, ineffective T cell triggering leads to much lower numbers of T cells, which are less likely to protect from disease [104]. Besides these quantitative aspects, the quality of T cell responses is likely important. For example, recent data suggest that T cell responses should include both effector and memory T cells [111]. Therefore, novel immune therapies should elicit substantial numbers of T cells, and profoundly impact on T cell differentiation such that effector cells become capable of destroying tumor cells, and lead to memory cells to assure long-term maintenance of responses.

Despite considerable efforts to date, T cell vaccination is still in an early phase of development. Unfortunately, only little therapeutic effect has yet been achieved with the available vaccines. To provide more information on the effects of experimental vaccination in early phase clinical trials, these studies are progressively exploited to investigate human immune responses in great detail. One of the aims is to determine whether those mechanisms that were established in basic models are actually functional in humans. This is much easier said than done. For example, dendritic cells (DCs) are difficult to assess, because they are infrequent, and it remains very difficult to trace activated DCs in vivo. Hopefully, future technologies will enable to identify DCs from individual patients, to characterize how they react to various stimuli, and how they subsequently impact on immune responses. By contrast, a field where great progress has already been made is for investigation of T cell responses in patients.

Assessment of T Cell Responses

Antigen-specific T cells can be detected based on TCR mediated binding to peptide–MHC (pMHC), or on cytokine production after short (4–6 h) triggering with antigen [6, 61, 63, 69]. For the former, the invention of fluorescent pMHC multimers [6] (formerly called tetramers) has opened a wide array of opportunities, i.e., to quantify T cells, to characterize their function, and to molecularly dissect cellular features down to the single cell level, as discussed in more detail below. A major disadvantage of pMHC multimers is that one can only identify T cells specific for known epitopes. Short-term (4–6 h) triggering of T cells reveals previously primed but not naïve T cells that can be detected either by flow cytometry (upon intracellular cytokine staining) or by Elispot assay [31, 61]. These techniques have the advantage that they detect T cells specific for known and unknown epitopes. However, one can only detect those T cells that have functional properties corresponding to the reagents used (e.g., anti-IFN-γ, anti-TNF-α, or anti-interleukin antibodies). Inhibitory T cells (e.g., Treg) or T cells producing other factors (e.g., inhibitory cytokines) are rarely detected. Inhibitory cells are more frequent among $CD4^+$ T cells. Unfortunately, the progress with pMHC multimers is much less advanced for the detection of $CD4^+$ T cells, a deficit that one needs to overcome for more comprehensive identification of activating and inhibitory T cell functions, and qualitative characterization (polarization) of T cell responses.

T cells with many different specificities can be analyzed simultaneously. Innovative assays use ten or more multimers, each labeled with different color combinations [52, 97]. They take advantage of novel fluorochromes and quantum dots, and multi-parameter flow cytometry. The approach can be further exploited by combining with phenotypic and functional analysis, enabling more comprehensive quantitative and qualitative assessment of a spectrum of antigen-specific T cells. The large amount of data provided with multi-parameter assays may also be analyzed and interpreted by specialized statistical tools, including new unsupervised analyses comparable to approaches developed for gene microarray studies.

High assay quality becomes increasingly important given the complexity and high precision requirements of sophisticated assays. Assay development generally has at least two phases, i.e., optimization and validation. Careful optimization may lead to useful results. Subsequently, the optimized assays require validation, which consists of the assessment of (1) precision (reproducibility, coefficient of variation), (2) accuracy or comparison with reference methods, and (3) robustness, i.e., the study of variations introduced by, e.g., different (batches of) reagents, different centers, etc. In case validation is not satisfactory, one needs to go back to further optimize the assay.

With the use of peptide MHC-I multimers, one can directly characterize phenotype and function of single antigen-specific T cells. The current limit of detection of specific cell populations using MHC-I multimers is approximately 0.01% of antigen-specific T cells. Less frequent populations cannot be detected ex vivo. The strategy to analyze T cells directly ex vivo enables immediate quantification of T cell numbers. Moreover, direct ex vivo analysis of phenotype and function allows concluding on T cell function in vivo. Finally, gene expression analysis can be done with T cells sorted directly ex vivo with pMHC multimers. With this approach, T cell responses can be dissected in great detail [7, 64, 110, 121, 136].

Many strategies require to culture T cells in vitro for one or several weeks, which introduces artifacts. Unfortunately, results are often overinterpreted. Nevertheless, in vitro cultured cells usually enable to distinguish presence from absence of T cell responses. Quantitative assessment of antigen-specific T cell numbers, however, are only possible when calculations are based on so-called "limiting dilution" cultures [145], which is rarely done. Analysis of limiting dilution cultures may be performed with multimers or by functional assays.

Particularly during acute disease phases, T cell function is highly dynamic. After priming or boosting, the first few days are characterized by extraordinary strong T cell proliferation, which is often followed by a steep decline of immune responses. Such acute T cell responses are better understood as opposed to T cells in chronic disease and cancer, which is perhaps one reason why it is frequently argued that effector T cell responses are short-lived. Indeed, in case of pathogen elimination, most T cells die and only a small number of memory T cells can persist. They are long-lived and proliferate at very low rates. In contrast, in malignant disease or chronic inflammation, numbers of T cells are larger, and the majority of them is constantly active and proliferates at relatively high rates.

As suggested by some studies, advanced patient age may be associated with decreased immune competence. It has been argued that T cells become increasingly senescent and progressively loose proliferative capacity [23, 53, 77, 81, 89, 99, 106]. Yet, prevention and particularly treatment of intracellular infections or cancer requires continued T cell proliferation, emphasizing the need to determine if and how T cells are capable for this task at medium and long term. Novel data indicate that clonotypic effector T cell populations can actually persist over many years in cancer patients, and that these T cells may be frequently and successfully induced, boosted, and maintained at high numbers and high effector activity by repetitive vaccination [58, 137]. Even in absence of antigen, CD8+ T cell clonotypes may not only persist as memory, but also as effector cells [41, 95, 146].

The number of T cell antigens in malignant disease is usually large, with potentially hundreds of unknown epitopes. Although difficult to achieve, it is necessary to assess the complete spectrum of antitumor antigen-specific T cell responses. Measuring cytokine production allows the detection of such T cells, provided that they are triggered with the relevant antigens. Autologous tumor cells are the most comprehensive source of antigens, but they are often not available. Alternatively, whole tumor antigenic proteins, and/or large numbers of (overlapping) peptides can be used.

An alternative strategy to identify reactive T cells is by staining for early activation membrane markers, expressed upon challenge in vitro with the antigen, e.g., sets of overlapping peptides. It has been proposed that the expression of CD154 on CD4+ T cells [26] and of CD137 on CD8+ T cells [154, 162] reliably reveal the majority of specific T cells in short-term stimulation assays (6–20 h). Major advantages of this assay format are the ability to simultaneously detect CD4+ and CD8+ T cell responses, the independence from previous knowledge of MHC restriction and/ or identity of the antigenic peptides and the ability to isolate responding viable cells by cell sorting.

Correlates of T Cell Mediated Protection from Disease

What are the most prominent biological features of T cells that correlate with protection? Many animal studies have allowed progress, but further knowledge is needed to fully characterize protective T cells, especially in humans. In infectious diseases, several T cell criteria have been established as correlates of protection. First, the capacity of T cells to efficiently interact with cognate antigen [4, 12, 36, 47, 86, 126, 139, 164, 167], a property which is often termed as "functional avidity" and which is controlled by TCRs and co-receptors. Functional avidity correlates with the capacity of T cells to recognize naturally expressed and processed tumor antigen [70]. High avidity CD4+ T cells would also be critical in determining tumor rejection mediated by CD8+ T cells [18]. However, a survey of oligo- or monoclonal

CD8$^+$ T cell responses to MAGE-A3 vaccination in melanoma patients who had objective tumor regression failed to show high avidity of antigen recognition [29]. Second, a central role is played by the precursor frequency of specific T cells [91, 100] [116]. Finally, protection depends on the functional capacity of T cells, likely influenced by functional avidity and many more properties, such as efficient proliferation, T cell survival, homing, effector function, and generation of immunological memory [7, 67, 158]. Recent attempts have focused on direct ex vivo functional profiling of T cells in order to identify multiple T cell functions [5, 14, 33, 78, 114]. Mouse models suggest that for tumor immunity, similar principles may apply as for infectious diseases. In the adoptive transfer setting, it is increasingly clear that T cells with the ability to persist for prolonged periods of time in vivo correlate with clinical efficacy [13, 55, 127, 168]. Improvement of immunotherapy may depend on careful optimization toward the generation of T cells fulfilling these criteria.

Outlook and Conclusions

Cancer vaccines are becoming a clinical reality. The first cancer vaccine to be approved by the FDA in 2009 involves the immunization via i.v. with autologous PBMCs loaded with the recombinant fusion protein comprising GM-CSF and the prostate acid phosphatase as fusion partners. This appears to lead to monocyte differentiation into dendritic cells, and has been explored in hormone refractory advanced prostate carcinoma patients [27]. Other promising cancer vaccine candidates are at advanced stages of testing in pivotal phase III randomized and placebo controlled clinical trials. Notably, the recombinant MAGE-A3 protein is one of them and is in phase III trial in patients with MAGE-A3$^+$ metastatic melanoma.

A very substantial part of the preclinical and clinical work leading to the rapid development of cancer vaccines has benefited from the unique human "model" that cutaneous melanoma has come to be. The experience accumulated thus allows one to draw some general conclusions. First, the learning curve for defined vaccines aimed at inducing tumor antigen-specific T cell responses in cancer patients has risen continuously during the last 15 years. Today, the success rate in terms of induction of specific T cell immunity nears 80–100%. The success rate in terms of clinical efficacy is around 5–10% based on conventional clinical response criteria, but reach 30–40% if other favorable clinical outcomes, including stable disease, mixed responses, and prolonged recurrence-free intervals, are taken into account. This has been the case in the several trials in melanoma patients using several different vaccine formulations.

Despite these modest advances, cancer vaccines will benefit from additional efforts in optimization. Antigen selection, dose, adjuvant composition, dose, route of injection, and vaccination schedule are the major parameters that are in need of systematic work to find the appropriate conditions for attaining maximal clinical activity. Further basic research is needed to understand the mechanisms of optimal dendritic cell activation and T cell memory formation in vivo.

A major set of hurdles that appear to limit the clinical efficacy of vaccine-based therapies lie at the level of the suppressive tumor microenvironment. Thus, future cancer vaccines likely need to be administered in combination with immunomodulators that can temporarily alleviate the counterregulatory mechanisms operating within tumor tissues. The recent demonstration of clinical benefit and the regulatory approval of humanized monoclonal antibody to block the coinhibitory receptor CTLA-4 [56] is a major source of optimism and should provide much needed impetus in the search of combinatorial immunotherapies that may effectively curb tumor growth in patients.

References

1. Adamina M, Rosenthal R, Weber WP, Frey DM, Viehl CT, Bolli M, et al. Intranodal immunization with a vaccinia virus encoding multiple antigenic epitopes and costimulatory molecules in metastatic melanoma. Mol Ther. 2010;18:651–9.
2. Adams S, O'Neill D, Bhardwaj N. Maturation matters: importance of maturation for antitumor immunity of dendritic cell vaccines. J Clin Oncol. 2004;22:3834–5; author reply 3835.
3. Adams S, O'Neill DW, Nonaka D, Hardin E, Chiriboga L, Siu K, et al. Immunization of malignant melanoma patients with full-length NY-ESO-1 protein using TLR7 agonist imiquimod as vaccine adjuvant. J Immunol. 2008;181:776–84.
4. Alexander-Miller MA, Leggatt GR, Berzofsky JA. Selective expansion of high- or low-avidity cytotoxic T lymphocytes and efficacy for adoptive immunotherapy. Proc Natl Acad Sci USA. 1996;93:4102–7.
5. Almeida JR, Price DA, Papagno L, Arkoub ZA, Sauce D, Bornstein E, et al. Superior control of HIV-1 replication by CD8+ T cells is reflected by their avidity, polyfunctionality, and clonal turnover. J Exp Med. 2007;204:2473–85.
6. Altman JD, Moss PAH, Goulder PJR, Barouch DH, McHeyzer-Williams MG, Bell JI, et al. Phenotypic analysis of antigen-specific T lymphocytes. Science. 1996;274:94–6.
7. Appay V, Douek DC, Price DA. CD8+ T cell efficacy in vaccination and disease. Nat Med. 2008;14:623–8.
8. Banchereau J, Ueno H, Dhodapkar M, Connolly J, Finholt JP, Klechevsky E, et al. Immune and clinical outcomes in patients with stage IV melanoma vaccinated with peptide-pulsed dendritic cells derived from CD34+ progenitors and activated with type I interferon. J Immunother. 2005;28:505–16.
9. Baumgaertner P, Rufer N, Devevre E, Derre L, Rimoldi D, Geldhof C, et al. Ex vivo detectable human CD8 T-cell responses to cancer-testis antigens. Cancer Res. 2006;66:1912–6.
10. Belli F, Testori A, Rivoltini L, Maio M, Andreola G, Sertoli MR, et al. Vaccination of metastatic melanoma patients with autologous tumor-derived heat shock protein gp96-peptide complexes: clinical and immunologic findings. J Clin Oncol. 2002;20:4169–80.
11. Bennaceur K, Chapman J, Brikci-Nigassa L, Sanhadji K, Touraine JL, Portoukalian J. Dendritic cells dysfunction in tumour environment. Cancer Lett. 2008;272:186–96.
12. Bennett MS, Ng HL, Dagarag M, Ali A, Yang OO. Epitope-dependent avidity thresholds for cytotoxic T-lymphocyte clearance of virus-infected cells. J Virol. 2007;81:4973–80.
13. Berger C, Jensen MC, Lansdorp PM, Gough M, Elliott C, Riddell SR. Adoptive transfer of effector CD8+ T cells derived from central memory cells establishes persistent T cell memory in primates. J Clin Invest. 2008;118:294–305.
14. Betts MR, Nason MC, West SM, De Rosa SC, Migueles SA, Abraham J, et al. HIV nonprogressors preferentially maintain highly functional HIV-specific CD8+ T cells. Blood. 2006;107:4781–9.
15. Beutler B. Inferences, questions and possibilities in Toll-like receptor signalling. Nature. 2004;430:257–63.

16. Birkholz K, Schwenkert M, Kellner C, Gross S, Fey G, Schuler-Thurner B, et al. Targeting of DEC-205 on human dendritic cells results in efficient MHC class II-restricted antigen presentation. Blood. 2010;116:2277–85.

17. Bonehill A, Van Nuffel AM, Corthals J, Tuyaerts S, Heirman C, Francois V, et al. Single-step antigen loading and activation of dendritic cells by mRNA electroporation for the purpose of therapeutic vaccination in melanoma patients. Clin Cancer Res. 2009;15:3366–75.

18. Brandmaier AG, Leitner WW, Ha SP, Sidney J, Restifo NP, Touloukian CE. High-avidity autoreactive CD4+ T cells induce host CTL, overcome Tregs and mediate tumor destruction. J Immunother. 2009;32:677–88.

19. Bronte V, Apolloni E, Cabrelle A, Ronca R, Serafini P, Zamboni P, et al. Identification of a CD11b(+)/Gr-1(+)/CD31(+) myeloid progenitor capable of activating or suppressing CD8(+) T cells. Blood. 2000;95:3838–46.

20. Brooks DG, Lee AM, Elsaesser H, McGavern DB, Oldstone MB. IL-10 blockade facilitates DNA vaccine-induced T cell responses and enhances clearance of persistent virus infection. J Exp Med. 2008;205:533–41.

21. Butterfield LH, Comin-Anduix B, Vujanovic L, Lee Y, Dissette VB, Yang JQ, et al. Adenovirus MART-1-engineered autologous dendritic cell vaccine for metastatic melanoma. J Immunother. 2008;31:294–309.

22. Butz EA, Bevan MJ. Massive expansion of antigen-specific CD8+ T cells during an acute virus infection. Immunity. 1998;8:167–75.

23. Cambier J. Immunosenescence: a problem of lymphopoiesis, homeostasis, microenvironment, and signaling. Immunol Rev. 2005;205:5–6.

24. Cassaday RD, Sondel PM, King DM, Macklin MD, Gan J, Warner TF, et al. A phase I study of immunization using particle-mediated epidermal delivery of genes for gp100 and GM-CSF into uninvolved skin of melanoma patients. Clin Cancer Res. 2007;13:540–9.

25. Chapman PB, Morrissey DM, Panageas KS, Hamilton WB, Zhan C, Destro AN, et al. Induction of antibodies against GM2 ganglioside by immunizing melanoma patients using GM2-keyhole limpet hemocyanin + QS21 vaccine: a dose-response study. Clin Cancer Res. 2000;6:874–9.

26. Chattopadhyay PK, Yu J, Roederer M. Live-cell assay to detect antigen-specific CD4+ T-cell responses by CD154 expression. Nat Protoc. 2006;1:1–6.

27. Cheever MA, Higano C. PROVENGE (Sipuleucel-T) in prostate cancer: the first FDA approved therapeutic cancer vaccine. Clin Cancer Res. 2011;17:3520–6.

28. Chianese-Bullock KA, Pressley J, Garbee C, Hibbitts S, Murphy C, Yamshchikov G, et al. MAGE-A1-, MAGE-A10-, and gp100-derived peptides are immunogenic when combined with granulocyte-macrophage colony-stimulating factor and montanide ISA-51 adjuvant and administered as part of a multipeptide vaccine for melanoma. J Immunol. 2005;174:3080–6.

29. Connerotte T, Van Pel A, Godelaine D, Tartour E, Schuler-Thurner B, Lucas S, et al. Functions of Anti-MAGE T-cells induced in melanoma patients under different vaccination modalities. Cancer Res. 2008;68:3931–40.

30. Cui W, Kaech SM. Generation of effector CD8+ T cells and their conversion to memory T cells. Immunol Rev. 2010;236:151–66.

31. Czerkinsky C, Andersson G, Ekre HP, Nillson LA, Klareskog L, Ouchterlony O. Reverse ELISPOT assay for clonal analysis of cytokine production. I. Enumeration of gamma-interferon-secreting cells. J Immunol Methods. 1988;110:29–36.

32. Dangoor A, Lorigan P, Keilholz U, Schadendorf D, Harris A, Ottensmeier C, et al. Clinical and immunological responses in metastatic melanoma patients vaccinated with a high-dose poly-epitope vaccine. Cancer Immunol Immunother. 2010;59:863–73.

33. Daucher M, Price DA, Brenchley JM, Lamoreaux L, Metcalf JA, Rehm C, et al. Virological outcome after structured interruption of antiretroviral therapy for human immunodeficiency virus infection is associated with the functional profile of virus-specific CD8+ T cells. J Virol. 2008;82:4102–14.

34. Davis ID, Chen W, Jackson H, Parente P, Shackleton M, Hopkins W, et al. Recombinant NY-ESO-1 protein with ISCOMATRIX adjuvant induces broad integrated antibody and

CD4(+) and CD8(+) T cell responses in humans. Proc Natl Acad Sci USA. 2004;101: 10697–702.

35. Day CL, Kaufmann DE, Kiepiela P, Brown JA, Moodley ES, Reddy S, et al. PD-1 expression on HIV-specific T cells is associated with T-cell exhaustion and disease progression. Nature. 2006;443:350–4.

36. Derby M, Alexander-Miller M, Tse R, Berzofsky J. High-avidity CTL exploit two complementary mechanisms to provide better protection against viral infection than low-avidity CTL. J Immunol. 2001;166:1690–7.

37. Derre L, Rivals JP, Jandus C, Pastor S, Rimoldi D, Romero P, et al. BTLA mediates inhibition of human tumor-specific CD8+ T cells that can be partially reversed by vaccination. J Clin Invest. 2010;120:157–67.

38. Eggermont AM. Therapeutic vaccines in solid tumours: can they be harmful? Eur J Cancer. 2009;45:2087–90.

39. Eggermont AM, Suciu S, Ruka W, Marsden J, Testori A, Corrie P, et al. EORTC 18961: postoperative adjuvant ganglioside GM2-KLH21 vaccination treatment vs observation in stage II (T3-T4N0M0) melanoma: 2nd interim analysis led to an early disclosure of the results. J Clin Oncol. 2008;26: [abstr 9004].

40. Epaulard O, Derouazi M, Margerit C, Marlu R, Filopon D, Polack B, et al. Optimization of a type III secretion system-based Pseudomonas aeruginosa live vector for antigen delivery. Clin Vaccine Immunol. 2008;15:308–13.

41. Ernst B, Lee DS, Chang JM, Sprent J, Surh CD. The peptide ligands mediating positive selection in the thymus control T cell survival and homeostatic proliferation in the periphery. Immunity. 1999;11:173–81.

42. Eton O, Kharkevitch DD, Gianan MA, Ross MI, Itoh K, Pride MW, et al. Active immunotherapy with ultraviolet B-irradiated autologous whole melanoma cells plus DETOX in patients with metastatic melanoma. Clin Cancer Res. 1998;4:619–27.

43. Franco JL, Ghosh P, Wiltrout RH, Carter CR, Zea AH, Momozaki N, et al. Partial degradation of T-cell signal transduction molecules by contaminating granulocytes during protein extraction of splenic T cells from tumor-bearing mice. Cancer Res. 1995;55:3840–6.

44. Frankenburg S, Elias O, Gelbart Y, Drize O, Lotem M, Ingber A, et al. Recombinant hydrophilic human gp100: uptake by dendritic cells and stimulation of autologous CD8+ lymphocytes from melanoma patients. Immunol Lett. 2004;94:253–9.

45. Freeman GJ, Wherry EJ, Ahmed R, Sharpe AH. Reinvigorating exhausted HIV-specific T cells via PD-1-PD-1 ligand blockade. J Exp Med. 2006;203:2223–7.

46. Gabrilovich DI, Nagaraj S. Myeloid-derived suppressor cells as regulators of the immune system. Nat Rev Immunol. 2009;9:162–74.

47. Gallimore A, Dumrese T, Hengartner H, Zinkernagel RM, Rammensee HG. Protective immunity does not correlate with the hierarchy of virus-specific cytotoxic T cell responses to naturally processed peptides. J Exp Med. 1998;187:1647–57.

48. Germain RN. An innately interesting decade of research in immunology. Nat Med. 2004;10:1307–20.

49. Ginsberg BA, Gallardo HF, Rasalan TS, Adamow M, Mu Z, Tandon S, et al. Immunologic response to xenogeneic gp100 DNA in melanoma patients: comparison of particle-mediated epidermal delivery with intramuscular injection. Clinical Cancer Res. 2010;16:4057–65.

50. Gnjatic S, Nishikawa H, Jungbluth AA, Gure AO, Ritter G, Jager E, et al. NY-ESO-1: review of an immunogenic tumor antigen. Adv Cancer Res. 2006;95:1–30.

51. Grunebach F, Erndt S, Hantschel M, Heine A, Brossart P. Generation of antigen-specific CTL responses using RGS1 mRNA transfected dendritic cells. Cancer Immunol Immunother. 2008;57:1483–91.

52. Hadrup SR, Bakker AH, Shu CJ, Andersen RS, van Veluw J, Hombrink P, et al. Parallel detection of antigen-specific T-cell responses by multidimensional encoding of MHC multimers. Nat Methods. 2009;6:520–6.

53. Hadrup SR, Strindhall J, Kollgaard T, Seremet T, Johansson B, Pawelec G, et al. Longitudinal studies of clonally expanded CD8 T cells reveal a repertoire shrinkage predicting mortality

and an increased number of dysfunctional cytomegalovirus-specific T cells in the very elderly. J Immunol. 2006;176:2645–53.

54. Hamid O, Solomon JC, Scotland R, Garcia M, Sian S, Ye W, et al. Alum with interleukin-12 augments immunity to a melanoma peptide vaccine: correlation with time to relapse in patients with resected high-risk disease. Clinical Cancer Res. 2007;13:215–22.

55. Heemskerk B, Liu K, Dudley ME, Johnson LA, Kaiser A, Downey S, et al. Adoptive cell therapy for patients with melanoma, using tumor-infiltrating lymphocytes genetically engineered to secrete interleukin-2. Hum Gene Ther. 2008;19:496–510.

56. Hodi FS, O'Day SJ, McDermott DF, Weber RW, Sosman JA, Haanen JB, et al. Improved survival with ipilimumab in patients with metastatic melanoma. N Engl J Med. 2010;363:711–23.

57. Hsueh EC, Essner R, Foshag LJ, Ollila DW, Gammon G, O'Day SJ, et al. Prolonged survival after complete resection of disseminated melanoma and active immunotherapy with a therapeutic cancer vaccine. J Clin Oncol. 2002;20:4549–54.

58. Iancu EM, Speiser DE, Rufer N. Assessing ageing of individual T lymphocytes: mission impossible? Mech Ageing Dev. 2008;129:67–78.

59. Jager E, Karbach J, Gnjatic S, Neumann A, Bender A, Valmori D, et al. Recombinant vaccinia/fowlpox NY-ESO-1 vaccines induce both humoral and cellular NY-ESO-1-specific immune responses in cancer patients. Proc Natl Acad Sci USA. 2006;103:14453–8.

60. Janeway Jr CA, Medzhitov R. Innate immune recognition. Annu Rev Immunol. 2002;20: 197–216.

61. Jung T, Schauer U, Heusser C, Neumann C, Rieger C. Detection of intracellular cytokines by flow cytometry. J Immunol Methods. 1993;159:197–207.

62. Kawabata R, Wada H, Isobe M, Saika T, Sato S, Uenaka A, et al. Antibody response against NY-ESO-1 in CHP-NY-ESO-1 vaccinated patients. Int J Cancer. 2007;120:2178–84.

63. Kearney ER, Pape KA, Loh DY, Jenkins MK. Visualization of peptide-specific T cell immunity and peripheral tolerance induction in vivo. Immunity. 1994;1:327–39.

64. Kedzierska K, La Gruta NL, Davenport MP, Turner SJ, Doherty PC. Contribution of T cell receptor affinity to overall avidity for virus-specific CD8+ T cell responses. Proc Natl Acad Sci USA. 2005;102:11432–7.

65. Kenter GG, Welters MJ, Valentijn AR, Lowik MJ, Berends-van der Meer DM, Vloon AP, et al. Vaccination against HPV-16 oncoproteins for vulvar intraepithelial neoplasia. N Engl J Med. 2009;361:1838–47.

66. Kirkwood JM, Ibrahim JG, Sosman JA, Sondak VK, Agarwala SS, Ernstoff MS, et al. High-dose interferon alfa-2b significantly prolongs relapse-free and overall survival compared with the GM2-KLH/QS-21 vaccine in patients with resected stage IIB-III melanoma: results of intergroup trial E1694/S9512/C509801. J Clin Oncol. 2001;19:2370–80.

67. Klebanoff CA, Gattinoni L, Restifo NP. CD8 T-cell memory in tumor immunology and immunotherapy. Immunol Rev. 2006;211:214–24.

68. Klein L, Trautman L, Psarras S, Schnell S, Siermann A, Liblau R, et al. Visualizing the course of antigen-specific CD8 and CD4 T cell responses to a growing tumor. Eur J Immunol. 2003;33:806–14.

69. Knabel M, Franz TJ, Schiemann M, Wulf A, Villmow B, Schmidt B, et al. Reversible MHC multimer staining for functional isolation of T-cell populations and effective adoptive transfer. Nat Med. 2002;8:631–7.

70. Kochenderfer JN, Gress RE. A comparison and critical analysis of preclinical anticancer vaccination strategies. Exp Biol Med (Maywood). 2007;232:1130–41.

71. Kreiter S, Diken M, Selmi A, Tureci O, Sahin U. Tumor vaccination using messenger RNA: prospects of a future therapy. Curr Opin Immunol. 2011;23(3):399–406.

72. Kruit WH, Suciu S, Dreno B, Chiarion-Sileni V, Mortier L, Robert C, et al. Immunization with recombinant MAGE-A3 protein combined with adjuvant systems AS15 or AS02B in patients with unresectable and progressive metastatic cutaneous melanoma: a randomized open-label phase II study of the EORTC Melanoma Group (16032–18031). J Clin Oncol. 2008;26: [abstract 9065].

73. Kruit WH, van Ojik HH, Brichard VG, Escudier B, Dorval T, Dreno B, et al. Phase 1/2 study of subcutaneous and intradermal immunization with a recombinant MAGE-3 protein in patients with detectable metastatic melanoma. Int J Cancer. 2005;117:596–604.
74. Kuhn AN, Diken M, Kreiter S, Selmi A, Kowalska J, Jemielity J, et al. Phosphorothioate cap analogs increase stability and translational efficiency of RNA vaccines in immature dendritic cells and induce superior immune responses in vivo. Gene Ther. 2010;17:961–71.
75. Kyte JA, Kvalheim G, Lislerud K, thor Straten P, Dueland S, Aamdal S, et al. T cell responses in melanoma patients after vaccination with tumor-mRNA transfected dendritic cells. Cancer Immunol Immunother. 2007;56:659–75.
76. Lai P, Rabinowich H, Crowley-Nowick PA, Bell MC, Mantovani G, Whiteside TL. Alterations in expression and function of signal-transducing proteins in tumor-associated T and natural killer cells in patients with ovarian carcinoma. Clin Cancer Res. 1996;2:161–73.
77. Lang A, Brien JD, Messaoudi I, Nikolich-Zugich J. Age-related dysregulation of CD8+ T cell memory specific for a persistent virus is independent of viral replication. J Immunol. 2008;180:4848–57.
78. Lichterfeld M, Yu XG, Mui SK, Williams KL, Trocha A, Brockman MA, et al. Selective depletion of high-avidity human immunodeficiency virus type 1 (HIV-1)-specific CD8+ T cells after early HIV-1 infection. J Virol. 2007;81:4199–214.
79. Lienard D, Rimoldi D, Marchand M, Dietrich PY, van Baren N, Geldhof C, et al. Ex vivo detectable activation of Melan-A-specific T cells correlating with inflammatory skin reactions in melanoma patients vaccinated with peptides in IFA. Cancer Immun. 2004;4:4.
80. Lindsey KR, Gritz L, Sherry R, Abati A, Fetsch PA, Goldfeder LC, et al. Evaluation of prime/boost regimens using recombinant poxvirus/tyrosinase vaccines for the treatment of patients with metastatic melanoma. Clin Cancer Res. 2006;12:2526–37.
81. Linton PJ, Dorshkind K. Age-related changes in lymphocyte development and function. Nat Immunol. 2004;5:133–9.
82. Livingston PO, Wong GY, Adluri S, Tao Y, Padavan M, Parente R, et al. Improved survival in stage III melanoma patients with GM2 antibodies: a randomized trial of adjuvant vaccination with GM2 ganglioside. J Clin Oncol. 1994;12:1036–44.
83. Lonchay C, van der Bruggen P, Connerotte T, Hanagiri T, Coulie P, Colau D, et al. Correlation between tumor regression and T cell responses in melanoma patients vaccinated with a MAGE antigen. Proc Natl Acad Sci USA. 2004;101 Suppl 2:14631–8.
84. Markovic SN, Dietz AB, Greiner CW, Maas ML, Butler GW, Padley DJ, et al. Preparing clinical-grade myeloid dendritic cells by electroporation-mediated transfection of in vitro amplified tumor-derived mRNA and safety testing in stage IV malignant melanoma. J Transl Med. 2006;4:35.
85. Mellor AL, Baban B, Chandler P, Marshall B, Jhaver K, Hansen A, et al. Cutting edge: induced indoleamine 2,3 dioxygenase expression in dendritic cell subsets suppresses T cell clonal expansion. J Immunol. 2003;171:1652–5.
86. Messaoudi I, Guevara Patino JA, Dyall R, LeMaoult J, Nikolich-Zugich J. Direct link between MHC polymorphism, T cell avidity, and diversity in immune defense. Science. 2002;298:1797–800.
87. Meyer RG, Britten CM, Siepmann U, Petzold B, Sagban TA, Lehr HA, et al. A phase I vaccination study with tyrosinase in patients with stage II melanoma using recombinant modified vaccinia virus Ankara (MVA-hTyr). Cancer Immunol Immunother. 2005;54:453–67.
88. Michiels A, Tuyaerts S, Bonehill A, Heirman C, Corthals J, Thielemans K. Delivery of tumor-antigen-encoding mRNA into dendritic cells for vaccination. Methods Mol Biol. 2008;423:155–63.
89. Miller RA. The aging immune system: primer and prospectus. Science. 1996;273:70–4.
90. Mitchell MS, Kan-Mitchell J, Kempf RA, Harel W, Shau HY, Lind S. Active specific immunotherapy for melanoma: phase I trial of allogeneic lysates and a novel adjuvant. Cancer Res. 1988;48:5883–93.

91. Moon JJ, Chu HH, Pepper M, McSorley SJ, Jameson SC, Kedl RM, et al. Naive CD4(+) T cell frequency varies for different epitopes and predicts repertoire diversity and response magnitude. Immunity. 2007;27:203–13.
92. Morton DL, Mozzillo N, Thompson JF, Kelley MC, Faries M, Wagner J, et al. An international, randomized, phase III trial of bacillus Calmette-Guerin (BCG) plus allogeneic melanoma vaccine (MCV) or placebo after complete resection of melanoma metastatic to regional or distant sites. J Clin Oncol. 2007;25: [abstract 8508].
93. Murali-Krishna K, Altman JD, Suresh M, Sourdive DJ, Zajac AJ, Miller JD, et al. Counting antigen-specific CD8 T cells: a reevaluation of bystander activation during viral infection. Immunity. 1998;8:177–87.
94. Murdoch C, Muthana M, Coffelt SB, Lewis CE. The role of myeloid cells in the promotion of tumour angiogenesis. Nat Rev Cancer. 2008;8:618–31.
95. Nesic D, Vukmanovic S. MHC class I is required for peripheral accumulation of CD8+ thymic emigrants. J Immunol. 1998;160:3705–12.
96. Nestle FO, Alijagic S, Gilliet M, Sun Y, Grabbe S, Dummer R, et al. Vaccination of melanoma patients with peptide- or tumor lysate-pulsed dendritic cells. Nat Med. 1998;4:328–32.
97. Newell EW, Klein LO, Yu W, Davis MM. Simultaneous detection of many T-cell specificities using combinatorial tetramer staining. Nat Methods. 2009;6:497–9.
98. Nicholaou T, Ebert LM, Davis ID, McArthur GA, Jackson H, Dimopoulos N, et al. Regulatory T-cell-mediated attenuation of T-cell responses to the NY-ESO-1 ISCOMATRIX vaccine in patients with advanced malignant melanoma. Clin Cancer Res. 2009;15:2166–73.
99. Nikolich-Zugich J. Ageing and life-long maintenance of T-cell subsets in the face of latent persistent infections. Nat Rev Immunol. 2008;8:512–22.
100. Obar JJ, Khanna KM, Lefrancois L. Endogenous naive CD8+ T cell precursor frequency regulates primary and memory responses to infection. Immunity. 2008;28:859–69.
101. Ochoa AC, Longo DL. Alteration of signal transduction in T cells from cancer patients. Important Adv Oncol. 1995;43–54.
102. Odunsi K, Qian F, Matsuzaki J, Mhawech-Fauceglia P, Andrews C, Hoffman EW, et al. Vaccination with an NY-ESO-1 peptide of HLA class I/II specificities induces integrated humoral and T cell responses in ovarian cancer. Proc Natl Acad Sci USA. 2007;104: 12837–42.
103. Ostrand-Rosenberg S, Sinha P. Myeloid-derived suppressor cells: linking inflammation and cancer. J Immunol. 2009;182:4499–506.
104. Pardoll D. Does the immune system see tumors as foreign or self? Annu Rev Immunol. 2003;21:807–39.
105. Paris RM, Kim JH, Robb ML, Michael NL. Prime-boost immunization with poxvirus or adenovirus vectors as a strategy to develop a protective vaccine for HIV-1. Expert Rev Vaccines. 2010;9:1055–69.
106. Pawelec G, Akbar A, Caruso C, Effros R, Grubeck-Loebenstein B, Wikby A. Is immunosenescence infectious? Trends Immunol. 2004;25:406–10.
107. Peterson AC, Harlin H, Gajewski TF. Immunization with Melan-A peptide-pulsed peripheral blood mononuclear cells plus recombinant human interleukin-12 induces clinical activity and T-cell responses in advanced melanoma. J Clin Oncol. 2003;21:2342–8.
108. Petrovas C, Casazza JP, Brenchley JM, Price DA, Gostick E, Adams WC, et al. PD-1 is a regulator of virus-specific CD8+ T cell survival in HIV infection. J Exp Med. 2006;203:2281–92.
109. Plog MS, Guyre CA, Roberts BL, Goldberg M, St George JA, Perricone MA. Preclinical safety and biodistribution of adenovirus-based cancer vaccines after intradermal delivery. Hum Gene Ther. 2006;17:705–16.
110. Price DA, Brenchley JM, Ruff LE, Betts MR, Hill BJ, Roederer M, et al. Avidity for antigen shapes clonal dominance in CD8+ T cell populations specific for persistent DNA viruses. J Exp Med. 2005;202:1349–61.
111. Pulendran B, Ahmed R. Translating innate immunity into immunological memory: implications for vaccine development. Cell. 2006;124:849–63.

112. Pullarkat V, Lee PP, Scotland R, Rubio V, Groshen S, Gee C, et al. A phase I trial of SD-9427 (progenipoietin) with a multipeptide vaccine for resected metastatic melanoma. Clin Cancer Res. 2003;9:1301–12.

113. Quaak SG, van den Berg JH, Toebes M, Schumacher TN, Haanen JB, Beijnen JH, et al. GMP production of pDERMATT for vaccination against melanoma in a phase I clinical trial. Eur J Pharm Biopharm. 2008;70:429–38.

114. Rehr M, Cahenzli J, Haas A, Price DA, Gostick E, Huber M, et al. Emergence of polyfunctional CD8+ T cells after prolonged suppression of human immunodeficiency virus replication by antiretroviral therapy. J Virol. 2008;82:3391–404.

115. Reyes-Sandoval A, Berthoud T, Alder N, Siani L, Gilbert SC, Nicosia A, et al. Prime-boost immunization with adenoviral and modified vaccinia virus Ankara vectors enhances the durability and polyfunctionality of protective malaria CD8+ T-cell responses. Infect Immun. 2010;78:145–53.

116. Rizzuto GA, Merghoub T, Hirschhorn-Cymerman D, Liu C, Lesokhin AM, Sahawneh D, et al. Self-antigen-specific CD8+ T cell precursor frequency determines the quality of the antitumor immune response. J Exp Med. 2009;206:849–66.

117. Romano E, Rossi M, Ratzinger G, de Cos MA, Chung DJ, Panageas KS, et al. Peptide-loaded langerhans cells, despite increased IL15 secretion and T-cell activation in vitro, elicit antitumor T-cell responses comparable to peptide-loaded monocyte-derived dendritic cells in vivo. Clin Cancer Res. 2011;17:1984–97.

118. Romero P, Cerottini JC, Speiser DE. Monitoring tumor antigen specific T-cell responses in cancer patients and phase I clinical trials of peptide-based vaccination. Cancer Immunol Immunother. 2004;53:249–55.

119. Rosenberg SA, Sherry RM, Morton KE, Scharfman WJ, Yang JC, Topalian SL, et al. Tumor progression can occur despite the induction of very high levels of self/tumor antigen-specific CD8+ T cells in patients with melanoma. J Immunol. 2005;175:6169–76.

120. Rosenberg SA, Yang JC, Restifo NP. Cancer immunotherapy: moving beyond current vaccines. Nat Med. 2004;10:909–15.

121. Rufer N. Molecular tracking of antigen-specific T-cell clones during immune responses. Curr Opin Immunol. 2005;17:441–7.

122. Russmann H, Shams H, Poblete F, Fu Y, Galan JE, Donis RO. Delivery of epitopes by the Salmonella type III secretion system for vaccine development. Science. 1998;281: 565–8.

123. Schadendorf D, Ugurel S, Schuler-Thurner B, Nestle FO, Enk A, Brocker EB, et al. Dacarbazine (DTIC) versus vaccination with autologous peptide-pulsed dendritic cells (DC) in first-line treatment of patients with metastatic melanoma: a randomized phase III trial of the DC study group of the DeCOG. Ann Oncol. 2006;17:563–70.

124. Schuler-Thurner B, Schultz ES, Berger TG, Weinlich G, Ebner S, Woerl P, et al. Rapid induction of tumor-specific type 1 T helper cells in metastatic melanoma patients by vaccination with mature, cryopreserved, peptide-loaded monocyte-derived dendritic cells. J Exp Med. 2002;195:1279–88.

125. Schwartzentruber DJ, Lawson D, Richards J, Conry RM, Miller D, Triesman J, et al. A phase III multi-institutional randomized study of immunization with the gp, 100:209–217(210 M) peptide followed by high-dose IL-2 compared with high-dose IL-2 alone in patients with metastatic melanoma. J Clin Oncol. 2009;27: [abstr CRA9011].

126. Sedlik C, Dadaglio G, Saron MF, Deriaud E, Rojas M, Casal SI, et al. In vivo induction of a high-avidity, high-frequency cytotoxic T-lymphocyte response is associated with antiviral protective immunity. J Virol. 2000;74:5769–75.

127. Shen X, Zhou J, Hathcock KS, Robbins P, Powell Jr DJ, Rosenberg SA, et al. Persistence of tumor infiltrating lymphocytes in adoptive immunotherapy correlates with telomere length. J Immunother. 2007;30:123–9.

128. Slingluff Jr CL, Petroni GR, Chianese-Bullock KA, Smolkin ME, Hibbitts S, Murphy C, et al. Immunologic and clinical outcomes of a randomized phase II trial of two multipeptide vaccines for melanoma in the adjuvant setting. Clin Cancer Res. 2007;13:6386–95.

129. Slingluff Jr CL, Petroni GR, Yamshchikov GV, Barnd DL, Eastham S, Galavotti H, et al. Clinical and immunologic results of a randomized phase II trial of vaccination using four melanoma peptides either administered in granulocyte-macrophage colony-stimulating factor in adjuvant or pulsed on dendritic cells. J Clin Oncol. 2003;21:4016–26.

130. Smith CL, Dunbar PR, Mirza F, Palmowski MJ, Shepherd D, Gilbert SC, et al. Recombinant modified vaccinia Ankara primes functionally activated CTL specific for a melanoma tumor antigen epitope in melanoma patients with a high risk of disease recurrence. Int J Cancer. 2005;113:259–66.

131. Smith CL, Mirza F, Pasquetto V, Tscharke DC, Palmowski MJ, Dunbar PR, et al. Immunodominance of poxviral-specific CTL in a human trial of recombinant-modified vaccinia Ankara. J Immunol. 2005;175:8431–7.

132. Smith 2nd JW, Walker EB, Fox BA, Haley D, Wisner KP, Doran T, et al. Adjuvant immunization of HLA-A2-positive melanoma patients with a modified gp100 peptide induces peptide-specific CD8+ T-cell responses. J Clin Oncol. 2003;21:1562–73.

133. Sondak VK, Liu PY, Tuthill RJ, Kempf RA, Unger JM, Sosman JA, et al. Adjuvant immunotherapy of resected, intermediate-thickness, node-negative melanoma with an allogeneic tumor vaccine: overall results of a randomized trial of the Southwest Oncology Group. J Clin Oncol. 2002;20:2058–66.

134. Sosman JA, Unger JM, Liu PY, Flaherty LE, Park MS, Kempf RA, et al. Adjuvant immunotherapy of resected, intermediate-thickness, node-negative melanoma with an allogeneic tumor vaccine: impact of HLA class I antigen expression on outcome. J Clin Oncol. 2002;20:2067–75.

135. Spaner DE, Astsaturov I, Vogel T, Petrella T, Elias I, Burdett-Radoux S, et al. Enhanced viral and tumor immunity with intranodal injection of canary pox viruses expressing the melanoma antigen, gp100. Cancer. 2006;106:890–9.

136. Speiser DE. Immunological techniques: ex vivo characterization of T cell-mediated immune responses in cancer. Curr Opin Immunol. 2005;17:419–22.

137. Speiser DE, Baumgaertner P, Barbey C, Rubio-Godoy V, Moulin A, Corthesy P, et al. A novel approach to characterize clonality and differentiation of human melanoma-specific T cell responses: spontaneous priming and efficient boosting by vaccination. J Immunol. 2006;177:1338–48.

138. Speiser DE, Baumgaertner P, Voelter V, Devevre E, Barbey C, Rufer N, et al. Unmodified self antigen triggers human CD8 T cells with stronger tumor reactivity than altered antigen. Proc Natl Acad Sci USA. 2008;105:3849–54.

139. Speiser DE, Kyburz D, Stübi U, Hengartner H, Zinkernagel RM. Discrepancy between in vitro measurable and in vivo virus neutralizing cytotoxic T cell reactivities: low T cell receptor specificity and avidity sufficient for in vitro proliferation or cytotoxicity to peptide coated target cells but not for in vivo protection. J Immunol. 1992;149:972–80.

140. Speiser DE, Lienard D, Rufer N, Rubio-Godoy V, Rimoldi D, Lejeune F, et al. Rapid and strong human CD8+ T cell responses to vaccination with peptide, IFA and CpG oligodeoxynucleotide 7909. J Clin Invest. 2005;115:739–46.

141. Speiser DE, Lienard D, Rufer N, Rubio-Godoy V, Rimoldi D, Lejeune F, et al. Rapid and strong human CD8+ T cell responses to vaccination with peptide, IFA, and CpG oligodeoxynucleotide 7909. J Clin Invest. 2005;115:739–46.

142. Staveley-O'Carroll K, Sotomayor E, Montgomery J, Borrello I, Hwang L, Fein S, et al. Induction of antigen-specific T cell anergy: an early event in the course of tumor progression. Proc Natl Acad Sci USA. 1998;95:1178–83.

143. Tacken PJ, de Vries IJ, Torensma R, Figdor CG. Dendritic-cell immunotherapy: from ex vivo loading to in vivo targeting. Nat Rev Immunol. 2007;7:790–802.

144. Takeda K, Kaisho T, Akira S. Toll-like receptors. Annu Rev Immunol. 2003;21:335–76.

145. Taswell C. Limiting dilution assays for the determination of immunocompetent cell frequencies. J Immunol. 1981;126:1614–9.

146. Touvrey C, Derre L, Devevre E, Corthesy P, Romero P, Rufer N, et al. Dominant human CD8 T cell clonotypes persist simultaneously as memory and effector cells in memory phase. J Immunol. 2009;182:6718–26.

147. Trautmann L, Janbazian L, Chomont N, Said EA, Gimmig S, Bessette B, et al. Upregulation of PD-1 expression on HIV-specific CD8+ T cells leads to reversible immune dysfunction. Nat Med. 2006;12:1198–202.

148. Uenaka A, Wada H, Isobe M, Saika T, Tsuji K, Sato E, et al. T cell immunomonitoring and tumor responses in patients immunized with a complex of cholesterol-bearing hydrophobized pullulan (CHP) and NY-ESO-1 protein. Cancer Immun. 2007;7:9.

149. Valmori D, Dutoit V, Ayyoub M, Rimoldi D, Guillaume P, Lienard D, et al. Simultaneous CD8+ T cell responses to multiple tumor antigen epitopes in a multipeptide melanoma vaccine. Cancer Immun. 2003;3:15.

150. Valmori D, Souleimanian NE, Tosello V, Bhardwaj N, Adams S, O'Neill D, et al. Vaccination with NY-ESO-1 protein and CpG in Montanide induces integrated antibody/Th1 responses and CD8 T cells through cross-priming. Proc Natl Acad Sci USA. 2007;104:8947–52.

151. van Baren N, Bonnet MC, Dreno B, Khammari A, Dorval T, Piperno-Neumann S, et al. Tumoral and immunologic response after vaccination of melanoma patients with an ALVAC virus encoding MAGE antigens recognized by T cells. J Clin Oncol. 2005;23:9008–21.

152. Verdijk P, Aarntzen EH, Lesterhuis WJ, Boullart AC, Kok E, van Rossum MM, et al. Limited amounts of dendritic cells migrate into the T-cell area of lymph nodes but have high immune activating potential in melanoma patients. Clin Cancer Res. 2009;15:2531–40.

153. Walker EB, Haley D, Miller W, Floyd K, Wisner KP, Sanjuan N, et al. gp100(209-2 M) peptide immunization of human lymphocyte antigen-A2+ stage I-III melanoma patients induces significant increase in antigen-specific effector and long-term memory CD8+ T cells. Clin Cancer Res. 2004;10:668–80.

154. Wehler TC, Karg M, Distler E, Konur A, Nonn M, Meyer RG, et al. Rapid identification and sorting of viable virus-reactive CD4(+) and CD8(+) T cells based on antigen-triggered CD137 expression. J Immunol Methods. 2008;339:23–37.

155. Weide B, Pascolo S, Scheel B, Derhovanessian E, Pflugfelder A, Eigentler TK, et al. Direct injection of protamine-protected mRNA: results of a phase 1/2 vaccination trial in metastatic melanoma patients. J Immunother. 2009;32:498–507.

156. Wherry EJ, Blattman JN, Murali-Krishna K, van der Most R, Ahmed R. Viral persistence alters CD8 T-cell immunodominance and tissue distribution and results in distinct stages of functional impairment. J Virol. 2003;77:4911–27.

157. Wherry EJ, Ha SJ, Kaech SM, Haining WN, Sarkar S, Kalia V, et al. Molecular signature of CD8+ T cell exhaustion during chronic viral infection. Immunity. 2007;27:670–84.

158. Wherry EJ, Teichgraber V, Becker TC, Masopust D, Kaech SM, Antia R, et al. Lineage relationship and protective immunity of memory CD8 T cell subsets. Nat Immunol. 2003;4:225–34.

159. Whiteside TL. Down-regulation of zeta-chain expression in T cells: a biomarker of prognosis in cancer? Cancer Immunol Immunother. 2004;53:865–78.

160. Willimsky G, Czeh M, Loddenkemper C, Gellermann J, Schmidt K, Wust P, et al. Immunogenicity of premalignant lesions is the primary cause of general cytotoxic T lymphocyte unresponsiveness. J Exp Med. 2008;205:1687–700.

161. Wolchok JD, Yuan J, Houghton AN, Gallardo HF, Rasalan TS, Wang J, et al. Safety and immunogenicity of tyrosinase DNA vaccines in patients with melanoma. Mol Ther. 2007;15:2044–50.

162. Wolfl M, Kuball J, Ho WY, Nguyen H, Manley TJ, Bleakley M, et al. Activation-induced expression of CD137 permits detection, isolation, and expansion of the full repertoire of CD8+ T cells responding to antigen without requiring knowledge of epitope specificities. Blood. 2007;110:201–10.

163. Wood LM, Guirnalda PD, Seavey MM, Paterson Y. Cancer immunotherapy using Listeria monocytogenes and listerial virulence factors. Immunol Res. 2008;42:233–45.

164. Yee C, Savage PA, Lee PP, Davis MM, Greenberg PD. Isolation of high avidity melanoma-reactive CTL from heterogeneous populations using peptide-MHC tetramers. J Immunol. 1999;162:2227–34.

165. Yewdall AW, Drutman SB, Jinwala F, Bahjat KS, Bhardwaj N. CD8+ T cell priming by dendritic cell vaccines requires antigen transfer to endogenous antigen presenting cells. PLoS One. 2010;5:e11144.
166. Yi JS, Cox MA, Zajac AJ. T-cell exhaustion: characteristics, causes and conversion. Immunology. 2010;129:474–81.
167. Zeh 3rd HJ, Perry-Lalley D, Dudley ME, Rosenberg SA, Yang JC. High avidity CTLs for two self-antigens demonstrate superior in vitro and in vivo antitumor efficacy. J Immunol. 1999;162:989–94.
168. Zhou J, Shen X, Huang J, Hodes RJ, Rosenberg SA, Robbins PF. Telomere length of transferred lymphocytes correlates with in vivo persistence and tumor regression in melanoma patients receiving cell transfer therapy. J Immunol. 2005;175:7046–52.
169. Zhu X, Zhou P, Cai J, Yang G, Liang S, Ren D. Tumor antigen delivered by Salmonella III secretion protein fused with heat shock protein 70 induces protection and eradication against murine melanoma. Cancer Sci. 2010;101:2621–8.
170. Zippelius A, Batard P, Rubio-Godoy V, Bioley G, Lienard D, Lejeune F, et al. Effector function of human tumor-specific CD8 T cells in melanoma lesions: a state of local functional tolerance. Cancer Res. 2004;64:2865–73.

Chapter 13
Adoptive Cell Therapy for the Treatment of Metastatic Melanoma

Jessica Ann Chacon, Patrick Hwu, and Laszlo G. Radvanyi

Abstract Adoptive transfer of autologous tumor-reactive T cells as an immunotherapy for melanoma patients has been evaluated in various forms over the past two decades. Major therapeutic successes have emerged recently as methods to improve T cell culture techniques, optimize host conditioning, and augment persistence of transferred T cells have been pursued. A major leap forward occurred when lymphodepleting regimens were introduced for host conditioning, which liberates availability of homeostatic cytokines and depletes regulatory cell populations. Clinical response rates of over 50% have been observed in patients eligible for this therapy. Newer approaches of transduction of antigen-specific TCR or chimeric receptor constructs, use of better functionally defined T cell clones, and artificial antigen-presenting cells to expand specific T cells from peripheral blood cells are all showing promise. The time may be ripe for organizing a multicenter trial to establish the efficacy of this therapy and hopefully elevate it to a standard of care in specialized centers.

Keywords Melanoma • Adoptive T-cell therapy • Tumor-infiltrating lymphocyte • Interleukin-2 • Chimeric antigen receptor • T-cell receptor transduced

Introduction

Skin cancer is currently the most frequent type of cancer in the USA, and melanoma accounts for the most skin cancer-related deaths [1–3]. Treating patients with melanoma is dependent upon three major factors: the age of the patient, the general health of the patient, and the stage of the disease [1–3]. While surgery is the primary

J.A. Chacon, MSc • P. Hwu, MD • L.G. Radvanyi, PhD (✉)
Department of Melanoma Medical Oncology, Immunology Program of the University
of Texas Health Science Center, Graduate School of Biomedical Sciences,
The University of Texas M.D. Anderson Cancer Center, Box 904,
1515 Holcombe Boulevard, Houston, TX 77030, USA
e-mail: lradvanyi@mdanderson.org

T.F. Gajewski and F.S. Hodi (eds.), *Targeted Therapeutics in Melanoma*,
Current Clinical Oncology, DOI 10.1007/978-1-61779-407-0_13,
© Springer Science+Business Media, LLC 2012

233

treatment for early stages of melanoma, more advanced stages are treated with systemic therapies, either in the adjuvant or the metastatic settings [1–3]. Dacarbazine has been traditionally used for the treatment of metastatic melanoma, and along with high-dose Interleukin-2 (IL-2), has represented the only FDA-approved therapies for this disease – until the recent FDA approval of anti-CTLA-4 mAb (ipilimumab) and the mutant B-REF inhibitor, PLX4032 in 2011. Dacarbazine and other chemotherapy-based regimens have had no major impact in improving overall survival due to the highly resistant nature of melanoma cells to cytotoxic agents and radiation.

Owing to the refractoriness of metastatic melanoma to chemotherapy and other traditional therapies, immunotherapy using antigen-specific vaccines, cytokines, and expanded lymphocytes [4–11, 17] has been a major focus of research over the last 2 decades. In fact, the first tumor-associated HLA-restricted T cell antigen (from MAGE-A1), discovered by Boon and colleagues in the early 1990s, was cloned from a melanoma [12].

The first major form of immunotherapy that was developed for melanoma was IL-2 [11, 13–15]. IL-2 therapy is given in high-dose bolus infusions (600,000–720,000 IU/kg) intravenously every 8 h, with multiple cycles of these bolus infusions given 3–5 weeks apart. Almost 20 years of clinical history with high-dose (HD) IL-2 has found that it induces clinical responses (according to RECIST) in 10–15% of patients with one or more visceral lesions, while patients with solely cutaneous disease typically have a more impressive 50% objective response rate [16]. One remarkable feature, however, of HD IL-2 therapy is that a small number of treated patients with visceral metastasis (5–6%) undergo complete disease remission lasting for many years (>10 years) [15, 16]. These features have motivated continued use of this therapy in a number of oncology centers despite the toxicities associated with IL-2, such as capillary leak syndrome [11, 13–15, 18, 19].

The success of HD IL-2 therapy prompted researchers initially at the National Cancer Institute (NCI) in Bethesda, Maryland (the USA) to combine it with another form of therapy called adoptive T cell therapy (ACT) [8, 20–22]. Adoptive cell therapy (in the context of solid tumor treatment) can simply be defined as a passive form of immunotherapy that takes autologous peripheral blood or tumor-derived lymphocytes from cancer patients and expands these cells ex vivo using a growth factor (outside the immunosuppressive host environment) and reinfuses these cells into the patient in large numbers. The infused lymphocytes can consist of T cells, NK cells, or combinations of T cells and NK cells. During the expansion process, methods to boost the frequency of tumor-specific cells are sometimes included, such as pulsing in tumor antigens during the expansion process, or adding in antigen-presenting cells (APC) expressing a selected tumor antigen to stimulate an antigen-specific T cell subpopulation [4, 23–25]. The most common form of ACT now in use for melanoma uses tumor-infiltrating lymphocytes (TIL) expanded ex vivo from small fragments of excised metastatic lesions that are infused intravenously followed by a course of HD IL-2 therapy. This form of ACT has now been fine-tuned over the years and now consistently leads to objective clinical responses in 50% or more of patients [7, 26–28]. A number of clinical centers are now endeavoring to adopt this methodology with similar success. We are now at the point where

Table 13.1 Advantages and disadvantages of the different adoptive cell therapies for melanoma

Expansion of tumor-infiltrating lymphocytes (TIL)

Advantages

- Able to expand antigen specific or bulk TIL to billions
- Currently the most efficient treatment for melanoma patients that have failed other first and second line therapies

Disadvantages

- Antigen specificity of most TIL unknown (many may be nonspecific)
- TIL cannot be isolated/expanded for all melanoma patients
- TIL may be too highly differentiated at time of infusion
- TIL persistence in vivo is limited

T-cell receptor transduced peripheral blood lymphocytes

Advantages

- Generation of TCR transduced PBL is relatively efficient and practical
- High-affinity or very high-avidity antigen-specific TCR can be selected or generated and used to engineer T cells

Disadvantages

- Targeting tumor associated antigens (TAA) using high-avidity TCRs can lead to damaging normal tissue that express the TAA
- Limited antigen recognition compared to TIL

Chimeric antigen receptor T lymphocytes

Advantages

- Expansion of melanoma antigen specific T lymphocytes
- CAR recognition is independent from MHC antigen presentation
- Fusion of costimulatory molecule endodomains (CD28, 4-1BB, OX40)

Disadvantages

- Expression of transgene for long periods in vivo is limited
- Too much costimulation – cytokine storm can occur?
- Cross-reactivity with self-antigens on normal tissue may occur

ACT using expanded TIL has proven itself to be a powerful therapy for metastatic melanoma in a number of Phase II clinical trials conducted at the NCI and other clinical centers around the World, including the Sheba Cancer Center (Jerusalem, Israel) [13, 27, 29–31], and unpublished work conducted at our center in Houston, Texas (USA).

The development of ACT using TIL has also sparked a new era in T cell therapy using gene therapy tools that allow activated T cells to be transduced via retroviral and lentiviral vectors with TCR genes encoding variable regions with high-affinity for melanoma-associated antigens. T cell therapy using these "TCR-transduced" peripheral blood T cells expanded to high numbers has also entered the clinic recently with promising results. Together with TCR transduction, another promising technology involving combining antibody recognition of cell surface antigens on melanoma cells with T cell activating molecules in chimeric antigen receptors (CARs) has also entered on to the stage of cell therapy for melanoma. These CAR vectors combine antibody recognition domains against key melanoma antigens with endodomains of TCR activation chains as well as costimulatory molecules [32–38]. Clinical testing of CAR-transduced and expanded peripheral blood T cells is also beginning [34, 35, 39–42].

In this chapter, we provide an overview of ACT. Table 13.1 reviews the advantages and disadvantages of the different areas of Adoptive T-cell therapy used for melanoma treatment. We then detail the current state-of-the-art in ACT using ex vivo expanded TIL together with some of the outstanding technical and biological issues that still need to be resolved in the upcoming years. A description of some of the new TCR and CAR transduction technologies for ACT is also included. Finally, we make a case for why ACT using TIL for melanoma needs to begin to be seriously considered as a mainstream therapy along with the newer and exciting therapies such as monoclonal antibodies against CTLA-4 and targeted inhibitor drugs (B-RAF and MEK inhibitors) that have made a meaningful impact recently in the clinic [43–50]. We suggest that ACT will represent a major therapeutic option, especially for relapsed patients, and that combination therapies along with ACT may provide an even more powerful treatment option. A roadmap is presented by which ACT for melanoma can be tested in pivotal Phase II/III clinical trials to establish this therapy as a standard treatment modality.

History of the Development of ACT for Melanoma

A flowchart tracing the history of ACT development is shown in Fig. 13.1. The origins of modern ACT trace back to 1926 when J.B. Murphy first suggested that lymphoid cells had an essential role in rejecting solid tumors that were transplanted in animal models [51]. It was not until 1958, however, that Sir Peter Medawar defined the term "immunological competent cell" to describe a cell that is "fully qualified to undertake an immunological response" [51, 52]. Before the advent of ACT in humans and knowledge of the T cell receptor and T cell and NK subtypes, many studies were done using the transfer of immune cells to treat rodent tumors [51–53]. In the mid-1960s, administering a high number of lymphocytes from immunized syngeneic animals, Alexander and colleagues demonstrated that sarcomas in rats could be successfully treated [11, 53]. In 1969, Fefer and colleagues demonstrated that the intraperitoneal infusion of lymphocytes with chemotherapy, successfully treated mice containing intraperitoneal virus-induced lymphomas [11, 54]. It wasn't until the mid-1970s that the opportunity to expand antitumor immune cells in vitro emerged starting with Eberlein and colleagues who demonstrated that immune cells grown with T cell growth factor (IL-2) and injected intravenously in mice could eradicate implanted tumors [11, 55–58].

In 1982, Grimm and colleagues reported on a new cytolytic cell type that was different from the conventional natural killer (NK) system [59–61]. This cell, later described as the "lymphokine-activated killer" cell (LAK cell), was able to kill fresh human tumor cells resistant to NK cells in about 95% of patients [59–61]. The LAK cells were generated from peripheral blood lymphocytes from cancer patients and normal donors by culture in medium with IL-2 [59–63]. Together with HD IL-2 infusion, LAK cell infusion was able to induce the regression of melanoma metastases in animal models [62–64]. Later, Rosenberg and colleagues at the NCI in 1985

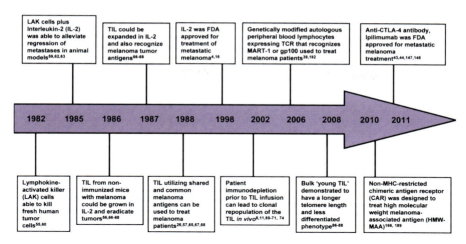

Fig. 13.1 Historical timeline and milestones in the development of modern adoptive-T-cell therapy for melanoma

demonstrated that LAK cells together with IL-2 had a significant impact on patients with advanced cancers in the first serious ACT clinical trials [62–64]. In 1987, a follow-up study was done that confirmed that LAK cells plus IL-2 treatment was more effective in metastatic melanoma patients than IL-2 alone [62–64]. During the first NCI clinical trial, melanoma patients received HD IL-2 for 3–5 days, followed by the infusion of HD IL-2 together with autologous LAK cells that were previously grown ex vivo in IL-2 for 2–4 days [62–64]. This treatment yielded about a 21% response rate (partial responses mostly according to RECIST) in the treated patients that was not much higher than HD IL-2 alone, however [62–64], but nonetheless generated interest in the approach.

The modest efficacy observed with LAK cells led investigators to seek out alternative cell sources, such as TIL, that had been shown to mediate more efficient antitumor effects than LAK cells [85]. In 1986, it was demonstrated that TIL from nonimmunized mice with melanoma could be productively grown with IL-2 in vitro and partially eradicate established tumors after adoptive transfer [11, 26, 31]. In 1987, it was demonstrated that freshly isolated melanoma TIL could be expanded with IL-2 and display major HLA-restricted recognition of the autologous tumor cells [57, 65–68]. In a phase II trial, metastatic melanoma patients treated with TIL and IL-2 had a response rate of 39% [8, 69–71]. Then, in 2002, Dudley et al. performed a series of seminal Phase II clinical trials in humans combining a preparative lymphodepleting chemotherapy regimen using cyclophosphamide and fludarabine in melanoma patients prior to infusing the TIL and HD IL-2 [69, 72]. They showed that this regimen facilitated the clonal repopulation of the TIL in vivo and improved the clinical response rate to approximately 50% according to RECIST [8, 69, 70, 72–74]. The TIL also demonstrated better persistence with lymphodepletion prior to infusion [8, 69, 70, 72–74]. Since then, the lymphodepletion regimen prior to adoptive transfer of T cells has become an essential component of most ACT protocols. It is thought that lymphodepleting regimens eliminate lymphocytes that would compete with the infused TIL for homeostatic cytokines, such as Interleukin-7 (IL-7) and Interleukin-15 (IL-15) [8, 69, 70, 73, 74]. Lymphodepletion also eliminates endogenous CD4+Foxp3+ T regulatory cells (Tregs) that can inhibit effector T cell function and the continued proliferation of infused TIL in vivo after adoptive transfer [75–77].

Current Methods of ACT for Melanoma

One major advantage of ACT is the opportunity to select in vitro for the desired T-cell functionality, avidity, phenotype, antigen specificity, and expand the selected populations prior to infusion back into the patient [7, 9–11]. Lymphodepletion has been found to be a critical component for most ACT protocols because, as mentioned earlier, it eliminates other cells in vivo that might compete with the infused TIL for critical cytokines, such as IL-7 and IL-15 [7, 8, 10, 11, 69]. Lymphodepletion usually involves the use of chemotherapy drugs cyclophosphamide and fludarabine [7, 8, 10, 11, 69, 74, 78]. There are also a number of protocols that involve the use of total body irradiation (TBI) in addition to cyclophosphamide and fludarabine [7, 8, 10, 11, 69, 74, 78]. The major types of ACT for melanoma are shown in Fig. 13.2. Below, we describe these major forms of melanoma ACT in more detail.

ACT Using Expanded, "Selected" TIL

As mentioned above, a group of seminal Phase II clinical trials at the NCI was the first to demonstrate the power of TIL adoptive transfer therapy for metastatic melanoma in lymphodepleted patients [69, 72]. These clinical trials first achieved a 40–50% clinical response rate with a significant number of patients (about 10%) achieving durable long-term complete remissions [69, 72]. The TIL expansion protocol used these studies has become known as the "selected" TIL protocol because it involved the initial expansion of TIL from melanoma tumors and the testing of these cells for antitumor reactivity followed by selection of the reactive TIL lines for further large-scale expansion for infusion [69, 72].

The "selected" TIL protocol is the prototype procedure with which all current TIL expansion studies are based with some variations. The procedure has two major phases or parts. The initial phase begins with the extraction of the tumor from the patient [6, 7, 20, 79]. The tumor is then cut into 3–5 mm² fragments that are placed in multiple minicultures (e.g., in wells of a 24-well plate) in culture medium with added IL-2 (usually 1,000–6,000 IU/mL). TIL migrate out of these tumor fragments and divide for a period of 4–5 weeks with periodic feeding with culture medium and IL-2 and subculturing as the cells become confluent [6, 7, 20, 79]. In the "selected" TIL ACT protocol that has been used mostly over the past decade, after the TIL have grown for 4–5 weeks, they are tested for autologous antitumor reactivity or

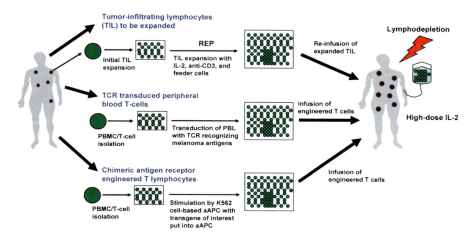

Fig. 13.2 Summary of different methods currently used to perform adoptive T cell therapy for metastatic melanoma

reactivity against HLA-A matched allogeneic melanoma cell lines using an IFN-γ secretion assay [8, 10, 11]. TIL lines exhibiting adequate antitumor reactivity are then "selected" and subjected to a further large-scale accelerated growth phase that has been termed the "rapid expansion protocol" (REP), as originally devised by Riddell and colleagues [6, 7, 20, 79, 80]. This second phase of the TIL culture process is a 2-week process in which the TIL are activated using an anti-CD3 monoclonal antibody in the presence of a 200:1 ratio of γ-irradiated peripheral blood mononuclear cells that act as "feeders" to support the TIL and provide costimulation [6, 7, 20, 79]. IL-2 (usually at 3,000–6,000 IU/mL) is added after a few days to stimulate the rapid cell division of the activated T cells. After the 2-week period, the TIL are harvested, washed, concentrated into one infusion bag, and transferred intravenously back into the patient, along with a cycle of HD IL-2 therapy starting the following day [6, 7, 20, 79] (see Fig. 13.2). Prior to the TIL being infused, the patient is lymphodepleted [6, 7, 20, 79].

Newer TIL Expansion Protocols Using More Minimally Cultured "Young" TIL for ACT

Most current protocols for expanding TIL for ACT used to treat metastatic melanoma involve the selection of tumor-reactive populations for each patient [7]. Although expanding TIL using the conventional protocol has shown to be successful, there are many limitations to this current procedure [10, 81]. Generating the autologous TIL can be technically challenging, and the long periods of time needed

(5 weeks for initial TIL outgrowth from tumor fragments and the 2-week REP) has led to many patients becoming ineligible for TIL infusion due to rapidly progressing disease and change in performance status. Moreover, it has led to a criticism of these adoptive T cell studies due to the possible selection bias toward patients who may not have as aggressive disease. Thus, limiting the period of time between the surgical removal of the tumor and the actual TIL infusion has become a new goal in ACT for melanoma.

A number of biological issues have also pushed toward limiting TIL culture times. It has been suggested that minimal time in culture for the TIL may lead to higher proliferative capacity, and a more undifferentiated phenotype [82, 83]. From the first report of TIL ACT in 1994, it was observed that the duration of ex vivo TIL culture correlated with clinical response where TIL cultured for shorter time generated better clinical responses in patients [27, 29, 84]. In addition, studies at the NCI found that TIL with longer telomeres may persist longer in vivo after adoptive transfer into patients and correlate with improved clinical response [84]. TIL expansion in IL-2 (giving an increased number of cell divisions) also has been shown to drive CD8+ T-cell differentiation toward a terminally differentiated phenotype with shorter telomeres [84]. Thus, another rationale for shortening TIL expansion time is that the less time the TIL spend in culture with IL-2 alone, the "younger" the T cells will be before transfer, yielding a more effective TIL product. To speed up the process and limit the initial phase of culture, the "young" TIL approach uses enzymatic single cell digests of excised tumors rather than cultured tumor fragments. The single cell suspensions are cultured under the same conditions with IL-2 as before, but then the nonadherent cells (T cells) are removed from adherent cells (tumor cells and stromal cells) within a few days. This approach has been found to generate the minimal numbers of TIL needed for the large-scale REP by 3 weeks, rather than the 5-week period needed for outgrowth from tumor fragments [86–89]. Another important difference with the minimally cultured, "young" TIL protocol is that the TIL are not tested or selected for antitumor reactivity. This decision was based on accumulating data indicating that that there was no significant correlation between positive antitumor reactivity of TIL expanded from tumor fragments and clinical response [82, 83].

The "young" TIL are subjected to the REP as usual and infused into the patient after lymphodepletion [82, 83]. "Young" TIL have been found to contain a more polyclonal population of CD4+ and CD8+ cells than the traditional antigen-specific TIL [82, 83]. "Young" TIL also have been shown to have longer telomere lengths and a less differentiated phenotype [82, 83]. Another positive point to the "young" TIL approach using tumor digests is that the success of initial pre-REP TIL expansion has been improved to over 80%, compared to the 55–60% rate achieved using the cultured tumor fragment method [82].

In 2010 Besser et al. announced the results of the first clinical trial using the "young" TIL protocol in conjunction with a cyclophosphamide and fludarabine preconditioning regimen in ACT for metastatic melanoma and reported 50% clinical response rate in a cohort of 20 patients (2 complete responses and 8 partial responses) [82, 88]. These results were very similar to previously reported clinical response for

TIL grown using traditional methods and confirm that TIL derived using the "young" TIL protocol are equally effective. However, unexpectedly, the shorter ex vivo culture period did not translate into better clinical response rate over the ~50% response rates observed in the "selected" TIL clinical trials originally by Dudley et al. [69, 72, 78]. Moreover, clinical trials of minimally cultured, unselected TIL at the NCI combining a CD8+ T-cell enrichment step, also did not reveal a higher clinical response rate [82, 86].

While the "young" TIL protocol has aimed to reduce the number of cell divisions and generate less differentiated cells with shorter telomere length, this biology needs to be confirmed by further careful phenotypic and functional studies. Although TIL in the "young" TIL protocol may be "younger" when placed into a REP situation, they may expand to a greater extent (more cell divisions) during the REP resulting ultimately in a spectrum of cells with similar biological properties for adoptive transfer as with current approaches using a longer "pre-REP" culture time. This may explain why the clinical response rates with the "young" TIL protocol have not improved. In the recently reported clinical trial by Besser et al. [82, 86] using the "young" TIL approach, it was found that clinical response was correlated with infusion of higher numbers of post-REP TIL (thus more extensively divided TIL). Despite this lack of apparent improvement in clinical response, from a practical standpoint, the decreased TIL product production time is an advantage. More studies will be needed to define markers of efficacy of the TIL product to tailor an expansion protocol preserving the desired characteristic.

ACT Using TCR-Transduced Peripheral Blood T Cells

Although using TIL for ACT to treat melanoma patients seems very promising, the major obstacle is that TIL cannot be expanded from resected tumors for every patient [7, 10]. Figure 13.3 highlights some of the major advantages and disadvantages of the different types of ACT. Owing to the fact that TIL cannot be adequately expanded from every patient, a number of groups are now focusing on infusing TCR-transduced peripheral T cells as an alternative, particularly for HLA-A2+ patients [90, 91].

This technique uses patient-derived peripheral blood lymphocytes that have been transduced with viral vectors expressing a TCR against a known melanoma antigen. So far, two antigens, MART-1 and gp100, have been targeted using this approach [90–93]. The first studies were done with T cells transduced to express an HLA-A0201-restricted gp100 epitope-specific TCR [94–96]. The TCR-transduced T lymphocytes were then infused into lymphodepleted melanoma patients, followed by IL-2 infusion [97–99]. Although the engineered T cells did persist and no toxicity was observed in the patient, the major setback of this pilot trial was that the cell-surface levels of gp100-specific TCR was relatively low, which resulted in minimal effector function of the engineered T cells [97–99]. More promising results have been obtained with a high-affinity TCR clone isolated from a melanoma patient

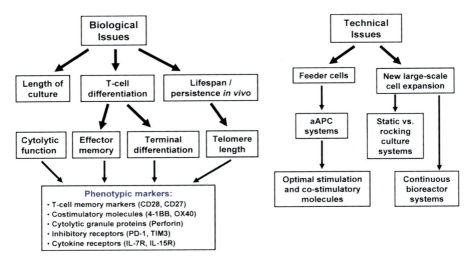

Fig. 13.3 Summary of important biological and technical issues under consideration for optimizing TIL expansion ex vivo and T cell persistence and anti-tumor function in vivo following adoptive transfer into patients

against an HLA-A0201-restricted MART-1 epitope (AAGIGILTV). This TCR has been cloned and transduced using a newer retroviral system that prevents mispairing of the recombinant TCR α and β chains with host α and β TCR chains, thus increasing the efficiency of the recombinant TCR expression in the T cells. Using this vector, 20–30% objective response rates have been achieved using expanded MART-1 TCR-transduced peripheral blood T cells [35, 39, 90–92].

A complicating issue with TCR transduction is that both activated and dividing CD8+ and CD4+ are transduced; this may be beneficial, as CD4+ T cells can provide "help" for CD8+ T cells. However, it may also pose a problem if the transduced CD4+ T cells are skewed into differentiation pathways in vivo (e.g., Th2 or induced regulatory T cells) that may inhibit antitumor responses by the transduced CD8+ T cells. Another issue at present is that TCR transduction can only address one antigen and one type of HLA restriction at any one time. Although one can envision a cocktail of different antigen-specific TCRs in the future, the system is still limited by the need to clone these TCRs and their specific HLA restrictions. Thus, TIL use, with a broader specificity of tumor antigen reactivity, still seems at present to be the optimal approach, at least for melanoma. However, for other solid tumors, such as epithelial cell-derived malignancies, where it has proven difficult to isolate and expand adequate number of TIL due to the nature of the tumor and the fact that surgical resection of metastases of the other tumor sites is not commonly practiced clinically, ACT using expanded T cells transduced with TCRs specific for overexpressed antigens is a feasible alternative. For example, cloned TCRs against CEA, MUC1, and HER2 are now being explored.

Generation of Antigen-Specific CD8+ T Cells from Peripheral Blood for ACT

CD8+ cells are able to bind to the HLA/MHC class I-peptide complexes and become specialized to kill after differentiation into CTL [100–101]. Using murine models, it has been demonstrated that a frequency of at least 1–10% of antigen-specific T cells is required for tumor regression in ACT melanoma models [84, 89, 102–106]. There have been a number of groups that have attempted to use antigen-specific (peptide-specific) CD8+ T cells in ACT clinical trials to treat metastatic melanoma [84, 89, 103–106]. One major approach has been the expansion of HLA-A0201-restricted CD8+ T cells from peripheral blood lymphocytes recognizing gp100, MART-1, or tyrosinase using peptide-pulsed autologous mature dendritic cells.

A phase I study in Stage IV metastatic melanoma patients was reported in which CD8+ T cell clones expanded to $10^{10}/m^2$ that targeted melanoma antigens MART-1 and gp100 were administered. These cells were shown to persist, traffic to tumor sites, and mediate an antigen-specific immune response leading to meaningful clinical responses, with about 30% of patients experiencing a CR, PR or disease stabilization for up to 11 months [84, 89, 103–106]. Mackensen et al. [104, 204] achieved favorable clinical responses in 3 of 10 melanoma patients after adoptive transfer of MART-1-specific T cells, which was associated with homing of the transferred T cells to tumor sites. Evidence for emergence of antigen-loss tumor variants was also found, suggesting that the infused MART-1-specific T cells mediated an antigen-specific response in the tumor that could have selected for the preferential survival of variants originally lacking MART-1 or losing MART-1 expression [104, 204]. In another study, Mitchell et al. [107] administered tyrosinase-specific CD8+ T cells (up to 5×10^8 cells with a frequency of 10–30% tetramer+ cells) expanded using an antigen-specific activation system employing insect cells pulsed with tyrosinase peptide after transduction with HLA-A2 and CD80. Although only modest clinical responses were observed, this clinical trial found that IL-2 infusion after adoptive transfer was essential to facilitate an enhanced persistence of the transferred T cells [107].

A more recent study by Butler and colleagues at Harvard Medical School involved the use of MART-1-transduced K562 artificial antigen-presenting cells (aAPC) expressing HLA-A0201 together with CD80 and CD83 to expand MART-1-specific CD8+ T cells from melanoma patient PBMC, along with IL-15 [108]. MART-1 peptide-specific tetramer+ CD8+ T cell frequencies ranging between 1 and 5% were achieved after expansion with these cells to >1,000-fold, with many retaining an effector-memory (CD27+CD62L−CD45RA−) phenotype [108]. They also used these K562 cells to express other tumor antigens, such as NY-ESO-1, HER-2/neu, and telomerase, to reproducibly expand antigen-specific CD8+ T cells from PBMC ranging between 4 and 10% tetramer+ T cells after a number of rounds of stimulations [108]. The K562 aAPC system is emerging to be an ideal system as it does not express endogenous HLA class I and class II and will elicit only minimal allogeneic T cell responses. As described in further detail below, these cells could be developed as an "off the shelf" APC to expand antigen-specific T cells of any desired HLA class I restriction, given the available of suitable expression vectors for gene transduction.

Use of Transferred Antigen-Specific CD4+ T Cells for Melanoma ACT

The role of antigen-specific CD4+ T cells used for ACT for metastatic melanoma patients has also been investigated. It has been shown that infusing tumor reactive CD4+ Th17 cells results in the complete shrinkage of a B16 tumor in C57BL/6 mice [109]. However, another type of CD4+ T cells, Tregs, can overpower the therapeutic effect of CD8+ transferred cells [77, 109]. There has been much controversy as to whether the infusion of CD4+ T cells correlates with tumor progression or shrinkage. Several studies suggest that the infusion of CD4+ is correlated with poor clinical prognosis, whereas other groups believe that polyclonal populations of CD4+ and CD8+ T cells are critical for a better clinical response [110–112].

For melanoma patients, the infusion of a polyclonal population consisting of CD4+ and CD8+ appears to be critical in obtaining clinical responses [104, 111, 113]. Tyrosinase, NY-ESO-1, and MAGE-1 are a few examples of a number of antigens containing well-defined HLA class II-restricted epitopes [68, 107, 114, 115]. In a first time trial using antigen-specific CD4+ T cells for ACT to treat melanoma, tyrosinase or NY-ESO-1-specific Th1 CD4+ T cell clones were used to treat nine metastatic melanoma patients at doses of up to 10^{10} cells/m^2 [107, 110, 114, 115]. It was observed that 3% of the CD4+ cells persisted for up to 2 months [107, 110, 114, 115]. In this study, one patient achieved a complete durable response of >3 years and four patients exhibited a partial response or stabilization of their disease. Notably, induction of T cell responses against nontargeted tumor antigens (a phenomenon called "antigen spreading") was observed in some patients that may have contributed to some of the clinical activity. Antigen spreading may circumvent the problem of selective outgrowth of antigen loss variants when targeting a single melanoma antigen.

Yee and colleagues also demonstrated the potential power of infusing cloned antigen-specific CD4+ T cells to treat metastatic melanoma. They developed an in vitro method for isolating and expanding autologous CD4+ T-cell clones with specificity for the melanoma-associated antigen NY-ESO-1 [196]. They infused these cells into a patient with refractory metastatic melanoma who had not undergone any previous conditioning or cytokine treatment and showed that the transferred CD4+ T cells mediated a durable clinical remission and led to endogenous responses against melanoma antigens other than NY-ESO-1 [196].

Current Biological and Technical Limitations of ACT for Melanoma

Currently, ACT using nonmyeloablative chemotherapy prior to infusing TIL has shown to have objective clinical responses in about 50% of melanoma patients [6, 10, 69]. Although expanding the T lymphocytes to large numbers prior to infusion has been beneficial, the functional characteristics, phenotype, and persistence in vivo have been found to be critical parameters, in addition to the infusion of adequate cell numbers, in determining clinical efficacy. These parameters also largely depend on the conditions under which TIL or antigen-specific peripheral blood T cells are expanded in vitro. Figure 13.3 summarizes some of the main outstanding biological and technical issues still facing TIL ACT that need to be addressed to improve not only the functionality of the transferred T cells but also to streamline the cell expansion technology to make it more technically feasible and easier to manage. It has been observed that there is a positive correlation between the long-term persistence of at least 1–2 major TCR clonotypes in the transferred TIL and objective clinical responses [116–118]. One of the main issues for the transferred T cells is once they are in vivo, the persistence is relatively short in most cases [116–118]. Persistence is critical in parallel to antitumor killing to ensure a long-term control of the melanoma [116–120]. Once the TIL are infused back into the body, they encounter many factors that affect their proliferation, effector function, and survival that may ultimately put the TIL in an anergic state or lead to their death upon reencounter with their specific antigen [116–120]. If the TIL are able to survive and persist for long periods in vivo, then the failures of ACT can be attributed to other aspects of the therapy, such as the actual characteristics and phenotypes of the TIL or resistance mechanisms at the level of the tumor microenvironment.

Telomere Shortening and Cellular Senescence in TIL

A critical parameter that has emerged in TIL ACT clinical trials is the possible issue of cellular senescence in TIL due to telomere shortening during extensive expansion in vitro. In humans, telomeres are DNA–protein structures that are located at the ends of all chromosomes [121–123]. During cell division, telomeres shorten. As T cells differentiate from the naïve to memory phase, they undergo extensive expansion and undergo such telomere shortening [121–123]. The enzyme telomerase, however, is able to synthesize terminal telomeric sequences and balance the telomere shortening process [121–123]. It has been shown that telomere length has been correlated with T cell survival and proliferation [8, 10, 83]. Therefore, many groups have further investigated whether the telomere length of TIL has any correlation with their persistence in vivo [8, 10, 83, 122]. It was found that after the extensive in vitro expansion of the TIL, the TIL had a shortened telomere length and a decrease in telomerase activity [8, 10, 83, 122]. It has also been observed that there was a correlation between telomere length and clonal persistence of infused TIL [8, 10, 83, 122] with TIL having longer telomere lengths reported to persist in vivo for longer periods of time, than those with shorter telomeres [8, 10, 83, 122]. Upon antigen stimulation, T cells show an increase in telomerase activity. However, with continued antigenic restimulation, telomerase activity may decrease, resulting in shorter telomeres [8, 10, 83, 122]. TIL with shorter telomere lengths may tend to enter a senescent state or undergo apoptosis [8, 10, 83, 122]. Telomere length has also been correlated with tumor regression, in addition to TIL persistence in vivo in melanoma patients [8, 10, 83, 122]. Thus, TIL expansion methods better able to preserve telomere length in the T cells should be explored.

Terminal Differentiation of CD8⁺ T Cells During Extensive TIL Expansion

One of the key issues during T cell expansion in vitro and in vivo is the induction of differentiation during multiple cell divisions associated with the appearance of end-stage effector cells and decreased proliferative potential due to extended culture with high-dose IL-2 [120, 124, 125]. The effector cell phenotype of the transferred T lymphocytes used for ACT to treat melanoma has been shown to be essential for clinical response [120, 124, 125]. The phenotype of the cells can be detected using surface markers to examine whether the cells are of CD4⁺ lineage or CD8⁺ lineage. Also, functional phenotypes can be examined using tumor cell killing analysis or TCR affinity experiments. Repeated antigenic stimulation of T cells has been shown to result in increased expression of different senescent markers, such as CD57 and killer cell lectin-like receptor G1 (KLRG1) [124–125]. CD57 has been associated with T cell end-stage differentiation and a loss of proliferative capacity [124–125]. However, CD8⁺CD57⁺ T cells also exhibit superior spontaneous antigen-specific cytolytic activity and proinflammatory cytokine secretion against virally infected cells and tumor cells [124–125]. Thus, the presence of these cells in TIL populations during ACT may be beneficial. However, we have found that a significant fraction of CD8⁺ T cells (up to 20%) in freshly isolated TIL from metastatic melanoma do express CD57, but upon long-term culture with IL-2 and following the REP, these CD57⁺ largely disappear (Wu et al., unpublished observations). Further study of this population of CD8⁺ TIL in our lab has found that it contains a high frequency of melanoma-specific CD8⁺ T cells (Wu et al., unpublished observations). Thus, the loss of this CD8⁺CD57⁺ originally found in fresh TIL may be detrimental due to the loss of melanoma-specificity in the final TIL product. This will need to be investigated further. Interestingly, we and other have not found appreciable numbers of CD8⁺CD56⁺ CTL infiltrating human melanomas.

Another biological issue in current TIL ACT protocols is the loss of critical costimulatory receptors during TIL expansion, such as CD28 and CD27, likely due to long-term culture with high doses of IL-2 [124–127]. The expression of these markers also delineates effector-memory cells vs. more end-stage effector cells that are more short-lived [124–128]. Infused TIL that persist for long periods in the peripheral blood have been associated with phenotypes expressing an effector-memory CD27[+] and CD28[+] with associated IL-7Rα reexpression [124–128]. The expression of CD28 has also been correlated with TIL having longer telomeres and better persistence in vivo [124–128]. In a recent study on MART-1-specific CD8[+] TIL, we found that only the CD8[+] T cells maintaining CD28 expression could respond to further antigenic stimulation following the REP [124]. This was not associated with decreased telomere length, however, but rather an overall change in the gene expression program in the CD8[+]CD28[-] TIL toward overexpression of cell cycle inhibitory genes and a series of killer-inhibitory receptors (KIR) [124]. Interestingly, in this study we did not find a role for sustained CD27 expression or signaling suggesting that maintenance of CD28 rather than CD27 in CD8[+] TIL may be more critical for better persistence [124]. Fortunately, there are ways to overcome the loss of CD28 and CD27 expression in extensively expanded melanoma TIL through their ability to still acquire expression of TNF-R family "alternative" costimulatory molecules. This possibility will be discussed in further detail below.

Technical Issues in Current TIL Expansion Methods for ACT

Figure 13.3 shows some of the technical issues we still face with TIL expansion protocols for ACT and some of the possible solutions. One key issue is the "feeder problem." At present, either autologous or allogeneic PBMC feeder cells are needed for the rapid expansion of TIL using anti-CD3 and IL-2 to prepare the final TIL infusion product. A 200:1 irradiated PBMC feeder-to-TIL ratio has been found to be optimal in the REP [7]. One of the main problems with using PBMC feeders is the variability in TIL expansion-supporting capacity of different PBMC lots. This has required the pooling of 4–6 different PBMC donor lots, but even these pooled lots can have batch-to-batch variation in activity. In addition, in many cases the numbers of autologous feeders, requiring leukopheresis of the patient prior to therapy, are difficult obtain, due to the immunosuppressed nature of many metastatic melanoma patients and the high numbers of myeloid-derived suppressor cells in the peripheral blood that cannot be separated by the apheresis machine. Many patients are also not healthy enough for a leukopheresis protocol to obtain at least 5–10 billion mononuclear cells needed for a typical large-scale clinical TIL REP. Allogeneic PBMC feeder cells are a reasonable alternative, but these are more difficult to obtain due to the need to recruit normal donors or the need to purchase expensive normal donor apheresis products from vendors. However, another alternative source of feeder cells is from normal donors using G-CSF-mobilized allogeneic stem cell products leftover because the intended recipients never received the product. These G-CSF-mobilized peripheral blood products can be successfully used to expand melanoma TIL (Radvanyi et al., unpublished observations). Nevertheless, it would be optimal to develop a universal-type of feeder cell or APC that can be established as a master cell bank and available for all TIL expansion protocols. As described below, such a solution is under development.

Other major technical limitations shown in Fig. 13.3 relate to the culture technology itself for T cell expansion (culture vessels and static vs. continuous fluid motion) and the high culture volumes needed to support the growth of the billions of TIL needed for infusion. Currently, the TIL REP is initiated in large T-175 up-right culture flasks (up to 50 flasks in some protocols) followed by transfer of the proliferating T cells into static gas-permeable culture bags midway through the growth period (usually on day 7 of the REP). However, the static nature of this system and the suboptimal gas exchange limits the maximum cell density that can be supported without compromising cell viability. The result is that total culture volumes can become very high (as much as 60 L by the end of the 2-week REP period). This also uses a large amount of recombinant IL-2 which further increases the expense above the culture medium costs. These shortcomings of the current static culture bag approach has led to the investigation of alternative technologies for TIL expansion, such as continual motion (rocking) bioreactor systems to improve gas exchange that are also described briefly in the section below.

Improvement of Current TIL Expansion Methods and ACT

Manipulating the Memory Phenotype of Adoptively Transferred T Cells to Improve Persistence and Effector Function

Recent studies have sought to augment the current methods for generating and infusing the lymphocytes that have been grown ex vivo. There are a number of ways to improve the durability of the transferred cells. For example, the role of alternative cytokines, such as IL-15 and IL-21, has been investigated. The conventional way to expand the T lymphocytes used for ACT to treat melanoma has been with IL-2 [13, 125, 126]. One key problem with IL-2 as a sole growth factor for T cell expansion (especially for TIL) is that it also can drive the terminal differentiation of CD8+ T cells into short-lived end-stage effector cells [124, 125, 127]. These effector cells (high spontaneous antitumor cytolytic and IFN-γ-secreting activity) may be ideal for short-term tumor control or a rapid regression of large, rapidly growing tumors, but may be much less ideal for more long-term tumor control to maintain durable responses. In this regard, other members of the common γ chain cytokine family, such as IL-15 and IL-21, can also be utilized to expand the T lymphocytes for ACT [124, 129, 130, 198]. IL-15 is crucial in the proliferation of CD8+ memory T cells and has been shown to better maintain both an effector-memory and in some cases a central memory phenotype of expanded T cells [124, 129, 130]. IL-21 has been shown to expand hematopoietic progenitors and regulate CD8+ T-cell proliferation [124, 129, 130]. Combining IL-21 with chemotherapy to treat B16 mice resulted in augmented frequencies of tumor-specific T cells and accelerated tumor control [130].

In combination, IL-15 and IL-21 can expand memory (CD44^{high}) and naïve (CD44^{low}) CD8$^+$ T cells and increase IFN-γ production in vitro [130–133, 197]. An in vivo study demonstrated that IL-21 plus IL-15 can increase the percentage of antigen-specific CD8$^+$ cells and result in tumor regression of established B16 melanomas [130–133]. It has been hypothesized that IL-15 and IL-21 may synergize through different receptors; with IL-15 playing a major role in cell division and inhibiting some loss if CD28, while IL-21 preserving CD28 expression and inhibiting cell differentiation [124, 130–133]. The combination of IL-15 and IL-21 has been shown to facilitate T-cell antitumor responses and increase cytokine production [128, 129, 131, 132]. The use of IL-15 and IL-21 has not yet been thoroughly tested for human TIL expansion. However, our laboratory has performed some investigation of these cytokines [124] in the TIL REP and found that IL-15 and IL-21 synergize in maintaining CD28 expression in CD8$^+$ TIL and improving post-REP TIL responses to antigenic restimulation. IL-15 alone induced a similar level of TIL expansion with concomitant loss of CD28, while IL-21 highly preserved CD28 and TIL responsiveness, but was poor at expanding the T cells. Interestingly, the combination of IL-15 and IL-21 seemed to combine the best properties of both cytokines and yields a TIL product with a "younger" phenotype [124].

Manipulation of T Cell Negative and Positive Costimulatory Pathways

ACT using TIL or TCR-transduced peripheral blood lymphocytes has the potential to eradicate large, established tumor burdens, but a number of factors in metastatic melanoma patients can impair the function of the transferred cells [134]. These include both local immunosuppressive factors in the tumor microenvironment as well as systemic T cell suppressive factors. Eradication of the tumor can be impaired by the expression of programmed death-ligand 1 (PD-L1/B7H1) expressed on tumor cells. High expression of PD-L1/B7H1 on tumors, including melanoma, has been correlated with poor clinical response. PD-L1/B7H1 interaction with its receptor programmed death-1 (PD-1) on CD8$^+$ T cells can lead to blunted T cell function and even apoptosis [134–135]. Inhibition of TCR-induced cytokine production, cytolytic activity, and proliferation has been observed [135–137]. In order to increase the function of tumor-reactive T lymphocytes, antibodies blocking the interaction between PD-1 and PD-L have been developed [134, 136–139]. Blocking the PD-1-PD-L1/B7H1 interaction may lead to improved TIL-mediated tumor control. It has been demonstrated that PD-1 expression is up regulated in melanoma NY-ESO-specific CD8$^+$ T cells, in comparison with MART-1 specific CD8$^+$ T cells [140]. TIL that express PD-1 can exhibit a more exhausted phenotype and decreased effector function [134–137]. A recent Phase I/II clinical trial of a human blocking anti-PD-1 in metastatic cancer patients (including melanoma) found that this agent was surprisingly nontoxic and, moreover, exhibited a significant response rate that has prompted additional Phase II/III testing [137–138]. We have found that blocking PD-1 signaling in melanoma TIL restimulated using antigen using anti-PD-1 antibodies could significantly enhance antigen-specific CD8+ TIL cell division in vitro (Radvanyi et al., unpublished observations). Although additional studies will need to be performed, these results together with the well-known negative effects of PD-1 signaling on CD8+ TIL function and the initial positive anti-PD-1 clinical trial results, suggest that blockade of PD-1 in vivo after TIL transfer into patients may be of therapeutic benefit in enhancing clinical responses.

There are two potent signals that drive T cell activation. The first signal is through the ligation of the TCR by MHC/peptide molecules located on APC [141–142]. The second signal occurs through the engagement of CD28 by the B7 family members CD80/CD86 located on the APC [141–142]. T cells also express other inhibitory members of the CD28/B7 family, such as Cytotoxic T-lymphocyte antigen-4 (CTLA-4) [143–145]. CTLA-4 is up-regulated following T cell activation and also binds to CD80/CD86 on APC [143–145]. This binding leads to the inhibition of cell proliferation and inhibition of cytokine production [144–145]. Blocking CTLA-4 using monoclonal antibodies has resulted in objective tumor regressions. A clinical response in 10–20% has been shown in melanoma and renal cancer patients in clinical trials [144–146]. A recent randomized Phase III clinical trial in melanoma patients found that the anti-CTLA-4 mAb ipilimumab almost doubled the overall survival of metastatic melanoma patients [144–146] compared to vaccination with gp100 peptide. This result, combined with data showing improved survival in comparison with historical controls, led to FDA approval of ipilimumab for metastatic melanoma [147–148]. The licensing of anti-CTLA-4 for melanoma has now opened up the exciting possibility of combining it with TIL adoptive cell therapy, although toxicities with this regimen will need to be carefully monitored due to the Grade III/IV events documented with anti-CTLA-4 therapy [143–148].

Another exciting area that can be exploited to improve TIL persistence and antitumor activity in vivo is engaging the TNF-R costimulatory pathways, such as 4-1BB and OX40. CD8+ T cells are especially critical during adoptive cell therapy against melanoma to kill tumor cells and maintain a recirculating effector-memory pool for long-term durable tumor control [10, 11, 124, 149, 150]. The 4-1BB pathway is emerging to be a potent "alternative" costimulatory pathway in TIL, especially if they have lost CD28 and CD27 expression during TIL expansion.

As mentioned earlier, a critical problem with current expansion protocols using TIL is that it yields highly differentiated effector cells that are susceptible to apoptosis and cannot persist well in vivo after the REP [124, 149]. In most cases, infused TIL (even in lymphodepleted patients) do not persist more than 2 weeks, with most TIL TCR clonotypes disappearing. We have found that post-REP TIL have enhanced CTL function, but this is associated with the downmodulation CD28 and CD27, making them highly susceptible to AICD when restimulated with antigen or anti-CD3 [124, 149]. This conundrum may explain why tumor regression in most patients is transient with loss of most infused TIL after only 1–2 weeks. CD28 costimulation has been shown to mediate antiapoptotic signaling in both naïve and effector-memory T cells. Compensating for the loss of CD28 with engagement of 4-1BB receptors on post-REP TIL may reverse this situation. In fact, we have found that 4-1BB is up-regulated on CD8+ TIL during the REP and after restimulation of post-REP CD8+ TIL with melanoma antigen or anti-CD3 mAb and that ligation of 4-1BB with agonistic fully human anti-41BB monoclonal antibody (BMS-663513 from Bristol Myers Squibb) potently protected CD8+ TIL from activation-induced apoptosis [149]. Moreover, 4-1BB costimulation also induced post-REP TIL to further expand and increased the expression of CTL granule proteins and induced the expression of antiapoptotic molecules (bcl-2 and bcl-xL), while downmodulating bim expression [149]. All this has translated into a significantly enhanced survival capacity and antitumor activity in vitro [149]. We have also found that addition of anti-4-1BB antibody (BMS-663513) during the REP can also improve the yield of CD8+ T cells with memory markers (CD28 and CD27), increased CTL granule proteins, and higher bcl-2 levels (Chacon et al., unpublished observations). Our results suggest that anti-4-1BB antibodies has the potential to significantly improve the clinical activity of TIL therapy for melanoma either by infusing it in vivo after TIL adoptive transfer into patients, or by using it strictly in vitro as a way of significantly improving the effector-memory phenotype and function of the infused CD8+ T cells.

Although OX40 has not been formally tested for its costimulatory role in melanoma TIL, a significant frequency of post-REP CD8+ T cells, including melanoma antigen-specific cells, do indeed express OX40 [149]. These cells may have unique properties and may respond to OX40 ligation in a similar or synergistic fashion with 4-1BB. This pathway should also be tested in TIL therapy, as clinical-grade human anti-OX40 antibodies are now becoming available.

Vaccination with Tumor Antigens to Boost TIL Function and Persistence After Adoptive Transfer

In addition to the provision of costimulatory signals or blocking negative signaling molecules on T cells using agonistic monoclonal antibodies or blocking antibodies, respectively, another avenue to improve upon the outcome TIL ACT for melanoma is by covaccinating patients with melanoma antigens recognized by the TIL population. One method being explored is using autologous antigen or peptide-pulsed DC infusion at the time of T cell adoptive transfer. We are currently conducting a randomized Phase II TIL ACT clinical trial testing the effects of an autologous MART-1 peptide-pulsed mature DC vaccine infused intravenously 4 h after TIL infusion (before the start of HD IL-2 therapy) and again 21 days after TIL infusion. This clinical trial is being conducted with HLA-A0201+ patients with MART-1 peptide-reactive (tetramer+) CD8+ T cells above 0.1% of the TIL population. The control arm is receiving TIL and IL-2 without DC. This study was based on preclinical data in a C57BL/6 mouse melanoma model using the transfer gp100

TCR transgenic CD8+ T cells (pmel T cells) showing that covaccination with gp100 peptide-pulsed mature DC increased the expansion of the gp100-specific T cells after adoptive transfer in vivo and greatly boosted their killing of established subcutaneous B16 tumors [151]. So far, we have treated three patients with TIL plus MART-1 peptide-pulsed DC, with two of the patients experiencing rapid and durable near complete responses within 12 weeks of TIL transfer (Radvanyi et al., unpublished observations).

Addressing the Problem of TIL Migration into Tumors

One of the main problems plaguing the field of TIL ACT is that most of the transferred T cells do not home to, and penetrate into, the metastatic lesions to manifest their antitumor killing and cytokine secretion function [152–153]. There is no easy solution to this problem as many TIL accumulate in the lung and liver after intravenous infusion [152– 153]. One possible solution is using intra-arterial delivery of TIL, but this is technically more challenging and may have increased risk. An alternative approach that we are currently investigating at the MD Anderson Cancer Center is transducing TIL with chemokine receptors that should facilitate intratumoral homing. Currently, we are targeting the CXCL1-CXCR2 interaction. CXCL1 is a chemokine produced by most human melanomas that acts as an autocrine growth/survival factor and can stimulate angiogenesis. CXCR2 is one of the key receptors for CXCL1, but T cells do not naturally express this receptor. Activated gp100-specific pmel T cells engineered to express CXCR2 had significantly increased homing ability into B16 melanomas expressing CXCL1 in an adoptive cell transfer model in C57BL/6 mice and mediated enhanced tumor control [153]. Based on these encouraging preclinical data, we are embarking on a Phase II ACT trial testing the efficacy of TIL retrovirally transduced with CXCR2 vs. TIL transduced with a control retroviral vector encoding a truncated nerve growth factor receptor (NGFR). Tracking of TIL in vivo both in the blood and in tumor biopsies can be easily accomplished by staining for either CXCR2 or the truncated NGFR, both expressed on the cell surface.

Targeting TGF-β

Transforming growth factor-beta 1 (TGF-β) is a cytokine that regulates cell proliferation, differentiation, and apoptosis [154–156, 202]. Tumors secrete TGF-β which can act to inhibit T cell proliferation and cytokine production [154–156]. This effect of TGF-β may have a negative impact on the transferred T cells used in immunotherapy for melanoma. TGF-β has been demonstrated to be a pleiotropic cytokine depending on the concentration of TGF-β used [155–157]. At lower concentrations,

TGF-β inhibits the cytokine secretion and proliferation of CD8+ T cells [154–156]. However, at higher concentrations of TGF-β, the cytokine can act to sustain the viability and proliferation of CD8+ T lymphocytes when they are activated with costimulatory signals boosting T cell activation and proliferation [154–156, 200]. In a recent study by Liu and colleagues, adding TGF-β while expanding TIL used for melanoma ACT maintained the CD8+ and antigen-specific population and prevented the overgrowth of CD4+ T cells sometimes seen when rapidly expanding TIL from some patients [158].

Nevertheless, in most situations in vivo, especially within the tumor microenvironment, TGF-β has been found to detrimental to CD8+ T cells by being a potent suppressor of CTL differentiation by downmodulating perforin and eomesodermin expression, and by inhibiting specific CD8+ T cell proliferation in the draining lymph nodes [159– 160]. Moreover, TGF-β is a key cytokine driving the differentiation of induced or adaptive CD4+ Tregs and is expressed on the surface of some suppressive Treg populations where it plays a role in inhibiting the proliferation of effector T cells [156–157, 201]. Thus, ways of making adoptively transferred T cells and TIL resistant to the effects of TGF-β is an interesting possibility to improve T-cell persistence and objective clinical responses during ACT.

One possible approach to inhibit TGF-β signaling in ACT being actively pursued is the introduction of a dominant-negative TGF-β-receptor II (DNRII) in TIL during the REP [157, 161, 203]. The hypothesis behind this work is that this will safely augment the proliferation of TIL in melanoma patients and their cytolytic function in the tumor microenvironment. Recently, researchers at the Baylor College of Medicine (Houston, TX) have generated clinical grade retroviral vector encoding a dominant negative TGF-β receptor (DNRII) and found that T cells expressing this receptor become resistant to the antiproliferative and anticytolytic effects induced by TGF-β both in vitro and in vivo [157, 161] and is now being explored in a clinical trial for patients with relapsed lymphoma [157, 161].

Newer Methods for the Clinical-Grade Expansion of Melanoma TIL for ACT

Technical as well as biological problems with the current TIL expansion technologies using IL-2 for extended periods of time and feeder cells to rapidly expand TIL to generate the final infusion product have sparked an interest in using novel approaches to expand melanoma using aAPC and new culture technology using different types of bioreactors.

In addition to potentially poor persistence of transferred T cells and the limitations of undefined feeder cells, a third major issue is that TIL do not grow from at least 35% of melanoma patients [8, 10, 162]. Therefore, we and others are beginning to study new ways of expanding melanoma TIL for therapy using aAPC.

The use of aAPCs in generating T cells for adoptive therapy has come a long way. Initially, dendritic cells (DC) were the APC of choice to expand T cells used for adoptive transfer [7, 10, 11, 150, 63]. However, DC are difficult expensive to generate in large numbers for most ACT applications. The first generation of aAPC consisted of antibodies linked to CD3 and CD28 bound to beads [164–170]. Although these beads successfully generated CD4+ T cells, they did not support the extended proliferation of CD8+, leaving researchers to investigate alternative and potentially more efficient methods. Moreover, we have found that TIL are highly susceptible to activation-induced apoptosis [149], and the bead method is not conducive to the "fine tuning" of the strength of the TCR ligation needed; this has resulted in an initial "die off" of activated TIL after bead-based activation, followed by the expansion of the remaining live T cells. However, T cell numbers never recover to the levels found in the traditional REP with feeders and soluble anti-CD3 antibody.

The second generation of aAPC, based on the erythromyeloid cell line K562, has shown more promise and versatility for the expansion of clinical-grade T cells for adoptive therapy [166–169]. K562 cells lack mostly all human HLA class I and class II molecules and therefore generate only minimal alloreactivity [166–169]. They can be uniformly propagated to high numbers very easily and are robust cells that survive large-scale culture very well. The current generation K562 aAPC have been induced to express CD64 (human high-affinity FcgR1); this allows for loading of TCR-activating antibodies, such as anti-CD3, to stimulate TIL for rapid expansion [165, 166, 168, 171]. K562 cells can also be transduced to stably express a number of cell surface or intracellular proteins (e.g., melanoma tumor antigens) and have largely retained their antigen processing and presentation machinery on HLA molecules and can present peptide epitopes from these melanoma antigens [165, 166, 168, 171]. Both lentivirus transduction and transduction with a new transposon-transposase expression system called the "Sleeping Beauty" system [172–175] can be used to efficiently transducer K562 cells for use as aAPC. Currently, a number of groups, including our own, have developed master cell banks of K562 cells meeting regulatory guidelines that can be used to establish clinical-grade TIL expansion protocols. These K562 aAPC have been engineered to express different combinations of costimulatory molecules (e.g., CD86, 4-1BBL, OX40L and other TNF-R superfamily members such as LIGHT), and membrane-bound cytokines (e.g., IL-15, IL-21, IL-7, and IL-12) [175–177]. The ability to engineer these cells in express active, membrane-bound version of these cytokines also solves the current problem of the lack of availability of IL-15, IL-21, and IL-7 for clinical use and the high expense that would be incurred when contemplating their use in large-scale TIL expansion regimens. We have begun test different versions of K562 aAPC for use in large-scale TIL expansion with promising results suggesting an improved maintenance of an effector-memory phenotype with high CD28 expression using aAPC expressing IL-21 and IL-15 (Radvanyi et al., unpublished observations). Overall, the K562 aAPC promises to solve many of technical and biological issues with our current TIL expansion processes. Phase II TIL therapy trials in melanoma patients using optimal blends of aAPC will be initiated in the near future.

Although the phenotype and characteristics of the transferred T lymphocytes used for melanoma ACT are crucial, the culture vessel technology itself used for expanding the T cells should not be overlooked. Over the past 10 years, several companies launched disposable, gas-permeable bag technology in an effort to decrease the risk of cross-contamination when expanding cells for immunotherapy, transplantation, and cellular therapy [178–183]. Recently, bioreactors with a presterile cultivation bag are being utilized to handle animal and human cells [178–183] such as the "WAVE™" bioreactor marketed by GE Technologies. This apparatus has a continuous slow back and forth rocking motion on a heated platform and a perfusion system for gas exchange and medium feeding. The rocking motion of the WAVE™ bioreactor allows the cells to obtain optimal nutrient distribution, and improved O_2 transfer and CO_2 removal [178–183]. The continuous motion and improved gas and nutrient exchange can increase the cell densities of TIL cultures over static culture systems, while maintaining growth and viability [178–183]. This can greatly decrease culture volumes reducing both culture medium and cytokine costs as well as processing time of the final TIL product.

The Prospect of CD4+ T-Helper 17 (Th17) Cells

Th17 cells have been shown to be important in autoimmune diseases and inflammation, but have hardly been studied in their role in immunotherapy. Th17 cells are elevated in melanoma TIL [184–185]. It has been shown through mice models that using tumor-specific Th17 cells for melanoma ACT stopped tumor development and activated CD8+ T cells [184–185]. IFN-γ has been shown to contribute to the ability of transferred Th17-liked cells eradicate B16 melanoma tumors [184–185]. The prospect of using expanded Th17 cells for melanoma ACT is an interesting new avenue for exploration. In murine models, transferred tumor antigen-specific Th17 cells trafficked into tumors and facilitated the migration of activated effector CD8+ T cells into the tumor [184–188]. One question with Th17 ACT in human cancer is whether antigen-specific (tumor-specific) Th17 cells would be required to home into tumor beds and establish a proinflammatory environment attracting other effector cells to the site. There are few HLA class II-presented antigens identified and some of these can cross-react with Tregs. However, this issue may be bypassed by transducing activated peripheral blood CD4+ T cells with tumor antigen-specific TCR genes or CARs. TCR and CAR transduction could be considered during the activation and expansion of CD4+ T cells under Th17-polarizing conditions (IL-1β, TGF-β, IL-6, and IL-23). It would be an exciting prospect to test this type of cell product for melanoma ACT due to the powerful antitumor-initiating characteristics of Th17 cells recently shown. One can also envision a synergistic scenario where TCR-transduced or chimeric antigen-receptor-transduced (see below) Th17 cells specific for melanoma antigen are infused together with expanded TIL or before TIL to home into the tumors and alter the tumor microenvironment to be conducive for effector CD8+ T cell entry and function.

Making Use of B-Cell Antigen Recognition to Drive T-Cell Antitumor Responses Using Chimeric Antigen Receptors (CARs)

Although using TIL for melanoma patients has been successful, there are still some patients from whom TIL cannot be expanded and cannot be treated using this type of therapy. Patients who have not been able to be treated using TIL can alternatively be treated using autologous peripheral blood T-cells transduced with high avidity HLA class I antigen-restricted TCR genes, as described earlier [189–192]. One major hurdle using TCR transduced T cells is that each transduced TCR is restricted to a specific class I or class II HLA subtype and therefore are restricted to patients not only expressing these HLA subtypes, but also expressing the processed and HLA-presented peptide epitopes from the tumor antigen in question [189–192, 195]. One clever way that has overcome this problem is the engineering of non-HLA-restricted CARs [165–168]. CARs are hybrid receptors composed of an immuno-globulin (Ig) variable region fused to the transmembrane and intracytoplasmic domains (endodomains) of either TCR signaling molecules, such as the ζ or ε chain that can trigger T-cell activation or CTL activity once the Ig domain on the cell surface binds to a cell surface tumor antigen on tumor cells [189–192]. The antigen-recognizing Ig variable domain can also be fused with signaling endodomains of costimulatory molecules, such as CD28, 4-1BB, and OX40 [177, 189–192]. An example of a melanoma-specific CAR construct under study currently is one recognizing the high molecular weight melanoma-associated antigen (HMW-MAA) also known as melanoma-associated chondroitin sulfate proteoglycan-1 (MCSP-1) [189]. Introduction of the HMW-MAA-specific CARs into T cells has been shown to result in cytokine production, proliferation, and other antigen-specific effector functions [189, 192]. Another melanoma-specific CAR of interest recognizes the ganglioside GD2 overexpressed on 50–60% of human melanomas [191].

Improvements in Lymphodepleting Preconditioning Regimens for ACT

Conditioning regimens also modulate the persistence of adoptively transferred CD8$^+$ T cells and TIL in vivo. In one study, adoptively transferred CD8$^+$ CTL clones infused following a regimen of DTIC persisted for more than 30 days following infusion and produced a response rate of 43% in metastatic melanoma patients [116]. To better define a well-tolerated conditioning regimen to improve T cell persistence, Yee et al. [74, 81] evaluated in sequential fashion, the influence of fludarabine lymphodepletion, using the identical CD8$^+$ T cell clone administered first without and then with fludarabine conditioning. A threefold increase in persistence in vivo was observed among transferred clones following fludarabine compared with no conditioning; this was associated with a rise in serum IL-15 [74, 81]. However clinical responses were not substantially better over previous studies. This may be attributed to the rapid increase in the proportion of Foxp3+ regulatory T cells arising after lymphocyte reconstitution [74, 81].

In another companion study, a nonmyeloablative regimen of high-dose cyclo-phosphamide (4 g/m^2) as a single conditioning agent was explored, prior to the adoptive transfer of antigen-specific CD8+ T cell clones then low-dose IL-2. This regimen was capable of achieving T cell frequencies of 1–3% more than 12 months after T-cell infusion. Four of six patients with refractory metastatic melanoma in this study exhibited an objective tumor regression, including one patient that had a durable complete response, and four experiencing partial or mixed responses [116].

Overall, these studies further emphasize the importance of the type and duration of the preconditioning regimens used to transiently deplete lymphocytes and how they alter the "cytokine landscape" in the patient and the rate at which endogenous T cells reemerge (e.g., Tregs) in the host. All these can greatly affect the persistence and function of the transferred T cells and will also need to be studied more carefully.

One more important question that has been addressed in melanoma ACT is whether the cyclophosphamide and fludarabine preconditioning regimen is "strong" enough to create an optimal environment for TIL persistence and expansion in vivo after transfer. As mentioned above, de novo T-cell recovery, especially the reappearance of Tregs after lymphodepletion may interfere with antitumor activity of the transferred TIL. One way this question has been addressed is by intensifying the preconditioning regimen to include TBI in addition to preparative chemotherapy. This is a myeloablative as well as lymphoablative preconditioning regimen. Two TBI plus chemo preparative regimens for TIL have been tested in the clinic at the NCI; one involving TBI of 2 Gy, and the other using a more intensive TBI of 12 Gy [8, 10, 11]. Patients were given stem cell support using an autologous CD34+ progenitor cell-mobilized product in addition to the TIL. The results have been very encouraging showing a significant clinical response rate of 72% with the 12 Gy TBI regimen, including an impressive 40% rate of complete responses [8, 10, 11].

Future of ACT for Melanoma

Many questions remain when considering how ACT might be optimized. It is not yet known what the optimal in vivo cytokines or synergistic immunomodulatory therapies (e.g., PD-1 blockade or stimulation of 4-1BB or OX40) are for patients receiving adoptively transferred T cells. The precise subpopulation of the effector T cells or effector-memory T cells that mediate tumor killing and promote objective clinical responses is still unclear. Identification, isolation, expansion, and specific infusion of these most effective TIL subpopulations could lead to more personalized therapy having greater efficacy, instead of a bulk population. Although ACT using expanded TIL has shown to mediate regression in around 50% of patients, there remain the other 50% of patients that do not respond to the therapy, and complete durable responses with the nonmyeloablative lymphodepleting preparative regimen protocols is still at a modest 8–10%. Do nonresponding patients have systemic host-related factors that make them resistant to the therapy, or are they within the tumor microenvironment? Are there still issues with the migration of TIL into the tumors based on earlier Indium labeling studies showing that most TIL still get "trapped" in the lungs after intravenous infusion [65, 193]? What is the optimal TIL memory phenotype driving the clinical responses in the responding patients? These and other questions need to be addressed in future studies to make ACT a more successful therapy.

Another critical issue now facing ACT using expanded TIL for melanoma is the appearance of newer targeted therapies with tyrosine kinase inhibitors (TKIs) that are poised to take center stage in the therapy of metastatic melanoma diverting attention away adoptive T-cell therapy. However, there is an emerging strong argument to combine these targeted therapies with TIL adoptive cell therapy to further improve both the extent and especially the durability of responses.

Combination of ACT with Targeted Therapy Using TKIs

Mitogen-activated protein kinase (MAPK) pathways are key signal transduction pathways that regulate cell proliferation and apoptosis [194]. The major pathway involves the RAS-RAF-MEK-ERK cascade and plays a key role in cell differentiation, proliferation, development, and survival [194]. Most melanoma cells seem to be "addicted" to enhanced or uncontrolled MAPK activation driving their proliferation and survival. In melanoma, the main activating mutation in the B-RAF gene (V600E) occurs in 60% of melanomas [50, 194, 205]. Drugs that inhibit B-RAF, such as PLX4032 (from Genentech), have undergone phase I, II, and III clinical trials [50, 194, 205]. PLX4032 has been shown to arrest melanoma cell cycle progression and can induce cause apoptosis in certain B-RAF-mutated melanoma cell lines. Recently, PLX4032 has been FDA- approved for the treatment of metastatic melanoma. More direct inhibition of the MEK 1/2 pathway is also being tested using MEK inhibitors, such as AZD6244. Overall, these drugs are showing great promise in arresting metastatic melanoma growth with rapid clinical effects after initiation of treatment with up to 80–85% of patients exhibiting partial responses [50, 194, 205].

Although B-RAF inhibitors have generated high percentages of clinical responses at a rapid rate, an unfortunate reality that is emerging is that in most cases the responses are transient in nature. In addition, at the time of disease progression, resistant and more aggressive tumors develop rapidly, leaving few treatment options open. However, ACT using antigen-specific peripheral blood T cells or TIL is still an option in this circumstance. We predict that although these new targeted drugs are becoming the therapy of choice for eligible patients, ACT will still have an important place for the treatment of the high numbers of patients that will ultimately relapse. In addition, mouse studies in our group at MD Anderson Cancer Center are beginning to show that ACT can synergize with B-RAF inhibitor therapy to enhance tumor eradication

(Hwu et al., unpublished observations). In fact, data now coming in on tumor biopsies from B-RAF inhibitor-treated patients is showing brisk lymphocytic infiltrates in these tumors that might be associated with higher and more durable response rates (David Fisher, Dana Farber Cancer Center, personal communication). Thus, it would be exciting to test a combination of B-RAF or MEK inhibitor therapy preceding or concomitant with TIL ACT for melanoma. Antigens released from dying melanoma cells following treatment with B-Raf inhibitors may also help further activate the transferred TIL. These clinical trials will surely be performed as soon as the first generation of B-RAF inhibitors becomes FDA-approved.

Toward Regulatory Approval of TIL Adoptive Therapy: Prospects for a Pivotal Multicenter Clinical Trial

There have been over 20 years of clinical experience with adoptive cell therapy using ex vivo expanded TIL for metastatic melanoma. During this time, continual improvements in cell culture technology and standardization of TIL expansion protocols have been achieved. In addition, considerable gains in clinical efficacy have been attained to the point that TIL therapy is perhaps emerging as the most powerful potential curative regimen for late stage melanoma. A number of published Phase II clinical trials at the NCI [10, 11, 27, 30] and at other sites around the world [13, 82, 86, 88] using TIL expanded from tumor fragments or with the "young" TIL protocol have consistently demonstrated about a 50% clinical response rate (RECIST) with about 10% of patients experiencing durable complete responses. New data emerging from the NCI also shows a significant increase in long-term survival in patients receiving adoptive cell therapy with TIL. At MD Anderson Cancer Center, we have also recently concluded a Phase II clinical trial with 33 melanoma patients finding about a 50% clinical response rate (partial and complete responders) with these patients clearly surviving longer than historical controls. This rich clinical experience and evidence of efficacy has resulted in a major push recently among the melanoma immunotherapy community to work toward achieving regulatory approval of this therapy. This would likely require greater clinical experience outside the NCI, a multicenter clinical trial design, and possibly a randomized phase III trial done on an intent-to-treat basis.

A number of possibilities could be considered for executing a multicenter clinical trial based on either single-arm Phase II or dual-arm randomized Phase III design [10, 11, 82, 86, 199, 206]. The nonrandomized Phase II approach could be considered for patients who are refractory to current treatment regimens, especially high-dose IL-2, ipilimumab (anti-CTLA-4), and B-RAF and MEK inhibitors, with treatment consisting of expanded TIL infused after lymphodepletion. The aim would be to demonstrate a robust durable or response rate beyond a critical threshold to convince regulators of efficacy in this late-stage patient population. Although this approach toward licensing of TIL therapy could be executed faster and with fewer patients than a randomized Phase III clinical trial, there are a number of risks. Firstly,

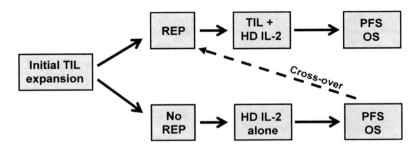

Fig. 13.4 Possible scheme for a pivotal randomized Phase III clinical trial demonstrated the superiority of TIL therapy vs. high-dose IL-2 (*REP* rapid expansion protocol; *HD* high-dose; *PFS* progression-free survival; *OS* overall survival)

the high degree of refractoriness of the disease after failing multiple therapies (including immunotherapies) is a concern since we do not have much experience, especially outside of the NCI, in treating these types of patients with TIL, especially the population of up and coming B-Raf inhibitor failures. Secondly, the threshold for durable complete response for a nonrandomized trial needs to be fairly high, and it is unclear whether clinical centers outside of the NCI can easily attain such a high goal given the different nature of the patient populations at different sites. Thirdly, to ensure reaching the high complete response rates needed to convince the FDA, most likely the chemo plus TBI preconditioning approach will need to be adopted with stem cell support. Only very few clinical centers would attempt such a protocol for TIL at present and such a protocol is not readily translatable to many clinical centers if the specific TIL therapy protocol would indeed get licensed.

Perhaps a less risky and more definitive approach at determining the efficacy of TIL therapy for melanoma would be the randomized Phase III approach [116]. A proposed scheme for a Phase III clinical trial is shown in Fig. 13.4. In this schema, Stage IIIc–IV melanoma patients eligible for high-dose IL-2 therapy would have a tumor resected and TIL expanded from tumor digests using the "young" TIL protocol described earlier [86–88]. Patients that have successful initial (pre-REP) TIL expansion would be randomized to receive high-dose IL-2 therapy alone or high-dose IL-2 plus TIL. In the latter situation, the TIL would be subjected to the large-scale REP and infused following chemotherapy-induced lymphodepletion followed by the IL-2 therapy. The end point of the clinical trial would a statistically significant increase in partial and complete response rates over IL-2 alone and increased relapse-free survival (RFS) as shown in Fig. 13.4. The clinical trial should could have built-in a crossover option for patients failing IL-2 therapy alone to receive expanded TIL as they will also have had a successful initial pre-REP TIL outgrowth that would have been cryopreserved and ready for further expansion [86–88]. In such a case, the overall survival (OS), however, could not be considered an end point of the clinical trial.

The other major issue that needs to be tackled when considering pivotal clinical trials aimed at licensing TIL therapy for melanoma is centered on logistics. Multiple issues need to be considered, including where and how the TIL culture and expansion will be done, which centers have the capability to perform clinical grade TIL expansion, and which centers have the capability of doing TIL infusion and high-dose IL-2 therapy. There are two main possibilities for this consideration. In the first scenario, different centers would each perform all aspects of the protocol using a unified set of SOPs (TIL expansion, infusion, and high-dose IL-2 therapy) and together the data could be combined across sites and submitted for regulatory approval. In that case, each site would likely apply for a separate license to treat their melanoma patients with their autologous TIL products. In the second scenario, a centralized facility would be established that would receive tumor samples from multiple sites and perform all the TIL culture and expansion according to a single set of SOPs [116]. The final expanded TIL product would be shipped by courier back to each respective treatment site for infusion. This latter approach may be more conducive for a randomized Phase III clinical trial and would also avoid site-to-site variations in sample handling and TIL culture and final TIL product processing. A number of parameters might need to be tested in a smaller Phase II setting to develop an optimized set of methods for tumor harvest and shipping followed by TIL expansion and shipping of an intact and viable TIL product back to each treatment site.

Many of the obstacles mentioned above have already been overcome (e.g., standardized methods to expand melanoma TIL) and shipping of tumors overnight maintaining sterility before processing and the capacity to successfully generate TIL for therapy has also been achieved (Mark Dudley, personal communication). There is also now considerable experience in overnight shipping of cell therapy products for infusion, for example for Dendreon's Provenge™ cell therapy product that has been licensed by the FDA for hormone refractory prostate cancer [201–208]. Thus, there are many reasons to be optimistic that a multicenter pivotal Phase III clinical trial can be achieved that, if positive, could ultimately lead to regulatory approval of TIL adoptive therapy as a standard-of-care for metastatic melanoma.

Conclusions

ACT used to treat melanoma has progressively advanced throughout the years, expanding from mice models to current clinical trials. Although melanoma ACT using transferred T lymphocytes appears to be promising in many respects, significant work needs to be done to further optimize this approach and increase clinical efficacy. One key setback is the lack of persistence of the transferred TIL and the loss of key costimulatory signals and telomere shortening in TIL that have been extensively expanded ex vivo. One approach that helped increased the viability and longevity of the transferred T cells is the lymphodepletion of the patients prior to infusion of the T cells. This allowed for "space" in the patient for the transferred T cells and the elimination of any suppressive cells or sinks that might compete with the transferred T cells for homeostatic cytokines, such as IL-7 and IL-15.

The in vitro expansion of the transferred T cells can also be optimized to improve persistence and increase effector function. Different cytokines such as IL-15 and IL-21 in combination have shown to be superior to IL-2 for cell growth, cytokine production, and effector function, and combining these cytokines with an optimal blend of T cell costimulatory ligands (e.g., through the TNF-R pathways) is showing great promise. New methods of expanding melanoma-specific T cells from peripheral blood using TCR transduction and transduction with CARs have now reached center stage and undoubtedly will have a major impact in the field of melanoma ACT in the near future. Another major developing area in melanoma ACT is the use of genetically engineered aAPC that can express any blend of costimulatory molecule and membrane-bound cytokine for T cell expansion that promises an "off-the-shelf" powerful APC technology for TIL and peripheral blood T cell expansion. Overall, the future of ACT for melanoma patients is very bright and has accelerated in the past few years with now multiple sites demonstrating the clinical efficacy of TIL adoptive therapy. This has spearheaded a movement to finally pursue regulatory approval for TIL therapy for metastatic melanoma that is gaining rapid momentum.

References

1. Geller AC, Annas GD. Epidemiology of melanoma and nonmelanoma skin cancer. Semin Oncol Nurs. 2003;19(1):2–11.
2. Hansson J. Familial cutaneous melanoma. Adv Exp Med Biol. 2010;685:134–45.
3. Hersey P. Immunotherapy of melanoma. Asia Pac J Clin Oncol. 2010;6 Suppl 1:S2–8.
4. Bordignon C, Carlo-Stella C, Colombo MP, De Vincentiis A, Lanata L, Lemoli RM, et al. Cell therapy: achievements and perspectives. Haematologica. 1999;84(12):1110–49.
5. Grange JM, Krone B, Stanford JL. Immunotherapy for malignant melanoma – tracing Ariadne's thread through the labyrinth. Eur J Cancer. 2009;45(13):2266–73.
6. Dudley ME, Rosenberg SA. Adoptive cell transfer therapy. Semin Oncol. 2007;34(6):524–31.
7. Dudley ME, Wunderlich JR, Shelton TE, Even J, Rosenberg SA. Generation of tumor-infiltrating lymphocyte cultures for use in adoptive transfer therapy for melanoma patients. J Immunother. 2003;26(4):332–42.
8. Dudley ME, Yang JC, Sherry R, Hughes MS, Royal R, Kammula U, et al. Adoptive cell therapy for patients with metastatic melanoma: evaluation of intensive myeloablative chemoradiation preparative regimens. J Clin Oncol. 2008;26(32):5233–9.
9. Huye LE, Dotti G. Designing T cells for cancer immunotherapy. Discov Med. 2010;9(47): 297–303.
10. Rosenberg SA, Dudley ME. Adoptive cell therapy for the treatment of patients with metastatic melanoma. Curr Opin Immunol. 2009;21(2):233–40.
11. Rosenberg SA, Restifo NP, Yang JC, Morgan RA, Dudley ME. Adoptive cell transfer: a clinical path to effective cancer immunotherapy. Nat Rev Cancer. 2008;8(4):299–308.
12. Gaugler B, Van den Eynde B, van der Bruggen P, Romero P, Gaforio JJ, De Plaen E, et al. Human gene MAGE-3 codes for an antigen recognized on a melanoma by autologous cytolytic T lymphocytes. J Exp Med. 1994;179(3):921–30.
13. Besser MJ, Schallmach E, Oved K, Treves AJ, Markel G, Reiter Y, et al. Modifying interleukin-2 concentrations during culture improves function of T cells for adoptive immunotherapy. Cytotherapy. 2009;11(2):206–17.
14. Dillman RO, Oldham RK, Barth NM, Cohen RJ, Minor DR, Birch R, et al. Continuous interleukin-2 and tumor-infiltrating lymphocytes as treatment of advanced melanoma. A national biotherapy study group trial. Cancer. 1991;68(1):1–8.

15. Geertsen PF, Hermann GG, Claesson MH, Steven K, Zeuthen J, von der Maase H. Interleukin-2 based immunotherapy of cancer. Ugeskr Laeger. 1990;152(47):3513–7.

16. Chang E, Rosenberg SA. Patients with melanoma metastases at cutaneous and subcutaneous sites are highly susceptible to interleukin-2-based therapy. J Immunother. 2001;24(1): 88–90.

17. Lee SM, Betticher DC, Thatcher N. Melanoma: chemotherapy. Br Med Bull. 1995;51(3): 609–30.

18. Baars JW, Fonk JC, Scheper RJ, von Blomberg-van der Flier BM, Bril H, von Valk P, et al. Treatment with tumour infiltrating lymphocytes and interleukin-2 in patients with metastatic melanoma: a pilot study. Biotherapy. 1992;4(4):289–97.

19. Moschos SJ, Mandic M, Kirkwood JM, Storkus WJ, Lotze MT. Focus on FOCIS: interleukin 2 treatment associated autoimmunity. Clin Immunol. 2008;127(2):123–9.

20. Eggermont AM, Schadendorf D. Melanoma and immunotherapy. Hematol Oncol Clin North Am. 2009;23(3):547–64, ix–x.

21. Faries MB, Morton DL. Melanoma: is immunotherapy of benefit? Adv Surg. 2003;37: 139–69.

22. Straten P, Becker JC. Adoptive cell transfer in the treatment of metastatic melanoma. J Invest Dermatol. 2009;129(12):2743–5.

23. Clark JW, Longo DL. Adoptive therapies: quo vadis? Pathol Immunopathol Res. 1988;7(6):442–58.

24. June CH. Principles of adoptive T cell cancer therapy. J Clin Invest. 2007;117(5):1204–12.

25. June CH. Adoptive T cell therapy for cancer in the clinic. J Clin Invest. 2007;117(6): 1466–76.

26. Rosenberg SA, Packard BS, Aebersold PM, Solomon D, Topalian SL, Toy ST, et al. Use of tumor-infiltrating lymphocytes and interleukin-2 in the immunotherapy of patients with metastatic melanoma. A preliminary report. N Engl J Med. 1988;319(25):1676–80.

27. Rosenberg SA, Yannelli JR, Yang JC, Topalian SL, Schwartzentruber DJ, Weber JS, et al. Treatment of patients with metastatic melanoma with autologous tumor-infiltrating lymphocytes and interleukin 2. J Natl Cancer Inst. 1994;86(15):1159–66.

28. Yannelli JR, Hyatt C, McConnell S, Hines K, Jacknin L, Parker L, et al. Growth of tumor-infiltrating lymphocytes from human solid cancers: summary of a 5-year experience. Int J Cancer. 1996;65(4):413–21.

29. Goedegebuure PS, Douville LM, Li H, Richmond GC, Schoof DD, Scavone M, et al. Adoptive immunotherapy with tumor-infiltrating lymphocytes and interleukin-2 in patients with metastatic malignant melanoma and renal cell carcinoma: a pilot study. J Clin Oncol. 1995;13(8):1939–49.

30. Khammari A, Nguyen JM, Pandolfino MC, Quereux G, Brocard A, Bercegeay S, et al. Long-term follow-up of patients treated by adoptive transfer of melanoma tumor-infiltrating lymphocytes as adjuvant therapy for stage III melanoma. Cancer Immunol Immunother. 2007;56(11):1853–60.

31. Rosenberg SA, Spiess P, Lafreniere R. A new approach to the adoptive immunotherapy of cancer with tumor-infiltrating lymphocytes. Science. 1986;233(4770):1318–21.

32. Berry LJ, Moeller M, Darcy PK. Adoptive immunotherapy for cancer: the next generation of gene-engineered immune cells. Tissue Antigens. 2009;74(4):277–89.

33. Davies DM, Maher J. Adoptive T-cell immunotherapy of cancer using chimeric antigen receptor-grafted T cells. Arch Immunol Ther Exp (Warsz). 2010;58(3):165–78.

34. Morgan RA, Dudley ME, Rosenberg SA. Adoptive cell therapy: genetic modification to redirect effector cell specificity. Cancer J. 2010;16(4):336–41.

35. Morgan RA, Dudley ME, Wunderlich JR, Hughes MS, Yang JC, Sherry RM, et al. Cancer regression in patients after transfer of genetically engineered lymphocytes. Science. 2006;314(5796):126–9.

36. Ngo MC, Rooney CM, Howard JM, Heslop HE. Ex vivo gene transfer for improved adoptive immunotherapy of cancer. Hum Mol Genet. 2011;20:R93–9.

37. Sadelain M. T-cell engineering for cancer immunotherapy. Cancer J. 2009;15(6):451–5.

38. Westwood JA, Kershaw MH. Genetic redirection of T cells for cancer therapy. J Leukoc Biol. 2010;87(5):791–803.
39. Johnson LA, Heemskerk B, Powell Jr DJ, Cohen CJ, Morgan RA, Dudley ME, et al. Gene transfer of tumor-reactive TCR confers both high avidity and tumor reactivity to nonreactive peripheral blood mononuclear cells and tumor-infiltrating lymphocytes. J Immunol. 2006;177(9):6548–59.
40. Kershaw MH, Westwood JA, Parker LL, Wang G, Eshhar Z, Mavroukakis SA, et al. A phase I study on adoptive immunotherapy using gene-modified T cells for ovarian cancer. Clin Cancer Res. 2006;12(20 Pt 1):6106–15.
41. Pule MA, Savoldo B, Myers GD, Rossig C, Russell HV, Dotti G, et al. Virus-specific T cells engineered to coexpress tumor-specific receptors: persistence and antitumor activity in individuals with neuroblastoma. Nat Med. 2008;14(11):1264–70.
42. Till BG, Jensen MC, Wang J, Chen EY, Wood BL, Greisman HA, et al. Adoptive immunotherapy for indolent non-Hodgkin lymphoma and mantle cell lymphoma using genetically modified autologous CD20-specific T cells. Blood. 2008;112(6):2261–71.
43. Eggermont AM, Testori A, Maio M, Robert C. Anti-CTLA-4 antibody adjuvant therapy in melanoma. Semin Oncol. 2010;37(5):455–9.
44. Hoos A, Ibrahim R, Korman A, Abdallah K, Berman D, Shahabi V, et al. Development of ipilimumab: contribution to a new paradigm for cancer immunotherapy. Semin Oncol. 2010;37(5):533–46.
45. Julia F, Thomas L, Dumontet C, Dalle S. Targeted therapies in metastatic melanoma: toward a clinical breakthrough? Anticancer Agents Med Chem. 2010;10(9):661–5.
46. Aziz SA, Jilaveanu LB, Zito C, Camp RL, Rimm DL, Conrad P, et al. Vertical targeting of the phosphatidylinositol-3 kinase pathway as a strategy for treating melanoma. Clin Cancer Res. 2010;16(24):6029–39.
47. Jiang CC, Lai F, Tay KH, Croft A, Rizos H, Becker TM, et al. Apoptosis of human melanoma cells induced by inhibition of B-RAFV600E involves preferential splicing of bimS. Cell Death Dis. 2010;1(9):e69.
48. Jiang CC, Lai F, Thorne RF, Yang F, Liu H, Hersey P, et al. MEK-independent survival of B-RAFV600E melanoma cells selected for resistance to apoptosis induced by the RAF inhibitor PLX4720. Clin Cancer Res. 2010;17(4):721–30.
49. Kaplan FM, Shao Y, Mayberry MM, Aplin AE. Hyperactivation of MEK-ERK1/2 signaling and resistance to apoptosis induced by the oncogenic B-RAF inhibitor, PLX4720, in mutant N-RAS melanoma cells. Oncogene. 2010;30(3):366–71.
50. Villanueva J, Vultur A, Lee JT, Somasundaram R, Fukunaga-Kalabis M, Cipolla AK, et al. Acquired resistance to BRAF inhibitors mediated by a RAF kinase switch in melanoma can be overcome by cotargeting MEK and IGF-1R/PI3K. Cancer Cell. 2010;18(6):683–95.
51. Silverstein AM. The lymphocyte in immunology: from James B. Murphy to James L. Gowans. Nat Immunol. 2001;2(7):569–71.
52. Miller JF. Discovering the origins of immunological competence. Annu Rev Immunol. 1999;17:1–17.
53. Baldwin RW. Tumour-specific immunity against spontaneous rat tumours. Int J Cancer. 1966;1(3):257–64.
54. Fass L, Fefer A. Factors related to therapeutic efficacy in adoptive chemoimmunotherapy of a Friend virus-induced lymphoma. Cancer Res. 1972;32(11):2427–31.
55. Eberlein TJ, Rosenstein M, Spiess P, Wesley R, Rosenberg SA. Adoptive chemoimmunotherapy of a syngeneic murine lymphoma with long-term lymphoid cell lines expanded in T cell growth factor. Cancer Immunol Immunother. 1982;13(1):5–13.
56. Kradin RL, Kurnick JT. Adoptive immunotherapy of cancer with activated lymphocytes and interleukin-2. Pathol Immunopathol Res. 1986;5(3–5):193–202.
57. Kradin RL, Kurnick JT, Lazarus DS, Preffer FI, Dubinett SM, Pinto CE, et al. Tumour-infiltrating lymphocytes and interleukin-2 in treatment of advanced cancer. Lancet. 1989;1(8638):577–80.
58. Oliver RT. The clinical potential of interleukin-2. Br J Cancer. 1988;58(4):405–9.

59. Grimm EA, Mazumder A, Zhang HZ, Rosenberg SA. Lymphokine-activated killer cell phenomenon. Lysis of natural killer-resistant fresh solid tumor cells by interleukin 2-activated autologous human peripheral blood lymphocytes. J Exp Med. 1982;155(6):1823–41.

60. Mazumder A, Grimm EA, Zhang HZ, Rosenberg SA. Lysis of fresh human solid tumors by autologous lymphocytes activated in vitro with lectins. Cancer Res. 1982;42(3):913–8.

61. Rosenberg SA, Eberlein TJ, Grimm EA, Lotze MT, Mazumder A, Rosenstein M. Development of long-term cell lines and lymphoid clones reactive against murine and human tumors: a new approach to the adoptive immunotherapy of cancer. Surgery. 1982;92(2):328–36.

62. Koretz MJ, Lawson DH, York RM, Graham SD, Murray DR, Gillespie TM, et al. Randomized study of interleukin 2 (IL-2) alone vs IL-2 plus lymphokine-activated killer cells for treatment of melanoma and renal cell cancer. Arch Surg. 1991;126(7):898–903.

63. Rosenberg SA, Lotze MT, Yang JC, Topalian SL, Chang AE, Schwartzentruber DJ, et al. Prospective randomized trial of high-dose interleukin-2 alone or in conjunction with lymphokine-activated killer cells for the treatment of patients with advanced cancer. J Natl Cancer Inst. 1993;85(8):622–32.

64. Atkins MB, Mier JW, Parkinson DR, Gould JA, Berkman EM, Kaplan MM. Hypothyroidism after treatment with interleukin-2 and lymphokine-activated killer cells. N Engl J Med. 1988;318(24):1557–63.

65. Griffith KD, Read EJ, Carrasquillo JA, Carter CS, Yang JC, Fisher B, et al. In vivo distribution of adoptively transferred indium-111-labeled tumor infiltrating lymphocytes and peripheral blood lymphocytes in patients with metastatic melanoma. J Natl Cancer Inst. 1989;81(22): 1709–17.

66. Spiess PJ, Yang JC, Rosenberg SA. In vivo antitumor activity of tumor-infiltrating lymphocytes expanded in recombinant interleukin-2. J Natl Cancer Inst. 1987;79(5):1067–75.

67. Topalian SL, Solomon D, Avis FP, Chang AE, Freerksen DL, Linehan WM, et al. Immunotherapy of patients with advanced cancer using tumor-infiltrating lymphocytes and recombinant interleukin-2: a pilot study. J Clin Oncol. 1988;6(5):839–53.

68. Topalian SL, Solomon D, Rosenberg SA. Tumor-specific cytolysis by lymphocytes infiltrating human melanomas. J Immunol. 1989;142(10):3714–25.

69. Dudley ME, Wunderlich JR, Yang JC, Sherry RM, Topalian SL, Restifo NP, et al. Adoptive cell transfer therapy following non-myeloablative but lymphodepleting chemotherapy for the treatment of patients with refractory metastatic melanoma. J Clin Oncol. 2005;23(10): 2346–57.

70. Klebanoff CA, Khong HT, Antony PA, Palmer DC, Restifo NP. Sinks, suppressors and antigen presenters: how lymphodepletion enhances T cell-mediated tumor immunotherapy. Trends Immunol. 2005;26(2):111–7.

71. Wang LX, Shu S, Plautz GE. Host lymphodepletion augments T cell adoptive immunotherapy through enhanced intratumoral proliferation of effector cells. Cancer Res. 2005;65(20): 9547–54.

72. Dudley ME, Wunderlich JR, Robbins PF, Yang JC, Hwu P, Schwartzentruber DJ, et al. Cancer regression and autoimmunity in patients after clonal repopulation with antitumor lymphocytes. Science. 2002;298(5594):850–4.

73. Lake RA, Robinson BW. Immunotherapy and chemotherapy – a practical partnership. Nat Rev Cancer. 2005;5(5):397–405.

74. Wallen H, Thompson JA, Reilly JZ, Rodmyre RM, Cao J, Yee C. Fludarabine modulates immune response and extends in vivo survival of adoptively transferred CD8 T cells in patients with metastatic melanoma. PLoS One. 2009;4(3):e4749.

75. Poehlein CH, Haley DP, Walker EB, Fox BA. Depletion of tumor-induced Treg prior to reconstitution rescues enhanced priming of tumor-specific, therapeutic effector T cells in lymphopenic hosts. Eur J Immunol. 2009;39(11):3121–33.

76. Powell Jr DJ, de Vries CR, Allen T, Ahmadzadeh M, Rosenberg SA. Inability to mediate prolonged reduction of regulatory T Cells after transfer of autologous CD25-depleted PBMC and interleukin-2 after lymphodepleting chemotherapy. J Immunother. 2007;30(4): 438–47.

77. Turk MJ, Guevara-Patino JA, Rizzuto GA, Engelhorn ME, Sakaguchi S, Houghton AN. Concomitant tumor immunity to a poorly immunogenic melanoma is prevented by regulatory T cells. J Exp Med. 2004;200(6):771–82.
78. Dudley ME, Wunderlich J, Nishimura MI, Yu D, Yang JC, Topalian SL, et al. Adoptive transfer of cloned melanoma-reactive T lymphocytes for the treatment of patients with metastatic melanoma. J Immunother. 2001;24(4):363–73.
79. Rosenberg SA, Yang JC, Restifo NP. Cancer immunotherapy: moving beyond current vaccines. Nat Med. 2004;10(9):909–15.
80. Riddell SR, Greenberg PD. The use of anti-CD3 and anti-CD28 monoclonal antibodies to clone and expand human antigen-specific T cells. J Immunol Methods. 1990;128(2): 189–201.
81. Yee C. Adoptive T cell therapy: addressing challenges in cancer immunotherapy. J Transl Med. 2005;3(1):17.
82. Besser MJ, Shapira-Frommer R, Treves AJ, Zippel D, Itzhaki O, Hershkovitz L, et al. Clinical responses in a phase II study using adoptive transfer of short-term cultured tumor infiltration lymphocytes in metastatic melanoma patients. Clin Cancer Res. 2010;16(9):2646–55.
83. Tran KQ, Zhou J, Durflinger KH, Langhan MM, Shelton TE, Wunderlich JR, et al. Minimally cultured tumor-infiltrating lymphocytes display optimal characteristics for adoptive cell therapy. J Immunother. 2008;31(8):742–51.
84. Shen X, Zhou J, Hathcock KS, Robbins P, Powell Jr DJ, Rosenberg SA, et al. Persistence of tumor infiltrating lymphocytes in adoptive immunotherapy correlates with telomere length. J Immunother. 2007;30(1):123–9.
85. Chakraborty NG, Sporn JR, Pasquale DR, Ergin MT, Mukherji B. Suppression of lymphokine-activated killer cell generation by tumor-infiltrating lymphocytes. Clin Immunol Immunopathol. 1991;59(3):407–16.
86. Besser MJ, Shapira-Frommer R, Treves AJ, Zippel D, Itzhaki O, Schallmach E, et al. Minimally cultured or selected autologous tumor-infiltrating lymphocytes after a lymphodepleting chemotherapy regimen in metastatic melanoma patients. J Immunother. 2009;32(4): 415–23.
87. Dudley ME, Gross CA, Langhan MM, Garcia MR, Sherry RM, Yang JC, et al. CD8+ enriched "young" tumor infiltrating lymphocytes can mediate regression of metastatic melanoma. Clin Cancer Res. 2010;16(24):6122–31.
88. Itzhaki O, Hovav E, Ziporen Y, Levy D, Kubi A, Zikich D, et al. Establishment and large-scale expansion of minimally cultured "young" tumor infiltrating lymphocytes for adoptive transfer therapy. J Immunother. 2011;34(2):212–20.
89. Prieto PA, Durflinger KH, Wunderlich JR, Rosenberg SA, Dudley ME. Enrichment of CD8+ cells from melanoma tumor-infiltrating lymphocyte cultures reveals tumor reactivity for use in adoptive cell therapy. J Immunother. 2010;33(5):547–56.
90. Adamina M. When gene therapy meets adoptive cell therapy: better days ahead for cancer immunotherapy? Expert Rev Vaccines. 2010;9(4):359–63.
91. Clay TM, Custer MC, Sachs J, Hwu P, Rosenberg SA, Nishimura MI. Efficient transfer of a tumor antigen-reactive TCR to human peripheral blood lymphocytes confers anti-tumor reactivity. J Immunol. 1999;163(1):507–13.
92. Coccoris M, de Witte MA, Schumacher TN. Prospects and limitations of T cell receptor gene therapy. Curr Gene Ther. 2005;5(6):583–93.
93. Leslie MC, Bar-Eli M. Regulation of gene expression in melanoma: new approaches for treatment. J Cell Biochem. 2005;94(1):25–38.
94. Marcu-Malina V, van Dorp S, Kuball J. Re-targeting T-cells against cancer by gene-transfer of tumor-reactive receptors. Expert Opin Biol Ther. 2009;9(5):579–91.
95. Roszkowski JJ, Lyons GE, Kast WM, Yee C, Van Besien K, Nishimura MI. Simultaneous generation of CD8+ and CD4+ melanoma-reactive T cells by retroviral-mediated transfer of a single T-cell receptor. Cancer Res. 2005;65(4):1570–6.
96. Coccoris M, Swart E, de Witte MA, van Heijst JW, Haanen JB, Schepers K, et al. Long-term functionality of TCR-transduced T cells in vivo. J Immunol. 2008;180(10):6536–43.

97. Dalgleish AG. The role of IL-2 in gene therapy. Gene Ther. 1994;1(2):83–7.
98. Jorritsma A, Gomez-Eerland R, Dokter M, van de Kasteele W, Zoet YM, Doxiadis II, et al. Selecting highly affine and well-expressed TCRs for gene therapy of melanoma. Blood. 2007;110(10):3564–72.
99. Kessels HW, Wolkers MC, van den Boom MD, van der Valk MA, Schumacher TN. Immunotherapy through TCR gene transfer. Nat Immunol. 2001;2(10):957–61.
100. Kamphorst AO, Guermonprez P, Dudziak D, Nussenzweig MC. Route of antigen uptake differentially impacts presentation by dendritic cells and activated monocytes. J Immunol. 2010;185(6):3426–35.
101. Valkenburg SA, Gras S, Guillonneau C, La Gruta NL, Thomas PG, Purcell AW, et al. Protective efficacy of cross-reactive CD8+ T cells recognising mutant viral epitopes depends on peptide-MHC-I structural interactions and T cell activation threshold. PLoS Pathog. 2010;6(8):e1001039.
102. Barth Jr RJ, Mule JJ, Spiess PJ, Rosenberg SA. Interferon gamma and tumor necrosis factor have a role in tumor regressions mediated by murine CD8+ tumor-infiltrating lymphocytes. J Exp Med. 1991;173(3):647–58.
103. Evans R, Duffy TM, Kamdar SJ. Differential in situ expansion and gene expression of CD4+ and CD8+ tumor-infiltrating lymphocytes following adoptive immunotherapy in a murine tumor model system. Eur J Immunol. 1991;21(8):1815–9.
104. Mackensen A, Meidenbauer N, Vogl S, Laumer M, Berger J, Andreesen R. Phase I study of adoptive T-cell therapy using antigen-specific CD8+ T cells for the treatment of patients with metastatic melanoma. J Clin Oncol. 2006;24(31):5060–9.
105. Overwijk WW, Theoret MR, Finkelstein SE, Surman DR, de Jong LA, Vyth-Dreese FA, et al. Tumor regression and autoimmunity after reversal of a functionally tolerant state of self-reactive CD8+ T cells. J Exp Med. 2003;198(4):569–80.
106. van Oijen M, Bins A, Elias S, Sein J, Weder P, de Gast G, et al. On the role of melanoma-specific CD8+ T-cell immunity in disease progression of advanced-stage melanoma patients. Clin Cancer Res. 2004;10(14):4754–60.
107. Mitchell MS, Darrah D, Yeung D, Halpern S, Wallace A, Voland J, et al. Phase I trial of adoptive immunotherapy with cytolytic T lymphocytes immunized against a tyrosinase epitope. J Clin Oncol. 2002;20(4):1075–86.
108. Butler MO, Lee JS, Ansen S, Neuberg D, Hodi FS, Murray AP, et al. Long-lived antitumor CD8+ lymphocytes for adoptive therapy generated using an artificial antigen-presenting cell. Clin Cancer Res. 2007;13(6):1857–67.
109. Muranski P, Boni A, Antony PA, Cassard L, Irvine KR, Kaiser A, et al. Tumor-specific Th17-polarized cells eradicate large established melanoma. Blood. 2008;112(2):362–73.
110. Hodi FS, Fisher DE. Adoptive transfer of antigen-specific CD4+ T cells in the treatment of metastatic melanoma. Nat Clin Pract Oncol. 2008;5(12):696–7.
111. Hu HM, Winter H, Urba WJ, Fox BA. Divergent roles for CD4+ T cells in the priming and effector/memory phases of adoptive immunotherapy. J Immunol. 2000;165(8):4246–53.
112. Muranski P, Restifo NP. Adoptive immunotherapy of cancer using CD4(+) T cells. Curr Opin Immunol. 2009;21(2):200–8.
113. Hanson HL, Donermeyer DL, Ikeda H, White JM, Shankaran V, Old LJ, et al. Eradication of established tumors by CD8+ T cell adoptive immunotherapy. Immunity. 2000;13(2):265–76.
114. Johannsen A, Genolet R, Legler DF, Luther SA, Luescher IF. Definition of key variables for the induction of optimal NY-ESO-1-specific T cells in HLA transgene mice. J Immunol. 2010;185(6):3445–55.
115. Topalian SL, Gonzales MI, Parkhurst M, Li YF, Southwood S, Sette A, et al. Melanoma-specific CD4+ T cells recognize nonmutated HLA-DR-restricted tyrosinase epitopes. J Exp Med. 1996;183(5):1965–71.
116. Weber J, Atkins M, Hwu P, Radvanyi L, Sznol M, Yee C. White paper on adoptive cell therapy for cancer with tumor-infiltrating lymphocytes: a report of the CTEP subcommittee on adoptive cell therapy. Clin Cancer Res. 2011;17(7):1664–73.

117. Melioli G, Guastella M, Semino C, Meta M, Pietra G, Ponte M, et al. Proliferative, phenotypic and functional and molecular characteristics of tumour-infiltrating lymphocytes obtained from unselected patients with malignant melanomas and expanded in vitro in the presence of recombinant interleukin-2. Melanoma Res. 1994;4(2):127–33.

118. Pisarra P, Mortarini R, Salvi S, Anichini A, Parmiani G, Sensi M. High frequency of T cell clonal expansions in primary human melanoma. Involvement of a dominant clonotype in autologous tumor recognition. Cancer Immunol Immunother. 1999;48(1):39–46.

119. Zhou J, Shen X, Huang J, Hodes RJ, Rosenberg SA, Robbins PF. Telomere length of transferred lymphocytes correlates with in vivo persistence and tumor regression in melanoma patients receiving cell transfer therapy. J Immunol. 2005;175(10):7046–52.

120. Huang J, Khong HT, Dudley ME, El-Gamil M, Li YF, Rosenberg SA, et al. Survival, persistence, and progressive differentiation of adoptively transferred tumor-reactive T cells associated with tumor regression. J Immunother. 2005;28(3):258–67.

121. Coleman C, Levine D, Kishore R, Qin G, Thorne T, Lambers E, et al. Inhibition of melanoma angiogenesis by telomere homolog oligonucleotides. J Oncol. 2010;2010:928628.

122. Goldkorn A, Blackburn EH. Assembly of mutant-template telomerase RNA into catalytically active telomerase ribonucleoprotein that can act on telomeres is required for apoptosis and cell cycle arrest in human cancer cells. Cancer Res. 2006;66(11):5763–71.

123. Puri N, Eller MS, Byers HR, Dykstra S, Kubera J, Gilchrest BA. Telomere-based DNA damage responses: a new approach to melanoma. FASEB J. 2004;18(12):1373–81.

124. Li Y, Liu S, Hernandez J, Vence L, Hwu P, Radvanyi L. MART-1-specific melanoma tumor-infiltrating lymphocytes maintaining CD28 expression have improved survival and expansion capability following antigenic restimulation in vitro. J Immunol. 2010;184(1):452–65.

125. Powell Jr DJ, Dudley ME, Robbins PF, Rosenberg SA. Transition of late-stage effector T cells to CD27+ CD28+ tumor-reactive effector memory T cells in humans after adoptive cell transfer therapy. Blood. 2005;105(1):241–50.

126. Boyman O, Surh CD, Sprent J. Potential use of IL-2/anti-IL-2 antibody immune complexes for the treatment of cancer and autoimmune disease. Expert Opin Biol Ther. 2006;6(12):1323–31.

127. Cheever MA, Greenberg PD, Fefer A, Gillis S. Augmentation of the anti-tumor therapeutic efficacy of long-term cultured T lymphocytes by in vivo administration of purified interleukin 2. J Exp Med. 1982;155(4):968–80.

128. Joshi NS, Kaech SM. Effector CD8 T cell development: a balancing act between memory cell potential and terminal differentiation. J Immunol. 2008;180(3):1309–15.

129. Pouw N, Treffers-Westerlaken E, Kraan J, Wittink F, ten Hagen T, Verweij J, et al. Combination of IL-21 and IL-15 enhances tumour-specific cytotoxicity and cytokine production of TCR-transduced primary T cells. Cancer Immunol Immunother. 2010;59(6):921–31.

130. Huarte E, Fisher J, Turk MJ, Mellinger D, Foster C, Wolf B, et al. Ex vivo expansion of tumor specific lymphocytes with IL-15 and IL-21 for adoptive immunotherapy in melanoma. Cancer Lett. 2009;285(1):80–8.

131. Overwijk WW, Schluns KS. Functions of gammaC cytokines in immune homeostasis: current and potential clinical applications. Clin Immunol. 2009;132(2):153–65.

132. Petersen CC, Diernaes JE, Skovbo A, Hvid M, Deleuran B, Hokland M. Interleukin-21 restrains tumor growth and induces a substantial increase in the number of circulating tumor-specific T cells in a murine model of malignant melanoma. Cytokine. 2010;49(1):80–8.

133. Zeng R, Spolski R, Finkelstein SE, Oh S, Kovanen PE, Hinrichs CS, et al. Synergy of IL-21 and IL-15 in regulating CD8+ T cell expansion and function. J Exp Med. 2005;201(1):139–48.

134. Pilon-Thomas S, Mackay A, Vohra N, Mule JJ. Blockade of programmed death ligand 1 enhances the therapeutic efficacy of combination immunotherapy against melanoma. J Immunol. 2010;184(7):3442–9.

135. Hodi FS, Dranoff G. The biologic importance of tumor-infiltrating lymphocytes. J Cutan Pathol. 2010;37 Suppl 1:48–53.

136. Hino R, Kabashima K, Kato Y, Yagi H, Nakamura M, Honjo T, et al. Tumor cell expression of programmed cell death-1 ligand 1 is a prognostic factor for malignant melanoma. Cancer. 2010;116(7):1757–66.
137. Ahmadzadeh M, Johnson LA, Heemskerk B, Wunderlich JR, Dudley ME, White DE, et al. Tumor antigen-specific CD8 T cells infiltrating the tumor express high levels of PD-1 and are functionally impaired. Blood. 2009;114(8):1537–44.
138. Brahmer JR, Drake CG, Wollner I, Powderly JD, Picus J, Sharfman WH, et al. Phase I study of single-agent anti-programmed death-1 (MDX-1106) in refractory solid tumors: safety, clinical activity, pharmacodynamics, and immunologic correlates. J Clin Oncol. 2010;28(19):3167–75.
139. Ascierto PA, Streicher HZ, Sznol M. Melanoma: a model for testing new agents in combination therapies. J Transl Med. 2010;8:38.
140. Fourcade J, Kudela P, Sun Z, Shen H, Land SR, Lenzner D, et al. PD-1 is a regulator of NY-ESO-1-specific CD8+ T cell expansion in melanoma patients. J Immunol. 2009;182(9):5240–9.
141. Bertram EM, Dawicki W, Sedgmen B, Bramson JL, Lynch DH, Watts TH. A switch in costimulation from CD28 to 4-1BB during primary versus secondary CD8 T cell response to influenza in vivo. J Immunol. 2004;172(2):981–8.
142. Watts TH. TNF/TNFR family members in costimulation of T cell responses. Annu Rev Immunol. 2005;23:23–68.
143. Fong L, Small EJ. Anti-cytotoxic T-lymphocyte antigen-4 antibody: the first in an emerging class of immunomodulatory antibodies for cancer treatment. J Clin Oncol. 2008;26(32):5275–83.
144. Phan GQ, Yang JC, Sherry RM, Hwu P, Topalian SL, Schwartzentruber DJ, et al. Cancer regression and autoimmunity induced by cytotoxic T lymphocyte-associated antigen 4 blockade in patients with metastatic melanoma. Proc Natl Acad Sci USA. 2003;100(14):8372–7.
145. Phan GQ, Weber JS, Sondak VK. CTLA-4 blockade with monoclonal antibodies in patients with metastatic cancer: surgical issues. Ann Surg Oncol. 2008;15(11):3014–21.
146. Maker AV, Attia P, Rosenberg SA. Analysis of the cellular mechanism of antitumor responses and autoimmunity in patients treated with CTLA-4 blockade. J Immunol. 2005;175(11):7746–54.
147. Pennock GK, Waterfield W, Wolchok JD. Patient responses to ipilimumab, a novel immuno-potentiator for metastatic melanoma: how different are these from conventional treatment responses? Am J Clin Oncol. 2011 Feb 17. [Epub ahead of print].
148. Thumar JR, Kluger HM. Ipilimumab: a promising immunotherapy for melanoma. Oncology (Williston Park). 2011;24(14):1280–8.
149. Hernandez-Chacon JA, Li Y, Wu RC, Bernatchez C, Wang Y, Weber JS, et al. Costimulation through the CD137/4-1BB pathway protects human melanoma tumor-infiltrating lymphocytes from activation-induced cell death and enhances antitumor effector function. J Immunother. 2011;34(3):236–50.
150. Nguyen LT, Yen PH, Nie J, Liadis N, Ghazarian D, Al-Habeeb A, et al. Expansion and characterization of human melanoma tumor-infiltrating lymphocytes (TILs). PLoS One. 2010;5(11):e13940.
151. Lou Y, Wang G, Lizee G, Kim GJ, Finkelstein SE, Feng C, et al. Dendritic cells strongly boost the antitumor activity of adoptively transferred T cells in vivo. Cancer Res. 2004;64(18):6783–90.
152. Economou JS, Belldegrun AS, Glaspy J, Toloza EM, Figlin R, Hobbs J, et al. In vivo trafficking of adoptively transferred interleukin-2 expanded tumor-infiltrating lymphocytes and peripheral blood lymphocytes. Results of a double gene marking trial. J Clin Invest. 1996;97(2):515–21.
153. Peng W, Ye Y, Rabinovich BA, Liu C, Lou Y, Zhang M, et al. Transduction of tumor-specific T cells with CXCR2 chemokine receptor improves migration to tumor and antitumor immune responses. Clin Cancer Res. 2010;16(22):5458–68.

154. Esser P, Grisanti S, Bartz-Schmidt K. TGF-beta in uveal melanoma. Microsc Res Tech. 2001;52(4):396–400.
155. Javelaud D, Alexaki VI, Mauviel A. Transforming growth factor-beta in cutaneous melanoma. Pigment Cell Melanoma Res. 2008;21(2):123–32.
156. Kaminska B, Wesolowska A, Danilkiewicz M. TGF beta signalling and its role in tumour pathogenesis. Acta Biochim Pol. 2005;52(2):329–37.
157. Bollard CM, Rossig C, Calonge MJ, Huls MH, Wagner HJ, Massague J, et al. Adapting a transforming growth factor beta-related tumor protection strategy to enhance antitumor immunity. Blood. 2002;99(9):3179–87.
158. Liu S, Etto T, Rodriguez-Cruz T, Li Y, Wu C, Fulbright OJ, et al. TGF-beta1 induces preferential rapid expansion and persistence of tumor antigen-specific CD8+ T cells for adoptive immunotherapy. J Immunother. 2010;33(4):371–81.
159. Arens R, Schoenberger SP. Plasticity in programming of effector and memory CD8 T-cell formation. Immunol Rev. 2010;235(1):190–205.
160. Atreya I, Schimanski CC, Becker C, Wirtz S, Dornhoff H, Schnurer E, et al. The T-box transcription factor eomesodermin controls CD8 T cell activity and lymph node metastasis in human colorectal cancer. Gut. 2007;56(11):1572–8.
161. Bollard CM, Dotti G, Gottschalk S, Liu E, Sheehan A, et al. Administration of tumor-specific cytotoxic T lymphocytes engineered to resist TGF-b to patients with EBV-associated lymphomas. American Association of Hematologists meeting; 2010. p. Abstract 560.
162. Klapper JA, Thomasian AA, Smith DM, Gorgas GC, Wunderlich JR, Smith FO, et al. Single-pass, closed-system rapid expansion of lymphocyte cultures for adoptive cell therapy. J Immunol Methods. 2009;345(1–2):90–9.
163. Mandruzzato S, Rossi E, Bernardi F, Tosello V, Macino B, Basso G, et al. Large and dissimilar repertoire of Melan-A/MART-1-specific CTL in metastatic lesions and blood of a melanoma patient. J Immunol. 2002;169(7):4017–24.
164. Morgan RA, Anderson WF. Human gene therapy. Annu Rev Biochem. 1993;62:191–217.
165. Chang J. Efficient amplification of melanoma-specific CD8+ T cells using artificial antigen presenting complex. Exp Mol Med. 2006;38(6):591–8.
166. Eshhar Z. Adoptive cancer immunotherapy using genetically engineered designer T-cells: first steps into the clinic. Curr Opin Mol Ther. 2010;12(1):55–63.
167. Eshhar Z, Waks T, Bendavid A, Schindler DG. Functional expression of chimeric receptor genes in human T cells. J Immunol Methods. 2001;248(1–2):67–76.
168. Grube M, Melenhorst JJ, Barrett AJ. An APC for every occasion: induction and expansion of human Ag-specific CD4 and CD8 T cells using cellular and non-cellular APC. Cytotherapy. 2004;6(5):440–9.
169. Singh H, Manuri PR, Olivares S, Dara N, Dawson MJ, Huls H, et al. Redirecting specificity of T-cell populations for CD19 using the Sleeping Beauty system. Cancer Res. 2008;68(8): 2961–71.
170. Loskog A, Giandomenico V, Rossig C, Pule M, Dotti G, Brenner MK. Addition of the CD28 signaling domain to chimeric T-cell receptors enhances chimeric T-cell resistance to T regulatory cells. Leukemia. 2006;20(10):1819–28.
171. Leong SP, Zhou YM, Granberry ME, Wang TF, Grogan TM, Spier C, et al. Generation of cytotoxic effector cells against human melanoma. Cancer Immunol Immunother. 1995;40(6): 397–409.
172. Aronovich EL, McIvor RS, Hackett PB. The Sleeping Beauty transposon system – a non-viral vector for gene therapy. Hum Mol Genet. 2011;20(R1):R14–20.
173. Hackett PB, Largaespada DA, Cooper LJ. A transposon and transposase system for human application. Mol Ther. 2010;18(4):674–83.
174. Izsvak Z, Chuah MK, Vandendriessche T, Ivics Z. Efficient stable gene transfer into human cells by the Sleeping Beauty transposon vectors. Methods. 2009;49(3):287–97.
175. Izsvak Z, Hackett PB, Cooper LJ, Ivics Z. Translating Sleeping Beauty transposition into cellular therapies: victories and challenges. Bioessays. 2010;32(9):756–67.

176. Jin Z, Maiti S, Huls H, Singh H, Olivares S, Mates L, et al. The hyperactive Sleeping Beauty transposase SB100X improves the genetic modification of T cells to express a chimeric antigen receptor. Gene Ther. 2011;18(9):849–56.

177. Sharma RK, Yolcu ES, Elpek KG, Shirwan H. Tumor cells engineered to codisplay on their surface 4-1BBL and LIGHT costimulatory proteins as a novel vaccine approach for cancer immunotherapy. Cancer Gene Ther. 2010;17(10):730–41.

178. Eibl R, Eibl D. Application of disposable bag-bioreactors in tissue engineering and for the production of therapeutic agents. Adv Biochem Eng Biotechnol. 2009.

179. Eibl R, Kaiser S, Lombriser R, Eibl D. Disposable bioreactors: the current state-of-the-art and recommended applications in biotechnology. Appl Microbiol Biotechnol. 2010;86(1):41–9.

180. Eibl R, Werner S, Eibl D. Bag bioreactor based on wave-induced motion: characteristics and applications. Adv Biochem Eng Biotechnol. 2010;115:55–87.

181. Bilgen B, Chang-Mateu IM, Barabino GA. Characterization of mixing in a novel wavy-walled bioreactor for tissue engineering. Biotechnol Bioeng. 2005;92(7):907–19.

182. Oncul AA, Kalmbach A, Genzel Y, Reichl U, Thevenin D. Characterization of flow conditions in 2 L and 20 L wave bioreactors using computational fluid dynamics. Biotechnol Prog. 2010;26(1):101–10.

183. Singh V. Disposable bioreactor for cell culture using wave-induced agitation. Cytotechnology. 1999;30(1–3):149–58.

184. Martin-Orozco N, Muranski P, Chung Y, Yang XO, Yamazaki T, Lu S, et al. T helper 17 cells promote cytotoxic T cell activation in tumor immunity. Immunity. 2009;31(5):787–98.

185. Soudja SM, Wehbe M, Mas A, Chasson L, de Tenbossche CP, Huijbers I, et al. Tumor-initiated inflammation overrides protective adaptive immunity in an induced melanoma model in mice. Cancer Res. 2010;70(9):3515–25.

186. Su X, Ye J, Hsueh EC, Zhang Y, Hoft DF, Peng G. Tumor microenvironments direct the recruitment and expansion of human Th17 cells. J Immunol. 2010;184(3):1630–41.

187. Hirata T, Osuga Y, Takamura M, Kodama A, Hirota Y, Koga K, et al. Recruitment of CCR6-expressing Th17 cells by CCL 20 secreted from IL-1 beta-, TNF-alpha-, and IL-17A-stimulated endometriotic stromal cells. Endocrinology. 2010;151(11):5468–76.

188. Hirota K, Yoshitomi H, Hashimoto M, Maeda S, Teradaira S, Sugimoto N, et al. Preferential recruitment of CCR6-expressing Th17 cells to inflamed joints via CCL20 in rheumatoid arthritis and its animal model. J Exp Med. 2007;204(12):2803–12.

189. Burns WR, Zhao Y, Frankel TL, Hinrichs CS, Zheng Z, Xu H, et al. A high molecular weight melanoma-associated antigen-specific chimeric antigen receptor redirects lymphocytes to target human melanomas. Cancer Res. 2010;70(8):3027–33.

190. Sadelain M, Riviere I, Brentjens R. Targeting tumours with genetically enhanced T lymphocytes. Nat Rev Cancer. 2003;3(1):35–45.

191. Yvon E, Del Vecchio M, Savoldo B, Hoyos V, Dutour A, Anichini A, et al. Immunotherapy of metastatic melanoma using genetically engineered GD2-specific T cells. Clin Cancer Res. 2009;15(18):5852–60.

192. Khammari A, Labarriere N, Vignard V, Nguyen JM, Pandolfino MC, Knol AC, et al. Treatment of metastatic melanoma with autologous Melan-A/MART-1-specific cytotoxic T lymphocyte clones. J Invest Dermatol. 2009;129(12):2835–42.

193. Fisher B, Packard BS, Read EJ, Carrasquillo JA, Carter CS, Topalian SL, et al. Tumor localization of adoptively transferred indium-111 labeled tumor infiltrating lymphocytes in patients with metastatic melanoma. J Clin Oncol. 1989;7(2):250–61.

194. Shepherd C, Puzanov I, Sosman JA. B-RAF inhibitors: an evolving role in the therapy of malignant melanoma. Curr Oncol Rep. 2010;12(3):146–52.

195. Abad JD, Wrzensinski C, Overwijk W, De Witte MA, Jorritsma A, Hsu C, et al. T-cell receptor gene therapy of established tumors in a murine melanoma model. J Immunother. 2008;31(1):1–6.

196. Hunder NN, Wallen H, Cao J, Hendricks DW, Reilly JZ, Rodmyre R, et al. Treatment of metastatic melanoma with autologous CD4+ T cells against NY-ESO-1. N Engl J Med. 2008;358(25):2698–703.

197. Pouw N, Treffers-Westerlaken E, Mondino A, Lamers C, Debets R. TCR gene-engineered T cell: limited T cell activation and combined use of IL-15 and IL-21 ensure minimal differentiation and maximal antigen-specificity. Mol Immunol. 2010;47(7–8):1411–20.

198. Krasagakis K, Garbe C, Zouboulis CC, Orfanos CE. Growth control of melanoma cells and melanocytes by cytokines. Recent Results Cancer Res. 1995;139:169–82.

199. Rodeck U, Herlyn M. Growth factors in melanoma. Cancer Metastasis Rev. 1991;10(2): 89–101.

200. Fan TM, Kranz DM, Flavell RA, Roy EJ. Costimulatory strength influences the differential effects of transforming growth factor beta1 for the generation of CD8+ regulatory T cells. Mol Immunol. 2008;45(10):2937–50.

201. Fu S, Zhang N, Yopp AC, Chen D, Mao M, Chen D, et al. TGF-beta induces Foxp3 + T-regulatory cells from CD4+ CD25-precursors. Am J Transplant. 2004;4(10):1614–27.

202. Wan YY, Flavell RA. TGF-beta and regulatory T cell in immunity and autoimmunity. J Clin Immunol. 2008;28(6):647–59.

203. Foster AE, Dotti G, Lu A, Khalil M, Brenner MK, Heslop HE, et al. Antitumor activity of EBV-specific T lymphocytes transduced with a dominant negative TGF-beta receptor. J Immunother. 2008;31(5):500–5.

204. Meidenbauer N, Marienhagen J, Laumer M, Vogl S, Heymann J, Andreesen R, et al. Survival and tumor localization of adoptively transferred Melan-A-specific T cells in melanoma patients. J Immunol. 2003;170(4):2161–9.

205. Smalley KS, Flaherty KT. Integrating BRAF/MEK inhibitors into combination therapy for melanoma. Br J Cancer. 2009;100(3):431–5.

206. Sznol M. Molecular markers of response to treatment for melanoma. Cancer J. 2011;17(2): 127–33.

207. DeFrancesco L. Landmark approval for Dendreon's cancer vaccine. Nat Biotechnol. 2010;28(6):531–2.

208. Rini BI. Technology evaluation: APC-8015, Dendreon. Curr Opin Mol Ther. 2002;4(1): 76–9.

Chapter 14
Anti-CTLA-4 Monoclonal Antibodies

Arvin S. Yang and Jedd D. Wolchok

Abstract The discovery of checkpoint proteins which regulate T cell activation and proliferation through inhibitory or stimulatory receptors has led to a new class of anti-tumor therapies. The goal of modulating these checkpoints is to overcome pathologic inhibition of T-cell activity which develops during tumorigenesis. The monoclonal antibody mediated blockade of cytotoxic T-lymphocyte antigen-4 (CTLA-4), a co-inhibitory molecule present on the surface of an activated T cell, has been a prototype for demonstration that augmentation of T cell activity can effectively treat malignant melanoma. In this review, we first describe the proposed mechanism of action and preclinical data for CTLA-4 blockade which led to its clinical development. Subsequently, we review the pivotal clinical trials which led to the characterization of inflammatory side effects and also the novel kinetics of anti-tumor response associated with CTLA-4 blockade. Finally, we discuss a panel of potential biomarkers for response to anti-CTLA-4 therapy. CTLA-4 monoclonal antibody blockade has demonstrated the ability to provide durable clinical benefit. With increasing knowledge of how to effectively manipulate this and other T cell checkpoints, cancer immunotherapies are emerging as an attractive therapeutic option in the treatment of melanoma and other malignancies.

Keywords ctla-4 • Anti-ctla-4 • Ipilimumab • Tremelimumab • Cytotoxic t-lymphocyte antigen-4 • Immuno-inhibitory • Checkpoint blockade • Immunotherapy • co-inhibitory molecule

A.S. Yang, MD, PhD
Oncology Medical Strategy-Ipilimumab, US Pharmaceuticals Medical,
Bristol-Myers Squibb Company, Plainsboro, NJ 08536, USA

J.D. Wolchok, MD, PhD (✉)
Department of Medicine, Memorial Sloan-Kettering Cancer Center,
New York, NY 10065, USA
e-mail: wolchokj@mskcc.org

T.F. Gajewski and F.S. Hodi (eds.), *Targeted Therapeutics in Melanoma*,
Current Clinical Oncology, DOI 10.1007/978-1-61779-407-0_14,
© Springer Science+Business Media, LLC 2012

Introduction

The incidence of melanoma continues to rise with almost 70,000 new cases in 2009 [33]. The FDA approved treatments for melanoma have been limited to adjuvant use of high-dose interferon-α, and in the metastatic setting, high-dose IL-2 and dacarbazine. None of the FDA approved agents have demonstrated an improvement in overall survival in a randomized phase III trial for patients with measurable metastatic disease. Consequently there has been significant interest in pursuing novel treatment strategies.

Recent advances in immunology have led to a profound insight into the function of co-stimulatory and co-inhibitory receptors expressed on T lymphocytes and provide a novel approach to optimize tumor immunotherapies through immunomodulation. Cytotoxic T-lymphocyte antigen-4 (CTLA-4) has been the prototype co-inhibitory molecule present on T lymphocytes targeted in recent tumor immunotherapeutic strategies. The development of monoclonal antibodies to harness the immuno-stimulatory and immuno-inhibitory checkpoints has been revolutionary. For the first time, targeting immunoregulatory pathways has resulted in the control of cancer in patients. The anti-CTLA-4 blocking antibody, ipilimumab, is the only anti-cancer therapy currently to have demonstrated increased overall survival in metastatic melanoma in a randomized phase III trial [28]. This pivotal result validates a new category of anti-neoplastic therapy aimed at "treating the patient" and not the tumor directly. This review will summarize the mechanism of action of anti-CTLA-4 monoclonal antibodies, preclinical evaluation, and key clinical trials that focus on distinct patterns of immune-related response, immune-related adverse events (irAEs), and potential biomarkers associated with response to anti-CTLA-4 therapy.

Mechanism of Immune Potentiation Through CTLA-4 Inhibition

The primary activation of a naïve T lymphocyte requires two signals. First, antigen specific recognition occurs through interactions between the T cell receptor (TCR) and a peptide-MHC complex. The second signal serves as an immunologic checkpoint to maintain balance between activation and tolerance to antigens. This second signal provides co-stimulation through CD28 present on the T lymphocyte binding to B7-1 (CD80) or B7-2 (CD86) expressed on the antigen presenting cell [23]. One determinant of T cell activation is the number of TCRs activated. Ligation of the co-stimulatory molecule CD28 appears to lower this TCR activation threshold [66]. In fact, mouse models deficient for CD28 (CD28$^{-/-}$ mice) demonstrated significant reduction in the ability to maintain T cell activation [41, 58]. This critical role CD28-B7 binding in T lymphocytes was further validated by the demonstration of blunted T lymphocyte activation in B7-1 and B7-2 double knockout mice [6].

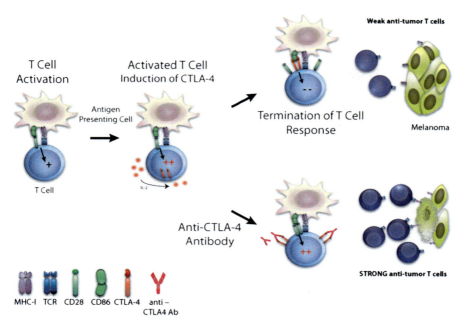

Fig. 14.1 T cell activation requires two signals including binding of the T-cell receptor to antigen bound to major histocompatibility complex on an antigen-presenting cell. Subsequently, full activation required binding of costimulatory receptors CD80/CD86 on the antigen-presenting cell to the CD28 receptor on the T cell. Intracellular stores of CTLA-4 are translocated with this activation and compete for binding to CD80/CD86 which results in downregulation of T cell activation. Anti-CTLA-4 blocking antibodies prevent this T cell downregulation

In addition to the initial signaling events driving T cell activation, other levels of regulation are required during normal immune homeostasis to prevent auto-immunity. Co-inhibitory receptors serve as additional checkpoints to control T cell activation. One such co-inhibitory molecule is CTLA-4, identified as a homolog of CD28, which is a major receptor that contributes to this negative regulation [63] (Fig. 14.1).

T Cell-Intrinsic Suppression

The critical role of CTLA-4 in inhibiting T cell activation was demonstrated through the generation of CTLA-4$^{-/-}$ mice, in which lymphoproliferation and tissue destruction were observed that resulted in death within 3–4 weeks of birth [61, 68]. There are currently multiple theories explaining CTLA-4 inhibition of T cell activation, which are not mutually exclusive. CTLA-4 has a 10–100 fold greater affinity to both B7-1 and B7-2 compared to CD28 [12]. One theory suggests that CTLA-4 out-competes CD28 for CD80/CD86 and thereby accounts for the inhibitory function of CTLA-4. Co-crystallization of CTLA-4 and B7-1 revealed a lattice-like structure which may exclude CD28 from binding to CD80/CD86 [21, 59]. Support for the CD80/CD86 competition theory includes experiments where inhibitory function was largely preserved even with truncation of the CTLA-4 cytoplasmic tail [44]. Additional studies with a mutant non-signaling CTLA-4 revealed that competition was a dominant mode of T cell inhibitory function when CTLA-4 and B7 were highly expressed [8].

CTLA-4 mediated negative signaling has been proposed as another mechanism underlying its inhibitory function. CTLA-4 does not have traditional immune tyrosine inhibitory motifs (ITIMs); however it does possess other tyrosine motifs which recruit phosphatases, including SHP-2, which can be involved in negative regulation of the TCR signaling cascade [4, 39]. Studies where B7-nonbinding CTLA-4 mutant T cells retained the ability to inhibit T cell proliferation, cytokine production, and TCR signaling support an important role for CTLA-4 negative signaling in T cell regulation [11].

Additional immunosuppressive effects of CTLA-4 may involve limiting antigen presenting cell (APC) function and/or T cell cytoskeletal events. Engagement of a T cell by an APC typically results in TCR signaling and also the delivery of a stop signal, causing decreased motility in lymph nodes. Antibody-mediated ligation of CTLA-4 reverses this stop signal and has been shown to inhibit the immune response of TCR transgenic T cells to antigen, resulting in decreased cytokine production and proliferation [57]. In fact, CTLA-4 has been shown to inhibit TCR lipid raft generation within the plasma membrane of T cells which may then serve to terminate T cell activation [43].

T Cell-Extrinsic Suppression

In addition to cell-intrinsic CTLA-4-mediated suppression, additional cell-extrinsic mechanisms were supported by a series of elegant adoptive transfer studies. Transfer of CTLA-4$^{-/-}$ T cells into RAG1$^{-/-}$ mice resulted in lymphoproliferation and tissue damage which could then be reversed by administration of wildtype T cells [2, 62]. Further analysis revealed that this T cell-extrinsic CTLA-4 inhibitory function was in part mediated by regulatory T cells. CD4$^+$CD25$^+$ T cells, but not CD8$^+$ T cells nor NKT cells, were involved in mediating this CTLA-4-dependent immune suppression [19]. In a different model, conditional deletion of CTLA-4 specifically in the regulatory T cell population resulted in spontaneous T cell activation and autoimmunity [72]. Additional immune suppressive effects of CTLA-4 function may be mediated through reverse signaling to dendritic cells. CTLA-4 binding to CD80/CD86 on dendritic cells has been reported to induce indoleamine 2,3-dixogenase (IDO) activity, which degrades tryptophan. The reduced tryptophan then causes inhibition of T cell proliferation and apoptosis [17]. In summary, the mechanism of CTLA-4 mediated suppression is complex and likely related to both effector

T cell-intrinsic and -extrinsic mechanisms. Regardless of the mechanism, CTLA-4 clearly plays a critical role in regulating lymphocyte activation and therefore offers a rational target for immune modulation as a cancer therapeutic.

Preclinical Studies of CTLA-4 Blocking Antibodies

The potential for effective tumor immunotherapy through application of CTLA-4 blocking antibodies was first demonstrated in transplantable models of colon carcinoma and fibrosarcoma. Anti-CTLA-4 therapy not only caused tumor regression but protection against subsequent tumor challenge [38]. Additional studies using the poorly immunogenic B16 melanoma model required the combination of both anti-CTLA-4 antibody and a GM-CSF-expressing whole cell vaccine in order to successfully treat established tumors [64]. In this same model, the anti-tumor effects were found to be dependent on CD8[+] T cells as well as perforin and Fas/FasL interactions [65]. Further analysis of tumor infiltrating lymphocytes from mice receiving the combined anti-CTLA-4 antibody and a GM-CSF secreting vaccine revealed a direct correlation between tumor rejection and increase in the ratio of effector T cells to regulatory T cells within the tumor [49]. These encouraging preclinical results paved the groundwork for clinical trials.

Clinical Trial Testing of Anti-CTLA-4 Antibodies

Two fully human monoclonal CTLA-4 blocking antibodies have been developed for clinical use: ipilimumab (MDX-010) and tremelimumab (CP-675,206). Both antibodies were developed from human immunoglobulin gene transgenic mice. Tremelimumab is an IgG2 antibody and ipilimumab is an IgG1 antibody [48, 51, 52, 69]. Given that both antibodies appear to have comparable spectra of clinical response and immune related adverse events (irAEs) their activity does not appear to be dependent on isotype.

Tremelimumab

In a phase I dose escalation trial (0.01–15 mg/kg), 34 melanoma patients were treated with tremelimumab with a 29% (8/28 patients with evaluable disease) objective response rate, with two complete responses (CRs), two partial responses (PRs), and four patients with stable disease (SD) observed. The duration of clinical responses was greater than 34+ months. Interestingly, one individual who obtained a CR had previously received ipilimumab, consistent with the efficacy of re-induction therapy later shown in the ipilimumab phase III trial [28, 52]. Three additional phase I/II trials followed with treatment at either 10 mg/kg monthly or 15 mg/kg every 3 months, in total there was a clinical benefit rate of 22.9% (79/345). Decreased frequency of grade 3/4 adverse events was noted in patients receiving the 15 mg/kg every 3 months (13%) schedule compared with patients in the 10 mg/kg monthly cohort (27%) [7, 34, 50]. Therefore, the 15 mg/kg every 3 months schedule was selected phase III testing. At the ASCO 2008 Annual Meeting, the results of a phase III trial, in which tremelimumab was compared with DTIC or temozolomide in 665 metastatic melanoma patients with a primary endpoint of overall survival, were presented. In the second interim analysis, tremelimumab failed to show improved overall survival compared to chemotherapy, with the median overall survival being 11.8 and 10.7 months in the tremelimumab and chemotherapy arms, respectively. Consequently, the trial was halted [54]. In the final efficacy results published in abstract form in 2010, the median overall survival increased to 12.6 months in the tremelimumab arm, while the chemotherapy arm remained at 10.7 months; however, this difference was not statistically significant [55].

Ipilimumab Monotherapy

In an initial pilot study, ipilimumab monotherapy was administered to 17 patients with unresectable melanoma as a 3 mg/kg single dose administration. A 12% objective response rate was noted with two partial responses (PRs) and only mild reversible pruritus observed as an adverse event [60]. Following this, a phase I/II safety and pharmacokinetic trial of ipilimumab was performed in 88 patients with unresectable stage III or IV melanoma. Both dose escalation (2.8–20 mg/kg) and number of doses (1–4) were examined in separate arms of the trial. Responses were noted in all groups, with a clinical benefit rate of 20% including one complete response (CR) and three PRs. Fourteen additional patients experienced durable stabilization of disease. Unique characteristics of response were noted including a median time to response of 123 days, and long duration of response (greater than 638 days) in the objective responders [71]. A separate multi-institutional dose escalation phase II trial of ipilimumab administered at 0.3, 3 or 10 mg/ kg every 3 weeks for four doses (induction) and if eligible, followed by ipilimumab administered every 12 weeks starting at week 24 (maintenance), established the 10 mg/kg cohort as the group with the greatest response rate. In the 217 unresectable stage III/IV melanoma patients treated with ipilimumab monotherapy, the best overall response rate was 11.1% in the 10 mg/kg cohort and 4.2% in the 3 mg/kg cohort while no responses were noted in the 0.3 mg/kg cohort. The 10 mg/kg vs. 3 mg/kg cohort had a 24 month median survival of 29.8 and 24.2% respectively, and a clinical benefit rate of 29.2 and 26.4% respectively [74]. In a separate multicenter phase II trial, an additional 155 patients were treated with 10 mg/kg ipilimumab every 3 weeks for four doses, and if eligible were followed by 10 mg/kg ipilimumab every 3 months starting at week 24. This study was consistent with the dose escalation study with a clinical benefit rate of 27.1% and best overall response rate of 5.8% [46].

Combination Trials: Peptide Vaccines

Given the preclinical support and immunological rationale for combining vaccination with immunomodulatory antibodies, a clinical trial combining treatment of ipilimumab at 3 mg/kg every 3 weeks and a gp100 peptide vaccine was conducted in 14 patients with metastatic melanoma. Two complete responses and an additional partial response were noted for an objective response rate of 21.4% [48]. As follow up to this trial, a larger series of patients (56) was treated with two dosing schedules of either 3 mg/kg ipilimumab every 3 weeks or an initial dose of 3 mg/kg ipilimumab with subsequent doses reduced to 1 mg/kg every 3 weeks, with both arms receiving concomitant gp100 vaccination. The objective response rate was 13% in this trial with two CRs, and five PRs, with all responses being durable. There appeared to be no difference between the response rate and toxicity rate between the two dosing schedules [1]. Dosing schedules were further evaluated in an intra-patient dose escalation study of ipilimumab with or without the addition gp100 vaccination based on HLA typing. Patients who did not develop objective tumor responses or dose limiting toxicity after one course of their starting dose had the ipilimumab dose increased on their next course of treatment. A 19% (16/85) objective response rate was noted, with no statistical difference in response rate between the combined gp100 peptide vaccine and ipilimumab arm vs. the ipilimumab alone arm [15].

In addition to combination with vaccines, a phase I/II trial of 0.1–3 mg/kg of ipilimumab given every 3 weeks combined with IL-2 has also been conducted in 36 metastatic melanoma patients. There was a reasonable object tumor response rate of 22% with three CRs and five PRs; however statistical analysis did not support a synergistic effect of the agents [42].

Immune Related Adverse Events

The side effects associated with anti-CTLA-4 therapy represent a unique panel of mechanism-based, tissue-specific inflammatory events that have been termed irAEs. They appear to be class-specific, occurring with both tremelimumab and ipilimumab administration [7, 74]. The most common irAEs in decreasing incidence include pruritus/rash, diarrhea, colitis, hepatitis, endocrinopathies and uveitis [3, 5, 56]. Early in clinical development, rare (2%) occurrences of colon perforations were noted; however the majority of irAEs appear to be reversible by systemic corticosteroids using well defined treatment algorithms [3].

For those irAEs that are refractory to standard corticosteroid administration, anti-tumor necrosis factor antibody (infliximab) or other immune suppressants have effectively reversed the irAEs [46]. Initial studies suggested a dose dependency for the development of irAEs, with 70% (50/71) of patients receiving 10 mg/kg ipilimumab vs. 26% (19/72) of patients receiving 0.3 mg/kg of ipilimumab developing irAEs [74]. However, the 10 mg/kg of ipilimumab has been safely tolerated with 47% of the irAEs being grade 1/2 in a multicenter phase II trial with 155 patients. The additional grade 3/4 irAEs observed included gastrointestinal (8.4%), hepatobiliary (7.1%), skin (3.2%) and endocrine (1.3%) toxicities [45].

Prophylactic administration of budesonide, a non-absorbed oral corticosteroid, was studied in 115 stage IV melanoma patients in a randomized phase II trial of 10 mg/kg of ipilimumab with or without budesonide. Similar response rates were noted in both the (12.1%) budesonide and (15.8%) placebo controlled arm, but there was no impact on the development of grade 2/3 diarrhea [70]. Budesonide is a non-absorbed steroid and therefore less likely to impact immune functions. However, multiple studies have also demonstrated that systemic corticosteroids do not appear to impact efficacy of ipilimumab, particularly when corticosteroid therapy is administered after initiation of ipilimumab treatment [3, 15].

Immune Related Response Criteria

Given that CTLA-4 blocking antibodies are the prototype for a new class of therapeutics, there are many unique characteristics of responses that have been observed, that differ from traditional response criteria seen with cytotoxic therapies. Response to anti-CTLA-4 therapy appears independent of traditional prognostic indicators including prior systemic therapies, gender, and LDH [73]. In addition, the response durations with ipilimumab therapy have been more durable than those seen with conventional agents [36, 47]. As the radiographic patterns of response to anti-CTLA-4 therapy were recognized, there became a need to establish novel criteria to appropriately capture individuals that were benefitting from ipilimumab therapy.

The traditional radiographic standards for evaluating anti-tumor responses in the cytotoxic chemotherapeutic era were either by Response Evaluation Criteria in Solid Tumors (RECIST) or the World Health Organization (WHO) criteria. Effective chemotherapy causes direct cytotoxic effects which results in rapid radiological decreases in tumor size. Therefore, radiographic images which show increases in tumor size are traditionally interpreted as progression of disease, especially when new lesions appear. However, anti-CTLA-4 therapy responses require activation of the immune system, which may occur in a few weeks or several months after initiating therapy. As such, radiographic evidence of progression of disease may actually reflect a mixture of progression in advance of response or inflammation, edema, and lymphocytic infiltration as opposed to true persistent tumor progression. Serial biopsies of regressing metastases in anti-CTLA-4-treated patients demonstrated infiltration with CD8$^+$ T cells associated with tumor necrosis [26].

To avoid premature termination of effective therapy and to capture the novel radiographic response kinetics, a set of immune related response criteria (irRC) was proposed by the Cancer Vaccine Clinical Trial Working Group [29, 74]. The irRC utilizes bidimensional tumor measurements according to the WHO criteria, and total tumor burden is then calculated by the summation of the individual sizes similar to the RECIST criteria. However, in the irRC, new transient lesions or increases in tumor size less than 25% are not considered progression of disease, which is different than that defined by the WHO criteria. The irRC were retrospectively validated utilizing phase II clinical trial data from 227 patients treated with ipilimumab in the 10 mg/kg ipilimumab phase II single-arm study CA184-008 and the dose-ranging study Phase II trial CA184-022. Interestingly, 9.7% (22 of 227) patients characterized as having progressive disease (PD) by the WHO criteria had evidence of clinical response to ipilimumab by the irRC. In fact, those individuals classified as PD by the WHO criteria but with immune related partial response (irPR) or immune related stable disease (irSD) by the irRC had an overall survival that was similar to those showing clinical benefit defined by the standard WHO criteria [74]. The irRC is being further prospectively validated in current anti-CTLA-4 clinical trials.

Phase III Clinical Testing of Ipilimumab

A phase III trial with 676 enrolled HLA-A*0201 positive patients receiving ipilimumab in the refractory disease setting was recently reported. There were three arms: ipilimumab alone, gp100 peptide vaccine alone, or the combination of both ipilimumab and gp100 vaccine, randomized in a 1:1:3 ratio. Ipilimumab was administered at 3 mg/kg every 3 weeks for a total of four doses. The primary endpoint of the trial was changed from best overall response rate to overall survival prior to unblinding. A statistical improvement in overall survival was observed in patients receiving ipilimumab with or without gp100 peptide vaccine compared with the gp100 peptide vaccine alone. The median overall survival for the ipilimumab plus gp100 and ipilimumab alone groups was 10.0 months ($p < 0.001$) and 10.1 months, respectively ($p = 0.003$) compared with 6.4 months in the patients receiving gp100 alone. There was no statistically significant difference in overall survival between the gp100 peptide vaccine combined with ipilimumab vs. the ipilimumab alone group. Twelve month overall survival for both ipilimumab groups (±gp100) was 43.6–45.6 vs. 25.3% in the gp100 alone group, while the 24 month survival was 21.6–23.5% in the ipilimumab groups compared with 13.7% in the gp100 alone group. These results highlight the durability of clinical response in those patients who benefited from ipilimumab. The disease control rate was 20.1% and 28.5% in the ipilimumab plus gp100, and ipilimumab alone groups respectively, compared with 11.0% in the gp100 alone group, which was consistent with results from multiple prior phase II clinical trials. It should be noted that the disease control rate may underestimate the actual benefit as it utilized the modified (WHO) criteria for tumor assessments, and did not account for patients that may have the appearance radiological tumor progression followed by ultimate clinical benefit [28].

Ipilimumab Plus Chemotherapy

In addition to combinations with other immunotherapeutic agents, combining ipilimumab with standard cancer therapies, including chemotherapy, has been evaluated. Preclinical studies have suggested the potential for chemotherapy to enhance immune responses through direct tumor lysis and increased antigen presentation and additional modulation of the immune repertoire by depletion of regulatory T cells. A phase II trial compared 3 mg/kg of ipilimumab every 3 weeks for four doses with or without dacarbazine in the treatment of 72 chemotherapy-naïve, advanced stage melanoma patients. The clinical benefit rate was 31.4 vs. 21.6%, favoring the combination arm [25]. Notably, the duration of response appeared to be enhanced by the addition of dacarbazine with a 23 vs. 10% 3-year survival rate in the combination vs. ipilimumab alone arm [24]. Other combinational trials are still accruing data, including a three arm clinical trial with 60 patients evaluating ipilimumab alone, combined with carboplatin and paclitaxel, or with dacarbazine. Finally, a phase III registration trial in treatment-naïve patients of 10 mg/kg of ipilimumab with maintenance ipilimumab combined with dacarbazine, vs. dacarbazine alone, has completed accrual. An estimated 500 patients have been enrolled in this trial with the primary endpoint being overall survival. We still await unblinding and analysis of these data.

Adjuvant Therapy

In adjuvant therapy setting, anti-CTLA-4 antibody therapy is aimed at augmenting the anti-tumor immune response in the setting of minimal tumor antigen available to prime immune responses against any remaining microscopic tumor. While in the metastatic setting, there is a high tumor burden and therefore greater tumor antigen available for presentation, but also increased tumor associated immune suppression. Therefore, the safety and efficacy of ipilimumab has been investigated in the adjuvant setting. A small clinical trial of ipilimumab in the adjuvant setting for resected stage III and IV melanoma patients with no evidence of disease has been completed. Three cohorts received escalating doses of ipilimumab at 0.3, 1 or 3 mg/kg every 4 weeks combined with a vaccine consisting of gp100, MART-1, and tyrosinase peptides. The goals of this adjuvant trial were to evaluate for toxicity and to determine a maximum tolerated dose. The five patients in the highest cohort all had some degree of diarrhea with grade 3 toxicity noted in three of the five patients, with all irAEs medically reversible. The secondary endpoints which evaluated relapse free survival in the nineteen patients demonstrated that 63% of the total treated patients relapsed, with 38% (3/8) of patients with evidence of irAEs relapsing while 82% (9/11) of patients without irAEs relapsing [56].

An additional adjuvant clinical trial was subsequently performed with 25 resected stage III/IV melanoma patients receiving the same combination peptide vaccine plus ipilimumab at 3 mg/kg every 8 weeks. There were grade 2/3 irAEs noted in

48% (12/25) of patients, with 20% (5/25) being dose limiting, but all irAEs were successfully treated with systemic corticosteroids. These encouraging preliminary data have led to a large ongoing EORTC-sponsored phase III double-blind, placebo-controlled, adjuvant ipilimumab trial for high risk, completely resected stage III melanoma patients, with an estimated target enrollment of 950 patients. This phase III EORTC trial will hopefully provide a definitive statement regarding the benefit of ipilimumab in adjuvant treatment of high risk stage III melanoma patients and additional insight into the association of clinical benefit with the development of irAEs. Given that the risk:benefit ratio of anti-CTLA-4 therapy is likely to be different for patients being treated in the adjuvant vs. in the metastatic setting, careful analysis of the clinical response and frequency and quality of toxicities will be studied carefully. This will include a panel of investigational biomarkers for this study.

Biomarkers of Response

In parallel with defining the irRC, there have been additional efforts to establish biomarkers of response to ipilimumab. As described in the irRC, a delayed response pattern can be noted with anti-CTLA-4 antibody therapy; therefore it is even more important to identify biomarkers which rapidly detect individuals likely to benefit in order to adjust therapy accordingly.

We and others have found detailed analysis of peripheral blood lymphocyte after two doses of ipilimumab to correlate with overall survival. Those patients with an absolute lymphocyte count (ALC) greater or equal to 1,000 cells/μL had both an improved clinical benefit rate (51 vs. 0% $p=0.01$) and median OS (11.9 vs. 1.4 months $p<0.001$) compared with those patients with an ALC <1,000 cells/μL [37]. Further subset analysis of the lymphocyte populations has suggested that increases in CD8[+] T cells may specifically correlate with clinical benefit [75].

Increases in peripheral blood antigen-specific T cells responses have also been shown, in preliminary analyses, to correlate with clinical benefit. Fifteen melanoma patients treated with ipilimumab were evaluated for antigen specific T cell responses. Five of the eight clinical responders developed antibody, CD4[+], and CD8[+] T cell responses to NY-ESO-1, a cancer testis antigen. This was in contrast to one out of the seven non-responders developing any such immune response [76]. Detailed analysis of an ipilimumab-treated melanoma patient having a complete clinical response provided further evidence that increased antigen-specific T cells responses may correlate with clinical benefit. As described by Klein et al., Melan-A-specific CD8[+] T cells, both in the peripheral blood and in the tumor, were identified that exhibited potent in vitro killing activity of a Melan-A-expressing melanoma [35]. It is important to note that, peripheral blood T cell responses may not always reflect intra-tumoral immune events. Three of 12 melanoma patients treated with tremelimumab experienced clinical benefit and were monitored for reactivity to gp100, MART1, and tyrosinase antigens. Within the peripheral blood, there was no significant change in antigen-specific CD8[+] T cells or in regulatory T cell numbers [13]. In contrast, there did appear to be in an increase in intratumoral gp100 specific T cells in a responding lesion. The complexity in evaluating the relevance of intratumoral biomarkers include the paradoxical association of increased expression of FOXP3 and indoleamine 2,3-dioxygenase (IDO) in tumor infiltrating lymphocytes from ipilimumab treated clinical responders. In addition, while marked CD8[+] T cell infiltration was noted in intratumoral samples from responders to tremelimumab therapy, no significant changes were noted in FOXP3 or IDO [22, 53].

Detailed analysis of the cellular phenotype and polyfunctionality of the T cell populations may further identify biomarkers for clinical response to anti-CTLA-4 therapy. Polyfunctional T cell subsets capable of generating multiple cytokines are a hallmark of a robust immune response. Polyfunctional T cells were initially found to correlate with clinical response in the infectious disease model including HIV and hepatitis [14, 16]. Polyfunctional NY-ESO-1 specific T cells producing IFN-γ, MIP-1β, and TNF-α, have recently been found in melanoma patients treated with ipilimumab who demonstrated clinical benefit [76].

Recently, inducible costimulator (ICOS) has also emerged as a potential biomarker of immune activation associated with anti-CTLA-4 therapy. ICOS, a T cell-expressed surface protein structurally related to CD28 and CTLA-4, is commonly expressed on the cell surface after T cell activation [31]. An increased frequency of CD4[+]ICOS[hi] T cells that also produced IFN-γ was noted in six bladder cancer patients treated with neoadjuvant ipilimumab [40]. In a follow-up study, sustained increases in both CD4[+]ICOS[hi] and CD8[+]ICOS[hi] T cells in 14 ipilimumab-treated melanoma patients was found to correlate with greater clinical benefit [9]. In a separate study with tremelimumab-treated breast cancer patients, increases in both CD4[+] and CD8[+] ICOS-expressing T cells were also noted, and there appeared to be a trend toward a greater percentage of ICOS[hi] T cells in patients with stable disease compared with those with progression of disease [67]. These results suggest that transient increase in CD4[+]ICOS[hi] T cells may reflect anti-CTLA-4 antibody activation of the immune response while a sustained elevation of CD4[+]or CD8[+]ICOS[hi] T cells may indicate clinical benefit.

Antibody Responses

In addition to T cell responses, there has been specific focus on correlating NY-ESO-1 antibody responses with the clinical outcome of anti-CTLA-4-treated melanoma patients. Melanoma differentiation antigens and cancer testis antigens have been associated with antigen-specific humoral responses [10, 30]. In fact, spontaneous high titer antibodies have been observed in subsets of patients with advanced melanoma [32]. In a detailed analysis of 15 metastatic melanoma patients treated with ipilimumab, 62% (5/8) of the patients experiencing clinical benefit were NY-ESO-1 seropositive compared with 0% (0/7) of the clinical non-responders.

Interestingly, the presence of NY-ESO-1 antibody responses in the clinical responders was also associated with NY-ESO-1-specific polyfunctional CD4$^+$ and CD8$^+$ T cells. This observation suggests that, in anti-CTLA-4-treated patients, both the humoral and cellular antigen-specific immune responses may be associated with clinical benefit [76]. A separate report presented conflicting results, indicating no correlation between clinical response and immune responses against NY-ESO-1; however, different definitions of clinical benefit, different treatment schedules, and different thresholds for definition of seropositivity may account for this discrepancy [20].

Conclusions

The success of CTLA-4-blocking antibodies in treating metastatic melanoma has established a promising new modality of anti-cancer therapy, through blockade of immune inhibitory pathways. Although most of the ipilimumab experience has been with melanoma, these immunomodulatory agents aim to enhance the patient's own immune system and do not appear to be restricted to specific tumor types. Thus, this therapeutic strategy will likely be applicable to multiple other cancer histologies. With increasing clinical experience utilizing these immunomodulatory agents, investigators have recognized unique characteristics including the patterns of response, durability of response, and the associated irAEs. These novel aspects of this therapeutic modality are important to consider as additional immunomodulatory antibodies, including those targeting PD-1, PDL-1, GITR, and others, enter clinical testing.

Anti-CTLA-4 monotherapy clearly does not benefit all melanoma patients. Therefore, CTLA-4 blocking antibodies will likely serve as solid foundation for additional complementary agents in order to improve overall efficacy. There is preclinical evidence supporting combinatorial strategies of anti-CTLA-4 therapy combined with additional means to enhance the "immunogenicity" of the tumor, such as tumor vaccines, chemotherapy, or radiation therapy. Small molecule targeted agents may also become a natural treatment partner to anti-CTLA-4 therapy. Recently, there has been clinical success in treating melanoma utilizing small molecular inhibitors targeting mutant B-RAF and KIT [18, 27]. Unfortunately, the benefit appears short-lived in many patients and thus provides incentive to pair them with immunological agents such as anti-CTLA-4 therapy in an attempt to attain a higher frequency of durable responses. Finally, there is clear need to define biomarkers both of negative and positive predictive value. Not only will biomarkers potentially help select individuals most likely to benefit from anti-CTLA-4 therapy, but also provide insight into the mechanisms of anti-CTLA-4 activity and methods to enhance its efficacy.

Acknowledgments The authors would like to thank Dr. David Schaer for his assistant in the preparation of Fig. 14.1 and Chrisann Kyi for editorial assistance.

References

1. Attia P, Phan GQ, Maker AV, Robinson MR, Quezado MM, Yang JC, et al. Autoimmunity correlates with tumor regression in patients with metastatic melanoma treated with anti-cytotoxic T-lymphocyte antigen-4. J Clin Oncol. 2005;23:6043–53.
2. Bachmann MF, Kohler G, Ecabert B, Mak TW, Kopf M. Cutting edge: lymphoproliferative disease in the absence of CTLA-4 is not T cell autonomous. J Immunol. 1999;163:1128–31.
3. Beck KE, Blansfield JA, Tran KQ, Feldman AL, Hughes MS, Royal RE, et al. Enterocolitis in patients with cancer after antibody blockade of cytotoxic T-lymphocyte-associated antigen 4. J Clin Oncol. 2006;24:2283–9.
4. Blank U, Launay P, Benhamou M, Monteiro RC. Inhibitory ITAMs as novel regulators of immunity. Immunol Rev. 2009;232:59–71.
5. Blansfield JA, Beck KE, Tran K, Yang JC, Hughes MS, Kammula US, et al. Cytotoxic T-lymphocyte-associated antigen-4 blockage can induce autoimmune hypophysitis in patients with metastatic melanoma and renal cancer. J Immunother. 2005;28:593–8.
6. Borriello F, Sethna MP, Boyd SD, Schweitzer AN, Tivol EA, Jacoby D, et al. B7-1 and B7-2 have overlapping, critical roles in immunoglobulin class switching and germinal center formation. Immunity. 1997;6:303–13.
7. Camacho LH, Antonia S, Sosman J, Kirkwood JM, Gajewski TF, Redman B, et al. Phase I/II trial of tremelimumab in patients with metastatic melanoma. J Clin Oncol. 2009;27:1075–81.
8. Carreno BM, Bennett F, Chau TA, Ling V, Luxenberg D, Jussif J, et al. CTLA-4 (CD152) can inhibit T cell activation by two different mechanisms depending on its level of cell surface expression. J Immunol. 2000;165:1352–6.
9. Carthon BC, Wolchok JD, Yuan J, Kamat A, Ng Tang DS, Sun J, et al. Preoperative CTLA-4 blockade: tolerability and immune monitoring in the setting of a presurgical clinical trial. Clin Cancer Res. 2010;16:2861–71.
10. Chen YT, Scanlan MJ, Sahin U, Tureci O, Gure AO, Tsang S, et al. A testicular antigen aberrantly expressed in human cancers detected by autologous antibody screening. Proc Natl Acad Sci USA. 1997;94:1914–8.
11. Chikuma S, Abbas AK, Bluestone JA. B7-independent inhibition of T cells by CTLA-4. J Immunol. 2005;175:177–81.
12. Collins AV, Brodie DW, Gilbert RJ, Iaboni A, Manso-Sancho R, Walse B, et al. The interaction properties of costimulatory molecules revisited. Immunity. 2002;17:201–10.
13. Comin-Anduix B, Lee Y, Jalil J, Algazi A, de la Rocha P, Camacho LH, et al. Detailed analysis of immunologic effects of the cytotoxic T lymphocyte-associated antigen 4-blocking monoclonal antibody tremelimumab in peripheral blood of patients with melanoma. J Transl Med. 2008;6:22.
14. De Rosa SC, Lu FX, Yu J, Perfetto SP, Falloon J, Moser S, et al. Vaccination in humans generates broad T cell cytokine responses. J Immunol. 2004;173:5372–80.
15. Downey SG, Klapper JA, Smith FO, Yang JC, Sherry RM, Royal RE, et al. Prognostic factors related to clinical response in patients with metastatic melanoma treated by CTL-associated antigen-4 blockade. Clin Cancer Res. 2007;13:6681–8.
16. Duvall MG, Precopio ML, Ambrozak DA, Jaye A, McMichael AJ, Whittle HC, et al. Polyfunctional T cell responses are a hallmark of HIV-2 infection. Eur J Immunol. 2008;38: 350–63.
17. Fallarino F, Grohmann U, Hwang KW, Orabona C, Vacca C, Bianchi R, et al. Modulation of tryptophan catabolism by regulatory T cells. Nat Immunol. 2003;4:1206–12.
18. Flaherty KT, Puzanov I, Kim KB, Ribas A, McArthur GA, Sosman JA, et al. Inhibition of mutated, activated BRAF in metastatic melanoma. N Engl J Med. 2010;363:809–19.
19. Friedline RH, Brown DS, Nguyen H, Kornfeld H, Lee J, Zhang Y, et al. CD4+ regulatory T cells require CTLA-4 for the maintenance of systemic tolerance. J Exp Med. 2009;206:421–34.
20. Goff SL, Robbins PF, El-Gamil M, Rosenberg SA. No correlation between clinical response to CTLA-4 blockade and presence of NY-ESO-1 antibody in patients with metastatic melanoma. J Immunother. 2009;32:884–5.

21. Greene JL, Leytze GM, Emswiler J, Peach R, Bajorath J, Cosand W, et al. Covalent dimerization of CD28/CTLA-4 and oligomerization of CD80/CD86 regulate T cell costimulatory interactions. J Biol Chem. 1996;271:26762–71.

22. Hamid O, Chasalow SD, Tsuchihashi Z, Alaparthy S, Galbraith S, Berman D. Association of baseline and on-study tumor biopsy markers with clinical activity in patients (pts) with advanced melanoma treated with ipilimumab (Meeting Abstracts). J Clin Oncol. 2009;27:9008.

23. Hathcock KS, Laszlo G, Pucillo C, Linsley P, Hodes RJ. Comparative analysis of B7-1 and B7-2 costimulatory ligands: expression and function. J Exp Med. 1994;180:631–40.

24. Hersh E, Weber J, Powderly J, Pavlik A, Nichol G, Yellin M, et al. Long-term survival of patients (pts) with advanced melanoma treated with ipilimumab with or without dacarbazine (Meeting Abstracts). J Clin Oncol. 2009;27:9038.

25. Hersh EM, Weber JS, Powderly JD, Khan K, Pavlick AC, Samlowski WE, et al. Disease control and long-term survival in chemotherapy-naive patients with advanced melanoma treated with ipilimumab (MDX- 010) with or without dacarbazine (Meeting Abstracts). J Clin Oncol. 2008;26:9022.

26. Hodi FS, Butler M, Oble DA, Seiden MV, Haluska FG, Kruse A, et al. Immunologic and clinical effects of antibody blockade of cytotoxic T lymphocyte-associated antigen 4 in previously vaccinated cancer patients. Proc Natl Acad Sci USA. 2008;105:3005–10.

27. Hodi FS, Friedlander P, Corless CL, Heinrich MC, Mac Rae S, Kruse A, et al. Major response to imatinib mesylate in KIT-mutated melanoma. J Clin Oncol. 2008;26:2046–51.

28. Hodi FS, O'Day SJ, McDermott DF, Weber RW, Sosman JA, Haanen JB, et al. Improved survival with ipilimumab in patients with metastatic melanoma. N Engl J Med. 2010;363:711–23.

29. Hoos A, Parmiani G, Hege K, Sznol M, Loibner H, Eggermont A, et al. A clinical development paradigm for cancer vaccines and related biologics. J Immunother. 2007;30:1–15.

30. Houghton AN, Eisinger M, Albino AP, Cairncross JG, Old LJ. Surface antigens of melanocytes and melanomas. Markers of melanocyte differentiation and melanoma subsets. J Exp Med. 1982;156:1755–66.

31. Hutloff A, Dittrich AM, Beier KC, Eljaschewitsch B, Kraft R, Anagnostopoulos I, et al. ICOS is an inducible T-cell co-stimulator structurally and functionally related to CD28. Nature. 1999;397:263–6.

32. Jager E, Stockert E, Zidianakis Z, Chen YT, Karbach J, Jager D, et al. Humoral immune responses of cancer patients against "cancer-testis" antigen NY-ESO-1: correlation with clinical events. Int J Cancer. 1999;84:506–10.

33. Jemal A, Siegel R, Ward E, Hao Y, Xu J, Thun MJ. Cancer statistics, 2009. CA Cancer J Clin. 2009;59:225–49.

34. Kirkwood JM, Lorigan P, Hersey P, Hauschild A, Robert C, McDermott DF, et al. A phase II trial of tremelimumab (CP-675,206) in patients with advanced refractory or relapsed melanoma (Meeting Abstracts). J Clin Oncol. 2008;26:9023.

35. Klein O, Ebert LM, Nicholaou T, Browning J, Russell SE, Zuber M, et al. Melan-A-specific cytotoxic T cells are associated with tumor regression and autoimmunity following treatment with anti-CTLA-4. Clin Cancer Res. 2009;15:2507–13.

36. Korn EL, Liu PY, Lee SJ, Chapman JA, Niedzwiecki D, Suman VJ, et al. Meta-analysis of phase II cooperative group trials in metastatic stage IV melanoma to determine progression-free and overall survival benchmarks for future phase II trials. J Clin Oncol. 2008;26:527–34.

37. Ku GY, Yuan J, Page DB, Schroeder SE, Panageas KS, Carvajal RD, et al. Single-institution experience with ipilimumab in advanced melanoma patients in the compassionate use setting: lymphocyte count after 2 doses correlates with survival. Cancer. 2010;116:1767–75.

38. Leach DR, Krummel MF, Allison JP. Enhancement of antitumor immunity by CTLA-4 blockade. Science. 1996;271:1734–6.

39. Lee KM, Chuang E, Griffin M, Khattri R, Hong DK, Zhang W, et al. Molecular basis of T cell inactivation by CTLA-4. Science. 1998;282:2263–6.

40. Liakou CI, Kamat A, Tang DN, Chen H, Sun J, Troncoso P, et al. CTLA-4 blockade increases IFNgamma-producing CD4+ICOShi cells to shift the ratio of effector to regulatory T cells in cancer patients. Proc Natl Acad Sci USA. 2008;105:14987–92.

41. Lucas PJ, Negishi I, Nakayama K, Fields LE, Loh DY. Naive CD28-deficient T cells can initiate but not sustain an in vitro antigen-specific immune response. J Immunol. 1995;154: 5757–68.
42. Maker AV, Phan GQ, Attia P, Yang JC, Sherry RM, Topalian SL, et al. Tumor regression and autoimmunity in patients treated with cytotoxic T lymphocyte-associated antigen 4 blockade and interleukin 2: a phase I/II study. Ann Surg Oncol. 2005;12:1005–16.
43. Martin M, Schneider H, Azouz A, Rudd CE. Cytotoxic T lymphocyte antigen 4 and CD28 modulate cell surface raft expression in their regulation of T cell function. J Exp Med. 2001;194:1675–81.
44. Nakaseko C, Miyatake S, Iida T, Hara S, Abe R, Ohno H, et al. Cytotoxic T lymphocyte antigen 4 (CTLA-4) engagement delivers an inhibitory signal through the membrane-proximal region in the absence of the tyrosine motif in the cytoplasmic tail. J Exp Med. 1999;190:765–74.
45. O'Day S, Weber J, Lebbe C, Maio M, Pehamberger H, Harmankaya K, et al. Effect of ipilimumab treatment on 18-month survival: Update of patients (pts) with advanced melanoma treated with 10 mg/kg ipilimumab in three phase II clinical trials (Meeting Abstracts). J Clin Oncol. 2009;27:9033.
46. O'Day SJ, Ibrahim R, DePril V, Maio M, Chiarion-Sileni V, Gajewski TF, et al. Efficacy and safety of ipilimumab induction and maintenance dosing in patients with advanced melanoma who progressed on one or more prior therapies (Meeting Abstracts). J Clin Oncol. 2008; 26:9021.
47. O'Day SJ, Maio M, Chiarion-Sileni V, Gajewski TF, Pehamberger H, Bondarenko IN, et al. Efficacy and safety of ipilimumab monotherapy in patients with pretreated advanced melanoma: a multicenter single-arm phase II study. Ann Oncol. 2010;21(8):1712–7.
48. Phan GQ, Yang JC, Sherry RM, Hwu P, Topalian SL, Schwartzentruber DJ, et al. Cancer regression and autoimmunity induced by cytotoxic T lymphocyte-associated antigen 4 blockade in patients with metastatic melanoma. Proc Natl Acad Sci USA. 2003;100:8372–7.
49. Quezada SA, Peggs KS, Curran MA, Allison JP. CTLA4 blockade and GM-CSF combination immunotherapy alters the intratumor balance of effector and regulatory T cells. J Clin Invest. 2006;116:1935–45.
50. Reuben JM, Lee BN, Li C, Gomez-Navarro J, Bozon VA, Parker CA, et al. Biologic and immunomodulatory events after CTLA-4 blockade with ticilimumab in patients with advanced malignant melanoma. Cancer. 2006;106:2437–44.
51. Ribas A. Overcoming immunologic tolerance to melanoma: targeting CTLA-4 with tremelimumab (CP-675,206). Oncologist. 2008;13 Suppl 4:10–5.
52. Ribas A, Camacho LH, Lopez-Berestein G, Pavlov D, Bulanhagui CA, Millham R, et al. Antitumor activity in melanoma and anti-self responses in a phase I trial with the anti-cytotoxic T lymphocyte-associated antigen 4 monoclonal antibody CP-675,206. J Clin Oncol. 2005;23:8968–77.
53. Ribas A, Comin-Anduix B, Economou JS, Donahue TR, de la Rocha P, Morris LF, et al. Intratumoral immune cell infiltrates, FoxP3, and indoleamine 2,3-dioxygenase in patients with melanoma undergoing CTLA4 blockade. Clin Cancer Res. 2009;15:390–9.
54. Ribas A, Hauschild A, Kefford R, Gomez-Navarro J, Pavlov D, Marshall MA. Phase III, open-label, randomized, comparative study of tremelimumab (CP-675,206) and chemotherapy (temozolomide [TMZ] or dacarbazine [DTIC]) in patients with advanced melanoma (Meeting Abstracts). J Clin Oncol. 2008;26:LBA9011.
55. Ribas A, Pavlov D, Marshall MA (2010) Final efficacy results of A3671009, A phase 3 study of tremelimumab vs chemotherapy (dacarbazine or temozolomide) in first line patients with unresectable melanoma. J Immunother. http://www.sitcancer.org/meetings/am10/47 (in press).
56. Sanderson K, Scotland R, Lee P, Liu D, Groshen S, Snively J, et al. Autoimmunity in a phase I trial of a fully human anti-cytotoxic T-lymphocyte antigen-4 monoclonal antibody with multiple melanoma peptides and Montanide ISA 51 for patients with resected stages III and IV melanoma. J Clin Oncol. 2005;23:741–50.
57. Schneider H, Downey J, Smith A, Zinselmeyer BH, Rush C, Brewer JM, et al. Reversal of the TCR stop signal by CTLA-4. Science. 2006;313:1972–5.

58. Shahinian A, Pfeffer K, Lee KP, Kundig TM, Kishihara K, Wakeham A, et al. Differential T cell costimulatory requirements in CD28-deficient mice. Science. 1993;261:609–12.
59. Stamper CC, Zhang Y, Tobin JF, Erbe DV, Ikemizu S, Davis SJ, et al. Crystal structure of the B7-1/CTLA-4 complex that inhibits human immune responses. Nature. 2001;410:608–11.
60. Tchekmedyian S, Glasby J, Korman A, Keler T, Deo Y, Davis TA. MDX-010 (human anti-CTLA4): a phase I trial in malignant melanoma. Proc Am Soc Clin Oncol. 2002;21:223; [abstr 56].
61. Tivol EA, Borriello F, Schweitzer AN, Lynch WP, Bluestone JA, Sharpe AH. Loss of CTLA-4 leads to massive lymphoproliferation and fatal multiorgan tissue destruction, revealing a critical negative regulatory role of CTLA-4. Immunity. 1995;3:541–7.
62. Tivol EA, Gorski J. Re-establishing peripheral tolerance in the absence of CTLA-4: complementation by wild-type T cells points to an indirect role for CTLA-4. J Immunol. 2002;169: 1852–8.
63. van der Merwe PA, Bodian DL, Daenke S, Linsley P, Davis SJ. CD80 (B7-1) binds both CD28 and CTLA-4 with a low affinity and very fast kinetics. J Exp Med. 1997;185:393–403.
64. van Elsas A, Hurwitz AA, Allison JP. Combination immunotherapy of B16 melanoma using anti-cytotoxic T lymphocyte-associated antigen 4 (CTLA-4) and Granulocyte/Macrophage colony-stimulating factor (GM-CSF)-producing vaccines induces rejection of subcutaneous and metastatic tumors accompanied by autoimmune depigmentation. J Exp Med. 1999;190: 355–66.
65. van Elsas A, Sutmuller RP, Hurwitz AA, Ziskin J, Villasenor J, Medema JP, et al. Elucidating the autoimmune and antitumor effector mechanisms of a treatment based on cytotoxic T lymphocyte antigen-4 blockade in combination with a B16 melanoma vaccine: comparison of prophylaxis and therapy. J Exp Med. 2001;194:481–9.
66. Viola A, Lanzavecchia A. T cell activation determined by T cell receptor number and tunable thresholds. Science. 1996;273:104–6.
67. Vonderheide RH, Lorusso P, Khalil M, Gartner EM, Khaira D, Soulieres D, et al. Tremelimumab in combination with exemestane in patients with advanced breast cancer and treatment-associated modulation of ICOS expression on patient t cells. Clin Cancer Res. 2010;16(13):3485–94.
68. Waterhouse P, Penninger JM, Timms E, Wakeham A, Shahinian A, Lee KP, et al. Lymphoproliferative disorders with early lethality in mice deficient in Ctla-4. Science. 1995; 270:985–8.
69. Weber J. Overcoming immunologic tolerance to melanoma: targeting CTLA-4 with ipilimumab (MDX-010). Oncologist. 2008;13 Suppl 4:16–25.
70. Weber J, Thompson JA, Hamid O, Minor D, Amin A, Ron I, et al. A randomized, double-blind, placebo-controlled, phase II study comparing the tolerability and efficacy of ipilimumab administered with or without prophylactic budesonide in patients with unresectable stage III or IV melanoma. Clin Cancer Res. 2009;15:5591–8.
71. Weber JS, O'Day S, Urba W, Powderly J, Nichol G, Yellin M, et al. Phase I/II study of ipilimumab for patients with metastatic melanoma. J Clin Oncol. 2008;26:5950–6.
72. Wing K, Onishi Y, Prieto-Martin P, Yamaguchi T, Miyara M, Fehervari Z, et al. CTLA-4 control over Foxp3+ regulatory T cell function. Science. 2008;322:271–5.
73. Wolchok JD, de Pril V, Linette G, Waterfield W, Gajewski T, Chiarion-Sileni V, et al. Efficacy of ipilimumab 10 mg/kg in advanced melanoma patients (pts) with good and poor prognostic factors (Meeting Abstracts). J Clin Oncol. 2009;27:9036.
74. Wolchok JD, Neyns B, Linette G, Negrier S, Lutzky J, Thomas L, et al. Ipilimumab monotherapy in patients with pretreated advanced melanoma: a randomised, double-blind, multicentre, phase 2, dose-ranging study. Lancet Oncol. 2009;11(2):155–64.
75. Yang A, Kendle RF, Ginsberg BA, Roman R, Heine AI, Pogoriler E, et al. CTLA-4 blockade with ipilimumab increases peripheral CD8+ T cells: Correlation with clinical outcomes (Meeting Abstracts). J Clin Oncol. 2010;28:2555.
76. Yuan J, Gnjatic S, Li H, Powel S, Gallardo HF, Ritter E, et al. CTLA-4 blockade enhances polyfunctional NY-ESO-1 specific T cell responses in metastatic melanoma patients with clinical benefit. Proc Natl Acad Sci USA. 2008;105:20410–5.

Chapter 15
Anti-PD-1 and Anti-B7-H1/PD-L1 Monoclonal Antibodies

Evan J. Lipson, Janis M. Taube, Lieping Chen, and Suzanne L. Topalian

Abstract Tumors can evade immune recognition by usurping regulatory pathways which, under normal circumstances, down-modulate immune activation and maintain tolerance to self. A key pathway operational in cancer-induced tolerance is composed of programmed death-1 (PD-1, CD279), a receptor expressed on activated T and B cells, and its ligands B7-H1/PD-L1 (hereafter B7-H1, CD274) and B7-DC/PD-L2 (hereafter B7-DC, CD273). PD-1 bears homology to CTLA-4 but transmits distinct inhibitory signals. B7-H1, which is homologous to other B7 family members, is constitutively expressed by many human cancers and is thought to be the major inhibitory ligand for PD-1; it is also expressed on activated hematopoietic cells, vascular endothelial cells, and cells inhabiting inflammatory microenvironments. Based on animal models implicating the importance of the B7-H1/PD-1 pathway in cancer-induced immunosuppression, and human studies correlating tumor expression of B7-H1 with unfavorable clinical outcomes, interest has recently focused on exploring B7-H1/PD-1 blockade as a new approach to cancer immunotherapy. Early results from clinical trials suggest that this may be an effective strategy for treating patients with advanced metastatic melanoma as well as malignancies of epithelial origin.

E.J. Lipson
Department of Oncology, The Johns Hopkins
University School of Medicine and the Sidney Kimmel Comprehensive Cancer Center,
Baltimore, MD, USA

J.M. Taube, MD
Departments of Dermatology and Pathology, Johns Hopkins Hospital, Baltimore, MD, USA

L. Chen, MD, PhD
Department of Immunobiology, Yale University School of Medicine, New Haven, CT, USA

S.L.Topalian, MD (✉)
Departments of Surgery and Oncology, The Johns Hopkins University School of Medicine
and the Sidney Kimmel Comprehensive Cancer Center, Baltimore, MD, USA
e-mail: stopali1@jhmi.edu

T.F. Gajewski and F.S. Hodi (eds.), *Targeted Therapeutics in Melanoma*,
Current Clinical Oncology, DOI 10.1007/978-1-61779-407-0_15,
© Springer Science+Business Media, LLC 2012

Keywords PD-1 • B7-H1 • PD-L1 • Monoclonal antibodies • Immunohistochemistry • Immune regulation • Tolerance • Immunotherapy

The B7-H1/PD-1 Pathway: Animal Models

Functionality Indicated by Phenotypes of B7-H1/PD-1 Deficient Mice

Studies in murine models have revealed important clues about the immune regulatory functions of the B7-H1/PD-1 pathway. The physiological functions of the B7-H1 molecule were elucidated by generating B7-H1-deficient mice with gene knockout technology. Although B7-H1-deficient mice do not develop spontaneous autoimmune diseases, mild-to-moderate levels of lymphocyte accumulation are evident in the kidneys, liver, and lung. This accumulation appears to be selective for peripheral but not lymphoid organs, with a predominant CD3$^+$CD8$^+$ component exhibiting significantly decreased apoptosis [20]. Although the mechanism underlying selective accumulation of CD8$^+$ T cells in B7-H1 knockout mice remains to be elucidated, these findings implicate a role for B7-H1 in the maintenance of T and cell homeostasis in peripheral organs. More recently, B7-H1 has been shown to interact not only with PD-1, but also with B7-1 at a distinct binding site [12]. This interaction appears to play an important role in inducing T cell tolerance in vivo, as shown using specific monoclonal antibodies (mAbs) to selectively block B7-H1/PD-1 or B7-H1/B7-1 ligation [49]. These new findings expand our understanding of the mechanisms by which B7-H1 may exert immune tolerance.

In contrast to B7-H1-deficient mice, PD-1-deficient mice spontaneously develop phenotypes of lymphoproliferative/autoimmune diseases, accompanied by a marked accumulation of inflammatory cells in affected organs, including CD4$^+$ and CD8$^+$ T cell subsets. These phenotypes have delayed onsets and are organ- and strain-specific. PD-1$^{-/-}$ mice on a C57BL/6 background develop a lupus-like arthritis [44], while PD-1 deficiency on a BALB/c background causes a cardiomyopathy secondary to the production of autoantibodies against cardiac troponin [45, 48]. Autoimmune manifestations in PD-1$^{-/-}$ mice are different from those observed in CTLA-4$^{-/-}$ mice, which die at 3–4 weeks of age from massive lymphocytic infiltration and tissue destruction in multiple organs [66, 74]. Collectively, these findings from murine models predict that autoimmune phenomena, if encountered in patients treated with B7-H1/PD-1 blockade, might be milder and less frequent than those observed following anti-CTLA-4 therapy.

B7-H1 appears to be the dominant ligand responsible for the suppressive function of PD-1 in vivo, as results obtained in PD-1 or B7-H1-deficient mice are often similar to those obtained with blocking antibodies against PD-1 or B7-H1. However, in some models, blockade of B7-H1 has a more profound effect than PD-1 blockade, perhaps reflecting the existence of other functional receptors for B7-H1, such as B7-1 [24, 69].

Regulation of PD-1 Expression

PD-1 expression is up-regulated on T lymphocytes within hours of exposure to cognate antigen, and is controlled by common gamma chain cytokines including IL-2, IL-7, IL-15, and IL-21 [37]. Upon antigen clearance, PD-1 expression wanes accordingly. However, persistent antigen exposure may prevent down-regulation of PD-1 and allow the delivery of suppressive signals, leading to loss of T cell function and a partially unresponsive state termed T cell exhaustion. These observations may be especially relevant to chronic maladies including infection, inflammation, and even malignant transformation, because persistent PD-1 expression has been documented in these disorders. In mice chronically infected with lymphocytic choriomeningitis virus (LCMV), PD-1 is up-regulated upon activation of antigen-specific T cells, and high levels are found on exhausted CD8$^+$ T cells [5]. As a consequence, activated T cells become dysfunctional and fail to become memory T cells. In vivo administration of mAbs blocking the interaction of B7-H1 with PD-1 restores the ability of exhausted LCMV-specific CD8$^+$ T cells to proliferate, secrete cytokines, kill infected targets, and decrease viral load in chronically infected animals. Correlates for these effects have been observed in humans with chronic infectious diseases. PD-1 is expressed at high levels on nonfunctional T cells during human immunodeficiency virus (HIV) infection, and anti-PD-1 or anti-B7-H1 mAbs can restore proliferative and effector T cell functions in vitro [17, 68]. Comparable findings have been observed in patients chronically infected with hepatitis B and C viruses [9, 52, 70], *Helicobacter pylori* [16], and *Mycobacterium tuberculosis* [33].

Functional Consequences of B7-H1/PD-1 Interactions

Murine models suggest a predominant role for B7-H1/PD-1 interactions in the establishment and/or maintenance of peripheral tolerance, including feto-maternal tolerance [25], and in the suppression of induced or ongoing immune responses, including alloreactive responses [55], graft-vs.-host disease [8], and various autoimmune diseases such as experimental autoimmune encephalopathy (EAE), diabetes, and collagen-induced arthritis [3, 41, 54, 71].

Our early observation that multiple murine and human tumor lines as well as freshly isolated malignant human tissues overexpress B7-H1[19, 26] has prompted the investigation of the potential role of the B7-H1/PD-1 pathway in regulating antitumor immunity. Up-regulation of B7-H1 appears to be associated with local inflammatory and immune responses often found at tumor sites, consistent with the observation that interferon (IFN) gamma is the most potent inducer of B7-H1 known [36]. In the murine P815 mastocytoma model, tumor cells transduced to express B7-H1 were significantly more resistant to immunotherapy with adoptively transferred preactivated T cells [19] or with anti-CD137 (a T cell agonist mAb), compared to mock transduced tumor cells [28]. Blockade of B7-H1 with a specific mAb restored T cell responses in this model. In a different model, overexpression of

B7-H1 on the murine squamous cell cancer line SCCVII resulted in diminished immune-mediated control that was restored upon B7-H1 blockade [60]. Similarly, tumor growth of the naturally B7-H1-expressing J558L myeloma cell line was diminished in syngeneic PD-1$^{-/-}$ mice and in wild-type mice treated with anti-B7-H1 mAb [31]. These studies demonstrate a critical role for the B7-H1/PD-1 pathway in resistance to antitumor immunity, and support a potential approach to enhancing immunity against human cancers by blocking this pathway.

In addition to T cell inhibition caused by direct interactions between B7-H1 on tumor cells and PD-1 on activated T cells, several other possible mechanisms contributing to the suppressive function of the B7-H1/PD-1 pathway in tumor immunity have been implicated in animal models. Preliminary results indicate that tumor cells expressing B7-H1 are intrinsically more resistant than B7-H1-negative cells to lysis by tumor-specific T lymphocytes. This resistance can be abrogated by blocking B7-H1 or PD-1, suggesting that B7-H1/PD-1 interaction activates a "molecular shield" through retrograde signaling into tumor cells, to prevent T cell lysis [4]. By transducing full-length or C-terminally truncated B7-H1 molecules into P815 tumor cells, it was shown that full-length B7-H1 can serve as receptor, delivering antiapoptotic signals into tumor cells, while B7-H1 without an intracellular tail cannot [4].

Tumor-associated antigen-presenting cells (APCs) can also utilize the B7-H1/PD-1 pathway to suppress antitumor immunity. In a human ovarian cancer xenograft model, anti-B7-H1 mAb augmented the effector functions of T cells stimulated in the presence of autologous tumor myeloid dendritic cells (MDCs) expressing high levels of B7-H1, leading to improved control of tumor growth in non-obese diabetic (NOD)/severe combined immunodeficiency (SCID) mice [15]. Furthermore, overexpression of B7-H1 on tumor stromal cells, including DCs, myeloid suppressor cells, and fibroblasts, has been shown to potentially inhibit immune responses and may contribute to the suppressive cancer microenvironment. B7-H1-expressing DCs may also mediate immune suppression by activating regulatory T cells (Tregs). In mice inoculated with B16 melanoma, plasmacytoid dendritic cells in tumor-draining lymph nodes expressed IDO, a potent activator of the suppressive activity of Tregs. Treg activation required cell contact with IDO-expressing DCs and was abrogated by B7-H1 blockade [57]. These results are consistent with recent findings that B7-H1 is required for inducing Tregs in mouse models[21] and reveal a potential new mechanism for the suppressive function of the B7-H1/PD-1 pathway. The role of B7-H1/PD-1-induced Tregs in the evasion of tumor immunity, however, remains to be confirmed in animal models.

Although information from animal models shows that the B7-H1/PD-1 pathway plays a critical role in the evasion of antitumor immunity, blockade of B7-H1 or PD-1 by individual mAbs is often not very effective in treating established transplanted tumors in murine models commonly used for immunotherapy studies. In several models using highly immunogenic murine tumors, only marginal-to-moderate therapeutic effects were observed with a "monotherapy" approach [28, 31, 32, 60, 75]. These findings are not totally unanticipated, because blockade of B7-H1 or PD-1 is not expected to stimulate de novo immune responses but rather to enhance ongoing immune responses against tumor antigens. In the majority of transplantable tumor models, rapid tumor growth in syngeneic mice might not allow time for the development of a significant antitumor immune response, and T cells in these models are often ignorant of tumor antigens [14]. However, combining B7-H1/PD-1 blockade with cancer vaccines [75], adoptive transfer of preactivated T cells, or T cell stimulation with anti-CD137 [28, 46, 60] often provides dramatic synergistic antitumor effects, in some cases eradicating well-established tumors. These observations highlight the importance of mechanism-based design of combinatorial treatment regimens with B7-H1/PD-1 blockade to maximize clinical efficacy.

B7-H1/PD-1 Expression and Function in Normal Human Tissues and Cancers

B7-H1 demonstrates limited constitutive cell-surface expression in normal human tissues, yet is expressed by a number of malignant neoplasms where it primarily serves as an inhibitory molecule when interacting with PD-1 [29]. While mRNA for B7-H1 has been detected in most human tissues, it is posttranscriptionally regulated such that constitutive protein expression is observed only in a proportion of cells from the activated monocyte/macrophage lineage, as well as by the endothelium in the placenta, thymus, and heart [11, 19, 40, 79]. Its expression can be induced in other normal cell types and in tumors by proinflammatory cytokines such as IFN-gamma and IL-10 [15, 19].

B7-H1 Expression in Solid Human Tumors

When B7-H1 is expressed aberrantly by human tumors, it presumably provides a selection advantage by inhibiting tumor-specific recognition and elimination by T cells. Several mechanisms have been proposed for this, including induction of T cell apoptosis through PD-1 signaling [19], and reverse transmission of B7-H1-mediated prosurvival signals [7, 18, 28]. Due to the fact that B7-H1 mRNA levels are not predictive of protein expression, most studies of B7-H1 expression employ immunohistochemistry-based methods on fresh frozen or paraffin-embedded tumor sections. In the majority of human studies conducted to date, tumors are considered "positive" for B7-H1 if cell surface ("membranous") expression is observed in greater than 5–10% of cells. B7-H1 expression has not been well studied in premalignant lesions, but has been identified in a broad spectrum of established solid human cancers. In addition to melanoma [27], other tumors expressing B7-H1 include urothelial carcinoma [42]; squamous cell carcinomas of the head and neck [60], esophagus [47], cervix [34], and lung [38]; adenocarcinomas of the breast [23], pancreas [22, 72], lung [38], and stomach;78] clear cell renal cell carcinoma (RCC) [64], Wilms tumor [53], and glioblastoma [76]. Importantly, B7-H1 expression in primary tumors is often associated with advanced clinicopathologic status [22, 23, 42, 53, 72, 78]. In some tumor types, including ovarian cancer [26], renal cancer [64, 65], pancreatic cancer [46], breast cancer [23], and bladder urothelial carcinoma [30, 42], retrospective studies have shown that intratumoral B7-H1 expression is an independent predictor of adverse patient outcomes [27, 47, 64, 78]. Interestingly, in ovarian cancer, the expression level of B7-H1 on tumor cells was found to correlate inversely with numbers of intraepithelial CD8+ T cells, while increased T cell infiltration was associated with improved clinical outcomes [26]. In melanoma, the correlation of B7-H1 expression with tumor progression and clinical outcomes is currently under study.

In addition to B7-H1 expression on tumor cells, primary human neoplasms often manifest B7-H1 on other cell types. Tumor infiltrating lymphocytes (TILs) and associated tissue macrophages express B7-H1 [18, 23, 27, 42, 64]. In some tumor types, high levels of B7-H1 expression by TILs have been shown to correlate with adverse patient outcomes [64]. Expression of B7-H1 by TILs in breast cancer was associated with larger tumor size and Her2/neu-positive status [23]. In renal cell cancer, overexpression of B7-H1 on both tumor cells and TILs correlated with aggressive tumor behavior and was associated with a 4.5-fold higher risk of cancer-related death [64]. Beyond the primary tumor, tumor cells and TILs in metastatic deposits also demonstrate B7-H1 expression [63]. This finding has potential clinical import, since patients with advanced disease are most likely to receive novel anti-B7-H1/PD-1 therapies. In such cases, the B7-H1 status of metastatic tumor cells and infiltrating immune cells holds special interest as a potential biomarker predictive of patient response to B7-H1/PD-1 targeted therapies.

PD-1 Expression on Hematopoietic Cells

PD-1 is a receptor for B7-H1 and is thought to play a role in maintaining self-tolerance. In addition to its expression on activated T cells, B cells, thymocytes, and myeloid cells [1, 13, 40, 43], PD-1 has been detected by immunohistochemistry on lymphocytes infiltrating RCC, non-small cell lung carcinoma, and cervical carcinoma [34, 38, 62]. In the cases of non-small cell lung carcinoma, a significant decrease in both the total number of TILs and the percentage of TILs expressing PD-1 was observed in B7-H1-positive tumor regions when compared to B7-H1-negative tumor regions [38]. In addition, PD-1 expression has been detected on TILs recovered from enzymatically digested metastatic melanoma lesions [2]. Similar to exhausted virus antigen-specific T cells observed in chronic viral infections, the majority of melanoma TILs express high levels of PD-1 compared with T cells from normal tissues and peripheral blood. One study showed that the majority of CD8+ TILs specific for the melanoma antigen MART-1 expressed significant levels of PD-1, compared with lower expression on MART-specific T cells from the peripheral blood of the same patients. PD-1 expression by melanoma TILs correlated with an exhausted T cell phenotype and impaired effector function [2]. These results suggest that the tumor microenvironment influences the phenotype of the surveying cells and potentially explain why tumor lesions may grow progressively despite the presence of tumor-reactive infiltrating lymphocytes.

B7-H1 and PD-1 Signaling and Associated Markers

B7-H1/PD-1 engagement impairs the functionality and proliferation of activated T cells. The signaling mechanisms leading to B7-H1 expression by tumors have not been well established, but local proinflammatory cytokines including IFN-gamma (a major effector cytokine released by activated T cells) have been shown to induce B7-H1 expression [19, 76]. There is evidence to suggest that this expression occurs through an AKT-mediated pathway in some tumor types [51]. The subsequent inhibition of T cell function triggered by B7-H1-mediated PD-1 ligation of tumor-infiltrating lymphocytes is better understood. PD-1 ligation causes immune paralysis of fully activated T cells by inhibiting T cell receptor-mediated proliferation and cytokine secretion. When the TCR and PD-1 are coligated, PD-1 delivers a negative signal through a tyrosine-based inhibitory motif contained in its cytoplasmic domain, leading to activation of Src homology region 2 domain-containing phosphatase-2 (SHP-2). Downstream effects include inhibition of the PI3-K/AKT and ERK/MAPK signaling pathways, which impair proliferation and IL-2 production [2, 50, 56, 58, 59].

TILs themselves may therefore paradoxically trigger their own down-regulation, i.e., TILs secrete proinflammatory cytokines leading to B7-H1 expression by tumor cells, which in turn causes T cell dysfunction via PD-1 ligation. A deeper understanding of the mechanisms influencing B7-H1 expression by tumors may suggest rational combinations of cytokines or small molecule inhibitors with B7-H1/PD-1 blockade to perturb these signaling pathways.

Application of B7-H1/PD-1 Blockade in Melanoma Therapy

Proof-of-principle for the important role of immunological checkpoint blockade in regulating antitumor immunity came from clinical experience with anti-CTLA-4 (tremelimumab, Pfizer; ipilimumab, Bristol-Myers Squibb). This set the stage for targeting other members of the CD28 superfamily, such as PD-1, or their ligands, such as B7-H1, in cancer immunotherapy. To date, results from clinical trials of two blocking antibodies against PD-1 have been reported. CT-011, a humanized IgG1 mAb, was raised by immunizing mice against human Daudi B cell lymphoma membrane extracts (CureTech Ltd., Yavne, Israel). MDX-1106 (BMS-936558/Ono-4358), a fully human IgG4 mAb, was generated in genetically modified mice immunized against Chinese hamster ovary (CHO) cell PD-1 transfectants and a recombinant PD-1 fusion protein (Medarex/Bristol-Myers Squibb, Princeton, NJ,

USA). These anti-PD-1 mAbs have been tested in patients with a variety of advanced solid and liquid tumors, but at this time, only MDX-1106 has been reported in treating melanoma. Two new anti-PD-1 blocking agents, MK-3475 (anti-PD-1 monoclonal antibody, Merck) and AMP-224 (B7-DC/IgG fusion protein, Amplimmune) have recently entered phase I clinical testing.

Preclinical Considerations

As mentioned above, our understanding of the effects of B7-H1/PD-1 pathway blockade comes, in part, from infectious disease models. Similar to malignant tumors, infectious pathogens can evade immune attack by co-opting immunoregulatory pathways designed to protect normal tissues. Preclinical studies in mice chronically infected with LCMV demonstrated overexpression of PD-1 on exhausted virus-specific CD8+ T cells, which regained proliferative and antiviral functions following B7-H1 antibody blockade [5]. Similarly, in vitro studies of immune cells from patients chronically infected with HIV have shown overexpression of PD-1 and B7-H1 on virus-specific T cells on APCs, respectively, and antivirus immune dysfunction can be reversed by blocking PD-1/B7-H1 interactions [35].

The immunology of cancer resembles chronic infection in that prolonged antigen exposure may activate immunosuppressive phenomena. Although melanoma is arguably the most immunogenic human cancer, studies of anti-melanoma immunity, including co-regulatory immunological pathways such as B7-H1/PD-1, have revealed findings which appear relevant to other forms of cancer. Antitumor T lymphocyte responses are readily demonstrated in the blood, lymph nodes, and tumors of most melanoma patients, and numbers of circulating melanoma-specific T cells can be boosted by peptide vaccines. CD8+ T cells infiltrating growing human melanomas have been shown to overexpress PD-1, compared to T cells in the blood or normal tissues [2]. While ineffective at controlling tumor growth in vivo, these cells nevertheless exhibit vigorous and specific antitumor activity (cytolysis, cytokine secretion, proliferation) when cultured in vitro [67]. These findings suggest that in vitro culture conditions bypass immunosuppressive factors present in situ in the tumor microenvironment. Such factors might include B7-H1 expression on tumor cells and intratumoral APCs. Furthermore, vaccine-induced peripheral CD8+ T cells specific for HLA-A2-restricted gp100 or MART-1/Melan-A peptides also express significant levels of PD-1. Wong and colleagues demonstrated enhanced proliferation and function of these cells following PD-1 blockade in vitro [77]. These investigators also demonstrated that PD-1 blockade interfered with Treg-based inhibition of CD8+ T cells, enhancing the generation of melanoma antigen-specific CD8+ T cells in vitro [73].

These in vitro laboratory findings, combined with evidence from in vivo murine tumor models, as described in the preceding sections, have provided a rationale for exploring the effects of B7-H1/PD-1 blockade in humans with melanoma and other cancers.

Early Clinical Experience

MDX-1106 is the only anti-PD-1 agent with reported clinical experience in melanoma. In a phase I, dose-escalation study conducted by Brahmer et al., 39 patients with treatment-refractory metastatic solid tumors, ten of whom had stage IV melanoma, received MDX-1106 therapy [10]. The objectives of this trial were to evaluate the safety and toxicity profile of MDX-1106, and to acquire preliminary information about antitumor activity. Eligible patients had good performance status, no active brain metastases, and no history of autoimmune disorders. MDX-1106 was administered as a single intravenous infusion in escalating doses to several patient cohorts, with an expansion cohort at the highest tolerated dose. Patients with stable disease or evidence of tumor regression 3 months after one infusion were eligible for repeated therapy.

MDX-1106 administered in this fashion was generally well-tolerated, and a maximum tolerated dose (MTD) was not defined, up to the highest planned dose of 10 mg/kg. The most common toxicities were decreased $CD4^+$ lymphocyte counts, lymphopenia, fatigue, and musculoskeletal complaints such as arthralgias, myalgias, or weakness. Immune-related adverse events included low-grade hypothyroidism and polyarticular arthropathies. One serious adverse event, a grade 3 inflammatory colitis, occurred in a patient with metastatic ocular melanoma after receiving multiple doses of MDX-1106. This event resembled cases of colitis observed with anti-CTLA-4 therapy, and responded to steroids and infliximab.

Among the 10 melanoma patients on this trial, one experienced a durable partial response (PR) to anti-PD-1 therapy. This 51-year-old female had lymph node and liver metastases which had progressed following high-dose interleukin-2 therapy and chemotherapy. A second melanoma patient experienced a significant but transient "mixed" tumor regression, with some lesions regressing while others progressed. Notably, among the non-melanoma study participants, a durable complete response in a patient with colorectal cancer and a PR in a patient with RCC were observed. Additionally, one patient with non-small cell lung cancer showed evidence of transient antitumor activity not meeting PR criteria. These findings suggest that in addition to its effects on melanoma, PD-1 blockade may have activity against some epithelial cancers which are typically considered to be poorly immunogenic. Two of the three objective responders from the first MDX-1106 study remain in remission 2.5 and 3 years later, respectively, without further therapy.

The pharmacokinetics of MDX-1106 were found to be dose-dependent, with a serum half-life of 12–20 days. However, the pharmacodynamic properties of PD-1 were unexpectedly discordant with pharmacokinetics. Despite decaying serum concentrations, circulating T cells displayed high levels of PD-1 receptor occupancy by MDX-1106, which were sustained for several weeks after a single dose. This effect was observed at all doses tested (0.3–10 mg/kg) and most likely reflects the high affinity of MDX-1106 for its target, suggesting a mechanism for prolonged drug activity which may be compatible with intermittent dosing.

Tumor biopsies from patients treated with MDX-1106 were also revealing. In one melanoma patient, new posttreatment CD8$^+$ (but not CD4$^+$) T cell infiltrates were observed in a regressing metastatic lesion. Additionally, in nine patients with melanoma or other solid tumors, pretreatment tumor cell surface expression of B7-H1 appeared to correlate with the likelihood of response to therapy. These preliminary results suggest that analysis of B7-H1 expression in tumor biopsies may provide a predictive biomarker of response to B7-H1/PD-1 blockade, and warrant further study in larger numbers of patients.

Anti-PD-1 therapy has also been tested in patients with advanced hematologic malignancies, using the mAb CT-011. Berger and colleagues administered CT-011 as a single intravenous dose to 17 patients [6]. The drug was generally well-tolerated and the MTD was not reached within the planned dose range of 0.2–6 mg/kg. Investigators examined percentages of circulating CD4$^+$, CD8$^+$, and CD69$^+$ lymphocytes, as well as serum levels of tumor necrosis factor (TNF) alpha and IFN-gamma, as potential markers of immune system activation following CT-011 infusion. A significant increase in the percentage of circulating CD4$^+$ T cells and decrease in CD8$^+$ T cells were observed in some dose cohorts. However, no significant changes in CD69$^+$ T cells, TNF-alpha, or IFN-gamma were reported. Of interest, one previously untreated patient with follicular B cell lymphoma experienced a complete response to CT-011 therapy, and a minor response was reported in a patient with refractory acute myeloid leukemia. CT-011 is currently undergoing further testing in next-generation clinical trials designed for patients with advanced hematologic malignancies, as well as melanoma and various solid tumors.

Future Clinical Development

Results from first-in-human clinical trials of two anti-PD-1 antibodies revealed early evidence of clinical activity and generally manageable toxicities in patients with melanoma and other cancers. These data, combined with information from preclinical studies, suggest considerable therapeutic potential for monotherapy and combinatorial therapy strategies incorporating B7-H1/PD-1 pathway blockade.

Current monotherapy studies include second generation trials with anti-PD-1 antibodies. Different dosing regimens of MDX-1106 are under investigation in expanded numbers of patients with advanced melanoma or cancers of the kidney, lung, colon, or prostate. A preliminary report of a phase I/II trial of MDX-1106 administered on a biweekly schedule appears to confirm the antitumor activity and manageable toxicity profile observed in the first-in-human trial. Notably, approximately one-third of patients with treatment refractory metastatic melanoma have experienced durable objective tumor regressions (Fig. 15.1) [61]. Significant responses were also reported in patients with non-small cell lung cancer and kidney cancer in this study. In addition, a first-in-human trial of anti-B7-H1 (MDX-1105, Medarex/Bristol-Myers Squibb) is underway and has already shown evidence of clinical activity in patients with melanoma and kidney cancer. It will be of interest

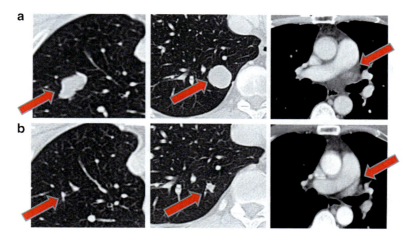

Fig. 15.1 Response of metastatic melanoma to PD-1 blockade (MDX-1106). This 50-year-old patient with stage IV treatment-refractory melanoma experienced regression of metastatic lesions in the lung and mediastinal lymph nodes (*arrows*) following biweekly anti-PD-1 therapy. (**a**) Pretreatment CT scans. (**b**) Partial tumor regression after 6 months of continuous therapy

to compare the clinical effects of PD-1 vs. B7-H1 antibody blockade, since these agents are predicted to have overlapping as well as unique spectra of activity.

Preclinical models suggest that achieving the true clinical potential of B7-H1/PD-1 blockade will depend on developing effective combinatorial therapies. Vaccine therapies designed to orient the immune response against specific tumor antigens, in combination with immunomodulatory antibodies, have yielded synergistic results in murine models. For example, in a study of B16 murine melanoma, Li et al. demonstrated synergy of PD-1 blockade with a GM-CSF-transduced melanoma cell vaccine [39]. Another intriguing strategy involves combining immunological checkpoint blockade with systemic tumoricidal therapies such as chemotherapy or targeted kinase inhibitors. These therapies may acutely release tumor antigens which could be presented endogenously by professional APCs for immune recognition, essentially creating an "autologous vaccine". Additional clinical strategies designed to liberate tumor antigens – especially in an inflammatory context providing "danger" signals for APC activation – may include localized radiofrequency ablation, stereotactic radiosurgery, or cryoablation. Finally, combining two immunomodulatory antibodies may also provide synergistic antitumor effects. An ongoing clinical trial is testing the combination of anti-CTLA-4 (ipilimumab) and anti-PD-1 (MDX-1106) in patients with advanced metastatic melanoma. These and other innovative and rational combinatorial treatment approaches, informed by preclinical models and a basic mechanistic understanding of the B7-H1/PD-1 pathway, are predicted to amplify the promising clinical results already observed with monotherapy approaches in melanoma and other cancers.

References

1. Agata Y, Kawasaki A, Nishimura H, Ishida Y, Tsubata T, Yagita H, et al. Expression of the PD-1 antigen on the surface of stimulated mouse T and B lymphocytes. Int Immunol. 1996;8: 765–72.
2. Ahmadzadeh M, Johnson LA, Heemskerk B, Wunderlich JR, Dudley ME, White DE, et al. Tumor antigen-specific CD8 T cells infiltrating the tumor express high levels of PD-1 and are functionally impaired. Blood. 2009;114:1537–44.
3. Ansari MJ, Salama AD, Chitnis T, Smith RN, Yagita H, Akiba H, et al. The programmed death-1 (PD-1) pathway regulates autoimmune diabetes in nonobese diabetic (NOD) mice. J Exp Med. 2003;198:63–9.
4. Azuma T, Yao S, Zhu G, Flies AS, Flies SJ, Chen L. B7-H1 is a ubiquitous antiapoptotic receptor on cancer cells. Blood. 2008;111:3635–43.
5. Barber DL, Wherry EJ, Masopust D, Zhu B, Allison JP, Sharpe AH, et al. Restoring function in exhausted CD8 T cells during chronic viral infection. Nature. 2006;439:682–7.
6. Berger R, Rotem-Yehudar R, Slama G, Landes S, Kneller A, Leiba M, et al. Phase I safety and pharmacokinetic study of CT-011, a humanized antibody interacting with PD-1, in patients with advanced hematologic malignancies. Clin Cancer Res. 2008;14:3044–51.
7. Blank C, Gajewski TF, Mackensen A. Interaction of PD-L1 on tumor cells with PD-1 on tumor-specific T cells as a mechanism of immune evasion: implications for tumor immunotherapy. Cancer Immunol Immunother. 2005;54:307–14.
8. Blazar BR, Carreno BM, Panoskaltsis-Mortari A, Carter L, Iwai Y, Yagita H, et al. Blockade of programmed death-1 engagement accelerates graft-versus-host disease lethality by an IFN-gamma-dependent mechanism. J Immunol. 2003;171:1272–7.
9. Boni C, Fisicaro P, Valdatta C, Amadei B, Di Vincenzo P, Giuberti T, et al. Characterization of hepatitis B virus (HBV)-specific T-cell dysfunction in chronic HBV infection. J Virol. 2007;81:4215–25.
10. Brahmer JR, Drake CG, Wollner I, Powderly JD, Picus J, Sharfman WH, et al. Phase I study of single-agent anti-programmed death-1 (MDX-1106) in refractory solid tumors: safety, clinical activity, pharmacodynamics, and immunologic correlates. J Clin Oncol. 2010;28: 3167–75.
11. Brown JA, Dorfman DM, Ma FR, Sullivan EL, Munoz O, Wood CR, et al. Blockade of programmed death-1 ligands on dendritic cells enhances T cell activation and cytokine production. J Immunol. 2003;170:1257–66.
12. Butte MJ, Keir ME, Phamduy TB, Sharpe AH, Freeman GJ. Programmed death-1 ligand 1 interacts specifically with the B7-1 costimulatory molecule to inhibit T cell responses. Immunity. 2007;27:111–22.
13. Carter L, Fouser LA, Jussif J, Fitz L, Deng B, Wood CR, et al. PD-1:PD-L inhibitory pathway affects both CD4(+) and CD8(+) T cells and is overcome by IL-2. Eur J Immunol. 2002;32: 634–43.
14. Chen L. Immunological ignorance of silent antigens as an explanation of tumor evasion. Immunol Today. 1998;19:27–30.
15. Curiel TJ, Wei S, Dong H, Alvarez X, Cheng P, Mottram P, et al. Blockade of B7-H1 improves myeloid dendritic cell-mediated antitumor immunity. Nat Med. 2003;9:562–7.
16. Das S, Suarez G, Beswick EJ, Sierra JC, Graham DY, Reyes VE. Expression of B7-H1 on gastric epithelial cells: its potential role in regulating T cells during *Helicobacter pylori* infection. J Immunol. 2006;176:3000–9.
17. Day CL, Kaufmann DE, Kiepiela P, Brown JA, Moodley ES, Reddy S, et al. PD-1 expression on HIV-specific T cells is associated with T-cell exhaustion and disease progression. Nature. 2006;443:350–4.
18. Dong H, Chen L. B7-H1 pathway and its role in the evasion of tumor immunity. J Mol Med. 2003;81:281–7.

19. Dong H, Strome SE, Salomao DR, Tamura H, Hirano F, Flies DB, et al. Tumor-associated B7-H1 promotes T-cell apoptosis: a potential mechanism of immune evasion. Nat Med. 2002;8:793–800.
20. Dong H, Zhu G, Tamada K, Flies DB, van Deursen JM, Chen L. B7-H1 determines accumulation and deletion of intrahepatic CD8(+) T lymphocytes. Immunity. 2004;20:327–36.
21. Francisco LM, Salinas VH, Brown KE, Vanguri VK, Freeman GJ, Kuchroo VK, et al. PD-L1 regulates the development, maintenance, and function of induced regulatory T cells. J Exp Med. 2009;206:3015–29.
22. Geng L, Huang D, Liu J, Qian Y, Deng J, Li D, et al. B7-H1 up-regulated expression in human pancreatic carcinoma tissue associates with tumor progression. J Cancer Res Clin Oncol. 2008;134:1021–7.
23. Ghebeh H, Mohammed S, Al-Omair A, Qattan A, Lehe C, Al-Qudaihi G, et al. The B7-H1 (PD-L1) T lymphocyte-inhibitory molecule is expressed in breast cancer patients with infiltrating ductal carcinoma: correlation with important high-risk prognostic factors. Neoplasia. 2006;8:190–8.
24. Goldberg MV, Maris CH, Hipkiss EL, Flies AS, Zhen L, Tuder RM, et al. Role of PD-1 and its ligand, B7-H1, in early fate decisions of CD8 T cells. Blood. 2007;110:186–92.
25. Guleria I, Khosroshahi A, Ansari MJ, Habicht A, Azuma M, Yagita H, et al. A critical role for the programmed death ligand 1 in fetomaternal tolerance. J Exp Med. 2005;202:231–7.
26. Hamanishi J, Mandai M, Iwasaki M, Okazaki T, Tanaka Y, Yamaguchi K, et al. Programmed cell death 1 ligand 1 and tumor-infiltrating CD8+ T lymphocytes are prognostic factors of human ovarian cancer. Proc Natl Acad Sci USA. 2007;104:3360–5.
27. Hino R, Kabashima K, Kato Y, Yagi H, Nakamura M, Honjo T, et al. Tumor cell expression of programmed cell death-1 ligand 1 is a prognostic factor for malignant melanoma. Cancer. 2010;116:1757–66.
28. Hirano F, Kaneko K, Tamura H, Dong H, Wang S, Ichikawa M, et al. Blockade of B7-H1 and PD-1 by monoclonal antibodies potentiates cancer therapeutic immunity. Cancer Res. 2005;65:1089–96.
29. Ichikawa M, Chen L. Role of B7-H1 and B7-H4 molecules in down-regulating effector phase of T-cell immunity: novel cancer escaping mechanisms. Front Biosci. 2005;10:2856–60.
30. Inman BA, Sebo TJ, Frigola X, Dong H, Bergstralh EJ, Frank I, et al. PD-L1 (B7-H1) expression by urothelial carcinoma of the bladder and BCG-induced granulomata: associations with localized stage progression. Cancer. 2007;109:1499–505.
31. Iwai Y, Ishida M, Tanaka Y, Okazaki T, Honjo T, Minato N. Involvement of PD-L1 on tumor cells in the escape from host immune system and tumor immunotherapy by PD-L1 blockade. Proc Natl Acad Sci USA. 2002;99:12293–7.
32. Iwai Y, Terawaki S, Honjo T. PD-1 blockade inhibits hematogenous spread of poorly immunogenic tumor cells by enhanced recruitment of effector T cells. Int Immunol. 2005;17:133–44.
33. Jurado JO, Alvarez IB, Pasquinelli V, Martinez GJ, Quiroga MF, Abbate E, et al. Programmed death (PD)-1:PD-ligand 1/PD-ligand 2 pathway inhibits T cell effector functions during human tuberculosis. J Immunol. 2008;181:116–25.
34. Karim R, Jordanova ES, Piersma SJ, Kenter GG, Chen L, Boer JM, et al. Tumor-expressed B7-H1 and B7-DC in relation to PD-1+ T-cell infiltration and survival of patients with cervical carcinoma. Clin Cancer Res. 2009;15:6341–7.
35. Kaufmann DE, Walker BD. PD-1 and CTLA-4 inhibitory cosignaling pathways in HIV infection and the potential for therapeutic intervention. J Immunol. 2009;182:5891–7.
36. Keir ME, Butte MJ, Freeman GJ, Sharpe AH. PD-1 and its ligands in tolerance and immunity. Annu Rev Immunol. 2008;26:677–704.
37. Kinter AL, Godbout EJ, McNally JP, Sereti I, Roby GA, O'Shea MA, et al. The common gamma-chain cytokines IL-2, IL-7, IL-15, and IL-21 induce the expression of programmed death-1 and its ligands. J Immunol. 2008;181:6738–46.
38. Konishi J, Yamazaki K, Azuma M, Kinoshita I, Dosaka-Akita H, Nishimura M. B7-H1 expression on non-small cell lung cancer cells and its relationship with tumor-infiltrating lymphocytes and their PD-1 expression. Clin Cancer Res. 2004;10:5094–100.

39. Li B, VanRoey M, Wang C, Chen TH, Korman A, Jooss K. Anti-programmed death-1 synergizes with granulocyte macrophage colony-stimulating factor–secreting tumor cell immunotherapy providing therapeutic benefit to mice with established tumors. Clin Cancer Res. 2009;15:1623–34.
40. Liang SC, Latchman YE, Buhlmann JE, Tomczak MF, Horwitz BH, Freeman GJ, et al. Regulation of PD-1, PD-L1, and PD-L2 expression during normal and autoimmune responses. Eur J Immunol. 2003;33:2706–16.
41. Matsumoto K, Inoue H, Nakano T, Tsuda M, Yoshiura Y, Fukuyama S, et al. B7-DC regulates asthmatic response by an IFN-gamma-dependent mechanism. J Immunol. 2004;172: 2530–41.
42. Nakanishi J, Wada Y, Matsumoto K, Azuma M, Kikuchi K, Ueda S. Overexpression of B7-H1 (PD-L1) significantly associates with tumor grade and postoperative prognosis in human urothelial cancers. Cancer Immunol Immunother. 2007;56:1173–82.
43. Nishimura H, Honjo T. PD-1: an inhibitory immunoreceptor involved in peripheral tolerance. Trends Immunol. 2001;22:265–8.
44. Nishimura H, Nose M, Hiai H, Minato N, Honjo T. Development of lupus-like autoimmune diseases by disruption of the PD-1 gene encoding an ITIM motif-carrying immunoreceptor. Immunity. 1999;11:141–51.
45. Nishimura H, Okazaki T, Tanaka Y, Nakatani K, Hara M, Matsumori A, et al. Autoimmune dilated cardiomyopathy in PD-1 receptor-deficient mice. Science. 2001;291:319–22.
46. Nomi T, Sho M, Akahori T, Hamada K, Kubo A, Kanehiro H, et al. Clinical significance and therapeutic potential of the programmed death-1 ligand/programmed death-1 pathway in human pancreatic cancer. Clin Cancer Res. 2007;13:2151–7.
47. Ohigashi Y, Sho M, Yamada Y, Tsurui Y, Hamada K, Ikeda N, et al. Clinical significance of programmed death-1 ligand-1 and programmed death-1 ligand-2 expression in human esophageal cancer. Clin Cancer Res. 2005;11:2947–53.
48. Okazaki T, Tanaka Y, Nishio R, Mitsuiye T, Mizoguchi A, Wang J, et al. Autoantibodies against cardiac troponin I are responsible for dilated cardiomyopathy in PD-1-deficient mice. Nat Med. 2003;9:1477–83.
49. Park JJ, Omiya R, Matsumura Y, Sakoda Y, Kuramasu A, Augustine MM, et al. B7-H1/CD80 interaction is required for the induction and maintenance of peripheral T cell tolerance. Blood. 2010;116(8):1291–8.
50. Parry RV, Chemnitz JM, Frauwirth KA, Lanfranco AR, Braunstein I, Kobayashi SV, et al. CTLA-4 and PD-1 receptors inhibit T-cell activation by distinct mechanisms. Mol Cell Biol. 2005;25:9543–53.
51. Parsa AT, Waldron JS, Panner A, Crane CA, Parney IF, Barry JJ, et al. Loss of tumor suppressor PTEN function increases B7-H1 expression and immunoresistance in glioma. Nat Med. 2007;13:84–8.
52. Penna A, Pilli M, Zerbini A, Orlandini A, Mezzadri S, Sacchelli L, et al. Dysfunction and functional restoration of HCV-specific CD8 responses in chronic hepatitis C virus infection. Hepatology. 2007;45:588–601.
53. Routh JC, Ashley RA, Sebo TJ, Lohse CM, Husmann DA, Kramer SA, et al. B7-H1 expression in Wilms tumor: correlation with tumor biology and disease recurrence. J Urol. 2008;179:1954–9; discussion 1959–60.
54. Salama AD, Chitnis T, Imitola J, Ansari MJ, Akiba H, Tushima F, et al. Critical role of the programmed death-1 (PD-1) pathway in regulation of experimental autoimmune encephalomyelitis. J Exp Med. 2003;198:71–8.
55. Sandner SE, Clarkson MR, Salama AD, Sanchez-Fueyo A, Domenig C, Habicht A, et al. Role of the programmed death-1 pathway in regulation of alloimmune responses in vivo. J Immunol. 2005;174:3408–15.
56. Saunders PA, Hendrycks VR, Lidinsky WA, Woods ML. PD-L2:PD-1 involvement in T cell proliferation, cytokine production, and integrin-mediated adhesion. Eur J Immunol. 2005; 35:3561–9.

57. Sharma MD, Baban B, Chandler P, Hou DY, Singh N, Yagita H, et al. Plasmacytoid dendritic cells from mouse tumor-draining lymph nodes directly activate mature Tregs via indoleamine 2,3-dioxygenase. J Clin Invest. 2007;117:2570–82.

58. Sheppard KA, Fitz LJ, Lee JM, Benander C, George JA, Wooters J, et al. PD-1 inhibits T-cell receptor induced phosphorylation of the ZAP70/CD3zeta signalosome and downstream signaling to PKCtheta. FEBS Lett. 2004;574:37–41.

59. Skeen JE, Bhaskar PT, Chen CC, Chen WS, Peng XD, Nogueira V, et al. Akt deficiency impairs normal cell proliferation and suppresses oncogenesis in a p53-independent and mTORC1-dependent manner. Cancer Cell. 2006;10:269–80.

60. Strome SE, Dong H, Tamura H, Voss SG, Flies DB, Tamada K, et al. B7-H1 blockade augments adoptive T-cell immunotherapy for squamous cell carcinoma. Cancer Res. 2003;63:6501–5.

61. Sznol, M., Powderly, J.D., Smith, D.C., Brahmer, J.R., Drake, C.G., McDermott, D.F., Lawrence, D.P., Wolchok, J.D., Topalian, S.L., and Lowy, I. (2010). Safety and antitumor activity of biweekly MDX-1106 (anti-PD-1, BMS-936558/ONO-4538) in patients with advanced refractory malignancies (Meeting Abstracts). J Clin Oncol 28 (suppl; abstr 2506).

62. Thompson RH, Dong H, Lohse CM, Leibovich BC, Blute ML, Cheville JC, et al. PD-1 is expressed by tumor-infiltrating immune cells and is associated with poor outcome for patients with renal cell carcinoma. Clin Cancer Res. 2007;13:1757–61.

63. Thompson RH, Gillett MD, Cheville JC, Lohse CM, Dong H, Webster WS, et al. Costimulatory molecule B7-H1 in primary and metastatic clear cell renal cell carcinoma. Cancer. 2005;104:2084–91.

64. Thompson RH, Gillett MD, Cheville JC, Lohse CM, Dong H, Webster WS, et al. Costimulatory B7-H1 in renal cell carcinoma patients: Indicator of tumor aggressiveness and potential therapeutic target. Proc Natl Acad Sci USA. 2004;101:17174–9.

65. Thompson RH, Kuntz SM, Leibovich BC, Dong H, Lohse CM, Webster WS, et al. Tumor B7-H1 is associated with poor prognosis in renal cell carcinoma patients with long-term follow-up. Cancer Res. 2006;66:3381–5.

66. Tivol EA, Borriello F, Schweitzer AN, Lynch WP, Bluestone JA, Sharpe AH. Loss of CTLA-4 leads to massive lymphoproliferation and fatal multiorgan tissue destruction, revealing a critical negative regulatory role of CTLA-4. Immunity. 1995;3:541–7.

67. Topalian SL, Solomon D, Rosenberg SA. Tumor-specific cytolysis by lymphocytes infiltrating human melanomas. J Immunol. 1989;142:3714–25.

68. Trautmann L, Janbazian L, Chomont N, Said EA, Gimmig S, Bessette B, et al. Upregulation of PD-1 expression on HIV-specific CD8+ T cells leads to reversible immune dysfunction. Nat Med. 2006;12:1198–202.

69. Tsushima F, Yao S, Shin T, Flies A, Flies S, Xu H, et al. Interaction between B7-H1 and PD-1 determines initiation and reversal of T-cell anergy. Blood. 2007;110:180–5.

70. Urbani S, Amadei B, Tola D, Massari M, Schivazappa S, Missale G, et al. PD-1 expression in acute hepatitis C virus (HCV) infection is associated with HCV-specific CD8 exhaustion. J Virol. 2006;80:11398–403.

71. Wang J, Yoshida T, Nakaki F, Hiai H, Okazaki T, Honjo T. Establishment of NOD-Pdcd1$^{-/-}$ mice as an efficient animal model of type I diabetes. Proc Natl Acad Sci USA. 2005;102: 11823–8.

72. Wang L, Ma Q, Chen X, Guo K, Li J, Zhang M. Clinical significance of b7-h1 and b7-1 expressions in pancreatic carcinoma. World J Surg. 2010;34:1059–65.

73. Wang W, Lau R, Yu D, Zhu W, Korman A, Weber J. PD1 blockade reverses the suppression of melanoma antigen-specific CTL by CD4+ CD25(Hi) regulatory T cells. Int Immunol. 2009;21:1065–77.

74. Waterhouse P, Penninger JM, Timms E, Wakeham A, Shahinian A, Lee KP, et al. Lymphoproliferative disorders with early lethality in mice deficient in Ctla-4. Science. 1995; 270:985–8.

75. Webster WS, Thompson RH, Harris KJ, Frigola X, Kuntz S, Inman BA, et al. Targeting molecular and cellular inhibitory mechanisms for improvement of antitumor memory responses reactivated by tumor cell vaccine. J Immunol. 2007;179:2860–9.
76. Wintterle S, Schreiner B, Mitsdoerffer M, Schneider D, Chen L, Meyermann R, et al. Expression of the B7-related molecule B7-H1 by glioma cells: a potential mechanism of immune paralysis. Cancer Res. 2003;63:7462–7.
77. Wong RM, Scotland RR, Lau RL, Wang C, Korman AJ, Kast WM, et al. Programmed death-1 blockade enhances expansion and functional capacity of human melanoma antigen-specific CTLs. Int Immunol. 2007;19:1223–34.
78. Wu C, Zhu Y, Jiang J, Zhao J, Zhang XG, Xu N. Immunohistochemical localization of programmed death-1 ligand-1 (PD-L1) in gastric carcinoma and its clinical significance. Acta Histochem. 2006;108:19–24.
79. Yamazaki T, Akiba H, Iwai H, Matsuda H, Aoki M, Tanno Y, et al. Expression of programmed death 1 ligands by murine T cells and APC. J Immunol. 2002;169:5538–45.

Chapter 16
Treatment of Melanoma with Agonist Immune Costimulatory Agents

Andrew Weinberg, Robert H. Vonderheide, and Mario Sznol

Abstract Immune therapy for melanoma is likely to be improved by better strategies to activate and expand tumor-specific T-cells, and to enhance their ability to infiltrate and function in the tumor microenvironment. In addition to or as an alternative to immunization with cancer antigens and administration of cytokines, antitumor T-cell responses can be positively modulated by activation of receptors that provide important dendritic cell (DC) maturation signals or T-cell costimulatory signals. At least three such stimulatory monoclonal antibodies, directed against OX40, CD137, and CD40, have been evaluated extensively in preclinical studies and have undergone at least preliminary evaluation in patients with metastatic melanoma. All three agents demonstrated limited but encouraging clinical antitumor activity in phase 1 trials. Future rational development of these agents will require a better understanding of the role of the receptors in evolving immune responses, the optimal timing and duration of administration in the context of the underlying host–tumor immune interactions, and the ability to combine the agents with each other and with other immunomodulators in appropriately selected patient populations.

Keywords IMMUNE Costimulation • Anti-CD137 • 4-1BB • OX40 • CD134 • ANTI-OX40 • ANTI-CD40 • CD40

A. Weinberg, PhD
Laboratory of Basic Immunology, Robert W. Franz Cancer Research Center,
Earle A. Chiles Research Institute, Portland, OR, USA

R.H. Vonderheide, MD, DPhil
Abramson Family Cancer Research Institute, University of Pennsylvania School of Medicine,
551 BRB II/III, 421 Curie Boulevard, Philadelphia, PA 19104, USA

M. Sznol, MD (✉)
Yale Cancer Center, 333 Cedar Street, FMP #126, PO Box 208032,
New Haven, CT 06520, USA
e-mail: Mario.sznol@yale.edu

T.F. Gajewski and F.S. Hodi (eds.), *Targeted Therapeutics in Melanoma*,
Current Clinical Oncology, DOI 10.1007/978-1-61779-407-0_16,
© Springer Science+Business Media, LLC 2012

Introduction

Metastatic disease in a subset of patients with disseminated melanoma will regress following administration of immunomodulatory agents, including cancer vaccines and various cytokines such as interferon(IFN)-α and interleukin-2. Responses can occur in patients with large tumor burdens, and can persist without relapse over many years, demonstrating the potential of an antitumor immune response to produce substantial clinical benefit. Although difficult to prove in humans, studies in animal models provide compelling evidence that tumor antigen-specific T-cells play a critical, nonredundant role in the tumor responses observed after administration of most immunomodulatory agents. Therefore, immune therapy for melanoma is likely to be improved by better strategies to activate and expand tumor-specific T-cells, and to enhance their ability to infiltrate and function in the tumor microenvironment.

Opportunities for development of novel immune therapy agents have come from a vast expansion of knowledge regarding signals controlling immune activation, expansion, and function of T-cells, prior and subsequent to T-cell receptor binding by the antigen-MHC complex. In addition to various cytokines produced by professional antigen-presenting cells (e.g., dendritic cells [DC]), stromal cells, and other immune cells, T-cells can be influenced by various ligand–receptor interactions between DC and T-cells, and between T-cells and their target cells. Among these ligand–receptor pairs, some have been found to provide positive costimulation to T-cells, while others were shown to transmit inhibitory signals. The ligand–receptor pairs between T-cells and DC or between T-cells and target cells can be blocked or activated by specific monoclonal antibodies. Several antibodies that provide activating or costimulating signals to DC or T-cells have been produced over the past several years, and have either entered clinical trials or are in preclinical development. Although multiple costimulatory ligand–receptor pairs have been identified and described in the literature, including CD80/CD86–CD28, CD137(4-1BB)-CD137L, OX40(CD134)-OX40L, CD27-CD70, and LIGHT-HVEM, we review in detail two of these, OX40 and CD137, and the related CD40-CD40L interactions, which have undergone at least Phase 1 testing in cancer patients and have greatest immediate relevance for treatment of melanoma [1].

General Principles

In manipulating immune responses for therapeutic purposes in cancer patients, several factors should be taken into consideration. Most important is the recognition of the immense complexity underlying control of immune responses to any antigen. For example, the response of T-cells to a costimulatory signal may depend on the differentiation state of the T-cell and the environmental milieu (presence or absence of other signals and cytokines) in which the signal is delivered. Moreover, different types of T-cells may be involved in antitumor immune responses, and signals through the same receptor may produce different biological effects in the different

T-cell subsets. The T-cell surface molecule targeted by the intervention may be expressed only during brief periods of T-cell differentiation or activation, or may be downregulated and rendered inactive by continuous stimulation.

Clinical evaluation of immune modulating antibodies is often based on results from animal models in which a similar antibody that binds to the analogous murine receptor is evaluated. However, the pattern and kinetics of receptor expression, and outcome after stimulation, may differ substantially between mice and humans. In addition, mouse tumor models, including genetically modified mice that develop spontaneous tumors, cannot fully reproduce the time-related interactions occurring between host and tumor in humans. For example, at the time of treatment, a human cancer has been present in its host for much longer than spontaneous or transplantable tumors in murine models. Thus, humans may have more extensive immune responses against their cancer, and more opportunities for development of mechanisms employed by tumor to suppress or evade those responses. These inhibitory signals may dominate over any activating or costimulatory signal.

Another complicating factor for clinical development of immune stimulatory antibodies is the heterogeneity of tumor biology and immune-tumor interactions between individual patients, all of whom have the same diagnosis of metastatic melanoma. The extent to which tumor antigen presentation is ongoing, or immune responses to tumor have developed, or tolerance to tumor antigens has been induced, or one or more of multiple possible systemic or local immune suppressive mechanisms are active is difficult to determine for any individual patient. Furthermore, there may be genetic variation between individuals that influences the effect, and magnitude of effect, for any specific immune intervention. Thus, for any targeted immune therapy, the underlying conditions necessary for generating a vigorous antitumor response may only be present in a small fraction of the population, and in most cases, this responsive subset cannot be prospectively identified with current technology. It is also likely that for most patients, multiple distinct agonist signals may be necessary to generate vigorous antitumor immune responses, and tumors may still not respond optimally unless the dominant immune suppressive factors in the tumor microenvironment are also inhibited concurrently.

OX40 (CD134)

Biology and Preclinical Studies

The original OX40 monoclonal antibody (Ab) bound activated CD4 T-cells and augmented their proliferation during the later stages of in vitro stimulation [2]. More recently, OX40 expression has also been demonstrated on CD8 T-cells and on T regulatory cells [3, 4]. The costimulatory function of OX40 on CD8 T-cells is important for their proliferation and survival [5], and a recent report suggests that anti-OX40 Abs can dampen Treg function in vivo [4]. When the biologic effects of anti-OX40 were originally described, the field of costimulation was in its infancy.

CD28 was the first costimulatory molecule described on T-cells; anti-CD28 was shown to augment T-cell stimulation when administered in combination with TCR signaling [6–8]. B7.1 (CD80) and B7.2 (CD86), which are expressed on antigen-presenting cells (APC), were identified as the ligands for CD28 and both molecules can stimulate T-cells through CD28. The CD28/B7 interaction is essential to achieve optimal activation of naïve T-cells; if a signal is delivered through the TCR receptor in the absence of CD28 ligation, the T-cell becomes anergic or dies prior to becoming a small resting T-cell [8]. There is another ligand for B7 on T-cells, termed CTLA-4, whose affinity for B7 is 100-fold greater than CD28 [9]. CTLA-4 is expressed on the T-cell surface after stimulation of naïve T-cells by antigen. Engagement of CTLA-4 puts the "brakes" on the initial wave of T-cell expansion [9]. T-cells stimulated through CD28 will proliferate for several divisions; however, the majority of cells will die prior to becoming small resting memory T-cells. OX40 was originally shown to have costimulatory activity on an Ag-specific CD4$^+$ T-cell line in vitro comparable to that of CD28 [10]. While interaction of B7/CD28 is required for the optimal stimulation of naïve T-cells [11], OX40-specific costimulation appears to be most important for the stimulation of effector T-cells [12, 13]. Since T-cells from OX40 knockout mice are more susceptible to apoptosis compared to their wild-type counterparts, it has been hypothesized that signaling through OX40 may save effector T-cells from activation-induced cell death (AICD), thereby leading to the generation of greater numbers of memory T-cells, and this was later shown to be the case [14]. Thus, both CD28 and OX40 appear to play important but distinct roles in the stimulation of Ag-activated peripheral T-cells; both signals are required for the optimal generation of memory T-cells [15].

Signaling through OX40 on T-cells occurs naturally through the OX40 ligand (OX40L), a TNF-family member that is a membrane-bound homotrimer expressed primarily on activated APC [16]. The OX40L trimer binds three OX40 molecules on the cell surface and the initial signaling process within T-cells occurs through the adapter proteins termed, TNF-associated factors (TRAFs). It was originally shown that TRAFs 2, 3, and 5 associated with the OX40 cytoplasmic tail [17], forming TRAF trimers just proximal to the cytoplasmic membrane. TRAF2 and 3 have been characterized as adapter proteins that can lead to the activation of NF-κB signaling pathways [17]. The increased signaling through OX40 within effector T-cells leads to increased proliferation, increased effector function (increased cytokines and cytotoxicity) and an increase in antiapoptotic pathways. These signaling events can be mimicked by adding exogenous OX40 agonists (anti-OX40 Abs or OX40L:Ig fusion protein) to T-cells both in vitro and in vivo in the absence of naturally expressed OX40L.

OX40 expression on recently activated naïve CD4 T-cells peaks 24–48 h after TCR engagement and returns to baseline levels 120 h later [12]. Effector CD4$^+$ T-cells upregulate OX40 expression more rapidly, expressing OX40 within 4 h of antigen stimulation [12]. The transient expression of OX40 is observed both in vitro and in vivo [12, 18]. OX40$^+$ T-cells are found preferentially at sites of inflammation and not normally found in the peripheral blood. In animal models for both autoimmunity and cancer, OX40$^+$ T-cells are enriched for the recently stimulated auto- or tumor antigen-specific T-cells [19–21]. Therefore, OX40 represents a convenient target by which the function in vivo stimulated T-cells can be modulated in various disease models, even without prior knowledge of the specific antigens involved [22]. In essence, manipulation of OX40+ T-cells in vivo targets the ongoing "endogenous" immune responses, without affecting the remainder of the peripheral T-cell repertoire. OX40+ T-cells have been detected at the inflammatory site in several human autoimmune diseases and in the following human cancers: melanoma, breast, colon, head and neck, prostate cancer, bladder cancer, lung cancer, and sarcoma ([22–24] and data not shown). Therefore, manipulation of OX40+ cells in patients with a variety of diseases including melanoma could have a wide range of clinical benefits.

The control point for OX40-dependent stimulation of T-cells during an immune response appears to be at the level of OX40L expression. While OX40 is expressed on all CD4+ and CD8+ T-cells after TCR engagement, OX40L expression is more tightly regulated. When T-cell activation occurs in the absence of a strong adjuvant, which is the usual case for tumor-derived antigens, the local expression of OX40L is minimal. Therefore, in the absence of adjuvant, the antigen-stimulated T-cells will express OX40, but because OX40L expression on APC is limiting, the majority of OX40+ T-cells will never engage their natural ligand. This may lead to apoptosis, decreased effector function, and limit the generation of memory T-cells. Evidence in support of this theory derives from two transgenic mouse models in which mice over express OX40L [25, 26]. In both models, the investigators noticed a large increase in the proportion of T-cells in the lymphoid compartments as the mice aged. The OX40L transgenic mice also showed a dramatic increase in memory T-cell generation and recall responses following immunization [26]. Therefore, it was hypothesized that the addition of OX40 agonists during immunization would greatly increase T-cell memory generation and effector T-cell responses in wild-type mice. When an OX40 agonist was administered following soluble Ag immunization, wild-type mice showed a large increase in effector cytokine production and memory T-cell survival [27, 28]. This was true for both CD4+ and CD8+ T-cells, although was more pronounced in the CD4+ T-cell compartment.

It was next tested whether the potent T-cell adjuvant properties of OX40 agonists would enhance antitumor immunity in cancer-bearing hosts leading to therapeutic efficacy. The initial study treated sarcoma-bearing mice 3 and 7 days after tumor inoculation with 100 μg of OX40L:Ig, a control fusion protein DR3:Ig (another TNF-R family member that does not bind OX40), or saline. Saline-treated and DR3:Ig treated mice all showed progressive tumor growth. By contrast, OX40L:Ig-treated mice experienced delayed tumor growth and 60% remained tumor free for >70 days. The OX40L:Ig treated mice that survived the initial tumor challenge rejected rechallenge with the MCA 303 tumor cells [21], which suggested that OX40L:Ig had increased tumor-specific T-cell memory. This OX40-based treatment regimen also showed efficacy in mice inoculated with the following tumors: melanoma (B16/F10), breast cancer (SM1, 4T1, EMT-6), colon cancer (CT26), glioma (GL261), sarcoma (MCA 203, 205, 207, 303), and lung cancer (Lewis lung carcinoma) [21, 29–33].

Several agents/techniques have been tested in combination with anti-OX40 to accentuate its antitumor activity. One study showed that anti-OX40 greatly enhanced adoptive immunotherapy, similar to and sometimes better than IL-2 [31]. A recent report has shown that anti-OX40 administered just after surgical removal of tumors can greatly decrease the recurrence of tumor [156]. This same manuscript also showed that combining focal radiation followed by anti-OX40 treatment had a synergistic therapeutic effect. There also been some success of combining tumor vaccines with OX40 agonist administration [22, 34–38]. In particular, a whole cell tumor vaccine secreting GM-CSF showed potent synergy with anti-OX40 administration in a breast cancer model where neither agent alone showed much efficacy [38]. The efficacy of tumor vaccines for melanoma and glioma was also enhanced by OX40 agonist stimulation in vivo [36, 39]. Anti-OX40 delivered in vivo has also been reported to upregulate the signaling subunit of the IL-12 receptor on antigen-stimulated CD4+ T-cells. This group subsequently combined anti-OX40 and IL-12 into tumor-bearing mice and showed therapeutic synergy [40]. Hence, there are clear pathways forward for OX40-specific combinations in future clinical trials, some of which are in the planning stages.

B16 melanoma is typically one of the most difficult mouse tumor models to cure with immunologic agents [41]. Initial reports indicated that OX40 agonists injected 3 days after B16/F10 tumor inoculation was able to cure 20% of mice. However, it has been reported more recently that a 75% cure rate of B16 melanoma occurred in mice with 6-day established tumors by injecting a single 250 mg/kg dose of cyclophosphamide followed by one OX40 agonist injection [41]. These results were striking as neither agent alone showed any significant tumor protection. This group compared the cyclophosphamide combination with other immune enhancing Abs (anti-CTLA-4 and anti-CD40) and found that the OX40 Ab was clearly superior in this combination format. This OX40/cyclophosphamide treatment combination was also effective in other poorly immunogenic models including lung cancer, breast cancer, and prostate cancer. This group found that this combination greatly increased tumor-specific T-cell responses when compared to either agent alone. They also found that this combination specifically induced regulatory T-cell depletion within the tumor microenvironment, which was accompanied by a large increase of CD8+ T-cells within the tumor. Thus, Treg depletion combined with OX40 agonists may be a particularly attractive approach to explore clinically.

OX40-Specific Nonhuman Primate Studies

The preclinical studies with OX40 agonists were so compelling that a group at Providence Portland Cancer Center (Oregon) decided to produce a GMP grade OX40 agonist antibody to deliver to cancer patients. Prior to performing a phase I study in cancer patients the mouse anti-human OX40 antibody was evaluated in nonhuman primates for toxicokinetics and immune stimulatory effects [42]. The initial study tested the OX40-specific immune adjuvant effects in monkeys immunized with the Simian Immunodeficiency Virus (SIV) protein, gp130. Anti-OX40 treatment (2 mg/kg) increased gp130 specific Ab titers and increased long-lived antigen-specific T-cell responses compared to controls. Following the immunization study a full toxicology study was performed at 0.4, 2.0, and 10 mg/kg. No clinical toxicity was observed, but acute splenomegaly and enlarged gut-associated lymph nodes were observed in various monkeys at all dose levels treated. The enlarged lymphoid organs resolved to base line levels by day 28 after the initial infusion. Upon histologic evaluation, there was an increase in lymphoblasts in both the spleen and the mesenteric lymph nodes 8 days after the initial OX40 infusion compared to controls, and this feature resolved by day 28. It was also noted that the histology did not exhibit any malignant features and normal architecture was maintained even in the enlarged spleen and lymph nodes. These preclinical monkey studies were submitted to the Food and Drug Administration and the Phase I trial was approved and started accruing cancer patients in March 2006.

Clinical Experience with Anti-OX40

The group at the Providence Cancer Center has recently completed a phase I study with the mouse anti-human OX40 antibody (Weinberg et al., manuscript in preparation). In this study, three doses of anti-OX40 were administered on days 1, 3, and 5. The murine anti-OX40 antibody induced a human anti-mouse antibody (HAMA) response in all patients by week 2 after antibody exposure. Thus, repetitive dosing was not feasible with this particular antibody. Thirty patients with stage IV disease were treated with anti-OX40 at 0.1, 0.4, and 2 mg/kg (ten patients per dose level). Toxicities were generally mild with grade 1–2 fatigue and transient lymphopenia as the most commonly observed side effects. A maximum tolerated dose (MTD) was not achieved. No patient achieved a complete or partial regression of their cancer using RECIST criteria, but 4 out of 7 melanoma patients showed regression of at least one tumor nodule in sites including lung, lymph node, and subcutaneous tissue. There was also evidence of increased tumor-specific responses within the melanoma patients after anti-OX40 treatment both in the T and B cell compartments. It was also found that anti-OX40 increased proliferation of T-cells within the peripheral blood as assessed by flow cytometry directly ex vivo, which generated a unique signature of T-cell activation after anti-OX40 treatment that could serve as a potential biomarker for activity.

These encouraging signs from a single treatment with the murine anti-OX40 antibody in cancer patients has prompted the group at the Providence Cancer Center to produce two fully human OX40 agonists; (1) A human OX40 ligand:Ig fusion protein, and (2) A humanized OX40-specific monoclonal antibody. The human OX40 ligand:Ig fusion protein has been tested in monkeys and is a potent stimulator of T-cell proliferation. Currently, the mouse monoclonal antibody used for the phase I study is being humanized and this Ab should be available for preclinical evaluation in 2011. During the time that the human OX40 agonists are being produced this group will be pursuing addition clinical trials with the murine OX40 antibody. In particular, they will be combining anti-OX40 with chemotherapy (cyclophosphamide) and focal radiation in patients with prostate cancer and breast cancer. Since the majority of patients that responded with some tumor shrinkage had metastatic melanoma, there will also be an exploratory clinical and immunologic assessment with the murine OX40 antibody in melanoma patients that should commence in 2011.

Anti-CD137 (4-1BB)

Biology and Preclinical Studies

There are remarkable parallels in the biology and immune functions of CD137 and OX40 (CD134). CD137, located on chromosome 1p36, is a member of the TNF receptor superfamily [43]. It is expressed, most often transiently and after cell activation, on CD4 and CD8 lymphocytes, NK cells, NKT cells, T-regulatory lymphocytes, dendritic cells, neutrophils, eosinophils, mast cells, and some endothelial cells, including tumor vasculature [44–52]. Expression of CD137 was also reported in basal epithelial cells of bronchial epithelium and in tumor cells including osteosarcoma and lung cancer [53, 54]. The ligand for CD137 is expressed by B-cells, macrophages, and dendritic cells and can be shed into the circulation [55, 56]. CD137L expression was also found in various tumor cell lines [52].

A large number of preclinical studies provide evidence for a role of CD137 and its ligand in regulation of immune responses, and for immune-enhancing effects of agonist anti-CD137 antibodies [57, 58]. During activation of naïve CD8$^+$ cells, CD137 expression is upregulated, and upon binding with its ligand, can provide a CD28-independent costimulatory signal [59, 60]. However, in several model systems, optimal activation of CD8$^+$ lymphocytes requires signals from both CD28 and CD137 [61]. The CD137 signal enhances cell survival, and in some experimental systems also increases cytokine secretion and effector function [62, 63]. CD137 signaling appears to have greater impact on T-cells recognizing nondominant or weak antigens [64, 65]. Agonist CD137 signals induce proliferation of memory CD8$^+$ cells in an antigen-independent manner, and enhance the recall response of CD8$^+$ T-cells to antigen challenge [66, 67]. CD137 signals also increase survival of CD4$^+$ T-cells late in a primary response, and promote the proliferation or survival of memory CD4$^+$ cells [67–69]. Agonist CD137 antibodies can directly stimulate the cytokine production and the ability of dendritic cells to activate T-cells [70]. In addition, CD137L is expressed by DC, and reverse signaling through CD137L can induce the production of IL-12. CD137 engagement has also been shown to costimulate NKT and NK cell activation [71–73], and to inhibit the suppressive function of CD4$^+$CD25$^+$ T-regulatory cells [49].

Although many or most of the biologic effects of agonist CD137 signals promote tumor immunity, several studies have shown potential immunosuppressive effects, for example, reversal or reduction of autoimmune disease in animal models, and in certain experimental systems, a detrimental effect on antitumor immune responses. Various mechanisms have been implicated, including B-cell depletion [74]; induction of CD4+ T-cell anergy during initial activation, and subsequent loss of T-cell-dependent antibody production [75]; expansion of a CD8+CD11c+ population capable of suppressing CD4+ T-cells, possibly by IFN-gamma-dependent induction of IDO in dendritic cells or by production of TGF-beta [76, 77]; inhibition of Th2 CD4+ responses [78]; enhancement of activation-induced cell death in T-cells; inhibition of human NK cell activity [79]; and increasing the CD11b-Gr-1 myeloid derived suppressor cell population capable of inhibiting both CD4+ and CD8+ T-cell function [80]. Enhancement vs. suppression of response may depend on timing of the agonist CD137 signal during T-cell activation; very early exposure may predispose to activation-induced cell death for both CD4+ and CD8+ cells, while delay of the agonist signal may improve survival and function of the cells. Recent data suggest that agonist CD137 signals concurrently in both T-cells and dendritic cells can result in activation-induced T-cell death through the induction of STAT3 in the dendritic cells [81]. In one model, an anti-human CD137 antibody that is capable of augmenting proliferation of lymphocytes in a mixed lymphocyte reaction (MLR) paradoxically inhibited the antitumor activity of adoptively transferred human lymphocytes against a xenograft in a SCID mouse [82]. Whether the suppression relates to timing of administration, the specific nature of the model, the unique characteristics of the particular antibody, or differences between mouse and human in response of cells remains unclear.

Agonist anti-CD137 antibodies cause delays in tumor growth or tumor regression in several mouse tumor models, suggesting that immune enhancing effects predominate in vivo over immune suppressive effects [83–86]. In some of the models, anti-CD137 causes regression of very large established tumors. Antitumor activity of the CD137 agonist antibodies requires the presence of CD8+ cells, and depending on the mouse tumor model, also CD4+ T-cells, NK cells, and dendritic cells [44, 83, 87]. Antitumor effects have been attributed in part to expansion of a CD8+CD11c+ population capable of producing large amounts of IFN-gamma, although definitive depletion experiments have not been reported [88]. In some models, the antitumor effects are abrogated in hosts lacking the CD40 or IFN-gamma genes, but not in mice lacking the IL-15 gene [85].

As expected from its biological effects, many different combinations of agonist anti-CD137 antibodies with other anticancer agents have shown additive or synergistic antitumor activity in murine models. The list includes 5-fluorouracil [89], cyclophosphamide [90], cisplatin [91], focal radiation [92], defined antigen vaccines including peptides in adjuvant and antigen-loaded dendritic cells [93, 94], whole cell vaccines expressing the GM-CSF gene, agonist OX40 antibodies [35, 95–97], agonist CD40 antibodies [98], depleting CD4 antibodies [99], antagonist anti-CTLA4 antibodies [100], antagonist antibodies against PD1 or B7-H1 (PD-L1) [101], intratumoral injection of IFN-alpha [102], intratumoral injection of TLR agonists [103], and adoptive transfer of antigen-specific CD8+ T-cells [84]. In an orthotopic renal cancer model, combination therapy with anti-DR5, anti-CD40, anti-CD137, and interleukin-2 was required for production of optimal antitumor immune responses [104].

Several of the potential combinations with agonist CD137 signals are noteworthy. The direct effects of chemotherapy or the process of T-cell homeostatic proliferation after lymphopenia may induce CD137 on lymphocytes. Administration of CD137 agonists concurrently or following chemotherapy has been shown to increase the speed and magnitude of lymphocyte recovery [90]. Cisplatin was shown to induce CD137 on kidney tubular epithelium, and combinations of cisplatin with agonist anti-CD137 reduced cisplatin nephrotoxicity in a mouse model [91]. The combination of agonist OX40 and CD137 antibodies resulted in a marked increase in antigen-specific CD8$^+$ T-cells after immunization, associated with increased CD8$^+$ expression of IL-7Rα and CD25 [96, 97]. Combinations of agonist CD137 and blocking anti-CTLA4 antibodies produced increased antitumor effect in some murine models that was CD8$^+$ T-cell-dependent. Interestingly, induction of autoimmune serologic responses by anti-CTLA4, and induction of liver inflammatory infiltrates by anti-CD137, were both reduced by the combination, possibly by increasing the activity of Tregs [100]. Expression of B7-H1 (PD-L1) by tumor was shown to produce resistance to the antitumor effects of agonist anti-CD137, which could be reversed by combining anti-CD137 with blocking antibodies against either B7-H1 or its ligand PD-1, the latter expressed by activated CD8$^+$ cytotoxic T-cells [101]. No studies of anti-CD137 combined with IDO inhibitors have been reported in the literature, although the preclinical data suggest that IDO inhibitors may abrogate part of the anti-CD137-induced immunosuppressive effects.

Various other uses have been found for the CD137-CD137L axis in development of antitumor immunotherapy. The intracellular signaling domain of CD137 has been included in the construction of chimeric antigen receptors for T-cells and imparts a powerful survival signal for the transfected cells [105–107]. Agonist anti-CD137 signals delivered by antibody or by antigen-presenting cells engineered to express CD137L, have been incorporated into the process for extracellular expansion of antigen-specific T-cells intended for adoptive immunotherapy into tumor-bearing hosts [108]. Introduction of CD137L into tumor cells or antigen-delivery vehicles can also enhance their immunogenicity and potential effectiveness as cancer vaccines [109, 110]. Finally, CD137-ligand has been attached to targeting moieties for specific delivery to the tumor microenvironment in the hope of avoiding both the toxicity related to immune activation and the potentially deleterious immune suppressive effects [111–113].

Clinical Experience with Anti-CD137

A fully human IgG4 monoclonal antibody to CD137 was developed for clinical trials by Bristol-Myers Squibb. The antibody did not block binding of the natural CD137-ligand and demonstrated costimulatory activity in vitro human lymphocyte cultures. Toxicology studies showed mild to moderate hepatic inflammation and liver mononuclear cell infiltrate that was IFN-gamma-dependent [114]. The initial phase 1 trial examined IV doses ranging from 0.3 to 15 mg/kg every 3 weeks [115].

After the phase 1 dose escalation was completed, expansion cohorts of approximately 30 patients in each of three disease types including melanoma were randomized to receive 1, 3, or 10 mg/kg. A MTD was not reached, and overall, the drug was well tolerated. The most common toxicities were fatigue (~23%), rash (~19%), pruritis (~12%), fever (~9%), and diarrhea (~9%). Of the latter, less than 5% percent of patients developed grade 3 toxicity, which was limited to fatigue and fever. Grade 3–4 laboratory abnormalities included elevations of transaminases (12–15%), lymphocytopenia (8%), neutropenia (6%), and thrombocytopenia (4%). One patient treated at 6 mg/kg developed severe but eventually reversible liver toxicity manifest as grade 3 transaminases and grade 4 hyperbilirubinemia. Dose-limiting reversible grade 3–4 neutropenia was reported in one patient each treated at 0.3 and 15 mg/kg, respectively.

The half-life of the antibody was estimated at 8–12 days. Peak concentrations ranged from approximately 1–300 μg/mL; trough concentrations at the 0.3 mg/kg dose level were in the range of 0.3 μg/mL, and were greater than 3 μg/mL for all higher dose levels. The investigators reported increases in activated (HLA-DR$^+$) CD4$^+$ and CD8$^+$ lymphocytes at day 8 for patients at dose levels from 1 to 10 mg/kg, increases in IFN-gamma-inducible genes in whole blood at day 8, and increases in serum neopterin at day 8 at all dose levels, but no increase in circulating IFN-gamma, IL-6, or TNFα.

Twenty-three patients with metastatic melanoma were treated in the dose escalation phase and 31 in the expansion cohorts. Twenty-two percent of the 54 total melanoma patients had noncutaneous primaries, 61% had stage M1C disease at study entry, and 80% had received one or more prior treatments. Three patients (6%) met partial response criteria, two of which had disease limited to lymph nodes. Response durations were 22 months, 10+ and 8+ months. Six other patients were progression-free for ≥6 months, including four patients with tumor regression ranging from 5 to 46%.

A four arm randomized phase 2 study in metastatic melanoma was initiated to determine the activity of 0.1, 1, and 5 mg/kg IV every 3 weeks and 1 mg/kg every 6 weeks. The study is listed as completed but results have not been reported to date. No other active melanoma studies are listed as of October, 2010.

CD40

Biology and Preclinical Studies

The cell-surface molecule CD40 is a member of the tumor necrosis factor receptor (TNF) superfamily and is broadly expressed by immune and other normal cells, as well as certain tumor cells [116]. CD40 is best appreciated as a critical regulator of cellular and humoral immunity via its expression on B cells, dendritic cells (DC), and monocytes [117, 118]. CD40-ligand (CD40L), also known as CD154, is the chief ligand for CD40 and is expressed primarily by activated T-cells [118, 119].

In addition, atherosclerosis, graft rejection, coagulation, infection control, and autoimmunity are all regulated by CD40-CD40L interactions [117, 118].

The physiological consequences of CD40 signaling are multifaceted, and potentially biologically opposed, depending on the type of cell expressing CD40 and the microenvironment in which the CD40 signal is provided [116]. Like some other members of the TNF receptor family, CD40 signaling is mediated by adapter molecules rather than by inherent signal-transduction activity of the CD40 cytoplasmic tail. Downstream kinases are activated when the receptor-assembled, multicomponent signaling complex translocates from CD40 to the cytosol [120] and a number of well-characterized signal transduction pathways are activated [121, 122]. These pathways, in turn, regulate alterations in gene expression that are themselves extensive, dynamic, and variable.

Signaling via CD40 activates APC both in vitro and in vivo. Physiologically, this signal represents a molecular prototype for T-cell "help" and mediates in large part the capacity of helper T-cells to "license" APC [123]. Ligation of CD40 on DC, for example, induces increased surface expression of costimulatory and MHC molecules, production of proinflammatory cytokines, and enhanced T-cell triggering [118, 124]. CD40 ligation on resting B cells increases antigen-presenting function and proliferation [118, 124, 125]. Patients with germ-line mutations in CD40 or CD40L are immunosuppressed, susceptible to infections, and have deficient T-dependent immune reactions including IgG and germinal center formation, and memory B cell induction [126–128].

In three separate reports, agonist CD40 antibodies were shown to mimic the signal of CD40L and substitute for the function of CD4+ helper T-cells in murine models of T-cell-mediated immunity [129–131]. A key mechanism of this effect was felt to be CD40/CD40L-mediated activation of host APC, suggesting that CD40 agonists rescue the function of APC in tumor-bearing hosts and restore effective immune responses against tumor-associated antigens. In 1999, three additional reports provided evidence for this hypothesis: agonist CD40 antibodies overcome T-cell tolerance in tumor-bearing mice, evoke effective cytotoxic T-cell responses, and enhance efficacy of antitumor vaccines [132–134].

Data from multiple preclinical models demonstrate synergistic enhancement from combining CD40 agonists with chemotherapy, radiotherapy, tumor vaccines, toll-like receptor agonists, cytokines, and other TNF receptor family agonists [133–138]. The rationale for these approaches is that combining strategies to induce tumor-cell apoptosis with T-cell activation results in greater antitumor responses. CD40-mediated tumor cell death appears at least additive and possibly synergic with chemotherapy both in vitro and in vivo [135, 139, 140]. In a mouse model of tumor implants, an anti-CD40 agonist antibody combined with gemcitabine cured most mice, which were resistant to tumor rechallenge [135]. This effect – dependent on CD8 T-cells and independent of CD4 T-cells – was only seen in vivo in the setting of tumor cell death and only when immunotherapy followed chemotherapy. Similar findings have been reported with cisplatin [141]. These findings fit well with a growing body of evidence demonstrating that chemotherapy can enhance tumor immunogenicity by promoting cross-presentation of tumor antigen [142–144], despite previous dogma that immunotherapy and chemotherapy are incompatible.

CD40 agonists have also been combined with agents that block negative immune checkpoints such as anti-CTLA4 mAb. CTLA-4 is a negative regulator of T-cell activation. Blockade of the CD80/86-CTLA-4 pathway with anti-CTLA-4 mAb enhances antitumor T-cell responses and leads to tumor rejection [145, 146]. In vivo animal studies have shown that the combination of anti-CD40 mAb and anti-CTLA-4 mAb can function as potent and safe immunomodulators that can enhance induction of CTL to tumor vaccines and significantly improve survival in a mouse tumor model [147].

Clinical Experience with CD40 Agonists for Cancer Therapy

Several drug formulations that target the CD40 pathway have undergone phase 1 clinical evaluation in advanced stage cancer patients, and initial results have been promising [116]. Most of these investigational drugs are designed as CD40 agonists, with a twofold rationale. First, CD40 agonists can trigger immune stimulation by activating host APC which then drive T-cell responses directed against tumors to cause tumor cell death. Second, CD40 ligation can impart direct tumor cytotoxicity on tumors that express CD40. Synergy develops if tumor antigens that are shed following a direct cytotoxic hit can be taken up by APCs during the activation process, resulting in tumor specificity to the T-cell response.

In the first test of the hypothesis that CD40 activation may be useful for cancer therapy, CD40 activation was studied in cancer patients using recombinant human CD40-ligand (rhCD40L) [148]. In a study of 32 patients with advanced tumors who received rhCD40L subcutaneously, two patients had an objective partial response (including one long term CR). Clinical efforts to target CD40 accelerated with the advent of agonist anti-CD40 monoclonal antibodies (mAb). Among them, CP-870,893 (Pfizer) is a fully human CD40 agonist mAb [149, 150], an IgG2 immunoglobulin (in contrast to most approved mAb which are IgG1), and is unlikely to activate complement or bind Fc receptors efficiently. Any potential biological effect is felt to be primarily related to CD40 signaling. Binding of CP-870,893 does not compete with ligation by CD154. In the first-in-human study, 29 patients with advanced solid tumors were treated with single i.v. doses of CP-870,893 [151]. Infusion was well tolerated and the MTD was estimated as 0.2 mg/kg [151]. The most common adverse event was transient, grade 1–2 cytokine release syndrome (CRS), associated with elevations in serum TNF-alpha and IL-6. Infusion of CP-870,893 was associated with dose-related, transient and clinically insignificant decreases in peripheral lymphocytes, monocytes, and platelets. Modest, transient elevations in serum D-dimer were observed in most patients treated at the two highest dose levels, but there were no signs of DIC.

Four patients, each with metastatic melanoma, were found to have a partial response (PR) after a single infusion of CP-870,893. PR was evident by regression of lesions in the liver, skin, lung, and muscle. Overall, 14% of all patients (and 27% of patients with melanoma) had objective responses. Seven patients (24%) had stable disease (SD), including one patient with melanoma at the 0.2 mg/kg dose level who had tumor regression that met criteria for SD but not PR. Seven patients with SD or PR were retreated with CP-870,893 without intervening anticancer therapy. One melanoma patient (0.2 mg/kg) had a sustained PR after the second dose and was subsequently treated with nine additional doses. Restaging after six doses showed a near complete resolution of metastatic disease on CT and complete resolution of abnormal FDG tracer activity without evidence for disease. Restaging after her tenth infusion showed complete resolution of preexisting disease on CT, but an isolated thigh lymph node recurrence was resected and CP-870,893 was discontinued. Since then, and without further therapy, the patient has been without evidence of disease, and an April 2010 PET/CT scan was negative (>4 years since the first dose of CP-870,893). These findings suggest potential utility of CP-870,893 in melanoma.

Single-dose pharmacodynamics of CP-870,893 was assessed by flow cytometry of peripheral blood. CP-870,893 infusion resulted in a rapid and dose-dependent decrease in the percentage and absolute count of $CD19^+$ B cells among peripheral blood lymphocytes, evident within 1 h of infusion and sustained for about 2 days. Moreover, there was a marked, rapid, and dose-related upregulation of CD86 on peripheral B cells after infusion. Both the percentage of $CD86^+$ cells among $CD19^+$ B cells and the mean fluorescence intensity (MFI) for CD86 among $CD86^+CD19^+$ B cells increased after infusion [151]. These data suggest that CP-870,893 is an immune activator in vivo, as had been shown in vitro [125, 152]. At the MTD, CP-870,893 was measurable in blood for only 8 h following dosing [151], indicating a short serum half-life in humans (compared to a 3-week half-life of CP-870,893 when injected in mice and suggesting a large in vivo sink of CP-870,893 target antigen). Human-anti-human antibodies were not detected in any patient receiving CP-870,893.

The $HLA-A24^+$ melanoma patient with a sustained PR after multiple doses of CP-870,893 was evaluated for the induction of melanoma-specific $CD8^+$ T-cells after treatment. HLA-A24-binding peptides derived from known melanoma tumor antigens (vs. control peptides from CMV and EBV) were used to stimulate T-cells obtained at baseline and after three infusions of CP-870,893. Cultures were evaluated for production of IFN-gamma in response to 5 h stimulation with peptide-loaded (vs. unloaded) autologous PHA blasts. IFN-gamma response was observed to melanoma peptides by $CD8^+$ T-cells obtained after but not before CP-870,893 treatment (RHV, unpublished). Responses to CMV/EBV peptides were present but unchanged before and after infusion. Overall, this result indicates the induction of functional, melanoma-specific T-cells in this patient with a prolonged clinical response to CP-870,893.

Repeated dosing of CP-870,893 was then evaluated in a phase I study of patients with advanced solid tumor malignancies who received weekly intravenous infusion of CP-870,893 in four dose level cohorts [153]. Twenty-seven patients, including 11 patients with metastatic melanoma, were treated. The most common adverse event was transient, infusion-related CRS, which again defined the MTD as 0.2 mg/kg.

Seven patients (26%) had SD as the best clinical response; no PR or CR were observed. Immunological analysis revealed rapid but transient depletion of CD19+ B cells with each dose of CP-870,893, with CD19+ cell counts returning to baseline by the time of the next infusion. Each weekly infusion also upregulated expression of CD86 and CD54 on B cells, but importantly, expression of CD86 or CD54 did not reset to baseline by the time of subsequent infusions. At the time of the fourth infusion of CP-870,893 (Day 22), for example, the percentage of B cells expressing CD86 was threefold higher than on Day 1, despite that the absolute number of CD19+ B cells was the same between Day 1 and 22. In mice, certain schedules of anti-CD40 monoclonal antibody administration, particularly frequent dosing, can result in deleterious effects on T-cells secondary to hyperstimulation [154, 155]. Subsets of peripheral blood T-cells before and after treatment were therefore studied in the CP-870,893 weekly trial and found that in up to 50% of patients, there were marked reductions of total CD3+ T-cells, involving decreases in both the CD4+ and CD8+ T-cells (median CD4+ decrease, 55%; median CD8+ decrease, 49%). In the majority of patients, CD4+ counts dropped below <200 cells/μL. These studies suggest that weekly CP-870,893 infusion is associated with chronic B cell activation and in some patients, T-cell depletion, suggesting that a longer dosing interval may be desirable for optimal immune pharmacodynamics.

CP-870,893 is also being tested in combination with chemotherapy. In one study, patients with advanced solid tumors, including metastatic melanoma, receive CP-870,893 either 2 or 7 days after carboplatin (AUC 6) and paclitaxel (175 mg/m²), with cycles of therapy repeated every 3 weeks in the absence of tumor progression or dose limiting toxicity. The rationale of the study is based on preclinical animal models demonstrating synergy of combining chemotherapy with CD40 agonist monoclonal antibody, if chemotherapy is delivered first to elicit release of tumor antigens following tumor cell death [135, 141].

Two other anti-CD40 monoclonal antibodies have also been tested in the clinic, as recently reviewed [116, 156]. One, dacetuzumab (formerly SGN-40), is a humanized IgG1 immunoglobulin and a weak agonist of CD40 signaling in blood mononuclear cells, including B cells [157]. Promising clinical results have been reported [158, 159]. A third monoclonal antibody, HCD 122 (formerly known as CHIR-12.12) (Novarits/XOMA) is a fully human IgG1 mAb that mediates ADCC and blocks CD40-ligand-induced cell survival and proliferation of normal and malignant B cells [160, 161].

Other clinical approaches targeting CD40 in cancer include gene therapy to achieve expression of CD40L in autologous tumor cells prior to reinfusion. Patients with chronic lymphocytic leukemia have been administered autologous leukemia cells transduced with adenovirus encoding recombinant CD40L without major toxicity [162, 163]. In another study, leukemic blasts administered with skin fibroblasts transduced with adenoviral vectors encoding human IL-2 and CD40L induced leukemic-specific T-cells and antibodies following repeated injection [164].

A clinical trial testing CP-870,893 in combination with the anti-CTLA-4 mAb tremelimumab for patients with metastatic melanoma is currently underway at the University of Pennsylvania.

Is Systemic CD40 Activation Too Much of a "Good Thing?"

Some concerns have been raised regarding the use of systemic *CD40* activation in humans [154, 165, 166]. As illustrated in mouse models, these include the prospect of inducing systemic autoimmunity [167, 168], accelerated tumor angiogenesis in light of *CD40* expression on endothelium [169], and abolishment of long-term T-cell responses against tumor or viral antigens [154, 155, 170, 171]. One alternative approach to address these concerns is to apply the "licensing" effect of *CD40* activation on APC in a controlled, ex vivo environment without systemic exposure. In this setting, licensed APC could be loaded with antigen and subsequently used as a cell-based vaccine. This approach conceivably would avoid toxic or undesirable effects of systemic in vivo administration of *CD40* monoclonal antibody such as CRS. Both *CD40*-activated, antigen-loaded DC and *CD40*-activated B cells have been studied, the latter of which represent alternative APCs that are able to both prime and boost T-cell responses and can be generated from small blood volumes [172]. For example, RNA as an antigenic payload can be introduced into *CD40*-activated B cells where it induces T-cell responses against tumor rejection antigens [173, 174]. A clinical trial is currently underway at the Veterinary School of the University of Pennsylvania to test the safety and efficacy of tumor RNA loaded *CD40*-activated B cells as a vaccine for privately owned dogs who present with lymphoma [175]. Positive results in this veterinary clinical trial would fuel efforts to test similar strategies in humans.

Conclusions

Several promising agents that provide agonist costimulatory signals to T-cells and DC are in development. Even in early Phase 1 trials, all of the agents have shown activity in patients with metastatic melanoma. While each individual agent may be effective in a small subset of patients, it seems likely that combinations of these agents with each other and with other cytokines, vaccines, chemotherapy, inhibitors of immune regulatory checkpoints, and/or inhibitors of tumor microenvironment immune suppressive factors will be necessary for optimal immune activation and antitumor effects. The careful dissection of the immunobiology of the ligand–receptor pairs, including the kinetics of expression during activation from naïve to memory and effector cells, and the expression and function on different cell subsets, will hopefully provide a rational basis and approach to clinical development.

References

1. Melero I, Hervas-Stubbs S, Glennie M, Pardoll DM, Chen L. Immunostimulatory monoclonal antibodies for cancer therapy. Nat Rev Cancer. 2007;7:95–106.
2. Paterson DJ, Jefferies WA, Green JR, Brandon MR, Corthesy P, Puklavec M, et al. Antigens of activated rat T lymphocytes including a molecule of 50,000 Mr detected only on CD4 positive T blasts. Mol Immunol. 1987;24:1281–90.

3. Baum PR, Gayle III RB, Ramsdell F, Srinivasan S, Sorensen RA, Watson ML, et al. Molecular characterization of murine and human OX40/OX40 ligand systems: identification of a human OX40 ligand as the HTLV-1-regulated protein gp34. EMBO J. 1994;13:3992–4001.
4. Valzasina B, Guiducci C, Dislich H, Killeen N, Weinberg AD, Colombo MP. Triggering of OX40 (CD134) on CD4(+)CD25+ T cells blocks their inhibitory activity: a novel regulatory role for OX40 and its comparison with GITR. Blood. 2005;105:2845–51.
5. Bansal-Pakala P, Halteman BS, Cheng MH, Croft M. Costimulation of CD8 T cell responses by OX40. J Immunol. 2004;172:4821–5.
6. Martin PJ, Ledbetter JA, Morishita Y, June CH, Beatty PG, Hansen JA. A 44 kilodalton cell surface homodimer regulates interleukin 2 production by activated human T lymphocytes. J Immunol. 1986;136:3282–7.
7. Jenkins MK, Mueller D, Schwartz RH, Carding S, Bottomley K, Stadecker MJ, et al. Induction and maintenance of anergy in mature T cells. Adv Exp Med Biol. 1991;292: 167–76.
8. Harding FA, McArthur JG, Gross JA, Raulet DH, Allison JP. CD28-mediated signalling co-stimulates murine T cells and prevents induction of anergy in T-cell clones. Nature. 1992;356:607–9.
9. Chambers CA, Kuhns MS, Egen JG, Allison JP. CTLA-4-mediated inhibition in regulation of T cell responses: mechanisms and manipulation in tumor immunotherapy. Annu Rev Immunol. 2001;19:565–94.
10. Kaleeba JA, Offner H, Vandenbark AA, Lublinski A, Weinberg AD. The OX-40 receptor provides a potent co-stimulatory signal capable of inducing encephalitogenicity in myelin-specific CD4+ T cells. Int Immunol. 1998;10:453–61.
11. Lenschow DJ, Walunas TL, Bluestone JA. CD28/B7 system of T cell costimulation. Annu Rev Immunol. 1996;14:233–58.
12. Gramaglia I, Weinberg AD, Lemon M, Croft M. Ox-40 ligand: a potent costimulatory molecule for sustaining primary CD4 T cell responses. J Immunol. 1998;161:6510–7.
13. Weinberg AD, Vella AT, Croft M. OX-40: life beyond the effector T cell stage. Semin Immunol. 1998;10:471–80.
14. Gramaglia I, Jember A, Pippig SD, Weinberg AD, Killeen N, Croft M. The OX40 costimulatory receptor determines the development of CD4 memory by regulating primary clonal expansion. J Immunol. 2000;165:3043–50.
15. Rogers PR, Song J, Gramaglia I, Killeen N, Croft M. OX40 promotes Bcl-xL and Bcl-2 expression and is essential for long-term survival of CD4 T cells. Immunity. 2001;15: 445–55.
16. Sugamura K, Ishii N, Weinberg AD. Therapeutic targeting of the effector T-cell co-stimulatory molecule OX40. Nat Rev Immunol. 2004;4:420–31.
17. Arch RH, Thompson CB. 4-1BB and Ox40 are members of a tumor necrosis factor (TNF)-nerve growth factor receptor subfamily that bind TNF receptor-associated factors and activate nuclear factor kappaB. Mol Cell Biol. 1998;18:558–65.
18. Weinberg AD, Celnik B, Vainiene M, Buenafe AC, Vandenbark AA, Offner H. The effect of TCR V beta 8 peptide protection and therapy on T cell populations isolated from the spinal cords of Lewis rats with experimental autoimmune encephalomyelitis. J Neuroimmunol. 1994;49:161–70.
19. Buenafe AC, Weinberg AD, Culbertson NE, Vandenbark AA, Offner H. V beta CDR3 motifs associated with BP recognition are enriched in OX-40+ spinal cord T cells of Lewis rats with EAE. J Neurosci Res. 1996;44:562–7.
20. Weinberg AD, Bourdette DN, Sullivan TJ, Lemon M, Wallin JJ, Maziarz R, et al. Selective depletion of myelin-reactive T cells with the anti-OX-40 antibody ameliorates autoimmune encephalomyelitis. Nat Med. 1996;2:183–9.
21. Weinberg AD, Rivera MM, Prell R, Morris A, Ramstad T, Vetto JT, et al. Engagement of the OX-40 receptor in vivo enhances antitumor immunity. J Immunol. 2000;164:2160–9.
22. Weinberg AD. OX40: targeted immunotherapy – implications for tempering autoimmunity and enhancing vaccines. Trends Immunol. 2002;23:102–9.

23. Ramstad T, Lawnicki L, Vetto J, Weinberg A. Immunohistochemical analysis of primary breast tumors and tumor-draining lymph nodes by means of the T-cell costimulatory molecule OX-40. Am J Surg. 2000;179:400–6.

24. Vetto JT, Lum S, Morris A, Sicotte M, Davis J, Lemon M, et al. Presence of the T-cell activation marker OX-40 on tumor infiltrating lymphocytes and draining lymph node cells from patients with melanoma and head and neck cancers. Am J Surg. 1997;174:258–65.

25. Brocker T, Gulbranson-Judge A, Flynn S, Riedinger M, Raykundalia C, Lane P. CD4 T cell traffic control: in vivo evidence that ligation of OX40 on CD4 T cells by OX40-ligand expressed on dendritic cells leads to the accumulation of CD4 T cells in B follicles. Eur J Immunol. 1999;29:1610–6.

26. Murata K, Nose M, Ndhlovu LC, Sato T, Sugamura K, Ishii N. Constitutive OX40/OX40 ligand interaction induces autoimmune-like diseases. J Immunol. 2002;169:4628–36.

27. Maxwell JR, Weinberg A, Prell RA, Vella AT. Danger and OX40 receptor signaling synergize to enhance memory T cell survival by inhibiting peripheral deletion. J Immunol. 2000;164:107–12.

28. Prell RA, Evans DE, Thalhofer C, Shi T, Funatake C, Weinberg AD. OX40-mediated memory T cell generation is TNF receptor-associated factor 2 dependent. J Immunol. 2003;171:5997–6005.

29. Kjaergaard J, Tanaka J, Kim JA, Rothchild K, Weinberg A, Shu S. Therapeutic efficacy of OX-40 receptor antibody depends on tumor immunogenicity and anatomic site of tumor growth. Cancer Res. 2000;60:5514–21.

30. Gri G, Gallo E, Di Carlo E, Musiani P, Colombo MP. OX40 ligand-transduced tumor cell vaccine synergizes with GM-CSF and requires CD40-Apc signaling to boost the host T cell antitumor response. J Immunol. 2003;170:99–106.

31. Kjaergaard J, Peng L, Cohen PA, Drazba JA, Weinberg AD, Shu S. Augmentation versus inhibition: effects of conjunctional OX-40 receptor monoclonal antibody and IL-2 treatment on adoptive immunotherapy of advanced tumor. J Immunol. 2001;167:6669–77.

32. Andarini S, Kikuchi T, Nukiwa M, Pradono P, Suzuki T, Ohkouchi S, et al. Adenovirus vector-mediated in vivo gene transfer of OX40 ligand to tumor cells enhances antitumor immunity of tumor-bearing hosts. Cancer Res. 2004;64:3281–7.

33. Morris A, Vetto JT, Ramstad T, Funatake CJ, Choolun E, Entwisle C, et al. Induction of anti-mammary cancer immunity by engaging the OX-40 receptor in vivo. Breast Cancer Res Treat. 2001;67:71–80.

34. Assudani DP, Ahmad M, Li G, Rees RC, Ali SA. Immunotherapeutic potential of DISC-HSV and OX40L in cancer. Cancer Immunol Immunother. 2006;55:104–11.

35. Cuadros C, Dominguez AL, Lollini PL, Croft M, Mittler RS, Borgstrom P, et al. Vaccination with dendritic cells pulsed with apoptotic tumors in combination with anti-OX40 and anti-4-1BB monoclonal antibodies induces T cell-mediated protective immunity in Her-2/neu transgenic mice. Int J Cancer. 2005;116:934–43.

36. Kuriyama H, Watanabe S, Kjaergaard J, Tamai H, Zheng R, Weinberg AD, et al. Mechanism of third signals provided by IL-12 and OX-40R ligation in eliciting therapeutic immunity following dendritic-tumor fusion vaccination. Cell Immunol. 2006;243:30–40.

37. Melero I, Martinez-Forero I, Dubrot J, Suarez N, Palazon A, Chen L. Palettes of vaccines and immunostimulatory monoclonal antibodies for combination. Clin Cancer Res. 2009;15:1507–9.

38. Murata S, Ladle BH, Kim PS, Lutz ER, Wolpoe ME, Ivie SE, et al. OX40 costimulation synergizes with GM-CSF whole-cell vaccination to overcome established CD8+ T cell tolerance to an endogenous tumor antigen. J Immunol. 2006;176:974–83.

39. Kjaergaard J, Wang LX, Kuriyama H, Shu S, Plautz GE. Active immunotherapy for advanced intracranial murine tumors by using dendritic cell-tumor cell fusion vaccines. J Neurosurg. 2005;103:156–64.

40. Ruby CE, Montler R, Zheng R, Shu S, Weinberg AD. IL-12 is required for anti-OX40-mediated CD4 T cell survival. J Immunol. 2008;180:2140–8.

41. Hirschhorn-Cymerman D, Rizzuto GA, Merghoub T, Cohen AD, Avogadri F, Lesokhin AM, et al. OX40 engagement and chemotherapy combination provides potent antitumor immunity with concomitant regulatory T cell apoptosis. J Exp Med. 2009;206:1103–16.

42. Weinberg AD, Thalhofer C, Morris N, Walker JM, Seiss D, Wong S, et al. Anti-OX40 (CD134) administration to nonhuman primates: immunostimulatory effects and toxicokinetic study. J Immunother. 2006;29:575–85.

43. Schwarz H, Arden K, Lotz M. CD137, a member of the tumor necrosis factor receptor family, is located on chromosome 1p36, in a cluster of related genes, and colocalizes with several malignancies. Biochem Biophys Res Commun. 1997;235:699–703.

44. Melero I, Johnston JV, Shufford WW, Mittler RS, Chen L. NK1.1 cells express 4-1BB (CDw137) costimulatory molecule and are required for tumor immunity elicited by anti-4-1BB monoclonal antibodies. Cell Immunol. 1998;190:167–72.

45. Heinisch IV, Daigle I, Knopfli B, Simon HU. CD137 activation abrogates granulocyte-macrophage colony-stimulating factor-mediated anti-apoptosis in neutrophils. Eur J Immunol. 2000;30:3441–6.

46. Broll K, Richter G, Pauly S, Hofstaedter F, Schwarz H. CD137 expression in tumor vessel walls. High correlation with malignant tumors. Am J Clin Pathol. 2001;115:543–9.

47. Heinisch IV, Bizer C, Volgger W, Simon HU. Functional CD137 receptors are expressed by eosinophils from patients with IgE-mediated allergic responses but not by eosinophils from patients with non-IgE-mediated eosinophilic disorders. J Allergy Clin Immunol. 2001;108:21–8.

48. Wilcox RA, Chapoval AI, Gorski KS, Otsuji M, Shin T, Flies DB, et al. Cutting edge: expression of functional CD137 receptor by dendritic cells. J Immunol. 2002;168:4262–7.

49. Choi BK, Bae JS, Choi EM, Kang WJ, Sakaguchi S, Vinay DS, et al. 4-1BB-dependent inhibition of immunosuppression by activated CD4+ CD25+ T cells. J Leukoc Biol. 2004;75:785–91.

50. Vinay DS, Choi BK, Bae JS, Kim WY, Gebhardt BM, Kwon BS. CD137-deficient mice have reduced NK/NKT cell numbers and function, are resistant to lipopolysaccharide-induced shock syndromes, and have lower IL-4 responses. J Immunol. 2004;173:4218–29.

51. Nishimoto H, Lee SW, Hong H, Potter KG, Maeda-Yamamoto M, Kinoshita T, et al. Costimulation of mast cells by 4-1BB, a member of the tumor necrosis factor receptor superfamily, with the high-affinity IgE receptor. Blood. 2005;106:4241–8.

52. Wang Q, Zhang P, Zhang Q, Wang X, Li J, Ma C, et al. Analysis of CD137 and CD137L expression in human primary tumor tissues. Croat Med J. 2008;49:192–200.

53. Boussaud V, Soler P, Moreau J, Goodwin RG, Hance AJ. Expression of three members of the TNF-R family of receptors (4-1BB, lymphotoxin-beta receptor, and Fas) in human lung. Eur Respir J. 1998;12:926–31.

54. Lisignoli G, Toneguzzi S, Cattini L, Pozzi C, Facchini A. Different expression pattern of cytokine receptors by human osteosarcoma cell lines. Int J Oncol. 1998;12:899–903.

55. Zhou Z, Kim S, Hurtado J, Lee ZH, Kim KK, Pollok KE, et al. Characterization of human homologue of 4-1BB and its ligand. Immunol Lett. 1995;45:67–73.

56. Salih HR, Schmetzer HM, Burke C, Starling GC, Dunn R, Pelka-Fleischer R, et al. Soluble CD137 (4-1BB) ligand is released following leukocyte activation and is found in sera of patients with hematological malignancies. J Immunol. 2001;167:4059–66.

57. Melero I, Murillo O, Dubrot J, Hervas-Stubbs S, Perez-Gracia JL. Multi-layered action mechanisms of CD137 (4-1BB)-targeted immunotherapies. Trends Pharmacol Sci. 2008;29:383–90.

58. Lynch DH. The promise of 4-1BB (CD137)-mediated immunomodulation and the immunotherapy of cancer. Immunol Rev. 2008;222:277–86.

59. Guinn BA, Bertram EM, DeBenedette MA, Berinstein NL, Watts TH. 4-1BBL enhances antitumor responses in the presence or absence of CD28 but CD28 is required for protective immunity against parental tumors. Cell Immunol. 2001;210:56–65.

60. Bukczynski J, Wen T, Watts TH. Costimulation of human CD28- T cells by 4-1BB ligand. Eur J Immunol. 2003;33:446–54.

61. Diehl L, van Mierlo GJ, den Boer AT, van der Voort E, Fransen M, van Bostelen L, et al. In vivo triggering through 4-1BB enables Th-independent priming of CTL in the presence of an intact CD28 costimulatory pathway. J Immunol. 2002;168:3755–62.

62. Laderach D, Movassagh M, Johnson A, Mittler RS, Galy A. 4-1BB co-stimulation enhances human CD8(+) T cell priming by augmenting the proliferation and survival of effector CD8(+) T cells. Int Immunol. 2002;14:1155–67.

63. May Jr KF, Chen L, Zheng P, Liu Y. Anti-4-1BB monoclonal antibody enhances rejection of large tumor burden by promoting survival but not clonal expansion of tumor-specific CD8+ T cells. Cancer Res. 2002;62:3459–65.

64. Halstead ES, Mueller YM, Altman JD, Katsikis PD. In vivo stimulation of CD137 broadens primary antiviral CD8+ T cell responses. Nat Immunol. 2002;3:536–41.

65. DeBenedette MA, Wen T, Bachmann MF, Ohashi PS, Barber BH, Stocking KL, et al. Analysis of 4-1BB ligand (4-1BBL)-deficient mice and of mice lacking both 4-1BBL and CD28 reveals a role for 4-1BBL in skin allograft rejection and in the cytotoxic T cell response to influenza virus. J Immunol. 1999;163:4833–41.

66. Bertram EM, Lau P, Watts TH. Temporal segregation of 4-1BB versus CD28-mediated costimulation: 4-1BB ligand influences T cell numbers late in the primary response and regulates the size of the T cell memory response following influenza infection. J Immunol. 2002;168:3777–85.

67. Zhu Y, Zhu G, Luo L, Flies AS, Chen L. CD137 stimulation delivers an antigen-independent growth signal for T lymphocytes with memory phenotype. Blood. 2007;109:4882–9.

68. Blazar BR, Kwon BS, Panoskaltsis-Mortari A, Kwak KB, Peschon JJ, Taylor PA. Ligation of 4-1BB (CDw137) regulates graft-versus-host disease, graft-versus-leukemia, and graft rejection in allogeneic bone marrow transplant recipients. J Immunol. 2001;166:3174–83.

69. Cannons JL, Lau P, Ghumman B, DeBenedette MA, Yagita H, Okumura K, et al. 4-1BB ligand induces cell division, sustains survival, and enhances effector function of CD4 and CD8 T cells with similar efficacy. J Immunol. 2001;167:1313–24.

70. Choi BK, Kim YH, Kwon PM, Lee SC, Kang SW, Kim MS, et al. 4-1BB functions as a survival factor in dendritic cells. J Immunol. 2009;182:4107–15.

71. Wilcox RA, Tamada K, Strome SE, Chen L. Signaling through NK cell-associated CD137 promotes both helper function for CD8+ cytolytic T cells and responsiveness to IL-2 but not cytolytic activity. J Immunol. 2002;169:4230–6.

72. Kim DH, Chang WS, Lee YS, Lee KA, Kim YK, Kwon BS, et al. 4-1BB engagement costimulates NKT cell activation and exacerbates NKT cell ligand-induced airway hyperresponsiveness and inflammation. J Immunol. 2008;180:2062–8.

73. Lin W, Voskens CJ, Zhang X, Schindler DG, Wood A, Burch E, et al. Fc-dependent expression of CD137 on human NK cells: insights into "agonistic" effects of anti-CD137 monoclonal antibodies. Blood. 2008;112:699–707.

74. Zhu G, Flies DB, Tamada K, Sun Y, Rodriguez M, Fu YX, et al. Progressive depletion of peripheral B lymphocytes in 4-1BB (CD137) ligand/I-E(alpha)-transgenic mice. J Immunol. 2001;167:2671–6.

75. Foell J, Strahotin S, O'Neil SP, McCausland MM, Suwyn C, Haber M, et al. CD137 costimulatory T cell receptor engagement reverses acute disease in lupus-prone NZB x NZW F1 mice. J Clin Invest. 2003;111:1505–18.

76. Kim YH, Choi BK, Kang WJ, Kim KH, Kang SW, Mellor AL, et al. IFN-gamma-indoleamine-2,3 dioxygenase acts as a major suppressive factor in 4-1BB-mediated immune suppression in vivo. J Leukoc Biol. 2009;85:817–25.

77. Vinay DS, Kim CH, Choi BK, Kwon BS. Origins and functional basis of regulatory CD11c+ CD8+ T cells. Eur J Immunol. 2009;39:1552–63.

78. Sun Y, Blink SE, Liu W, Lee Y, Chen B, Solway J, et al. Inhibition of Th2-mediated allergic airway inflammatory disease by CD137 costimulation. J Immunol. 2006;177:814–21.

79. Baessler T, Charton JE, Schmiedel BJ, Grunebach F, Krusch M, Wacker A, et al. CD137 ligand mediates opposite effects in human and mouse NK cells and impairs NK-cell reactivity against human acute myeloid leukemia cells. Blood. 2010;115:3058–69.

80. Lee JM, Seo JH, Kim YJ, Kim YS, Ko HJ, Kang CY. Agonistic anti-CD137 monoclonal antibody treatment induces CD11bGr-1 myeloid-derived suppressor cells. Immune Netw. 2010;10:104–8.

81. Zhang B, Zhang Y, Niu L, Vella AT, Mittler RS. Dendritic cells and Stat3 are essential for CD137-induced CD8 T cell activation-induced cell death. J Immunol. 2010;184:4770–8.

82. Sabel MS, Conway TF, Chen FA, Bankert RB. Monoclonal antibodies directed against the T-cell activation molecule CD137 (interleukin-A or 4-1BB) block human lymphocyte-mediated suppression of tumor xenografts in severe combined immunodeficient mice. J Immunother. 2000;23:362–8.

83. Melero I, Shuford WW, Newby SA, Aruffo A, Ledbetter JA, Hellstrom KE, et al. Monoclonal antibodies against the 4-1BB T-cell activation molecule eradicate established tumors. Nat Med. 1997;3:682–5.

84. Kim JA, Averbook BJ, Chambers K, Rothchild K, Kjaergaard J, Papay R, et al. Divergent effects of 4-1BB antibodies on antitumor immunity and on tumor-reactive T-cell generation. Cancer Res. 2001;61:2031–7.

85. Miller RE, Jones J, Le T, Whitmore J, Boiani N, Gliniak B, et al. 4-1BB-specific monoclonal antibody promotes the generation of tumor-specific immune responses by direct activation of CD8 T cells in a CD40-dependent manner. J Immunol. 2002;169:1792–800.

86. Murillo O, Arina A, Hervas-Stubbs S, Gupta A, McCluskey B, Dubrot J, et al. Therapeutic antitumor efficacy of anti-CD137 agonistic monoclonal antibody in mouse models of myeloma. Clin Cancer Res. 2008;14:6895–906.

87. Murillo O, Dubrot J, Palazon A, Arina A, Azpilikueta A, Alfaro C, et al. In vivo depletion of DC impairs the anti-tumor effect of agonistic anti-CD137 mAb. Eur J Immunol. 2009;39:2424–36.

88. Ju SA, Park SM, Lee SC, Kwon BS, Kim BS. Marked expansion of CD11c+ CD8+ T-cells in melanoma-bearing mice induced by anti-4-1BB monoclonal antibody. Mol Cells. 2007;24:132–8.

89. Ju SA, Cheon SH, Park SM, Tam NQ, Kim YM, An WG, et al. Eradication of established renal cell carcinoma by a combination of 5-fluorouracil and anti-4-1BB monoclonal antibody in mice. Int J Cancer. 2008;122:2784–90.

90. Kim YH, Choi BK, Oh HS, Kang WJ, Mittler RS, Kwon BS. Mechanisms involved in synergistic anticancer effects of anti-4-1BB and cyclophosphamide therapy. Mol Cancer Ther. 2009;8:469–78.

91. Kim YH, Choi BK, Kim KH, Kang SW, Kwon BS. Combination therapy with cisplatin and anti-4-1BB: synergistic anticancer effects and amelioration of cisplatin-induced nephrotoxicity. Cancer Res. 2008;68:7264–9.

92. Shi W, Siemann DW. Augmented antitumor effects of radiation therapy by 4-1BB antibody (BMS-469492) treatment. Anticancer Res. 2006;26:3445–53.

93. Wilcox RA, Flies DB, Zhu G, Johnson AJ, Tamada K, Chapoval AI, et al. Provision of antigen and CD137 signaling breaks immunological ignorance, promoting regression of poorly immunogenic tumors. J Clin Invest. 2002;109:651–9.

94. Li B, Lin J, Vanroey M, Jure-Kunkel M, Jooss K. Established B16 tumors are rejected following treatment with GM-CSF-secreting tumor cell immunotherapy in combination with anti-4-1BB mAb. Clin Immunol. 2007;125:76–87.

95. Dawicki W, Bertram EM, Sharpe AH, Watts TH. 4-1BB and OX40 act independently to facilitate robust CD8 and CD4 recall responses. J Immunol. 2004;173:5944–51.

96. Lee SJ, Myers L, Muralimohan G, Dai J, Qiao Y, Li Z, et al. 4-1BB and OX40 dual costimulation synergistically stimulate primary specific CD8 T cells for robust effector function. J Immunol. 2004;173:3002–12.

97. Lee SJ, Rossi RJ, Lee SK, Croft M, Kwon BS, Mittler RS, et al. CD134 costimulation couples the CD137 pathway to induce production of supereffector CD8 T cells that become IL-7 dependent. J Immunol. 2007;179:2203–14.

98. Gray JC, French RR, James S, Al-Shamkhani A, Johnson PW, Glennie MJ. Optimising antitumour CD8 T-cell responses using combinations of immunomodulatory antibodies. Eur J Immunol. 2008;38:2499–511.

99. Choi BK, Kim YH, Kang WJ, Lee SK, Kim KH, Shin SM, et al. Mechanisms involved in synergistic anticancer immunity of anti-4-1BB and anti-CD4 therapy. Cancer Res. 2007;67: 8891–9.
100. Kocak E, Lute K, Chang X, May Jr KF, Exten KR, Zhang H, et al. Combination therapy with anti-CTL antigen-4 and anti-4-1BB antibodies enhances cancer immunity and reduces autoimmunity. Cancer Res. 2006;66:7276–84.
101. Hirano F, Kaneko K, Tamura H, Dong H, Wang S, Ichikawa M, et al. Blockade of B7-H1 and PD-1 by monoclonal antibodies potentiates cancer therapeutic immunity. Cancer Res. 2005;65:1089–96.
102. Dubrot J, Palazon A, Alfaro C, Azpilikueta A, Ochoa MC, Rouzaut A, et al. Intratumoral injection of interferon-alpha and systemic delivery of agonist anti-CD137 monoclonal antibodies synergize for immunotherapy. Int J Cancer. 2011;128(1):105–18.
103. Westwood JA, Haynes NM, Sharkey J, McLaughlin N, Pegram HJ, Schwendener RA, et al. Toll-like receptor triggering and T-Cell costimulation induce potent antitumor immunity in mice. Clin Cancer Res. 2009;15:7624–33.
104. Westwood JA, Darcy PK, Guru PM, Sharkey J, Pegram HJ, Amos SM, et al. Three agonist antibodies in combination with high-dose IL-2 eradicate orthotopic kidney cancer in mice. J Transl Med. 2010;8:42.
105. Stephan MT, Ponomarev V, Brentjens RJ, Chang AH, Dobrenkov KV, Heller G, et al. T cell-encoded CD80 and 4-1BBL induce auto- and transcostimulation, resulting in potent tumor rejection. Nat Med. 2007;13:1440–9.
106. Milone MC, Fish JD, Carpenito C, Carroll RG, Binder GK, Teachey D, et al. Chimeric receptors containing CD137 signal transduction domains mediate enhanced survival of T cells and increased antileukemic efficacy in vivo. Mol Ther. 2009;17:1453–64.
107. Zhao Y, Wang QJ, Yang S, Kochenderfer JN, Zheng Z, Zhong X, et al. A herceptin-based chimeric antigen receptor with modified signaling domains leads to enhanced survival of transduced T lymphocytes and antitumor activity. J Immunol. 2009;183:5563–74.
108. Zhang H, Snyder KM, Suhoski MM, Maus MV, Kapoor V, June CH, et al. 4-1BB is superior to CD28 costimulation for generating CD8+ cytotoxic lymphocytes for adoptive immunotherapy. J Immunol. 2007;179:4910–8.
109. Kudo-Saito C, Hodge JW, Kwak H, Kim-Schulze S, Schlom J, Kaufman HL. 4-1BB ligand enhances tumor-specific immunity of poxvirus vaccines. Vaccine. 2006;24:4975–86.
110. Wiethe C, Dittmar K, Doan T, Lindenmaier W, Tindle R. Provision of 4-1BB ligand enhances effector and memory CTL responses generated by immunization with dendritic cells expressing a human tumor-associated antigen. J Immunol. 2003;170:2912–22.
111. Yang Y, Yang S, Ye Z, Jaffar J, Zhou Y, Cutter E, et al. Tumor cells expressing anti-CD137 scFv induce a tumor-destructive environment. Cancer Res. 2007;67:2339–44.
112. Zhang N, Sadun RE, Arias RS, Flanagan ML, Sachsman SM, Nien YC, et al. Targeted and untargeted CD137L fusion proteins for the immunotherapy of experimental solid tumors. Clin Cancer Res. 2007;13:2758–67.
113. Muller D, Frey K, Kontermann RE. A novel antibody-4-1BBL fusion protein for targeted costimulation in cancer immunotherapy. J Immunother. 2008;31:714–22.
114. Dubrot J, Milheiro F, Alfaro C, Palazon A, Martinez-Forero I, Perez-Gracia JL, et al. Treatment with anti-CD137 mAbs causes intense accumulations of liver T cells without selective antitumor immunotherapeutic effects in this organ. Cancer Immunol Immunother. 2010;59:1223–33.
115. Sznol M, Hodi FS, Margolin K, McDermott DF, Ernstoff MS, Kirkwood JM, et al. Phase I study of BMS-663513, a fully human anti-CD137 agonist monoclonal antibody, in patients (pts) with advanced cancer (CA). J Clin Oncol. 2008;26:abstr 3007.
116. Vonderheide RH. Prospect of targeting the CD40 pathway for cancer therapy. Clin Cancer Res. 2007;13:1083–8.
117. Grewal IS, Flavell RA. CD40 and CD154 in cell-mediated immunity. Annu Rev Immunol. 1998;16:111–35.
118. van Kooten C, Banchereau J. CD40-CD40 ligand. J Leukoc Biol. 2000;67:2–17.

119. Armitage RJ, Fanslow WC, Strockbine L, Sato TA, Clifford KN, Macduff BM, et al. Molecular and biological characterization of a murine ligand for CD40. Nature. 1992;357:80–2.
120. Matsuzawa A, Tseng PH, Vallabhapurapu S, Luo JL, Zhang W, Wang H, et al. Essential cytoplasmic translocation of a cytokine receptor-assembled signaling complex. Science. 2008;321:663–8.
121. Dadgostar H, Zarnegar B, Hoffmann A, Qin XF, Truong U, Rao G, et al. Cooperation of multiple signaling pathways in CD40-regulated gene expression in B lymphocytes. Proc Natl Acad Sci USA. 2002;99:1497–502.
122. Gallagher E, Enzler T, Matsuzawa A, Anzelon-Mills A, Otero D, Holzer R, et al. Kinase MEKK1 is required for CD40-dependent activation of the kinases Jnk and p38, germinal center formation, B cell proliferation and antibody production. Nat Immunol. 2007;8:57–63.
123. Lanzavecchia A. Immunology. Licence to kill. Nature. 1998;393:413–4.
124. Quezada SA, Jarvinen LZ, Lind EF, Noelle RJ. CD40/CD154 interactions at the interface of tolerance and immunity. Annu Rev Immunol. 2004;22:307–28.
125. Carpenter EL, Mick R, Ruter J, Vonderheide RH. Activation of human B cells by the agonist CD40 antibody CP-870,893 and augmentation with simultaneous toll-like receptor 9 stimulation. J Transl Med. 2009;7:93.
126. Allen RC, Armitage RJ, Conley ME, Rosenblatt H, Jenkins NA, Copeland NG, et al. CD40 ligand gene defects responsible for X-linked hyper-IgM syndrome. Science. 1993;259:990–3.
127. Ferrari S, Giliani S, Insalaco A, Al-Ghonaium A, Soresina AR, Loubser M, et al. Mutations of CD40 gene cause an autosomal recessive form of immunodeficiency with hyper IgM. Proc Natl Acad Sci USA. 2001;98:12614–9.
128. Etzioni A, Ochs HD. The hyper IgM syndrome – an evolving story. Pediatr Res. 2004;56: 519–25.
129. Bennett SR, Carbone FR, Karamalis F, Flavell RA, Miller JF, Heath WR. Help for cytotoxic-T-cell responses is mediated by CD40 signalling. Nature. 1998;393:478–80.
130. Ridge JP, Di Rosa F, Matzinger P. A conditioned dendritic cell can be a temporal bridge between a CD4+ T- helper and a T-killer cell. Nature. 1998;393:474–8.
131. Schoenberger SP, Toes RE, van der Voort EI, Offringa R, Melief CJ. T-cell help for cytotoxic T lymphocytes is mediated by CD40-CD40L interactions. Nature. 1998;393:480–3.
132. French RR, Chan HT, Tutt AL, Glennie MJ. CD40 antibody evokes a cytotoxic T-cell response that eradicates lymphoma and bypasses T-cell help. Nat Med. 1999;5:548–53.
133. Diehl L, den Boer AT, Schoenberger SP, van der Voort EI, Schumacher TN, Melief CJ, et al. CD40 activation in vivo overcomes peptide-induced peripheral cytotoxic T-lymphocyte tolerance and augments anti-tumor vaccine efficacy. Nat Med. 1999;5:774–9.
134. Sotomayor EM, Borrello I, Tubb E, Rattis FM, Bien H, Lu Z, et al. Conversion of tumor-specific CD4+ T-cell tolerance to T-cell priming through in vivo ligation of CD40. Nat Med. 1999;5:780–7.
135. Nowak AK, Robinson BW, Lake RA. Synergy between chemotherapy and immunotherapy in the treatment of established murine solid tumors. Cancer Res. 2003;63:4490–6.
136. Ahonen CL, Doxsee CL, McGurran SM, Riter TR, Wade WF, Barth RJ, et al. Combined TLR and CD40 triggering induces potent CD8+ T cell expansion with variable dependence on type I IFN. J Exp Med. 2004;199:775–84.
137. Uno T, Takeda K, Kojima Y, Yoshizawa H, Akiba H, Mittler RS, et al. Eradication of established tumors in mice by a combination antibody-based therapy. Nat Med. 2006;12:693–8.
138. Ahonen CL, Wasiuk A, Fuse S, Turk MJ, Ernstoff MS, Suriawinata AA, et al. Enhanced efficacy and reduced toxicity of multifactorial adjuvants compared with unitary adjuvants as cancer vaccines. Blood. 2008;111:3116–25.
139. Eliopoulos AG, Dawson CW, Mosialos G, Floettmann JE, Rowe M, Armitage RJ, et al. CD40-induced growth inhibition in epithelial cells is mimicked by Epstein-Barr Virus-encoded LMP1: involvement of TRAF3 as a common mediator. Oncogene. 1996;13:2243–54.
140. Ghamande S, Hylander BL, Oflazoglu E, Lele S, Fanslow W, Repasky EA. Recombinant CD40 ligand therapy has significant antitumor effects on CD40-positive ovarian tumor xeno-

grafts grown in SCID mice and demonstrates an augmented effect with cisplatin. Cancer Res. 2001;61:7556–62.

141. Nowak A, Mahendran S, Van der Most R, RA L. Cisplatin and pemetrexed synergizes with immunotherapy to result in cures in established murine malignant mesothelioma. Proc AACR meeting. 2008;2008:Abstract 2073.

142. Gabrilovich DI. Combination of chemotherapy and immunotherapy for cancer: a paradigm revisited. Lancet Oncol. 2007;8:2–3.

143. Zitvogel L, Apetoh L, Ghiringhelli F, Kroemer G. Immunological aspects of cancer chemotherapy. Nat Rev Immunol. 2008;8:59–73.

144. Zitvogel L, Apetoh L, Ghiringhelli F, Andre F, Tesniere A, Kroemer G. The anticancer immune response: indispensable for therapeutic success? J Clin Invest. 2008;118:1991–2001.

145. Leach DR, Krummel MF, Allison JP. Enhancement of antitumor immunity by CTLA-4 blockade. Science. 1996;271:1734–6.

146. Yang YF, Zou JP, Mu J, Wijesuriya R, Ono S, Walunas T, et al. Enhanced induction of antitumor T-cell responses by cytotoxic T lymphocyte-associated molecule-4 blockade: the effect is manifested only at the restricted tumor-bearing stages. Cancer Res. 1997;57:4036–41.

147. Ito D, Ogasawara K, Iwabuchi K, Inuyama Y, Onoe K. Induction of CTL responses by simultaneous administration of liposomal peptide vaccine with anti-CD40 and anti-CTLA-4 mAb. J Immunol. 2000;164:1230–5.

148. Vonderheide RH, Dutcher JP, Anderson JE, Eckhardt SG, Stephans KF, Razvillas B, et al. Phase I study of recombinant human CD40 ligand in cancer patients. J Clin Oncol. 2001;19:3280–7.

149. Gladue R, Cole S, Donovan C, Paradis T, Alpert R, Natoli E, et al. In vivo efficacy of the CD40 agonist antibody CP-870,893 against a broad range of tumor types: impact of tumor CD40 expression, dendritic cells, and chemotherapy. J Clin Oncol. 2006;24(18S):103s.

150. Bedian V, Donovan C, Garder J, Natoli E, Paradis T, Alpert R, et al. In vitro characterization and pre-clinical pharmacokinetics of CP-870,893, a human anti-CD40 agonist antibody. J Clin Oncol. 2006;24(18S):109s.

151. Vonderheide RH, Flaherty KT, Khalil M, Stumacher MS, Bajor DL, Hutnick NA, et al. Clinical activity and immune modulation in cancer patients treated with CP-870,893, a novel CD40 agonist monoclonal antibody. J Clin Oncol. 2007;25:876–83.

152. Hunter TB, Alsarraj M, Gladue RP, Bedian V, Antonia SJ. An agonist antibody specific for CD40 induces dendritic cell maturation and promotes autologous anti-tumour T-cell responses in an in vitro mixed autologous tumour cell/lymph node cell model. Scand J Immunol. 2007;65:479–86.

153. Ruter J, Antonia SJ, Burris III HA, Huhn RD, Vonderheide RH. Immune modulation with weekly dosing of an agonist CD40 antibody in a phase I study of patients with advanced solid tumors. Cancer Biol Ther. 2010;10(10):983–93.

154. Kedl RM, Jordan M, Potter T, Kappler J, Marrack P, Dow S. CD40 stimulation accelerates deletion of tumor-specific CD8(+) T cells in the absence of tumor-antigen vaccination. Proc Natl Acad Sci USA. 2001;98:10811–6.

155. Berner V, Liu H, Zhou Q, Alderson KL, Sun K, Weiss JM, et al. IFN-gamma mediates CD4+ T-cell loss and impairs secondary antitumor responses after successful initial immunotherapy. Nat Med. 2007;13:354–60.

156. Khalil M, Vonderheide RH. Anti-CD40 agonist antibodies: preclinical and clinical experience. Update Cancer Ther. 2007;2(2):61–5.

157. Law CL, Gordon KA, Collier J, Klussman K, McEarchern JA, Cerveny CG, et al. Preclinical antilymphoma activity of a humanized anti-CD40 monoclonal antibody, SGN-40. Cancer Res. 2005;65:8331–8.

158. Hussein M, Berenson JR, Niesvizky R, Munshi N, Matous J, Sobecks R, et al. A phase I multidose study of dacetuzumab (SGN-40; humanized anti-CD40 monoclonal antibody) in patients with multiple myeloma. Haematologica. 2010;95:845–8.

159. Furman RR, Forero-Torres A, Shustov A, Drachman JG. A phase I study of dacetuzumab (SGN-40, a humanized anti-CD40 monoclonal antibody) in patients with chronic lymphocytic leukemia. Leuk Lymphoma. 2010;51:228–35.
160. Tong X, Georgakis GV, Long L, O'Brien S, Younes A, Luqman M. In vitro activity of a novel fully human anti-CD40 antibody CHIR-12.12 in chronic lymphocytic leukemia: blockade of CD40 activation and induction of ADCC. Blood. 2005;106:Abstract 2504.
161. Luqman M, Klabunde S, Lin K, Georgakis GV, Cherukuri A, Holash J, et al. The antileukemia activity of a human anti-CD40 antagonist antibody, HCD122, on human chronic lymphocytic leukemia cells. Blood. 2008;112:711–20.
162. Wierda WG, Cantwell MJ, Woods SJ, Rassenti LZ, Prussak CE, Kipps TJ. CD40-ligand (CD154) gene therapy for chronic lymphocytic leukemia. Blood. 2000;96:2917–24.
163. Fukuda T, Chen L, Endo T, Tang L, Lu D, Castro JE, et al. Antisera induced by infusions of autologous Ad-CD154-leukemia B cells identify ROR1 as an oncofetal antigen and receptor for Wnt5a. Proc Natl Acad Sci USA. 2008;105:3047–52.
164. Rousseau RF, Biagi E, Dutour A, Yvon ES, Brown MP, Lin T, et al. Immunotherapy of high-risk acute leukemia with a recipient (autologous) vaccine expressing transgenic human CD40L and IL-2 after chemotherapy and allogeneic stem cell transplantation. Blood. 2006;107:1332–41.
165. Bergmann S, Pandolfi PP. Giving blood: a new role for CD40 in tumorigenesis. J Exp Med. 2006;203:2409–12.
166. Haanen JB, Schumacher TN. Vaccine leads to memory loss. Nat Med. 2007;13:248–50.
167. Roth E, Schwartzkopff J, Pircher H. CD40 ligation in the presence of self-reactive CD8 T cells leads to severe immunopathology. J Immunol. 2002;168:5124–9.
168. Ichikawa HT, Williams LP, Segal BM. Activation of APCs through CD40 or Toll-like receptor 9 overcomes tolerance and precipitates autoimmune disease. J Immunol. 2002;169:2781–7.
169. Chiodoni C, Iezzi M, Guiducci C, Sangaletti S, Alessandrini I, Ratti C, et al. Triggering CD40 on endothelial cells contributes to tumor growth. J Exp Med. 2006;203:2441–50.
170. Mauri C, Mars LT, Londei M. Therapeutic activity of agonistic monoclonal antibodies against CD40 in a chronic autoimmune inflammatory process. Nat Med. 2000;6:673–9.
171. Bartholdy C, Kauffmann SO, Christensen JP, Thomsen AR. Agonistic anti-CD40 antibody profoundly suppresses the immune response to infection with lymphocytic choriomeningitis virus. J Immunol. 2007;178:1662–70.
172. Schultze JL. Vaccination as immunotherapy for B cell lymphoma [in process citation]. Hematol Oncol. 1997;15:129–39.
173. Coughlin CM, Fleming MD, Carroll RG, Pawel BR, Hogarty MD, Shan X, et al. Immunosurveillance and survivin-specific T-cell immunity in children with high-risk neuroblastoma. J Clin Oncol. 2006;24:5725–34.
174. Coughlin CM, Vance BA, Grupp SA, Vonderheide RH. RNA-transfected CD40-activated B cells induce functional T-cell responses against viral and tumor antigen targets: implications for pediatric immunotherapy. Blood. 2004;103:2046–54.
175. Mason NJ, Coughlin CM, Overley B, Cohen JN, Mitchell EL, Colligon TA, et al. RNA-loaded CD40-activated B cells stimulate antigen-specific T-cell responses in dogs with spontaneous lymphoma. Gene Ther. 2008;15:955–65.
176. Gought MJ, Crittenden MR, Safff M, Pang P, Seung SK, Vetto JT, Hu Hm, Re mond WL, Holland J, Wesingere AD. Adjuvand Therapy with agonistic antibodies to CD134 (OX40) increase local control after surgical or radition Therapy of cancer in mice. I immunother 2010; 33(8):789–809.

Chapter 17
Novel Cytokines for Immunotherapy of Melanoma

Shailender Bhatia and John A. Thompson

Abstract Modulation of the immune system using cytokines, most notably interleukin-2 (IL-2) and interferon-α (IFN-α), has been the mainstay of immunotherapy of melanoma for more than a decade. High-dose IL-2 has been associated with durable complete responses (CR) in a subset of metastatic melanoma and renal cell carcinoma (RCC) patients, providing proof-of-concept for successful use of cytokine immunotherapy. IFN-α as adjuvant therapy of high-risk melanoma is associated with improved relapse-free survival and in some studies, a modest improvement in overall survival. However, the therapeutic utility of IL-2 and IFN-α is limited by low response rates, significant treatment-associated toxicities and the paucity of biomarkers predictive of response to therapy. With the recent advances in our understanding of tumor immunology, it is apparent that the tumor immune microenvironment is extremely complex with several obstacles to the successful use of immunotherapeutic modalities. The use of novel cytokines with unique immunomodulatory properties, as well as the investigation of novel methods of cytokine delivery, has the potential to circumvent some of these obstacles. This chapter focuses on some of the novel cytokine-based immunotherapeutic approaches that appear promising for the treatment of melanoma.

Keywords Cancer immunotherapy • Cytokine immunotherapy • Novel cytokines • Interleukin (IL) • IL-21 • IL-12 • IL-15 • Cytokine delivery • Intratumoral therapy • Melanoma immunotherapy • Tumor microenvironment

S. Bhatia, MD (✉) • J.A. Thompson, MD
Department of Medicine, Division of Medical Oncology, University of Washington
School of Medicine, Fred Hutchinson Cancer Research Center, Seattle Cancer Care Alliance,
825 Eastlake Ave E, Mailstop G4-830, Seattle, WA 98109, USA
e-mail: sbhatia@u.washington.edu

T.F. Gajewski and F.S. Hodi (eds.), *Targeted Therapeutics in Melanoma*,
Current Clinical Oncology, DOI 10.1007/978-1-61779-407-0_17,
© Springer Science+Business Media, LLC 2012

The Ideal Cytokine for Cancer Immunotherapy

The ideal cytokine for cancer immunotherapy should:

1. Possess potent immunostimulatory properties, so as to overcome the multiple mechanisms of immune-evasion by the tumors. These characteristics may lead not only to the stimulation of innate and adaptive immune responses against cancer, but also to the generation of memory responses for long-lasting immunity.
2. Not induce a paradoxical suppression of the immune system (such as proliferation of regulatory T-cells or activation-induced cell death [AICD] attributed to IL-2).
3. Have minimal acute as well as long-term toxicity, and should ideally be specific for cancer so as to avoid autoimmune toxicities.
4. Combine well with other cancer therapies, including chemotherapy, antiangiogenic therapies, targeted agents as well as alternative immunotherapeutic approaches such as cancer vaccines, adoptive cell therapy, or immune checkpoint blockade drugs.

The emerging novel cytokine therapies that are discussed below possess one or more of the characteristics described above and may lead to improved patient outcomes in melanoma and other cancers. We focus mainly on Interleukin-12 and Interleukin-21, both of which have been tested in several clinical trials in melanoma and other tumor types. We also briefly discuss other novel cytokines such as Interleukin-15 and cytokine-delivery approaches that appear promising for immunotherapy of cancers.

Interleukin-12

Interleukin-12 (IL-12) is a 70-kDa heterodimeric, multifunctional protein consisting of two subunits, a 35-kDa light chain (known as p35 or IL-12α) and a 40 kDa heavy chain (known as p35 or IL-12β) linked by a disulfide bond [40, 87]. It was first discovered in 1989 as "Natural killer cell stimulatory factor" and independently by another group in 1990 as "Cytotoxic lymphocyte maturation factor" [40, 80]. Soon afterward, it was recognized as a master regulator of adaptive type 1 cell-mediated immunity, as IL-12 production by innate immune cells in response to microbial pathogens was shown to polarize the naïve CD4$^+$ T-cells toward the T-helper-1 (T_H1) phenotype [33]. IL-12 was also found to induce the production of IFN-γ from, as well as increase the proliferation and cytotoxicity of, NK cells and T-cells [9].

Biological Properties of IL-12

IL-12 is produced primarily by activated inflammatory cells (monocytes, macrophages, neutrophils, and dendritic cells) [15, 49]. Both genes encoding the two subunits of IL-12 need to be expressed together in the same cell to lead to the secretion of the active heterodimeric form of IL-12. The mRNA of p35 is expressed widely, but the expression of p40 seems to be restricted to the phagocytic cells and dendritic cells (DCs). Microbial products such as CpG-containing oligonucleotides, double-stranded RNA, and bacterial DNA are strong inducers of IL-12 production by phagocytes and DCs, likely through the engagement of Toll-like receptors (TLRs) on these cells. The production of IL-12 heterodimer seems to be amplified by the presence of IFN-γ or other enhancing cytokines; this effect of IFN-γ on IL-12 production is more pronounced in phagocytic cells than in DCs and leads to a positive feedback mechanism during inflammatory and T_H1 responses [48].

The IL-12 receptor (IL-12R) is composed of two chains – IL-12Rβ1 and IL-12Rβ2; coexpression of both these chains is required for generation of high-affinity IL-12 binding sites [65]. The IL-12Rβ2 subunit functions as the signal-transducing component of the receptor complex; signal transduction occurs through the Janus kinase (JAK)–STAT (signal transducer and activator of transcription) pathways. Activation of STAT4 appears to be the dominant mechanism in relaying the specific cellular effects of IL-12 [36, 83]. IL-12R is expressed mainly by activated T cells and NK cells, but is also present on other cell types, such as DCs and B cells [65]. Low level expression of IL-12R on resting NK cells explains the ability of these cells to respond rapidly to IL-12. Most resting T cells do not have detectable levels of IL-12R. Activation of T cells through the T cell receptor (TCR) upregulates the transcription and expression of both chains of IL-12R, and this upregulation, particularly that of the β2-chain, is enhanced by the presence of other cytokines such as IFN-α, IFN-γ, tumor-necrosis factor (TNF), and IL-12 itself, and also by costimulation through CD28. In T cells, the expression of IL-12Rβ2 is confined to T_H1 cells, and its expression correlates with responsiveness to IL-12 [70, 82].

As would be expected from the IL-12R expression patterns, IL-12 does not induce the proliferation of resting T or NK cells, but has a direct proliferative effect on preactivated T cell and NK cells, and induces the production by these cells of IFN-γ and other cytokines [80]. It also enhances the cytolytic activity of cytotoxic T-lymphocytes (CTLs) and NK cells by inducing the transcription of genes that encode cytolytic effector molecules such as perforin and granzymes. IL-12 also appears to be a potent inducer of the T_H1-type immune responses by facilitating the optimal differentiation of naïve CD4$^+$ T cells into the T_H1 cells; these cells are irreversibly primed to produce high levels of IFN-γ upon restimulation [33].

Antitumor Activity of IL-12 in Preclinical Models

The biological properties of IL-12 described above led to an extensive investigation of the antitumor efficacy of IL-12 in many preclinical models, as well as in clinical trials. Many of the preclinical IL-12 studies for the treatment of cancer were conducted in poorly immunogenic and metastatic murine models such as the B16 melanoma model [1, 21, 32, 45, 46, 73]. Despite poor immunogenicity, limited regression of established, primary tumors and the prevention of new metastases were reported in these models [1, 74]. Tumor regression induced by IL-12 therapy likely involves multiple mechanisms. A direct action of IL-12 on tumor cells is unlikely as in vitro studies involving coincubation of tumor cells with IL-12 did not result in tumor cell death [9]. Regression of tumors after IL-12 therapy appears dependent on CD8+ T cells [9]. T cells have been implicated in other studies as the critical cell type for IL-12 induced tumor regression and memory responses [7, 23, 86]. In addition to the antigen specific effects of T cells, IL-12 immunotherapy results in the production of IFN-γ. Induction of IFN-γ plays a critical role in tumor rejection, but injection of IFN-γ alone may not be as potent for regression [9]. Recent studies have shown that IL-12 also acts to upregulate the expression of HLA class I and II, as well as ICAM-1 on human cancer cells (melanoma), which may increase their immunogenicity [96]. IL-12 immunotherapy also results in the inhibition of angiogenesis via mechanisms not thoroughly elucidated, although both IFN-γ and NK cells have been implicated [25, 76, 95]. IL-12 immunotherapy also combined effectively with both peptide-based and cell-based antitumor vaccines leading to regression of established tumors in murine models suggesting a potential role for the use of IL-12 as an adjuvant in vaccination strategies [57, 66].

Encouraged by these unique biological properties and the promising preclinical data mentioned above, recombinant IL-12 (rIL-12) was actively investigated in the treatment of advanced solid tumors and hematologic malignancies, both as a monotherapy and in combination with other therapies.

Clinical Investigation of IL-12 in Cancer Immunotherapy

Systemic administration of IL-12: In the first phase I dose escalation trial, a total of 40 patients, including 20 with renal cancer and 12 with melanoma, were enrolled; the patients received, starting 2 weeks after a single test dose of rIL-12, a regimen of once daily intravenous rIL-12 injections for 5 days repeated every 3 weeks [2]. The maximum tolerated dose (MTD) was 500 ng/kg. Common clinical toxicities included fever/chills, fatigue, nausea, vomiting, and headache; laboratory abnormalities included cytopenias, hypoalbuminemia, hyperglycemia, and hepatic function test abnormalities. Dose-limiting toxicities (DLTs) included oral stomatitis and hepatic dysfunction, mostly elevated transaminases. A transient complete response in a patient with melanoma and one partial response (PR) in a patient with renal cell cancer were documented. Biological effects included dose-dependent increases in circulating IFN-γ and neopterin levels and transient lymphopenia. IL-12-induced lymphopenia involved all of the major lymphocyte subsets, although NK cells seemed to be the most profoundly affected and CD4+ T cells were relatively spared [67]. The kinetics of lymphocyte recovery was different from those seen with IL-2, with a slower recovery and lack of rebound lymphocytosis. The data also suggested that rIL-12 could reverse the defects in NK cell and T-cell functions that are usually seen with advanced cancer [67].

In a subsequent phase II study, 17 RCC patients received the same daily IV dose of rIL-12 at the same schedule as the above trial, albeit without the test dose [14]. Shockingly, most patients had severe toxicities including treatment-related deaths in two patients; the toxicities affected multiple organ systems. These intriguing findings were confirmed in mice and cynomologus monkeys: the animals did not develop severe toxicity if they were given a single dose of IL-12, a rest period, and then multiple doses; however, multiple high doses of IL-12 were highly toxic if they were given without an initial single dose [14]. The profound difference in toxicity associated with relatively minor variation in the schedule of administration of IL-12 was thought to be due to down-modulation of the inflammatory response with sequential doses of rIL-12. Indeed, in the phase I trial, the peak IFN-γ levels tended to diminish with repetitive 5-day multiple dose cycles of rIL-12 [2].

Two separate phase I dose-escalation clinical trials investigated the subcutaneous (SC) administration of rIL-12 on days 1, 8, and 15 of a 28-day cycle in patients with RCC and melanoma, respectively. The RCC trial used a fixed-dose schedule initially and found the MTD to be 1 mcg/kg; DLTs included increase in transaminase concentration, pulmonary toxicity, and leukopenia. The toxicities were most pronounced after the first dose and attenuated rapidly with the subsequent cycles. Using an up-titration scheme, in which the doses were escalated weekly to the final stable dose, the MTD was 1.5 mcg/kg. One patient had a CR, and 34 patients had stable disease (SD). The second study enrolled ten patients with MM who were all treated with a fixed dose of 0.5 mcg/kg [3]. No partial or complete responses were documented, but tumor shrinkage involving subcutaneous metastases, superficial adenopathy, and hepatic metastases was observed. Correlative immune monitoring in the peripheral blood of these patients indicated that rIL-12 administration induced a striking burst of HLA-restricted CTL precursors directed to autologous tumors and to an immunogenic tumor-associated antigen (Melan-A/Mart-126-35 peptide) [55]. Most interestingly, infiltration of neoplastic tissue by CD8+ T cells with a memory and cytolytic phenotype was identified by immunohistochemistry in all available biopsies of the posttreatment metastatic lesions.

In another phase I study using a rIL-12 administration schedule based on twice-weekly IV injections for 6 weeks, the blood levels of IFN-γ, IL-15, and IL-18 were found to be elevated in treated patients [26]. Despite the immunological effects of rIL-12, the clinical efficacy was disappointing with no objective responses seen in the eight patients with MM. Interestingly, whereas IFN-γ and IL-15 induction was attenuated during the first cycle in patients with progressive disease (PD), those patients with tumor regression or stable disease (SD) showed sustained higher levels of IFN-γ, IL-15, and IL-18. This observation suggested the need for strategies to sustain the induction of IFN-γ; based on in vitro data, addition of IL-2 was proposed as one such strategy. In a subsequent study, 28 patients were treated with 6-week cycles of twice-weekly IV rIL-12 with the addition of SC IL-2 midway through cycle 1 [27]. There was one PR and two pathologic responses, all of which occurred in patients with melanoma. When administered at the MTD, IL-2 significantly augmented IFN-γ production by rIL-12 and led to a threefold expansion of NK cells.

Systemic administration of rIL-12 has also been used in combination with other approaches such as peptide vaccination with mixed results [11, 42, 63]. In a trial of 48 patients with resected stage III or IV melanoma who were immunized with peptides derived from tyrosinase and gp100, with or without SC administration of rIL-12, rIL-12 augmented peptide-specific delayed-type hypersensitivity reactivity to the gp100 antigen in 34 of 40 patients [42]. Further, the gp100-specific and tyrosinase-specific peripheral immune response, as measured by IFN-γ release were enhanced by the treatment in 37 of 42 patients. In another trial, 28 metastatic melanoma patients with Melan-A expressing tumors were enrolled to receive Melan-A$_{26-35}$ and influenza matrix$_{58-66}$ peptides intradermally in combination with various doses of rIL-12 SC or IV [11]. Clinical responses were mostly mixed, with only one CR in a patient with low volume subcutaneous disease and one PR in a patient with hepatic metastases. Tumor biopsies revealed infiltration of CD4$^+$ and CD8$^+$ T cells capable of lysing a Melan-A/Mart-1 peptide-pulsed target in vitro. In a phase II trial of 20 pretreated patients with advanced melanoma received autologous peripheral blood mononuclear cells pulsed with tumor-antigen peptides (Melan-A/Mart-1) plus SC rIL-12 [63]. Two patients with numerous metastases achieved a complete response and several other patients had minor or mixed responses or SD. A significant association was observed between an increased number of Melan-A-specific T cells and clinical outcome.

Local administration of IL-12: Systemic administration of rIL-12 in patients has been limited by considerable toxicity. In addition to the toxic side effects, high rIL-12 dosage levels have been linked to temporary immune suppression, which would be unfavorable for effective immunotherapy [26, 58]. Studies in a colon carcinoma model and a fibrosarcoma tumor model have shown that the amount of IFN-γ generated at the tumor site is the key in effecting tumor regression [12, 30, 53, 99]. These observations led to clinical trials designed to deliver IL-12 directly to the tumor, in forms other than recombinant protein. Localized delivery of IL-12 cDNA to the tumor site has been achieved through local administration of IL-12 cDNA via direct injection of IL-12 plasmid, of viral vectors, or of modified fibroblasts, autologous tumor cells, or dendritic cells that were engineered to secrete IL-12 [21, 31, 35, 45, 46, 50, 52, 53, 81, 88]. A recent clinical trial attempting local delivery of IL-12 involved intratumoral injection of IL-12 plasmid DNA followed by in vivo electroporation to enhance the efficiency of transfection [16]. Seven dose cohorts with a total of 24 patients were treated in this study at various doses of IL-12 plasmid (0.1–1.6 mg/mL) with treatment administered on days 1, 5, and 8. The experimental regimen was found to be safe and well tolerated, with minimal systemic toxicity and no significant IL-12 spillage into circulation. Most (76%) electroporated lesions demonstrated necrosis (>20%) at the time of follow-up biopsy or excision after the last injection. Four of 19 patients, who had distant disease, had evidence of distant responses including three CRs. All three CRs occurred in the setting of patients with disseminated progressive cutaneous lesions. An immune mechanism of action was suggested for these responses, which occurred over a span of 6–18 months and were associated with hypopigmentation and gradual regression of tumors at sites distinct from the electroporated sites. Six additional patients had stable disease lasting from 4–20 months at distant sites. A phase II trial is currently being developed in patients with melanoma.

In summary, IL-12 is a potent immunomodulatory cytokine with promising antitumor efficacy. The integration of IL-12 as a vaccine adjuvant has shown improved priming against tumor antigens. Local delivery of IL-12 in the vicinity of tumor cells may result in immune-stimulatory responses against tumor cells, while minimizing systemic side-effects.

Interleukin-21

Interleukin-21 (IL-21) is a type-I cytokine with close homology to IL-2, IL-4, and IL-15; the receptors of these cytokines (and other cytokines such as IL-7 and IL-9) share the common cytokine-receptor γ-chain (γ_c). The IL-21-receptor (IL-21R) and IL-21 system was discovered in 2000 [59, 60]. Since its discovery, a broad range of actions have been ascribed to the IL-21 system with important implications for several human diseases, including cancer. The biological characteristics of IL-21 and the data from clinical investigation of IL-21 for treatment of cancer are summarized below.

Biological Properties of IL-21

IL-21 is produced primarily by activated CD4[+] T cells [60]. IL-21 signals through the IL-21 receptor complex, which is a heterodimeric complex comprised of the IL-21R and the common γ_c chain. IL-21R is expressed preferentially by NK cells, B cells and activated T cells, which explains the major actions of IL-21 on these cell types [59, 60]. The IL-21 system distinguishes itself from the other γ_c-dependent cytokines by activating primarily STAT1 and STAT3 (and more weakly, STAT5A and STAT5B) for signal transduction; this is in contrast to the other γ_c cytokines which signal primarily through other STAT molecules (for example, STAT5A and STAT5B by IL-2, IL-7, IL-9, and IL-15, and STAT 6 by IL-4) [43, 59, 60].

IL-21 serves as a T-cell comitogen, augmenting the proliferation of T-cells in response to other primary signals [60]. IL-21 has a marked synergistic effect on the in vitro proliferation of CD8[+] T cells in combination with either IL-7 or IL-15; however, IL-21 alone had little effect [97]. This combination of cytokines also led to increases in the expression of granzyme B in CD8[+] T cells and in the number of IFN-γ-producing CD8[+] T cells, illustrating the effects of IL-21 on clonal expansion and effector function of CD8[+] T cells. The synergistic effects of these cytokines occur for both naïve and memory phenotype CD8[+] T cells [97]. These findings suggest the possible role of IL-21 in activation, expansion, and prolonged survival of antigen-specific CD8-cytotoxic T lymphocytes. Unlike IL-2, however, IL-21 does not result in AICD of antigen-specific CD8[+] T cells [54]. Rather, these antigen-specific CD8[+] T cells can survive long-term while maintaining effector activity, a property shared by IL-15. Hence, IL-21 likely has a unique role in initiation and maintenance of a CD8[+] T cell response that may be critical for achieving durable immunity. The functional effects of IL-21 on CD4[+] T cells are less well characterized and are probably more limited. Importantly, IL-21 (unlike IL-2) renders CD4[+] T cells resistant to regulatory T cell suppression and does not enhance proliferation of regulatory T cells [62].

IL-21 also appears to have important roles in the terminal differentiation and activation of natural killer cells [60, 61]. In combination with IL-7, IL-15, and other factors, IL-21 enhances the generation of NK cells from bone-marrow progenitors in vitro [77]. IL-21 augments the acquisition of a fully functional cytotoxic state by NK cells, by inducing the expression of killer inhibitory receptors (KIRs) and the production of IFN-γ by NK cells [77]. Interestingly, higher doses of IL-21 can induce apoptosis of NK cells coincident with the enhanced effector function of the cells, which is inhibited by the addition of IL-15 [8, 37]. Besides its effects on T-cells and NK-cells, IL-21 has also been associated with an enhancement of T cell-dependent B cell proliferation, plasma cell differentiation and immunoglobulin production [60]. IL-21 has also been associated with angiostatic activity [10].

Antitumor Activity of IL-21 in Preclinical Models

Potent antitumor effects of IL-21 have been reported in various preclinical cancer models [20, 54, 78, 92]. The antitumor activity of IL-21 may be mediated by its effects on either NK cells or CD8+ T-cells or both. Treatment of tumor-bearing mice with IL-21 plasmid DNA with subsequent generation of high levels of circulating IL-21 resulted in significant inhibition of growth of B16 melanoma or MCA205 fibrosarcoma [92]. This antitumor activity was considerably reduced by in vivo depletion of NK cells, but not by depletion of CD4+ or CD8+ T cells; importantly, the toxicity of the high systemic levels of IL-21 was markedly reduced as compared to the toxicity usually seen with the high levels of IL-2 required to activate NK cells. In another murine model, B16F1 and MethA fibrosarcoma tumor cells that were engineered to express IL-21 were completely rejected in vivo [47]. In this model, antitumor activity was dependent on the presence of both CD8+ T cells and NK cells. IL-21 supported the generation of IFN-γ-secreting Ag-specific T cells along with augmentation of the CTL activity. These effects were independent of IFN-γ and other cytokines, but required perforin, thus suggesting a critical role for perforin-mediated cytotoxicity. However, in another study using the IL-21 expressing murine mammary adenocarcinoma cells, the IL-21-mediated tumor rejection by CD8+ T-cells was dependent on IFN-γ, although, IFN-γ-independent effects were also evident [20]. In a comparative evaluation of IL-2, IL-15, and IL-21 in a syngeneic thymoma model, the antitumor benefit of IL-21 was completely lost with CD8+ T-cell depletion [54]. Interestingly, the depletion of NK cells significantly reduced the median survival time, but not the frequency of long-term survivors. This suggested that the innate immune responses may be more relevant in the initial stages of antitumor benefit from IL-21, but that CD8+ T-cells are indispensable for durable antitumor immunity. Similar to IL-2, IL-21 enhanced Ag-specific CD8+ T-cell activation and clonal expansion. Unlike IL-2, IL-21 did not result in AICD, but rather these IL-21-enhanced activated CD8+ T cells survived while maintaining effector activity [54]. Hence, IL-21 has a unique ability to behave in certain respects like both IL-2 and IL-15 and this special property could prove helpful in inducing durable immunity. This overlap in properties was also reflected by a demonstration of synergistic effects of IL-21 and IL-15 in a murine melanoma model treated with adoptively transferred CD8+ T cells [97]. In this model, IL-21 and IL-15 monotherapy after adoptive transfer of T cells induced partial tumor regressions, but combination therapy led to complete regressions and prolonged survival.

The encouraging results from the various preclinical models and the above-mentioned unique biological properties of IL-21 have generated considerable interest in the clinical investigation of recombinant IL-21 (rIL-21) for the treatment of melanoma as well as for other advanced solid tumors and hematologic malignancies, either as monotherapy, or in combination with other therapies.

Clinical Investigation of IL-21 in Cancer Immunotherapy

Recombinant IL-21 (rIL-21) therapy has been investigated in several human clinical trials [18, 19, 84]. A phase I trial of intravenous rIL-21 monotherapy was conducted in patients with metastatic MM and RCC; 43 patients (24MM; 19RCC) were treated at various dose-levels of rIL-21 ranging from 3 to 100 mcg/kg/day [84]. rIL-21 was administered as two 5-day cycles on days 1 through 5 and 15 through 19 of a treatment course by rapid daily IV infusion in an outpatient setting. Most clinical adverse events were mild during the dose-escalation phase of the study and DLTs primarily consisted of transient grade 3 laboratory abnormalities including hyponatremia, cytopenias, hyperbilirubinemia, and hypophosphatemia. The MTD was determined to be 30 mcg/kg/day; overall, a total of 34 patients were treated at this dose level. Common adverse events included transient and reversible flu-like symptoms, pruritus, and skin rash. No capillary leak syndrome was observed at any dose level. Common laboratory abnormalities were also mild and included cytopenias, elevation in hepatic transaminases, bilirubin, or triglycerides and decreases in albumin, calcium, magnesium, phosphorus, or sodium. Retreatment with rIL-21 was not associated with increased toxicity, with the exception of one patient who developed reversible toxic hepatonecrosis in the second treatment course. Pharmacodynamic effects of rIL-21 included dose-dependent increases in serum concentration of soluble CD25 (sCD25 or IL-2Rα); since sCD25 is cleaved from T and NK cells on activation, this suggests possible IL-21-mediated activation of these cells in patients [34]. Treatment was associated with promising antitumor effects. Among the 24 MM patients, the best responses were CR in 1 patient and SD in 11 patients. Among the 19 RCC patients, 17 patients had achieved SD or better on study (including 4 patients with PR, 13 with SD). In some patients, repeat treatment with rIL-21 was associated with progressive shrinkage of tumors. Responses were seen across all tumor sites including visceral metastases, and in patients who had received prior high-dose IL-2.

Another phase I study investigated two different schedules of IV administration of rIL-21 in patients with metastatic MM [19]. One schedule, the 5 + 9 schedule, used daily dosing of rIL-21 for 5 days in weeks 1, 3, and 5 of an 8-week-long cycle (total of 15 doses in one cycle). The other schedule, the 3/week schedule, consisted of administration of rIL-21 three times each week for the first 6 weeks of an 8-week-long cycle (total of 18 doses in a cycle). The first dose was administered in the hospital for safety evaluation, but the rest of the treatment was administered in the outpatient setting. The MTD for both schedules was determined to be 30 mcg/kg/day and was the recommended dose for future investigation, although some patients in the 5 + 9 schedule of administration were able to tolerate higher dose levels. The most common AEs were fatigue, fever, nausea, headaches, vomiting, rash, myalgias, and anorexia. There were no significant differences in the pharmacokinetic parameters and the safety profile of the two schedules. Pharmacodynamic assays revealed dose-dependent increases in sCD25 levels, and an upregulation of perforin-1 and granzyme B mRNA levels in purified peripheral blood CD8+ T cells and NK cells. These findings suggested an activation of the cytolytic CD8+ T-cells and NK cells. The clinical efficacy was modest with SD as the best outcome in nine patients, although one patient had a CR that was ongoing at 32 months at the last report.

The promising efficacy signals from phase I studies mentioned above have led to further investigation of rIL-21 monotherapy in melanoma. In a phase II trial, 24 patients with metastatic melanoma and no prior systemic therapy for metastatic disease were treated with rIL-21 monotherapy at the 30 mcg/kg/day dose per the 5 + 9 schedule mentioned above [18]. The objective response rate was a modest 8% including 1 CR and 1 PR, both of which lasted only a few weeks. Consistent with prior studies, serum sCD25 levels and mRNA expression levels of perforin, IFN-γ, and granzyme B in purified peripheral blood CD8+ T cells and NK cells were increased suggesting activation of these cell types. The proportion of CD25+ NK cells and CD25+CD8+ T cells also increased significantly suggesting activation of these cells. In the CD4+ T cell subpopulation, however, no increase in the percentage of CD25+ cells was seen. Notably, the frequency of CD4+CD25bright cells did not increase. This is consistent with the differential effects of rIL-21 on various lymphocytic subsets seen in preclinical studies.

Another phase II trial tested rIL-21 monotherapy in previously untreated patients with metastatic melanoma [64]. In this trial, patients with bulky disease (defines as ≥5 cm) or with brain metastases were excluded. The majority of the enrolled patients were treated at the 30 mcg/kg/day dose of rIL-21 according to the 5 + 9 schedule described above (daily dosing of rIL-21 for 5 days in weeks 1, 3, and 5 of an 8-week-long cycle, i.e., a total of 15 doses in one cycle). Toxicities were similar to those seen in previous trials. The efficacy was promising with 23% of evaluable patients achieving a PR and 40% with SD; the median progression-free survival was 4.3 months and the median duration of response was 5 months. Based on these results, a randomized phase II study comparing rIL-21 with dacarbazine is currently underway in treatment-naïve patients with metastatic melanoma who do not have bulky disease and brain metastases.

In light of the tolerability of rIL-21 monotherapy and evidence of antitumor activity, several combinations of rIL-21 with other emerging therapies have been explored as well. Our group has been involved in the investigation of rIL-21 in combination with sorafenib in patients with metastatic RCC. A total of 52 patients were treated in this phase 1/2 study [6]. Treatment was administered in the outpatient setting; rIL-21 was administered on days 1–5 and 15–19 of every 7-week cycle and sorafenib was self-administered daily at the standard dose (starting at 800 mg/day). The MTD of rIL-21 in combination with sorafenib was 30 mcg/kg/day. The safety profile of the combination was acceptable with majority of the AEs at the MTD of rIL-21 being grade 1 or 2. The toxicities were similar to those observed with either agent alone in previous trials. The antitumor efficacy of this combination appears promising with ORR of 24%, DCR of 82% and PFS of 5.7 months in a previously treated patient population; the results compare favorably to that seen with sorafenib monotherapy in treatment-naïve or pretreated patient populations. Two patients have had durable partial responses (near CR with persistent small residual masses) that are ongoing at 34+ months and 25+ months after treatment initiation (unpublished data).

Another clinical trial investigated the combination of rIL-21 and rituximab in subjects with relapsed, indolent CD20+ B cell lymphomas who had received at least one prior course of systemic therapy [85]. The combination rIL-21 with rituximab was well tolerated and associated with an ORR of 33% in a heavily pretreated patient population. These data suggest the potential feasibility of combination of rIL-21 with some of the emerging targeted therapies for metastatic melanoma, including BRAF inhibitors.

In summary, IL-21 is a novel cytokine with unique immunomodulatory properties that make it an attractive candidate for immunotherapy of cancer. Recombinant IL-21 has been safely administered in the outpatient setting with an acceptable toxicity profile. The preliminary investigations have revealed promising antitumor efficacy in several tumor types, including melanoma. The combinations of rIL-21 with other treatment modalities appear feasible and promising. Further investigation of this cytokine in cancer immunotherapy is ongoing and worth developing further.

Interleukin-15 (IL-15)

Interleukin-15 was independently discovered by two groups in 1994 as a 14–15 kDa cytokine, which interacted with the IL-2Rβ chain and possessed an ability to stimulate T-cell and NK-cell proliferation, just like IL-2 [4, 28]. Similar to IL-2, the receptor for IL-15 (IL-15R) is heterotrimeric; in fact, IL-2R and IL-15R share a common β chain (IL-2/15Rβ) and the common cytokine-receptor γ-chain (γ_c). This sharing of receptor subunits explains the redundancy in the actions of these two cytokines. Indeed, both cytokines stimulate the proliferation of T cells and the generation of CTLs, the proliferation and activation of NK cells, and the proliferation of, and synthesis of immunoglobulins by, B cells [41, 90, 91, 98]. However, the high-affinity receptors for IL-2 and IL-15 contain a unique third subunit for each cytokine: IL-2Rα and IL-15Rα, respectively; this difference in α subunit also explains, at least partially, the unique properties and functional differences of IL-15 as compared to IL-2. These differences have considerable implications for the optimal use of these cytokines in treatment of human diseases.

Biological Properties of IL-15

IL-15 mRNA is constitutively expressed by a large variety of tissues; however, the detection of IL-15 protein appears to be most restricted to monocytes, epithelial cells, DCs, and fibroblasts. In contrast to IL-2, IL-15 is only secreted in small quantities and is primarily membrane-bound. IL-15Rα is expressed primarily by activated monocytes and DCs (as compared to IL-2Rα, which is expressed primarily by activated T-cells and B-cells); the IL-15 and IL-15Rα expressed by these monocytes and DCs then become associated on the cell surface and can result in persistence of membrane-bound IL-15Rα associated with IL-15. This IL-15 is presented by IL-15Rα *in-trans* to cells that express IL-12/15Rβ and γ_c including NK cells and CD8[+] memory T-cells, hence explaining the important role of this cytokine in in vivo persistence of NK cells and mature CD8[+] memory T cells. This is an important distinction from IL-2 which inhibits the persistence of CD8[+] memory T cells [41]. IL-15 overexpressing mice have increased number of and activation of NK cells; since IL-15Rα is constitutively expressed in NK progenitor cells and IL-15Rα[-/-] mice are deficient in mature NK cells, IL-15 appears to play a critical role in NK cell development [44]. Also, in sharp contrast to the pivotal role of IL-2 in elimination of self-reactive T cells through AICD, IL-15 opposes IL-2 induced AICD [51]. These various properties of IL-15, including proliferation and activation of T-cells and NK cells, inhibition of AICD and facilitation of persistence of CD8[+] memory T cells, are especially appealing for the treatment of cancer and for vaccination against infectious pathogens.

Indeed, IL-15 has been reported to have promising antitumor activity in several preclinical investigations; this antitumor activity seems to be mediated through NK cells, CD8[+] T-cells, and possibly other independent mechanisms [17, 22, 24, 39, 72, 89, 94]. This encouraging preclinical data has led to considerable interest in clinical investigation of IL-15-based immunotherapeutic approaches. At a 2007 NCI immunotherapy workshop, IL-15 was considered as having the highest potential for successful use in cancer immunotherapy [13]. A phase-I dose-escalation trial of recombinant human IL-15 in patients with metastatic melanoma and RCC is ongoing (www.clinicaltrials.gov identifier # NCT01021059).

Other Promising Cytokines

Besides IL-12, IL-21, and IL-15, there is considerable interest in clinical investigation of several other cytokines for immunotherapy of cancer. Granulocyte-macrophage colony stimulating factor (GM-CSF) and IFN-α continue to be investigated extensively, either as monotherapy or as an adjuvant in vaccination and other approaches. Interleukin-7 (IL-7) has generated a lot of interest due to its unique roles in T cell development, and in survival and expansion of naive T cells in the periphery. IL-7 is particularly appealing as a vaccine adjuvant or as an immunorestorative T cell growth factor for naive T cells, especially in patients with prior lymphodepleting chemotherapy or elderly patients [13]. In two separate phase I clinical trials, treatment with recombinant human IL-7 (rhIL-7) led to a marked expansion in the number of CD4+ and CD8+ T-cells in the periphery; contrary to IL-2, the CD4+ T_{reg} cells were relatively decreased [71, 79]. Studies of rhIL-7, as monotherapy or in combination with vaccines, are ongoing in patients with malignancy and infectious diseases. Interleukin-18 (IL-18), a member of the interleukin-1 superfamily of cytokines, is an immunostimulatory cytokine that regulates innate as well as both Th1- and Th2-driven adaptive immune responses [29, 56]. IL-18 enhances IFN-γ production by, and augments the cytolytic activity of, T cells and NK cells, and promotes the differentiation of CD4+ T cells into helper effector cells; it acts synergistically with IL-12. Two clinical trials testing rhIL-18 have reported safety and feasibility of its administration, and evidence of biological activity, although antitumor responses have been disappointing [68, 69].

Novel Cytokine Delivery Approaches

In addition to exploration of new cytokines given systemically, there is also significant interest in optimizing the delivery of cytokines to the tumor microenvironment (TME). As evident from the use of high-dose bolus IL-2 and intravenous rIL-12, systemic administration of cytokines in patients is associated with considerable toxicity. The DLTs associated with systemic delivery of cytokines may result in suboptimal drug concentrations in the TME and may potentially compromise efficacy. Further, these toxicities may limit the application of cytokine immunotherapy to relatively younger patients with minimal comorbidities. As discussed above with IL-12, several approaches have been tried to target the delivery of the cytokines to the TME, where immune-stimulation is most needed. Effective local delivery of cytokines to the TME may overcome the immune-evasion mechanisms by the tumor cells and tilt the balance of the immune battle in the favor of the host, avoiding systemic toxicity at the same time. A recent murine study reported antitumor efficacy of local intratumoral production of IL-12 by adoptively transferred genetically engineered T cells; the therapeutic effect of IL-12 produced locally in the TME could not be mimicked with systemic administration of high doses of IL-12 [38]. As witnessed in the IL-12 plasmid electroporation trial that was described above, several patients with disseminated melanoma had complete regressions of distant nonelectroporated metastases demonstrating the potential of successful local immunostimulation to translate into systemic immune responses [16]. Another example of a targeted delivery approach is ALT-801, an IL-2 recombinant fusion protein consisting of the IL-2 fused to a humanized soluble TCR directed against an antigen derived from the tumor suppressor protein p53. The TCR moiety of IL-2 recombinant fusion protein ALT-801 binds to tumor cells displaying p53 epitope/MHC complexes; subsequently, the tumor cell-localized IL-2 moiety may stimulate natural killer (NK) cell and T cell cytotoxic immune responses against p53-expressing tumor cells [5, 93]. A phase I clinical trial of ALT-801 in patients with metastatic melanoma has been completed with encouraging safety and efficacy results; another clinical trial of ALT-801 in combination with cisplatin in melanoma patients is ongoing (www. clinicaltrials.gov identifier # NCT01029873). Another promising example of local delivery of an immunomodulatory cytokine locally is JS1/34.5-/47-/GM-CSF (OncoVEX^{GM-CSF}, BioVex, Woburn, MA); this is an immune-enhanced, oncolytic herpes simplex virus type 1 (HSV-1), which is engineered for tumor-selective replication and also contains the coding sequence for human GM-CSF to stimulate the maturation, proliferation, and differentiation of dendritic cells, with the expectation of amplifying the antitumor immune response generated by lysed tumor products. The phase II results in 50 patients with unresectable melanoma were encouraging with durable regressions in distant noninjected lesions, an overall response rate of 26% (CR-16%) and a 2-year survival rate of 52% [75]. A phase III trial, which is comparing this drug to subcutaneously administered GM-CSF in stages IIIb, IIIc, and IV melanoma, is now underway (www.clinicaltrials.gov identifier # NCT00769704).

In summary, new cytokines continue to be discovered at a rapid pace; many of these novel cytokines possess unique properties that may overcome the limitations of current immunotherapies. Immunotherapy will likely play a major role in advancing outcomes of cancer patients over the next few years. Investigation of rational combinations of cytokines with other immunotherapeutic modalities and of novel methods to optimize the delivery of cytokines will be critical to the achievement of major advances in cancer immunotherapy. Identification of predictive biomarkers will also be important, as it will enable selection of patients who are most likely to benefit from cytokine therapy, hence avoiding unnecessary toxicity.

References

1. Asada H, Kishida T, Hirai H, Satoh E, Ohashi S, Takeuchi M, et al. Significant antitumor effects obtained by autologous tumor cell vaccine engineered to secrete interleukin (IL)-12 and IL-18 by means of the EBV/lipoplex. Mol Ther. 2002;5:609–16.
2. Atkins MB, Robertson MJ, Gordon M, Lotze MT, DeCoste M, DuBois JS, et al. Phase I evaluation of intravenous recombinant human interleukin 12 in patients with advanced malignancies. Clin Cancer Res. 1997;3:409–17.
3. Bajetta E, Del Vecchio M, Mortarini R, Nadeau R, Rakhit A, Rimassa L, et al. Pilot study of subcutaneous recombinant human interleukin 12 in metastatic melanoma. Clin Cancer Res. 1998;4:75–85.
4. Bamford RN, Grant AJ, Burton JD, Peters C, Kurys G, Goldman CK, et al. The interleukin (IL) 2 receptor beta chain is shared by IL-2 and a cytokine, provisionally designated IL-T, that stimulates T-cell proliferation and the induction of lymphokine-activated killer cells. Proc Natl Acad Sci USA. 1994;91:4940–4.
5. Belmont HJ, Price-Schiavi S, Liu B, Card KF, Lee HI, Han KP, et al. Potent antitumor activity of a tumor-specific soluble TCR/IL-2 fusion protein. Clin Immunol. 2006;121:29–39.
6. Bhatia S, Heath E, Puzanov I, Miller W, Curti B, Gordon M, et al. Phase II study of recombinant IL-21 (rIL-21) plus sorafenib as second- or third-line therapy for metastatic renal cell cancer (mRCC): final results. J Clin Oncol. 2009;27:15s(Suppl; abstr 3023).
7. Bohm W, Thomas S, Leithauser F, Moller P, Schirmbeck R, Reimann J. T cell-mediated, IFN-facilitated rejection of murine B16 melanomas. J Immunol. 1998;161:897.

8. Brady J, Hayakawa Y, Smyth MJ, Nutt SL. IL-21 induces the functional maturation of murine NK cells. J Immunol. 2004;172:2048–58.

9. Brunda M, Luistro L, Warrier R, Wright R, Hubbard B, Murphy M, et al. Antitumor and antimetastatic activity of interleukin 12 against murine tumors. J Exp Med. 1993;178:1223.

10. Castermans K, Tabruyn SP, Zeng R, van Beijnum JR, Eppolito C, Leonard WJ, et al. Angiostatic activity of the antitumor cytokine interleukin-21. Blood. 2008;112:4940–7.

11. Cebon J, Jager E, Shackleton MJ, Gibbs P, Davis ID, Hopkins W, et al. Two phase I studies of low dose recombinant human IL-12 with Melan-A and influenza peptides in subjects with advanced malignant melanoma. Cancer Immun. 2003;3:7.

12. Chan SH, Perussia B, Gupta JW, Kobayashi M, Pospisil M, Young HA, et al. Induction of interferon gamma production by natural killer cell stimulatory factor: characterization of the responder cells and synergy with other inducers. J Exp Med. 1991;173:869–79.

13. Cheever MA. Twelve immunotherapy drugs that could cure cancers. Immunol Rev. 2008;222: 357–68.

14. Cohen J. IL-12 deaths: explanation and a puzzle. Science. 1995;270:908.

15. D'Andrea A, Rengaraju M, Valiante NM, Chehimi J, Kubin M, Aste M, et al. Production of natural killer cell stimulatory factor (interleukin 12) by peripheral blood mononuclear cells. J Exp Med. 1992;176:1387–98.

16. Daud AI, DeConti RC, Andrews S, Urbas P, Riker AI, Sondak VK, et al. Phase I trial of interleukin-12 plasmid electroporation in patients with metastatic melanoma. J Clin Oncol. 2008;26:5896–903.

17. Davies E, Reid S, Medina MF, Lichty B, Ashkar AA. IL-15 has innate anti-tumor activity independent of NK and CD8 T cells. J Leukoc Biol. 2010;88:529–36.

18. Davis ID, Brady B, Kefford RF, Millward M, Cebon J, Skrumsager BK, et al. Clinical and biological efficacy of recombinant human interleukin-21 in patients with stage IV malignant melanoma without prior treatment: a phase IIa trial. Clin Cancer Res. 2009;15:2123–9.

19. Davis ID, Skrumsager BK, Cebon J, Nicholaou T, Barlow JW, Moller NP, et al. An open-label, two-arm, phase I trial of recombinant human interleukin-21 in patients with metastatic melanoma. Clin Cancer Res. 2007;13:3630–6.

20. Di Carlo E, Comes A, Orengo AM, Rosso O, Meazza R, Musiani P, et al. IL-21 induces tumor rejection by specific CTL and IFN-gamma-dependent CXC chemokines in syngeneic mice. J Immunol. 2004;172:1540–7.

21. Dietrich A, Kraus K, Brinckmann U, Friedrich T, Muller A, Liebert UG, et al. Complex cancer gene therapy in mice melanoma. Langenbecks Arch Surg. 2002;387:177–82.

22. Dubois S, Patel HJ, Zhang M, Waldmann TA, Muller JR. Preassociation of IL-15 with IL-15R alpha-IgG1-Fc enhances its activity on proliferation of NK and CD8+/CD44high T cells and its antitumor action. J Immunol. 2008;180:2099–106.

23. Egilmez N, Jong Y, Sabel M, Jacob J, Mathiowitz E, Bankert R. In situ tumor vaccination with interleukin-12-encapsulated biodegradable microspheres: induction of tumor regression and potent antitumor immunity. Cancer Res. 2000;60:3832.

24. Epardaud M, Elpek KG, Rubinstein MP, Yonekura AR, Bellemare-Pelletier A, Bronson R, et al. Interleukin-15/interleukin-15R alpha complexes promote destruction of established tumors by reviving tumor-resident CD8+ T cells. Cancer Res. 2008;68:2972–83.

25. Gee M, Koch C, Evans S, Jenkins R, Pletcher C, Moore J, et al. Hypoxia-mediated apoptosis from angiogenesis inhibition underlies tumor control by recombinant interleukin 12. Cancer Res. 1999;59:4882.

26. Gollob JA, Mier JW, Veenstra K, McDermott DF, Clancy D, Clancy M, et al. Phase I trial of twice-weekly intravenous interleukin 12 in patients with metastatic renal cell cancer or malignant melanoma: ability to maintain IFN-gamma induction is associated with clinical response. Clin Cancer Res. 2000;6:1678–92.

27. Gollob JA, Veenstra KG, Parker RA, Mier JW, McDermott DF, Clancy D, et al. Phase I trial of concurrent twice-weekly recombinant human interleukin-12 plus low-dose IL-2 in patients with melanoma or renal cell carcinoma. J Clin Oncol. 2003;21:2564–73.

28. Grabstein KH, Eisenman J, Shanebeck K, Rauch C, Srinivasan S, Fung V, et al. Cloning of a T cell growth factor that interacts with the beta chain of the interleukin-2 receptor. Science. 1994;264:965–8.

29. Gracie JA, Robertson SE, McInnes IB. Interleukin-18. J Leukoc Biol. 2003;73:213–24.

30. Gri G, Chiodoni C, Gallo E, Stoppacciaro A, Liew FY, Colombo MP. Antitumor effect of interleukin (IL)-12 in the absence of endogenous IFN-gamma: a role for intrinsic tumor immunogenicity and IL-15. Cancer Res. 2002;62:4390–7.

31. Heinzerling L, Burg G, Dummer R, Maier T, Oberholzer PA, Schultz J, et al. Intratumoral injection of DNA encoding human interleukin 12 into patients with metastatic melanoma: clinical efficacy. Hum Gene Ther. 2005;16:35–48.

32. Heinzerling L, Dummer R, Pavlovic J, Schultz J, Burg G, Moelling K. Tumor regression of human and murine melanoma after intratumoral injection of IL-12-encoding plasmid DNA in mice. Exp Dermatol. 2002;11:232–40.

33. Hsieh CS, Macatonia SE, Tripp CS, Wolf SF, O'Garra A, Murphy KM. Development of TH1 CD4+ T cells through IL-12 produced by Listeria-induced macrophages. Science. 1993;260: 547–9.

34. Junghans RP, Waldmann TA. Metabolism of Tac (IL2Ralpha): physiology of cell surface shedding and renal catabolism, and suppression of catabolism by antibody binding. J Exp Med. 1996;183:1587–602.

35. Kang WK, Park C, Yoon HL, Kim WS, Yoon SS, Lee MH, et al. Interleukin 12 gene therapy of cancer by peritumoral injection of transduced autologous fibroblasts: outcome of a phase I study. Hum Gene Ther. 2001;12:671–84.

36. Kaplan MH, Sun YL, Hoey T, Grusby MJ. Impaired IL-12 responses and enhanced development of Th2 cells in Stat4-deficient mice. Nature. 1996;382:174–7.

37. Kasaian MT, Whitters MJ, Carter LL, Lowe LD, Jussif JM, Deng B, et al. IL-21 limits NK cell responses and promotes antigen-specific T cell activation: a mediator of the transition from innate to adaptive immunity. Immunity. 2002;16:559–69.

38. Kerkar SP, Muranski P, Kaiser A, Boni A, Sanchez-Perez L, Yu Z, et al. Tumor-specific CD8+ T cells expressing interleukin-12 eradicate established cancers in lymphodepleted hosts. Cancer Res. 2010;70:6725–34.

39. Kobayashi H, Dubois S, Sato N, Sabzevari H, Sakai Y, Waldmann TA, et al. Role of transcellular IL-15 presentation in the activation of NK cell-mediated killing, which leads to enhanced tumor immunosurveillance. Blood. 2005;105:721–7.

40. Kobayashi M, Fitz L, Ryan M, Hewick RM, Clark SC, Chan S, et al. Identification and purification of natural killer cell stimulatory factor (NKSF), a cytokine with multiple biologic effects on human lymphocytes. J Exp Med. 1989;170:827–45.

41. Ku CC, Murakami M, Sakamoto A, Kappler J, Marrack P. Control of homeostasis of CD8+ memory T cells by opposing cytokines. Science. 2000;288:675–8.

42. Lee P, Wang F, Kuniyoshi J, Rubio V, Stuges T, Groshen S, et al. Effects of interleukin-12 on the immune response to a multipeptide vaccine for resected metastatic melanoma. J Clin Oncol. 2001;19:3836–47.

43. Lin JX, Migone TS, Tsang M, Friedmann M, Weatherbee JA, Zhou L, et al. The role of shared receptor motifs and common Stat proteins in the generation of cytokine pleiotropy and redundancy by IL-2, IL-4, IL-7, IL-13, and IL-15. Immunity. 1995;2:331–9.

44. Lodolce JP, Boone DL, Chai S, Swain RE, Dassopoulos T, Trettin S, et al. IL-15 receptor maintains lymphoid homeostasis by supporting lymphocyte homing and proliferation. Immunity. 1998;9:669–76.

45. Lohr F, Lo D, Zaharoff D, Hu K, Zhang X, Yongping L, et al. Effective tumor therapy with plasmid-encoded cytokines combined with in vivo electroporation. Cancer Res. 2001;61: 3281–4.

46. Lucas ML, Heller L, Coppola D, Heller R. IL-12 plasmid delivery by in vivo electroporation for the successful treatment of established subcutaneous B16.F10 melanoma. Mol Ther. 2002;5:668–75.

47. Ma HL, Whitters MJ, Konz RF, Senices M, Young DA, Grusby MJ, et al. IL-21 activates both innate and adaptive immunity to generate potent antitumor responses that require perforin but are independent of IFN-gamma. J Immunol. 2003;171:608–15.
48. Ma X, Trinchieri G. Regulation of interleukin-12 production in antigen-presenting cells. Adv Immunol. 2001;79:55–92.
49. Macatonia SE, Hosken NA, Litton M, Vieira P, Hsieh CS, Culpepper JA, et al. Dendritic cells produce IL-12 and direct the development of Th1 cells from naive CD4+ T cells. J Immunol. 1995;154:5071–9.
50. Mahvi DM, Henry MB, Albertini MR, Weber S, Meredith K, Schalch H, et al. Intratumoral injection of IL-12 plasmid DNA–results of a phase I/IB clinical trial. Cancer Gene Ther. 2007;14:717–23.
51. Marks-Konczalik J, Dubois S, Losi JM, Sabzevari H, Yamada N, Feigenbaum L, et al. IL-2-induced activation-induced cell death is inhibited in IL-15 transgenic mice. Proc Natl Acad Sci USA. 2000;97:11445–50.
52. Mazzolini G, Alfaro C, Sangro B, Feijoo E, Ruiz J, Benito A, et al. Intratumoral injection of dendritic cells engineered to secrete interleukin-12 by recombinant adenovirus in patients with metastatic gastrointestinal carcinomas. J Clin Oncol. 2005;23:999–1010.
53. Mendiratta SK, Quezada A, Matar M, Wang J, Hebel HL, Long S, et al. Intratumoral delivery of IL-12 gene by polyvinyl polymeric vector system to murine renal and colon carcinoma results in potent antitumor immunity. Gene Ther. 1999;6:833–9.
54. Moroz A, Eppolito C, Li Q, Tao J, Clegg CH, Shrikant PA. IL-21 enhances and sustains CD8+ T cell responses to achieve durable tumor immunity: comparative evaluation of IL-2, IL-15, and IL-21. J Immunol. 2004;173:900–9.
55. Mortarini R, Borri A, Tragni G, Bersani I, Vegetti C, Bajetta E, et al. Peripheral burst of tumor-specific cytotoxic T lymphocytes and infiltration of metastatic lesions by memory CD8+ T cells in melanoma patients receiving interleukin 12. Cancer Res. 2000;60:3559–68.
56. Nakanishi K, Yoshimoto T, Tsutsui H, Okamura H. Interleukin-18 regulates both Th1 and Th2 responses. Annu Rev Immunol. 2001;19:423–74.
57. Noguchi Y, Richards EC, Chen YT, Old LJ. Influence of interleukin 12 on p53 peptide vaccination against established Meth A sarcoma. Proc Natl Acad Sci USA. 1995;92:2219–23.
58. Ohe Y, Kasai T, Heike Y, Saijo N. Clinical trial of IL-12 for cancer patients. Gan To Kagaku Ryoho. 1998;25:177–84.
59. Ozaki K, Kikly K, Michalovich D, Young PR, Leonard WJ. Cloning of a type I cytokine receptor most related to the IL-2 receptor beta chain. Proc Natl Acad Sci USA. 2000;97:11439–44.
60. Parrish-Novak J, Dillon SR, Nelson A, Hammond A, Sprecher C, Gross JA, et al. Interleukin 21 and its receptor are involved in NK cell expansion and regulation of lymphocyte function. Nature. 2000;408:57–63.
61. Parrish-Novak J, Foster DC, Holly RD, Clegg CH. Interleukin-21 and the IL-21 receptor: novel effectors of NK and T cell responses. J Leukoc Biol. 2002;72:856–63.
62. Peluso I, Fantini MC, Fina D, Caruso R, Boirivant M, MacDonald TT, et al. IL-21 counteracts the regulatory T cell-mediated suppression of human CD4+ T lymphocytes. J Immunol. 2007;178:732–9.
63. Peterson AC, Harlin H, Gajewski TF. Immunization with Melan-A peptide-pulsed peripheral blood mononuclear cells plus recombinant human interleukin-12 induces clinical activity and T-cell responses in advanced melanoma. J Clin Oncol. 2003;21:2342–8.
64. Petrella T, Tozer R, Belanger K, Savage K, Wong R, Kamel-Reid S, et al. Interleukin-21 (IL-21) activity in patients (pts) with metastatic melanoma (MM). J Clin Oncol. 2010;28:15s(Suppl; abstr 8507).
65. Presky DH, Yang H, Minetti LJ, Chua AO, Nabavi N, Wu CY, et al. A functional interleukin 12 receptor complex is composed of two beta-type cytokine receptor subunits. Proc Natl Acad Sci USA. 1996;93:14002–7.
66. Pulaski BA, Clements VK, Pipeling MR, Ostrand-Rosenberg S. Immunotherapy with vaccines combining MHC class II/CD80+ tumor cells with interleukin-12 reduces established metastatic

disease and stimulates immune effectors and monokine induced by interferon gamma. Cancer Immunol Immunother. 2000;49:34–45.

67. Robertson MJ, Cameron C, Atkins MB, Gordon MS, Lotze MT, Sherman ML, et al. Immunological effects of interleukin 12 administered by bolus intravenous injection to patients with cancer. Clin Cancer Res. 1999;5:9–16.

68. Robertson MJ, Kirkwood JM, Logan TF, Koch KM, Kathman S, Kirby LC, et al. A dose-escalation study of recombinant human interleukin-18 using two different schedules of administration in patients with cancer. Clin Cancer Res. 2008;14:3462–9.

69. Robertson MJ, Mier JW, Logan T, Atkins M, Koon H, Koch KM, et al. Clinical and biological effects of recombinant human interleukin-18 administered by intravenous infusion to patients with advanced cancer. Clin Cancer Res. 2006;12:4265–73.

70. Rogge L, Barberis-Maino L, Biffi M, Passini N, Presky DH, Gubler U, et al. Selective expression of an interleukin-12 receptor component by human T helper 1 cells. J Exp Med. 1997; 185:825–31.

71. Rosenberg SA, Sportes C, Ahmadzadeh M, Fry TJ, Ngo LT, Schwarz SL, et al. IL-7 administration to humans leads to expansion of CD8+ and CD4+ cells but a relative decrease of CD4+ T-regulatory cells. J Immunother. 2006;29:313–9.

72. Rowley J, Monie A, Hung CF, Wu TC. Inhibition of tumor growth by NK1.1+ cells and CD8+ T cells activated by IL-15 through receptor beta/common gamma signaling in trans. J Immunol. 2008;181:8237–47.

73. Schultz J, Heinzerling L, Pavlovic J, Moelling K. Induction of long-lasting cytokine effect by injection of IL-12 encoding plasmid DNA. Cancer Gene Ther. 2000;7:1557–65.

74. Schultz J, Pavlovic J, Strack B, Nawrath M, Moelling K. Long-lasting anti-metastatic efficiency of interleukin 12-encoding plasmid DNA. Human Gene Ther. 1999;10:407.

75. Senzer NN, Kaufman HL, Amatruda T, Nemunaitis M, Reid T, Daniels G, et al. Phase II clinical trial of a granulocyte-macrophage colony-stimulating factor-encoding, second-generation oncolytic herpesvirus in patients with unresectable metastatic melanoma. J Clin Oncol. 2009;27:5763–71.

76. Sgadari C, Angiolillo A, Tosato G. Inhibition of angiogenesis by interleukin-12 is mediated by the interferon-inducible protein-10. Blood. 1996;87:3877.

77. Sivori S, Cantoni C, Parolini S, Marcenaro E, Conte R, Moretta L, et al. IL-21 induces both rapid maturation of human CD34+ cell precursors towards NK cells and acquisition of surface killer Ig-like receptors. Eur J Immunol. 2003;33:3439–47.

78. Sondergaard H, Frederiksen KS, Thygesen P, Galsgaard ED, Skak K, Kristjansen PE, et al. Interleukin 21 therapy increases the density of tumor infiltrating CD8+ T cells and inhibits the growth of syngeneic tumors. Cancer Immunol Immunother. 2007;56:1417–28.

79. Sportes C, Babb RR, Krumlauf MC, Hakim FT, Steinberg SM, Chow CK, et al. Phase I study of recombinant human interleukin-7 administration in subjects with refractory malignancy. Clin Cancer Res. 2010;16:727–35.

80. Stern AS, Podlaski FJ, Hulmes JD, Pan YC, Quinn PM, Wolitzky AG, et al. Purification to homogeneity and partial characterization of cytotoxic lymphocyte maturation factor from human B-lymphoblastoid cells. Proc Natl Acad Sci USA. 1990;87:6808–12.

81. Sun Y, Jurgovsky K, Moller P, Alijagic S, Dorbic T, Georgieva J, et al. Vaccination with IL-12 gene-modified autologous melanoma cells: preclinical results and a first clinical phase I study. Gene Ther. 1998;5:481–90.

82. Szabo SJ, Dighe AS, Gubler U, Murphy KM. Regulation of the interleukin (IL)-12R beta 2 subunit expression in developing T helper 1 (Th1) and Th2 cells. J Exp Med. 1997;185: 817–24.

83. Thierfelder WE, van Deursen JM, Yamamoto K, Tripp RA, Sarawar SR, Carson RT, et al. Requirement for Stat4 in interleukin-12-mediated responses of natural killer and T cells. Nature. 1996;382:171–4.

84. Thompson JA, Curti BD, Redman BG, Bhatia S, Weber JS, Agarwala SS, et al. Phase I study of recombinant interleukin-21 in patients with metastatic melanoma and renal cell carcinoma. J Clin Oncol. 2008;26:2034–9.

85. Timmerman J, Byrd J, Andorsky D, Siadak M, DeVries T, Hausman D, et al. Efficacy and safety of recombinant interleukin-21 (rIL-21) and rituximab in relapsed/refractory indolent lymphoma. J Clin Oncol. 2008;26:(20 Suppl; abstr 8554).
86. Toda M, Martuza R, Kojima H, Rabkin S. In situ cancer vaccination: an IL-12 defective vector/ replication-competent herpes simplex virus combination induces local and systemic antitumor activity. J Immunol. 1998;160:4457.
87. Trinchieri G. Interleukin-12 and the regulation of innate resistance and adaptive immunity. Nat Rev. 2003;3:133–46.
88. Triozzi PL, Allen KO, Carlisle RR, Craig M, LoBuglio AF, Conry RM. Phase I study of the intratumoral administration of recombinant canarypox viruses expressing B7.1 and interleukin 12 in patients with metastatic melanoma. Clin Cancer Res. 2005;11:4168–75.
89. Ugen KE, Kutzler MA, Marrero B, Westover J, Coppola D, Weiner DB, et al. Regression of subcutaneous B16 melanoma tumors after intratumoral delivery of an IL-15-expressing plasmid followed by in vivo electroporation. Cancer Gene Ther. 2006;13:969–74.
90. Waldmann TA, Dubois S, Tagaya Y. Contrasting roles of IL-2 and IL-15 in the life and death of lymphocytes: implications for immunotherapy. Immunity. 2001;14:105–10.
91. Waldmann TA, Tagaya Y. The multifaceted regulation of interleukin-15 expression and the role of this cytokine in NK cell differentiation and host response to intracellular pathogens. Annu Rev Immunol. 1999;17:19–49.
92. Wang G, Tschoi M, Spolski R, Lou Y, Ozaki K, Feng C, et al. In vivo antitumor activity of interleukin 21 mediated by natural killer cells. Cancer Res. 2003;63:9016–22.
93. Wen J, Zhu X, Liu B, You L, Kong L, Lee HI, et al. Targeting activity of a TCR/IL-2 fusion protein against established tumors. Cancer Immunol Immunother. 2008;57:1781–94.
94. Yajima T, Nishimura H, Wajjwalku W, Harada M, Kuwano H, Yoshikai Y. Overexpression of interleukin-15 in vivo enhances antitumor activity against MHC class I-negative and -positive malignant melanoma through augmented NK activity and cytotoxic T-cell response. Int J Cancer. 2002;99:573–8.
95. Yao L, Sgadari C, Furuke K, Bloom E, Teruy-Feldstein J, Tosato G. Contribution of natural killer cells to inhibition of angiogenesis by interleukin-12. Blood. 1999;93:1612.
96. Yue F, Geertsen R, Hemmi S, Burg G, Pavlovic J, Laine E, et al. IL-12 directly up-regulates the expression of HLA class I, HLA class II, and ICAM-1 on human melanoma cells: a mechanism for its antitumor activity? Eur J Immunol. 1999;29:1762.
97. Zeng R, Spolski R, Finkelstein SE, Oh S, Kovanen PE, Hinrichs CS, et al. Synergy of IL-21 and IL-15 in regulating CD8+ T cell expansion and function. J Exp Med. 2005;201:139–48.
98. Zhang X, Sun S, Hwang I, Tough DF, Sprent J. Potent and selective stimulation of memory-phenotype CD8+ cells in vivo by IL-15. Immunity. 1998;8:591–9.
99. Zilocchi C, Stoppacciaro A, Chiodoni C, Parenza M, Terrazzini N, Colombo MP. Interferon gamma-independent rejection of interleukin 12-transduced carcinoma cells requires CD4+ T cells and granulocyte/macrophage colony-stimulating factor. J Exp Med. 1998;188:133–43.

Chapter 18
Modulating the Tumor Microenvironment

Carl E. Ruby and Howard L. Kaufman

Abstract Melanomas arise in a complex microenvironment composed of tumor cells, cellular and soluble stroma, and immune cells. The dynamic interactions and crosstalk between these elements drive tumor initiation, progression, invasiveness, and immunity. Melanoma is considered the prototypical "immunogenic" tumor since the immune system can often recognize and occasionally reject established tumors. There is now evidence that the complex tumor microenvironment often establishes an immune suppressive state that blocks tumor eradication. In this chapter we describe the cellular and noncellular factors within the tumor microenvironment that modulate local antitumor immunity. The chapter also highlights several current therapeutic strategies in clinical development that target various elements of the tumor microenvironment to restore effective antitumor immunity.

Keywords Tumor microenvironment • Stroma • Immune suppression • Tregs • PD-L1 • IDO • TGF-β • Costimulation

Introduction

Immunotherapy offers a highly specific and potentially durable means to treat malignant melanoma. Melanoma is generally considered the "prototypical" immunogenic tumor and the likely molecular basis for melanoma susceptibility to immune-mediated rejection has been identified. A broad number of T cell specific and associated melanoma antigens have been characterized and spontaneous and vaccine-induced T

C.E. Ruby, PhD
Department of General Surgery, Rush University Medical Center, Chicago, IL, USA

H.L. Kaufman, MD (✉)
Rush Medical College, Rush University Cancer Center, Rush University Medical Center, Chicago, IL, USA
e-mail: howard_kaufman@rush.edu

T.F. Gajewski and F.S. Hodi (eds.), *Targeted Therapeutics in Melanoma*,
Current Clinical Oncology, DOI 10.1007/978-1-61779-407-0_18,
© Springer Science+Business Media, LLC 2012

cell responses are frequently reported in the peripheral blood of melanoma patients. Tumor rejection, however, is an uncommon event following immunotherapy, and established tumors often escape immune-mediated rejection. A major obstacle to successful immunotherapy has been suggested by the observation that when activated effector T cells encounter a highly suppressive tumor microenvironment their function is often blocked allowing tumor cells to escape immune detection and control.

Tumor cells exist in a complex milieu of cellular and noncellular components that develop as a result of altered homeostatic regulation mediated by host tumor cells. The tumor microenvironment consists of tumor cells, stroma (microvessels, supporting tissue, and soluble factors) and immune cells, which interact to mediate the balance between tumor growth and regression. The complex changes that occur in the local microenvironment have profound implications not only for tumor growth, but also for the effectiveness of therapeutic interventions that may be influenced by the molecular and cellular composition of the microenvironment. This is especially true for tumor immunotherapy in which effector immune cells must be activated, traffic to sites of established tumors, and mediate antigen-specific cytotoxic functions.

The interactions between the tumor and immune system are clearly influenced by changes in the structure and components of the tumor microenvironment. While some tumors may be subject to immune-mediated regression, others have evolved to evade immunological detection and favor the emergence of a tumor better suited for survival. Thus, understanding the biology of the tumor microenvironment and how its components, the cells and noncellular factors that comprise the microenvironment, contribute to local immune suppression would provide the framework for designing complementary tumor microenvironment-targeted therapies for the treatment of malignant melanoma. This chapter will focus on the three primary components of the tumor microenvironment – the tumor cells, stroma, and immune cells – and describe how they can mediate immune suppression and also serve as potential targets for therapeutic intervention that promotes antitumor immunity.

Composition and Development of the Tumor Microenvironment

Tumor Cells

The development of the tumor microenvironment is ultimately dictated by changes in host tumor cells. A number of genetic and environmental changes have been reported to promote early changes in tumor morphology and growth. For example, chromosomal aberrations (gain or loss), changes in cell cycle protein expression (e.g., cyclin D1, Rb), and loss of E-cadherin expression, are needed to collectively change the early radial growth phase of melanoma to the more advanced vertical growth phase [35]. The loss of cell-to-cell adhesion control mediated by E-cadherin is a critical driver of tumor progression and emergence of an invasive phenotype. Additionally, the dysregulated growth of the melanoma cells upregulates the expression of vascular endothelial growth factor (VEGF) and its receptor, VEGF-R, to mediate angiogenesis and neovascularization. In concert with enhanced VEGF-mediated vascularization, melanoma cells change their pattern of chemokine secretion, resulting in the recruitment of immune and stromal cells that continue to shape the microenvironment [56]. Although a number of altered tumor-specific molecular pathways govern VEGF and chemokine production, activated STAT3 may act as a potential "master switch" exerting control on both of these processes [73]. Thus, the altered molecular patterns that set in motion melanoma tumor progression and growth, also furnish the blueprint for the development of the tumor microenvironment to favor immune suppression. The immunosuppressive conditions further allow the primary tumor to resist immune recognition and escape immune control to grow and metastasize [17].

Stroma

The stroma can be broadly defined by its cellular components and the soluble factors that permeate the developing microenvironment. Several key distinguishing morphologic features of the stroma from melanocytic lesions include the following: microvessels (endothelial cells), fibroblasts, keratinocytes, and extracellular matrix (fibrin, collagen, and hyaluronan). Arrangement of these stromal elements, which is ultimately determined by the developing tumor vasculature, varies between tumors and gives rise to different architectural patterns among melanoma lesions [61]. These elements are essential in providing physical support to the tumor, transport of nutrients that foster tumor growth, and production of growth factors and cytokines.

The ability of the stoma to provide physical support relies on fibroblasts that shape the architecture of the microenvironment as structural cells and through the production of the extracellular matrix. During the development of the tumor microenvironment, one of the early and important events of stromatogenesis is the recruitment of fibroblasts, either resident and/or mesenchymal stem cells (pre-fibroblast cells). Once recruited to the growing tumor microenvironment, the fibroblasts undergo multiple rounds of proliferation and become activated. The final phase of stromatogenesis, the differentiation of the fibroblast, triggers the secretion of extracellular matrix components to form the boundary of the tumor microenvironment with normal tissue [61]. In addition to fibroblast-associated "landscaping" the microenvironment, these cells are a rich source of growth factors, such as transforming growth factor-β (TGF-β), that act in both paracrine and autocrine fashion to drive the growth of melanoma cells. In fact, fibroblasts isolated from human cancers are more efficient than normal tissue fibroblasts to promote the growth of tumor cells, likely a result of augmented paracrine growth factor secretion [51].

The other two primary cell types that make up the melanoma tumor environment are vascular endothelial cells and keratinocytes. Vascular endothelial cells are associated with microvessel formation and neovascularization, and can also produce chemokines and indoleamine-2,3-dioxygenase (IDO), a tryptophan-catabolizing enzyme, that shape the composition and activation of the immune compartment within the developing microenvironment. Since T cells rely on tryptophan for their survival, the depletion of this amino acid in the tumor microenvironment may lead to functional tolerance even in the presence of antigen-specific T cells. Keratinocytes reside in normal skin in conjunction with melanocytes at ratio of 35:1 (keratinocytes to melanocytes). The interaction between keratinocytes and melanocytes is mediated by E-cadherin and the loss of these connections alters melanocyte gene expression patterns, leading to increased expression of melanoma-associated genes [65, 71].

Soluble factors play a critical role in the development of the tumor microenvironment through both a paracrine and autocrine network of signals established between the tumor, stroma, and immune cells. Early mediators of melanoma growth include basic fibroblast growth factor (bFGF), platelet derived growth factor (PDGF), and TGF-β. These factors activate fibroblasts, contribute to melanoma progression in an autocrine fashion, promote collagen production (ECM), and suppress adaptive T cell responses. Stromal cells in turn produce growth factors (e.g., TGF-β and VEGF) that support continued tumor growth. VEGF, in particular, has a wide range of effects on the cells of the microenvironment. Produced largely by stromal cells in response to PDGF, TNF-β, IL-1α, and hypoxia, VEGF influences tumor proliferation and invasiveness, increases microvessel growth, and suppresses T cell responses in part by downregulating dendritic cell maturation [23]. Melanoma tumor cells also produce chemokines (e.g., IL-8, MIP-1α/β RANTES, CCL2), stromal cell-derived factor-1 (SDF-1), and cytokines (e.g., IL-10) that recruit inflammatory immune cells and skew the differentiation of T cells toward a Th2 response. Chemokines and SDF-1 often exhibit dual functions in recruiting immune cells and also promoting angiogenesis [42, 59]. The increased presence of inflammatory immune cells within the microenvironment gives rise to a number of inflammatory cytokines found within the microenvironment that include TNF-α, IL-1β, IL-6, IL-10, and IL-12. The timing and local concentration of inflammatory cytokines in the tumor can alter immune responses. In some cases this may promote tumor rejection, for example when IL-12 mediates Th1 (cell mediated/cytotoxic) T cell differentiation. In other cases, the cytokine profile may promote tumor escape, as occurs when IL-6 and TNF-α recruit and pathogenic macrophages. The balance in local soluble factors may result in a critical inflection point within individual tumor microenvironments that changes the potential for effective antitumor immunity.

Immune Cells

Cells of the innate and adaptive immune system profoundly shape the tumor microenvironment via a paradoxical relationship between the growing tumor and infiltrating immune cells. Indeed, the presence of immune cells in the tumor microenvironment would be predicted to result in the eradication of tumor cells; yet it is the chronic involvement of innate immune cells that has been observed to support tumor development and survival. Inflammation appears to be a key feature in the immunological molding of the tumor microenvironment and levels of inflammation appear to be dependent on the cell type, activation status, and composition of the immune cells found within a given tumor microenvironment.

Two subsets of immune cells, innate inflammatory cells and T lymphocytes, are typically involved in development of the tumor microenvironment. Neutrophils, monocytes, and macrophages are the primary inflammatory cells recruited to the tumor. Neutrophils are among the first to infiltrate the melanocytic lesion to control tumor growth through the secretion of cytotoxic reactive compounds (reactive oxygen intermediates and hypochlorous acid); however they may inevitably initiate inflammatory conditions due in part to oxidative cellular death. Tumor-associated macrophages, the result of monocyte differentiation, promote angiogenesis (via VEGF) and produce TGF-β and IL-10, two potent immune suppressive factors [3]. More importantly, macrophages function to recruit additional immune cells to the microenvironment through the prodigious production of chemokines. In addition to inflammatory cells, T cells, both CD4+ and CD8+, infiltrate the microenvironment, but unlike inflammatory cells, the role of adaptive cells in the development of the tumor microenvironment is not fully understood, as these cells appear to differentially modulate the microenvironment in an organ- and etiology-dependent manner [13].

Mechanisms of Immune Escape: Role of the Tumor Microenvironment

The immune system can be highly effective and exquisitely capable of detecting and inducing regression of tumors. The induction of such a response against a tumor hinges on the ability of the immune system to produce a sufficient number of tumor-specific T cells that traffic and infiltrate the tumor, and also possess the machinery to generate cytotoxic mediators. In many instances these requisite criteria are often met. In fact, there is evidence that significant numbers of tumor-specific T cells are often found infiltrating regressing tumors and they exhibit an activated/cytotoxic phenotype [28, 77, 78]. Yet, infiltrated tumors frequently escape from the control of the immune system. An explanation for this paradox could be attributed to the various mechanism of immune modulation mediated by the various components of the tumor microenvironment that renders the infiltrating T cells ineffective or defective. A number of negative regulatory mechanisms have been identified in human cancers and mouse tumor models, and several highly relevant candidate mechanisms have been associated with human melanoma. These mechanisms may be mediated by tumor cells, stromal components, or the immune system and will be considered individually.

Tumor Cell-Mediated Suppression

Melanoma cells within the tumor microenvironment may escape immune detection and destruction by changes in immune recognition cell surface molecule expression. These changes include the loss or deficiency of antigen presentation via major histocompatibility complex proteins (MHC), or decreased co-stimulatory B7 protein expression [14, 25]. The loss of MHC class I expression on tumors is a frequent event, in some cases 70–96% of the tumors have been identified to be MHC class I deficient, depending on the tumor type [25]. The striking loss of MHC class I in these tumors can be the result of defects in antigen processing and presentation and includes changes in β2-microglobulin and MHC heavy chain [25]. Malignant melanoma tumors can also be deficient in the expression of B7.1 and B7.2 [14]. Insufficient B7.1/2 co-stimulation through interactions with T cell-associated CD28 has been shown to induce anergy, a state of T cell hyporesponsiveness, which in addition to loss of MHC allows tumors to evade early immune detection and rejection [19, 63].

Tumors can also express the co-inhibitory ligand PD-L1, a member of the B7-family of molecules, and deactivate an established T cell-mediated antitumor response [16, 32]. Most melanomas express PD-L1 constitutively or in response to IFN-γ and upon interaction with the T cell surface protein PD-1 mediates a potent inhibitory signal and represents an effective mechanism of immune escape [43]. Expression of PD-1 on T cells can be the consequence of constant antigen exposure, as seen in chronic viral infections, which results in the functional decline and exhaustion of antigen-specific T cells [4]. Chronic antigen exposure within the tumor microenvironment might also be expected to induce T cell exhaustion and subsequent PD-1 expression, thus, contributing to immune suppression.

Stroma-Mediated Suppression

Expression of the tryptophan-catabolizing enzyme, IDO by various cells of the tumor microenvironment (tumors, dendritic cells, and endothelial cells) mediates local metabolic dysregulation, and results in local immunosuppressive conditions [70]. IDO catalyzes the degradation of the essential amino acid L-tryptophan to N-formylkynurenine causing a depletion of tryptophan that has been implicated in immunologic tolerance, suppression of T cell proliferation, and T cell apoptosis [18, 49]. A second amino acid catabolizing enzyme, arginase, has also been implicated in causing T cell anergy and loss of antitumor immunity [57, 58]. Together IDO- and arginase-catalyzed metabolic dysregulation within the tumor microenvironment represents another mechanism of negative immune regulation.

The tumor microenvironment also elaborates a host of immune regulatory soluble growth factors and cytokines that permeate the tumor to facilitate immune escape. A key secreted factor, VEGF, previously described to direct angiogenesis and vascularization of the tumor, also has the ability to inhibit the maturation of dendritic cells, which results in defective antigen-presentation and T cell anergy [22–24]. The regulatory cytokine IL-10, expressed by many tumors, achieves negative regulation of immune response by several different pathways. IL-10 downregulates the expression of MHC and the intracellular adhesion molecules (ICAMs), diminishes antigen processing, alters dendritic cell maturation and function, and induces T cell anergy [6, 53, 60]. In addition to IL-10, the potent immune modulator TGF-β can also be found in abundance within some tumors. TGF-β has profound effects on immune cells in the tumor setting, by altering differentiation and function of these infiltrating cells [20]. TGF-β alters dendritic cell trafficking and downregulates expression of MHC class II and co-stimulatory molecules producing an immature dendritic cell phenotype [44, 74]. Cytotoxic CD8+ T cells can be inhibited through the TGF-β-mediated downregulation of critical cytolytic genes (e.g., granzymes) and blockade of T cell receptor signaling and activation [15, 68]. Still the most important effect of TGF-β appears to be on the differentiation of CD4+ T cells. Tumor microenvironment-derived TGF-β can drive the differentiation of CD4+ T cells toward a regulatory bias, by promoting and enforcing expression of the transcription factor FoxP3 to generate regulatory T cells (Tregs) [20]. Thus, by targeting three important immune populations (dendritic cells, CD8+ and CD4+ T cells) by soluble factors VEGF, IL-10, and TGF-β the tumor microenvironment is able to uncouple the generation of productive antitumor immune responses.

Immune Cell-Mediated Suppression

Polarization of CD4+ T helper responses (Th) that foster antibody/humoral responses (Th2) over cell-mediated/cytotoxic responses (Th1) has been considered to be a potential mechanism by which tumors evade immune destruction. Elevated levels of Th2 cytokines (IL-4, IL-10, and IL-13) are often found circulating in patients with advanced tumors and these levels correlate with poor prognosis [50]. The tumor microenvironment has been associated with Th2 polarization of T cells and subsequent overproduction of these Th2-related cytokines [48], however, the levels of Th2 and Th1 cytokine mRNA within melanoma tumors has been observed to be equal, thus the mechanism of polarization within the microenvironment is not well defined [50]. An interesting observation is that the predominance of tumor-specific Th2 cells in melanoma cancer patients can shift to a Th1 bias after tumor clearance [67]. These data suggest the microenvironment may not directly drive Th2 bias over Th1 directly, but more likely the tumor microenvironment dampens Th1 responses and differentiation by factors such as TGF-β and VEGF [20, 50]. In effect, it is the decrease in Th1 response that may be the basis for tumor immune escape, rather than the enhancement of a Th2 response.

Antitumor immune response can be suppressed in a "T cell-extrinsic fashion" by regulatory T cells (Tregs) that include CD4+CD25+FoxP3+ Tregs, CD4+CD122+CD25−FoxP3− Tregs, and a subpopulation of regulatory CD8+ T cells [11, 21, 27]. The impact of regulatory T cells is evident in patients with melanoma and other advanced solid tumors. These patients have been reported to experience an increase in both circulating Treg numbers and Treg accumulation in the tumor microenvironment. In many cases, the increase in Treg frequency has been correlated with decreased overall survival [10, 75]. As previously stated several different types of Tregs have been described, yet the CD4+CD25+FoxP3+ Treg population is the most abundant and studied type of regulatory T cell. This type of Treg forms a heterogeneous population containing two subsets, natural Tregs (nTregs) and inducible Tregs (iTregs). Development of nTregs occurs in the thymus to maintain self-tolerance and iTregs develop in the periphery in response to self or tumor antigen. Although absolute discrimination of these two subsets is difficult, it is thought that the increase in Tregs within tumors is in part the result of intratumoral iTreg development. In this scenario, infiltrating CD4$^+$ T cells encounter excess tumor antigen and elevated levels of TGF-β in the tumor microenvironment to drive inhibitory Treg differentiation over antitumor Th1 differentiation [46, 72]. Tregs may also suppress activated T cells in an antigen-independent manner, which could further increase negative regulation and lead to more profound immunosuppression within the tumor microenvironment. Tregs possess a number of mechanisms to mediate immune suppression. These include the production of the cytokines, such as IL-10 and TGF-β and the enzyme IDO, all previously described to mediate negative regulation and immune evasion and tumor escape.

Finally, emerging evidence suggests that intracellular signal transducers and activators of transcription-3 (STAT3) signaling in host tumor cells underlies several of the negative regulatory mechanism present in the tumor microenvironment. The constitutive activation of the transcription factor STAT3 within melanoma tumor cells regulates the pattern of cytokine expression, resulting in the inhibition of pro-inflammatory cytokines, such as IL-12. In addition to cytokine regulation, STAT3 activation has been associated with production of VEGF and other cytokines [73].

Targeting the Tumor Microenvironment for Immunotherapy

The involvement of multiple mechanisms of immune suppression mediated by the tumor microenvironment suggest that therapeutic intervention will be required to target one or more of these mechanisms with the goal of eliciting productive antitumor immune responses. Strategies that target the various components of the microenvironment to promote the effector phase of an antitumor response have been developed and are being applied clinically to treat melanoma. These strategies include: (1) induction of a pro-inflammatory response using cytokines, viruses and toll-like receptor (TLR) agonists, (2) blockade of immune suppressive factors via agents that neutralize local factors, cells or enzymes, and (3) enhancement of immune recognition and activation. These approaches are summarized in Fig. 18.1 and can be targeted to various components of the tumor microenvironment.

Targeting the Tumor

Several strategies have been tested for targeting tumor cells within the microenvironment to enhance the effectiveness of tumor immunotherapy. These approaches

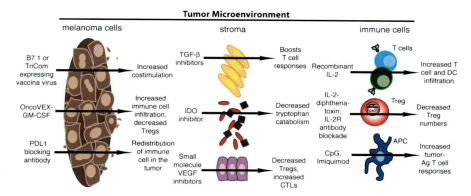

Fig. 18.1 Schematic diagram showing specific therapeutic strategies in clinical development by targeting tumor cells (*left panel*), stroma (*center panel*), and immune cells (*right panel*) within the tumor microenvironment

have sought to deliver local pro-inflammatory signals, replace host tumor co-stimulatory molecule expression, block host tumor co-inhibitory molecule expression, and directly lyse tumor cells to promote local and systemic melanoma-specific antitumor immunity. Although there are many other examples in preclinical development, this section will focus on those strategies that have shown therapeutic potential in clinical trials.

The direct intratumoral injection of recombinant vaccinia viruses expressing T cell co-stimulatory molecules has been explored and demonstrated significant tumor regression in patients with metastatic melanoma [37]. In a Phase I clinical trial, 12 patients with refractory metastatic melanoma were treated with three injections of a vaccinia virus expressing the human B7.1 co-stimulatory molecule [37]. There were minimal side effects reported, largely grade I injection site and constitutional symptoms. Two patients had stable disease and one patient demonstrated regression of both injected and non-injected lesions, and went on to have a complete response on-going 6 years after completing the trial. Those patients with therapeutic responses also displayed an increase in circulating gp100- and MART-1-specific T cell responses in the peripheral blood for up to 6 months after vaccination suggesting the development of systemic anti-melanoma immunity. The complete responder also developed vitiligo, which has correlated with successful tumor immunity in other trials. Serial sampling of injected tumor sites demonstrated a strong association between local interferon-γ expression and tumor regression. Similarly, local IL-10 expression was associated with progressive tumor growth.

In subsequent studies vaccinia virus expressing three T cell co-stimulatory molecules (B7.1, ICAM-1, and LFA-3) was performed using a similar patient population and study design [36]. In this trial, the toxicity profile was similar to the vaccinia-B7.1 study but an objective response rate of 38% was reported in injected lesions and 15% in non-injected lesions; an additional injected lesion and two non-injected lesions were stable. Thus, local injection of vaccinia viruses expressing T cell co-stimulatory molecules appears to be safe, can induce therapeutic responses in some patients and is associated with the induction of local and systemic antitumor immunity.

Melanoma tumor cell expression of PD-L1 is also being targeted since local expression may render tumor infiltrating T cells dysfunctional. A PD-1-specific monoclonal antibody has been tested in a Phase I clinical trial for patients with solid tumors to neutralize PDL1-PD-1 signals. Thirty-nine patients were treated and one episode of autoimmune colitis in a melanoma patient was observed. There was one complete response in a colorectal cancer patient and two partial responses that included one patient with melanoma. In this trial, circulating T cells continued to show >70% PD-1 expression but clinical responses did correlate with decreased levels of B7-H1 on tumor cells in the microenvironment [9]. This suggests that the predominant effect of the anti-PD-1 treatment may be on tumor cells within the microenvironment and not on peripheral T cells. A monoclonal antibody targeting CTLA-4 has also shown an improvement in overall survival in metastatic melanoma patients when used as a single agent and in combination with and HLA-A2-restricted gp100 peptide vaccine [30]. Although the mechanism of this effect is not clearly defined, the impact of CTLA-4 blockade could promote effector T cell activation, inhibit regulatory T cells, and alter the composition of T cells within the tumor microenvironment.

Another strategy that has shown particular promise is the use of an engineered oncolytic herpes simplex, type 1 virus encoding human GM-CSF (designated OncoVEX^{GMCSF}). The vector is injected directly into an established metastatic melanoma lesion and replicates selectively in melanoma cells. The local expression of GM-CSF and lytic death of tumor cells should promote a tumor-specific immune response. Early phase clinical trials confirmed the safety of this agent and only minor grade I adverse events were seen, including fever and local injection site pain. In a Phase II clinical trial in which patients with refractory Stage IV or unresectable Stage III melanoma were treated to maximum response, an objective clinical response of 28% was observed [64]. This included regression of injected and non-injected visceral disease. Further, evaluation of peripheral blood and tumor biopsy specimens suggested that regressing tumors were associated with the appearance of MART-1-specific effector T cells, a decrease in $CD4^+FoxP3^+$ Tregs and myeloid-derived suppressor cells [38]. These data demonstrated the potential therapeutic potential of local oncolytic virus treatment and a confirmatory Phase III clinical trial is in progress.

These studies highlight the potential benefit of targeting tumor cells with proinflammatory reagents designed to stimulate local immunity and block local suppressive mechanisms. These approaches need to be better evaluated but may also be combined with more potent adjuvants, additional therapeutic strategies, or with agents that target other elements of the tumor microenvironment.

Targeting the Stroma

Although several factors are expressed in the tumor microenvironment by stromal cells that might serve as targets for enhancing tumor immunotherapy, VEGF is an especially attractive target since it is widely expressed in many tumors, promotes tumor growth through several mechanisms (e.g., angiogenesis and immune suppression) and there are several available agents that target VEGF in clinical use. Limited data from clinical studies in ovarian cancer and adoptive T cell therapy in melanoma patients, suggest that blocking VEGF with anti-VEGF monoclonal antibodies resulted in decreased CD4+FoxP3+ Tregs and increased effector CD8+ T cell numbers and infiltration into the tumor [7, 66]. In addition to effects on T cells, anti-VEGF treatment was observed to induce an increase in circulating differentiated dendritic cells in the peripheral blood of treated patients [52]. In light of these favorable results, more studies are needed to determine the full effect of anti-VEGF treatment on tumor immune responses.

The enzyme IDO can be targeted through the administration of 1-methyl-tryptophan. Preclinical models have shown that 1-methyl-tryptophan in combination with chemotherapy induced regression of established tumors [31]. In addition to early phase I clinical trials using 1-methyl-tryptophan, an orally active hydroxyamidine small molecule inhibitor that has been proven to suppress IDO-catalyzed tryptophan metabolism in animals, is poised to start clinical trials [39].

TGF-β is found in abundance in the tumor microenvironment and local or systemic depletion of this regulatory growth factor may facilitate the expansion of anti-tumor immune responses. A number of TGF-β inhibitors, from monoclonal antibodies to small molecule inhibitors, are in the early stages of clinical testing after demonstrating they could be well tolerated in animal models [76]. One of these inhibitor molecules, a TGF-β2-specific antisense oligodeoxynucleotide (trabedersen), has been administered intra-tumorally for the treatment of malignant gliomas, resulting in a 15% response rate at 14 months (traditional chemotherapy response rate at 14 months was 0%) and generating several long-lasting remissions [8, 29]. The seemingly late timing of the antisense reagent-mediated response rate was hypothesized to be due to the gradual development of a tumor-specific immune response, but conclusive immunologic data is still needed. A second reagent of note, a TGF-β neutralizing antibody (fresolimumab (GC-1008)), has entered into clinical trial for the treatment of metastatic melanoma, but results from these studies are not complete [26]. Although TGF-β is a potent immunosuppressant in the tumor setting, it has other pleiotropic functions that could ultimately limit the application of these TGF-β inhibitors.

Target the Local Immune System

There are several strategies for local treatment that target the immune system in a specific or nonspecific manner. The direct injection of recombinant IL-2 into tumors (oral squamous cell and melanoma metastases) resulted in response rates that reached up to 85% and were correlated with an enhanced immune response [54, 69]. The immunological changes seen included an increased ratio of CD4+ T cells to CD8+ T cells, dendritic cell migration into the stroma of the tumor and a reduction in tumor-associated macrophages. These changes were accompanied by tumor cell apoptosis and eventual complete destruction of the tumor.

Another approach to inhibit extrinsic suppression of Tregs has been explored by using an IL-2 diphtheria toxin conjugate [12, 45, 55]. Administration of this agent (denileukin diflitox) was able to selectively eliminate CD25-expressing Tregs from the peripheral blood of cancer patients. The transient decrease in Tregs was associated with augmented T cell responses (as measured by T cell proliferation and cytotoxicity assays) after active immunization [12]. Early results from clinical trials in cancer patients, demonstrated an abrogation of the suppressive activity of Tregs in vivo and boosted tumor-specific T cell stimulation when used in combination with a dendritic cell vaccine [12]. Despite these data, further calibration of denileukin diflitox is needed as other studies failed to obtain similar results, which may be due to the depletion of effector cells as well as Tregs at the doses used [2]. In addition, other strategies to deplete Tregs are being developed. Low doses of cyclophosphamide have been reported to deplete Tregs and this agent is often used for this purpose prior to an active immunization, although some have questioned the effectiveness of cyclophosphamide for this purpose [47]. An anti-IL-2R monoclonal antibody (Daclizumab), originally developed to prevent organ transplant rejection, may also attenuate Treg immune suppression in melanoma patients and is being explored [33, 34].

The application of TLR agonists, potent immune stimulants, has also been suggested for the treatment of superficial cutaneous melanomas. The TLR family is a well-characterized group of innate cell receptors that recognize highly conserved molecular patterns from a diversity of pathogenic microorganisms. Ligation of TLRs by these pattern molecules induces a transcriptional cascade that activates antigen-presenting cells and initiates secretion of inflammatory mediators [5]. These features led to the clinical development of TLR agonists, such as the TLR 7/8 agonist imiquimod (Aldara) and the TLR9 agonist CpG (PF-3512676), for cancer therapy. Early clinical reports have documented regression of locally treated lesions with these agents [41, 62]. Tumors exhibiting regression following TLR agonist treatment have been associated with a significant immune response, as there is an upregulation of the pro-inflammatory cytokine IL-12, and an increase in CD8[+] T cell infiltration [41]. Imiquimod, which is formulated as a cream, has also been used in combination with tumor vaccines to elicit more potent systemic antitumor immune responses. In one study, imiquimod was applied topically, followed by vaccination with the tumor antigen NY-ESO-1 or melanoma peptides administered into the skin at the imiquimod-treated site. The endpoint of this study was induction of NY-ESO-1-specific T cell responses, which was observed in 44% of the treated patients [1].

The future of therapeutic strategies to mitigate the regulatory immunologic milieu generated by the tumor microenvironment may require creating reagents that simultaneously target multiple elements and cellular components at once. For example, a preclinical study combined agents that targeted both the tumor and the immune system through an engineered molecule containing a siRNA inhibitor of STAT3 conjugated to CpG [40]. The reagent was able to effectively silence constitutive activation of the transcription factor STAT3 within tumor cells, which likely underlies the negative regulation of pro-inflammatory cytokine expression. In addition, TLR activation of local antigen-presenting cells was also noted and this included an increase in mature dendritic cells and pro-inflammatory cytokine production. The sum of the effects of STAT3 inhibition and TLR activation in modulating the tumor microenvironment resulted in the increased infiltration of T cells and tumor regression in an animal tumor model [40].

Conclusions

Tumors are not homogeneous entities, but rather exist in a complex formation that includes tumor cells, immune, and stromal cells. These cells interact with each other and the host through a network of soluble factors that shape the local tumor microenvironment. The elaborate interplay between the components of the microenvironment governs the ability of the tumor to acquire numerous immune regulatory mechanisms that protect the tumor from immune recognition and destruction, thereby allowing continued survival and growth. The success of targeted therapy, like tumor immunotherapy, will ultimately depend on a better understanding of the complex interplay of components within the tumor microenvironment.

The tumor cells, stromal elements, immune cells, and soluble factors all contribute to the growth of a tumor and produce cell surface and soluble factors that are designed to block effective antitumor immunity. The identification of these factors has allowed a more directed manipulation of the tumor microenvironment through the use of agents that specifically target these factors to disrupt the immunosuppressive framework and communication of the microenvironment. There are now numerous clinical trials in development that have targeted the tumor cells, stromal factors, and immune cells to promote a more pro-inflammatory and effector T cell environment while blocking various suppressor pathways operative within established tumors. These strategies are beginning to yield promising results although further work is needed to better understand how tumors co-opt their local environment to escape immune detection and how best to combine targeted therapeutics to overcome the barriers found in the tumor microenvironment.

References

1. Adams S, O'Neill DW, Nonaka D, Hardin E, Chiriboga L, Siu K, et al. Immunization of malignant melanoma patients with full-length NY-ESO-1 protein using TLR7 agonist imiquimod as vaccine adjuvant. J Immunol. 2008;181:776–84.
2. Attia P, Maker AV, Haworth LR, Rogers-Freezer L, Rosenberg SA. Inability of a fusion protein of IL-2 and diphtheria toxin (Denileukin Diftitox, DAB389IL-2, ONTAK) to eliminate regulatory T lymphocytes in patients with melanoma. J Immunother. 2005;28:582–92.
3. Azenshtein E, Meshel T, Shina S, Barak N, Keydar I, Ben-Baruch A. The angiogenic factors CXCL8 and VEGF in breast cancer: regulation by an array of pro-malignancy factors. Cancer Lett. 2005;217:73–86.

4. Barber DL, Wherry EJ, Masopust D, Zhu B, Allison JP, Sharpe AH, et al. Restoring function in exhausted CD8 T cells during chronic viral infection. Nature. 2006;439:682–7.
5. Barton GM, Kagan JC. A cell biological view of Toll-like receptor function: regulation through compartmentalization. Nat Rev Immunol. 2009;9:535–42.
6. Beissert S, Hosoi J, Grabbe S, Asahina A, Granstein RD. IL-10 inhibits tumor antigen presentation by epidermal antigen-presenting cells. J Immunol. 1995;154:1280–6.
7. Bellati F, Napoletano C, Ruscito I, Pastore M, Pernice M, Antonilli M, et al. Complete remission of ovarian cancer induced intractable malignant ascites with intraperitoneal bevacizumab. Immunological observations and a literature review. Invest New Drugs. 2010;28:887–94.
8. Bogdahn U, Hau P, Stockhammer G, Venkataramana NK, Maapatra AK, Suri A, et al. Targeted therapy for high-grade glioma with the TGF-beta2 inhibitor trabedersen: results of a randomized and controlled phase IIb study, Neuro Oncol. First published 27 Oct 2010. doi:10.1093/neuonc/noq142.
9. Brahmer JR, Drake CG, Wollner I, Powderly JD, Picus J, Sharfman WH, et al. Phase I study of single-agent anti-programmed death-1 (MDX-1106) in refractory solid tumors: safety, clinical activity, pharmacodynamics, and immunologic correlates. J Clin Oncol. 2010;28:3167–75.
10. Curiel TJ, Coukos G, Zou L, Alvarez X, Cheng P, Mottram P, et al. Specific recruitment of regulatory T cells in ovarian carcinoma fosters immune privilege and predicts reduced survival. Nat Med. 2004;10:942–9.
11. Curotto de Lafaille MA, Lafaille JJ. Natural and adaptive foxp3+ regulatory T cells: more of the same or a division of labor? Immunity. 2009;30:626–35.
12. Dannull J, Su Z, Rizzieri D, Yang BK, Coleman D, Yancey D, et al. Enhancement of vaccine-mediated antitumor immunity in cancer patients after depletion of regulatory T cells. J Clin Invest. 2005;115:3623–33.
13. de Visser KE, Eichten A, Coussens LM. Paradoxical roles of the immune system during cancer development. Nat Rev Cancer. 2006;6:24–37.
14. Denfeld RW, Dietrich A, Wuttig C, Tanczos E, Weiss JM, Vanscheidt W, et al. In situ expression of B7 and CD28 receptor families in human malignant melanoma: relevance for T-cell-mediated anti-tumor immunity. Int J Cancer. 1995;62:259–65.
15. di Bari MG, Lutsiak ME, Takai S, Mostbock S, Farsaci B, Semnani RT, et al. TGF-beta modulates the functionality of tumor-infiltrating CD8+ T cells through effects on TCR signaling and Spred1 expression. Cancer Immunol Immunother. 2009;58:1809–18.
16. Dong H, Strome SE, Salomao DR, Tamura H, Hirano F, Flies DB, et al. Tumor-associated B7-H1 promotes T-cell apoptosis: a potential mechanism of immune evasion. Nat Med. 2002;8:793–800.
17. Dunn GP, Old LJ, Schreiber RD. The three Es of cancer immunoediting. Annu Rev Immunol. 2004;22:329–60.
18. Fallarino F, Grohmann U, Vacca C, Bianchi R, Orabona C, Spreca A, et al. T cell apoptosis by tryptophan catabolism. Cell Death Differ. 2002;9:1069–77.
19. Fields P, Fitch FW, Gajewski TF. Control of T lymphocyte signal transduction through clonal anergy. J Mol Med. 1996;74:673–83.
20. Flavell RA, Sanjabi S, Wrzesinski SH, Licona-Limon P. The polarization of immune cells in the tumour environment by TGFbeta. Nat Rev Immunol. 2010;10:554–67.
21. Fontenot JD, Rasmussen JP, Williams LM, Dooley JL, Farr AG, Rudensky AY. Regulatory T cell lineage specification by the forkhead transcription factor foxp3. Immunity. 2005;22:329–41.
22. Gabrilovich D, Ishida T, Oyama T, Ran S, Kravtsov V, Nadaf S, et al. Vascular endothelial growth factor inhibits the development of dendritic cells and dramatically affects the differentiation of multiple hematopoietic lineages in vivo. Blood. 1998;92:4150–66.
23. Gabrilovich DI, Chen HL, Girgis KR, Cunningham HT, Meny GM, Nadaf S, et al. Production of vascular endothelial growth factor by human tumors inhibits the functional maturation of dendritic cells. Nat Med. 1996;2:1096–103.
24. Gabrilovich DI, Ishida T, Nadaf S, Ohm JE, Carbone DP. Antibodies to vascular endothelial growth factor enhance the efficacy of cancer immunotherapy by improving endogenous dendritic cell function. Clin Cancer Res. 1999;5:2963–70.

25. Garcia-Lora A, Algarra I, Garrido F. MHC class I antigens, immune surveillance, and tumor immune escape. J Cell Physiol. 2003;195:346–55.
26. Grutter C, Wilkinson T, Turner R, Podichetty S, Finch D, McCourt M, et al. A cytokine-neutralizing antibody as a structural mimetic of 2 receptor interactions. Proc Natl Acad Sci USA. 2008;105:20251–6.
27. Han Y, Guo Q, Zhang M, Chen Z, Cao X. CD69+ CD4+ CD25- T cells, a new subset of regulatory T cells, suppress T cell proliferation through membrane-bound TGF-beta 1. J Immunol. 2009;182:111–20.
28. Harlin H, Kuna TV, Peterson AC, Meng Y, Gajewski TF. Tumor progression despite massive influx of activated CD8(+) T cells in a patient with malignant melanoma ascites. Cancer Immunol Immunother. 2006;55:1185–97.
29. Hau P, Jachimczak P, Schlingensiepen R, Schulmeyer F, Jauch T, Steinbrecher A, et al. Inhibition of TGF-beta2 with AP 12009 in recurrent malignant gliomas: from preclinical to phase I/II studies. Oligonucleotides. 2007;17:201–12.
30. Hodi FS, O'Day SJ, McDermott DF, Weber RW, Sosman JA, Haanen JB, et al. Improved survival with ipilimumab in patients with metastatic melanoma. N Engl J Med. 2010;363:711–23.
31. Hou DY, Muller AJ, Sharma MD, DuHadaway J, Banerjee T, Johnson M, et al. Inhibition of indoleamine 2,3-dioxygenase in dendritic cells by stereoisomers of 1-methyl-tryptophan correlates with antitumor responses. Cancer Res. 2007;67:792–801.
32. Iwai Y, Ishida M, Tanaka Y, Okazaki T, Honjo T, Minato N. Involvement of PD-L1 on tumor cells in the escape from host immune system and tumor immunotherapy by PD-L1 blockade. Proc Natl Acad Sci USA. 2002;99:12293–7.
33. Jacobs JF, Punt CJ, Lesterhuis WJ, Sutmuller RP, Brouwer HM, Scharenborg NM, et al. Dendritic cell vaccination in combination with anti-CD25 monoclonal antibody treatment: a phase I/II study in metastatic melanoma patients. Clin Cancer Res. 2010;16:5067–78.
34. Jones E, Dahm-Vicker M, Simon AK, Green A, Powrie F, Cerundolo V, et al. Depletion of CD25+ regulatory cells results in suppression of melanoma growth and induction of autoreactivity in mice. Cancer Immun. 2002;2:1.
35. Karim RZ, Li W, Sanki A, Colman MH, Yang YH, Thompson JF, et al. Reduced p16 and increased cyclin D1 and pRb expression are correlated with progression in cutaneous melanocytic tumors. Int J Surg Pathol. 2009;17:361–7.
36. Kaufman HL, Cohen S, Cheung K, DeRaffele G, Mitcham J, Moroziewicz D, et al. Local delivery of vaccinia virus expressing multiple costimulatory molecules for the treatment of established tumors. Hum Gene Ther. 2006;17:239–44.
37. Kaufman HL, Deraffele G, Mitcham J, Moroziewicz D, Cohen SM, Hurst-Wicker KS, et al. Targeting the local tumor microenvironment with vaccinia virus expressing B7.1 for the treatment of melanoma. J Clin Invest. 2005;115:1903–12.
38. Kaufman HL, Kim DW, DeRaffele G, Mitcham J, Coffin RS, Kim-Schulze S. Local and distant immunity induced by intralesional vaccination with an oncolytic herpes virus encoding GM-CSF in patients with stage IIIc and IV melanoma. Ann Surg Oncol. 2010;17:718–30.
39. Koblish HK, Hansbury MJ, Bowman KJ, Yang G, Neilan CL, Haley PJ, et al. Hydroxyamidine inhibitors of indoleamine-2,3-dioxygenase potently suppress systemic tryptophan catabolism and the growth of IDO-expressing tumors. Mol Cancer Ther. 2010;9:489–98.
40. Kortylewski M, Swiderski P, Herrmann A, Wang L, Kowolik C, Kujawski M, et al. In vivo delivery of siRNA to immune cells by conjugation to a TLR9 agonist enhances antitumor immune responses. Nat Biotechnol. 2009;27:925–32.
41. Krieg AM. Toll-like receptor 9 (TLR9) agonists in the treatment of cancer. Oncogene. 2008;27:161–7.
42. Kryczek I, Lange A, Mottram P, Alvarez X, Cheng P, Hogan M, et al. CXCL12 and vascular endothelial growth factor synergistically induce neoangiogenesis in human ovarian cancers. Cancer Res. 2005;65:465–72.
43. Kryczek I, Zou L, Rodriguez P, Zhu G, Wei S, Mottram P, et al. B7-H4 expression identifies a novel suppressive macrophage population in human ovarian carcinoma. J Exp Med. 2006;203:871–81.

44. Li MO, Wan YY, Sanjabi S, Robertson AK, Flavell RA. Transforming growth factor-beta regulation of immune responses. Annu Rev Immunol. 2006;24:99–146.
45. Litzinger MT, Fernando R, Curiel TJ, Grosenbach DW, Schlom J, Palena C. IL-2 immunotoxin denileukin diftitox reduces regulatory T cells and enhances vaccine-mediated T-cell immunity. Blood. 2007;110:3192–201.
46. Liu VC, Wong LY, Jang T, Shah AH, Park I, Yang X, et al. Tumor evasion of the immune system by converting CD4+ CD25- T cells into CD4+ CD25+ T regulatory cells: role of tumor-derived TGF-beta. J Immunol. 2007;178:2883–92.
47. Matsushita N, Pilon-Thomas SA, Martin LM, Riker AI. Comparative methodologies of regulatory T cell depletion in a murine melanoma model. J Immunol Methods. 2008;333:167–79.
48. McCarter M, Clarke J, Richter D, Wilson C. Melanoma skews dendritic cells to facilitate a T helper 2 profile. Surgery. 2005;138:321–8.
49. Munn DH, Zhou M, Attwood JT, Bondarev I, Conway SJ, Marshall B, et al. Prevention of allogeneic fetal rejection by tryptophan catabolism. Science. 1998;281:1191–3.
50. Nevala WK, Vachon CM, Leontovich AA, Scott CG, Thompson MA, Markovic SN. Evidence of systemic Th2-driven chronic inflammation in patients with metastatic melanoma. Clin Cancer Res. 2009;15:1931–9.
51. Orimo A, Gupta PB, Sgroi DC, Arenzana-Seisdedos F, Delaunay T, Naeem R, et al. Stromal fibroblasts present in invasive human breast carcinomas promote tumor growth and angiogenesis through elevated SDF-1/CXCL12 secretion. Cell. 2005;121:335–48.
52. Osada T, Chong G, Tansik R, Hong T, Spector N, Kumar R, et al. The effect of anti-VEGF therapy on immature myeloid cell and dendritic cells in cancer patients. Cancer Immunol Immunother. 2008;57:1115–24.
53. Petersson M, Charo J, Salazar-Onfray F, Noffz G, Mohaupt M, Qin Z, et al. Constitutive IL-10 production accounts for the high NK sensitivity, low MHC class I expression, and poor transporter associated with antigen processing (TAP)-1/2 function in the prototype NK target YAC-1. J Immunol. 1998;161:2099–105.
54. Radny P, Caroli UM, Bauer J, Paul T, Schlegel C, Eigentler TK, et al. Phase II trial of intralesional therapy with interleukin-2 in soft-tissue melanoma metastases. Br J Cancer. 2003;89:1620–6.
55. Rasku MA, Clem AL, Telang S, Taft B, Gettings K, Gragg H, et al. Transient T cell depletion causes regression of melanoma metastases. J Transl Med. 2008;6:12.
56. Richmond A, Yang J, Su Y. The good and the bad of chemokines/chemokine receptors in melanoma. Pigment Cell Melanoma Res. 2009;22:175–86.
57. Rodriguez PC, Quiceno DG, Zabaleta J, Ortiz B, Zea AH, Piazuelo MB, et al. Arginase I production in the tumor microenvironment by mature myeloid cells inhibits T-cell receptor expression and antigen-specific T-cell responses. Cancer Res. 2004;64:5839–49.
58. Rodriguez PC, Zea AH, DeSalvo J, Culotta KS, Zabaleta J, Quiceno DG, et al. L-arginine consumption by macrophages modulates the expression of CD3 zeta chain in T lymphocytes. J Immunol. 2003;171:1232–9.
59. Rofstad EK, Halsor EF. Vascular endothelial growth factor, interleukin 8, platelet-derived endothelial cell growth factor, and basic fibroblast growth factor promote angiogenesis and metastasis in human melanoma xenografts. Cancer Res. 2000;60:4932–8.
60. Rohrer JW, Coggin Jr JH. CD8 T cell clones inhibit antitumor T cell function by secreting IL-10. J Immunol. 1995;155:5719–27.
61. Ruiter D, Bogenrieder T, Elder D, Herlyn M. Melanoma-stroma interactions: structural and functional aspects. Lancet Oncol. 2002;3:35–43.
62. Schulze HJ, Cribier B, Requena L, Reifenberger J, Ferrandiz C, Garcia Diez A, et al. Imiquimod 5% cream for the treatment of superficial basal cell carcinoma: results from a randomized vehicle-controlled phase III study in Europe. Br J Dermatol. 2005;152:939–47.
63. Schwartz RH. T cell clonal anergy. Curr Opin Immunol. 1997;9:351–7.
64. Senzer NN, Kaufman HL, Amatruda T, Nemunaitis M, Reid T, Daniels G, et al. Phase II clinical trial of a granulocyte-macrophage colony-stimulating factor-encoding, second-generation

oncolytic herpesvirus in patients with unresectable metastatic melanoma. J Clin Oncol. 2009; 27:5763–71.

65. Shih IM, Elder DE, Hsu MY, Herlyn M. Regulation of Mel-CAM/MUC18 expression on melanocytes of different stages of tumor progression by normal keratinocytes. Am J Pathol. 1994;145:837–45.

66. Shrimali RK, Yu Z, Theoret MR, Chinnasamy D, Restifo NP, Rosenberg SA. Antiangiogenic agents can increase lymphocyte infiltration into tumor and enhance the effectiveness of adoptive immunotherapy of cancer. Cancer Res. 2010;70:6171–80.

67. Tatsumi T, Kierstead LS, Ranieri E, Gesualdo L, Schena FP, Finke JH, et al. Disease-associated bias in T helper type 1 (Th1)/Th2 CD4(+) T cell responses against MAGE-6 in HLA-DRB10401(+) patients with renal cell carcinoma or melanoma. J Exp Med. 2002;196: 619–28.

68. Thomas DA, Massague J. TGF-beta directly targets cytotoxic T cell functions during tumor evasion of immune surveillance. Cancer Cell. 2005;8:369–80.

69. Timar J, Ladanyi A, Forster-Horvath C, Lukits J, Dome B, Remenar E, et al. Neoadjuvant immunotherapy of oral squamous cell carcinoma modulates intratumoral CD4/CD8 ratio and tumor microenvironment: a multicenter phase II clinical trial. J Clin Oncol. 2005;23: 3421–32.

70. Uyttenhove C, Pilotte L, Theate I, Stroobant V, Colau D, Parmentier N, et al. Evidence for a tumoral immune resistance mechanism based on tryptophan degradation by indoleamine 2,3-dioxygenase. Nat Med. 2003;9:1269–74.

71. Valyi-Nagy IT, Hirka G, Jensen PJ, Shih IM, Juhasz I, Herlyn M. Undifferentiated keratinocytes control growth, morphology, and antigen expression of normal melanocytes through cell-cell contact. Lab Invest. 1993;69:152–9.

72. Valzasina B, Piconese S, Guiducci C, Colombo MP. Tumor-induced expansion of regulatory T cells by conversion of CD4+ CD25- lymphocytes is thymus and proliferation independent. Cancer Res. 2006;66:4488–95.

73. Wang T, Niu G, Kortylewski M, Burdelya L, Shain K, Zhang S, et al. Regulation of the innate and adaptive immune responses by Stat-3 signaling in tumor cells. Nat Med. 2004;10:48–54.

74. Weber F, Byrne SN, Le S, Brown DA, Breit SN, Scolyer RA, et al. Transforming growth factor-beta1 immobilises dendritic cells within skin tumours and facilitates tumour escape from the immune system. Cancer Immunol Immunother. 2005;54:898–906.

75. Woo EY, Chu CS, Goletz TJ, Schlienger K, Yeh H, Coukos G, et al. Regulatory CD4(+) CD25(+) T cells in tumors from patients with early-stage non-small cell lung cancer and late-stage ovarian cancer. Cancer Res. 2001;61:4766–72.

76. Wrzesinski SH, Wan YY, Flavell RA. Transforming growth factor-beta and the immune response: implications for anticancer therapy. Clin Cancer Res. 2007;13:5262–70.

77. Yu P, Fu YX. Tumor-infiltrating T lymphocytes: friends or foes? Lab Invest. 2006;86: 231–45.

78. Zippelius A, Batard P, Rubio-Godoy V, Bioley G, Lienard D, Lejeune F, et al. Effector function of human tumor-specific CD8 T cells in melanoma lesions: a state of local functional tolerance. Cancer Res. 2004;64:2865–73.

Index

A

Activation-induced cell death (AICD), 310
Adjuvant therapy, 282–283
Adoptive cell therapy
  ACT, 234
  advantages and disadvantages, 235–236
  biological and technical limitations
    long-term persistence, 245
    technical issues, 242, 247–248
    telomere shortening and cellular
      senescence, 245–246
    terminal differentiation, CD8+ T Cells,
      246–247
  capillary leak syndrome, 234
  CARs, B-cell antigen recognition,
    235, 256
  CD4+ T-Helper 17/Th17 cells, 255
  clinical-grade expansion
    adoptive therapy, 253–254
    erythromyeloid cell, 254
    gas-permeable bag technology, 255
    sleeping beauty system, 254
  costimulatory pathways, negative and
      positive
    CTLA-4, 250
    phase II/III testing, 250
    TNF-R costimulatory pathways, 250
    tumor eradication, 249
  dacarbazine, 234
  factors, melanoma patients, 233–234
  function and persistence, TIL, 251–252
  future perspective
    cytokines/synergistic
      immunomodulatory, 257–258
    pivotal multicenter clinical trial,
      259–261
    TIL adoptive therapy, 259–261
    TKIs therapy, 258–259
  IL-2 therapy, 234
  lymphodepleting, 256–257
  melanoma development
    cyclophosphamide and fludarabine,
      237–238
    historical timeline and milestones, 236,
      237
    immunological competent cell, 236
    NK cells, 236–237
  melanoma methods
    ACT and TIL, 238–239
    antigen-specific CD4 + T cells, 244
    antigen-Specific CD8 + T cells,
      243–244
    TCR-transduced peripheral blood T
      cells, 241–242
    TIL expansion protocols, 239–241
  persistence and effector function, 248–249
  targeting TGF-., 252–253
  TIL methods and ACT, 234–235, 248
  tumor migration, 252
Adoptive T cell therapy (ACT), 234
Agonist immune costimulatory agents
  anti-CD137/4-1BB
    cisplatin, 316
    clinical experience, 316–317
    enhancement *vs.* suppression, 315
    immune-enhancing effects, 314
    osteosarcoma and lung cancer, 314
    proliferation/survival, 314
    tumor growth/regression, delays, 315
  antitumor immune responses, 308–309
  CD40, 319–321
  clinical experience, anti-OX40, 313–314

Agonist immune costimulatory agents (*cont.*)
  endothelium, 322
  human, host and tumor interaction, 309
  IFN-α and interleukin-2, 308
  licensing effect, 322
  ligand–receptor interactions, 308
  OX40/CD134
    AICD, 310
    breast cancer model, 312
    CD28/B7 interaction, 310
    cyclophosphamide treatment, 312
    proliferation and survival, 309–310
    sarcoma-bearing mice, 311
    synergistic therapeutic effect, 312
    transgenic mouse models, 311
  OX40-specific nonhuman, 312–313
Anti-angiogenesis therapy
  agents, completed trials, 163–167
  axitinib, 163
  biologic/cytotoxic agents, 171–174
  chemotherapy theories, 171
  clinical activity, 162
  clinical trials, 169
  combinations chemotherapy, 171
  components, therapies, 169–170
  disease progression, 156–158
  EGFL7, 170
  highly vascular malignancy, 155–156
  immunotherapy, 176
  indirect effects, 169
  inhibitors *vs.* combinations, 171, 175
  integrins, 170
  lymphangiogenesis, 171
  mediators of angiogenesis
    immunohistochemical analysis, 158
    soluble angiogenic factors, 158–162
    VEGF/VEGF-A, 158
  monocyte maturation and activation, 175
  prognostic significance, 162
  sorafenib, 168
  tumor-infiltrating myeloid cells, 170
  vascular normalization, 171
  VEGF ligand, 167–168
  VEGFR TKIs, 168–169
Anti-CTLA-4 monoclonal antibodies
  blocking antibodies, 277
  checkpoint immuno-inhibitory, 274
  clinical trial testing
    adjuvant therapy, 282–283
    antibody responses, 284–285
    biomarkers, 283–284
    immune, adverse events, 279–280
    ipilimumab monotherapy, 278
    ipilimumab plus chemotherapy, 282

    peptide vaccines, 279
    phase III, ipilimumab, 281
    response criteria, 280–281
    tremelimumab, 277–278
  co-inhibitory molecule, 275
  immune potentiation mechanism, 274–275
  immuno-inhibitory, 274
  T cell-extrinsic suppression, 276–277
  T cell-intrinsic suppression, 275–276
  tumor immunotherapy, 277
Apoptotic pathways
  Bcl-2 protein
    cancer cells, 132
    cell damage, BH3 domains, 128
    family proteins, targeting, 132
    gossypol, 132–133
    immunohistochemical, 129
    loss expression, 128–129
    Mcl-1 expression, 129–130
    melanoma metastasis, 128–129
    MITF, 128
    mitochondria, 127
    neutralization model, 128
    OMM interaction, 127–128
    PFS and ORR, 132
    structure and role, 126–127
  BH3 mimetics, 133–134
  cancer therapy, smac mimetics, 139–140
  extrinsic pathway, 126
  IAPs negative regulation, 138–139
  intrinsic/mitochondrial cell death, 126
  melanoma proteins, 137–138
  microRNAs, 142–143
  upregulation, BH3-only, 131
  RAS/RAF/MEK/ERK
    blocks apoptosis, 134–135
    BRAF mutation, 134
    carboplatin/paclitaxel effects, 136
    CREB activation, 135
    farnesyltransferase inhibitors, 135
    G protein-coupled receptors, 134
    GRP78, 135
    SCCs toxicity and induction, 137
    signal pathway inhibitors, 135–136
    tanespimycin, 137
  TRAIL induction, 141–142
  tumorigenesis, 125–126
  tumor suppressors, Rb and P53, 130–131

B
Basic fibroblast growth factor receptor
    (bFGFR), 91
B7-H1/PD-1 pathway, monoclonal antibodies

APCs, 294
EAE, 293
hematopoietic cells, 296–297
immune tolerance, 292
immunohistochemistry, 295, 296
immunotherapy, 293, 294, 297
interferon gamma observation, 293–294
melanoma therapy application
    early clinical experience, 299–300
    future clinical development, 300–301
    preclinical considerations, 298
murine models, 294–295
PD-1 expression, 293
phenotypes, deficient mice, 292
signaling and associated markers, 297
solid human tumors, 295–296
T cell inhibition interaction, 294
BRAF, 5–7
B-Raf, targeted inhibition
clinical trials
    broad-spectrum features, 70
    GSK2118436, 70–71
    resistance mechanism, 72–73
    sorafenib agent, 70
future perspective, 73–74
MAPK pathway, 64–65
MEK inhibition, 71–72
melanoma mutations, 65
PLX4032/RO5185426, clinical studies
    dose-response relationship and
        escalation, 68
    immunohistochemistry, 69
    keratoacanthoma (KA), 68
    lesions, dose escalation cohorts, 68
    phase II trial, 69
    tumor cells inhibition, 67
    untreated patients, phase III trial, 69–70
preclinical studies
    mutated melanoma causes, cell death,
        66–67
    wild-type cells, MAPK pathway
        activation, 65–66
signaling pathway, MAPK, 63–64

C
Cancer Therapy Evaluation Program (CTEP),
    81
Central nervous system (CNS), 50
Chimeric antigen receptors (CARs), 256
Chronic sun damage (CSD), 44
Comparative genome hybridization (CGH), 6
Cytotoxic T-lymphocyte antigen-4
    (CTLA-4), 274

D
Death-inducing signaling complexes
    (DISC), 126
Disease-specific survival (DSS), 21
Dose-limiting toxicities (DLTs), 336

E
Epidermal growth factor receptor (EGFR), 91
Epithelial-mesenchymal transition (EMT), 93
Experimental autoimmune encephalopathy
    (EAE), 293

F
Fluorescent in situ hybridization (FISH), 46

G
Gamma secretase inhibitors (GSIs), 30
Gangliosides, 211–212
Gastrointestinal stromal tumors (GIST), 47
GNAQ, 11
Granulocytemacrophage colony stimulating
    factor (GM-CSF), 344

H
Haemophilus influenza, 214
Hematopoietic cells, PD-1 expression,
    296–297
Herpes simplex virus type 1 (HSV-1), 346

I
Indoleamine-2,3-dioxygenase (IDO), 32
Inhibitor of apoptosis protein (IAP), 126
Ipilimumab monotherapy, 278
Ipilimumab plus chemotherapy, 282

K
c-KIT, 9–10
KIT therapeutic target
    acral melanoma, 46, 47
    amplification/mutation, 56
    cancer role, 47–48
    dasatinib, 47, 52
    imatinib, 48
    inhibition, melanomas harboring
        activation, 44, 49
    mucosal melanoma, 48–50
    nilotinib, 47
    proto-oncogene

KIT therapeutic target (*cont.*)
    MAPK and PI3K, 44
    signaling pathways, 44, 46
    type III trans-membrane RTK, 44
  sunitinib, 47
  tyrosine kinase inhibitors
    CD117, immunohistochemistry, 48
    chronic sun-damaged skin, 53
    clinical trials, melanoma subtypes,
      53–54
    CNS metastases, 50
    first-line treatment, 52
    immunohistochemistry, 48
    masatinib, 56
    mucosal and acral melanomas, 52–54
    multi-kinase inhibitor, 52
    mutation/amplification, 48–50
    mutation analysis, 50–51
    nilotinib, 53
    nodal and lung metastases, 50
    overcoming resistance, 52, 55–56
    patient CT images, 51–52
    proliferation and progression, 44, 48
    sunitinib, 52

M
Malignant melanoma initiating cells (MMICs),
    94
Mammalian target of rapamycin (mTOR), 107
Melanoma genomics, gene expression
    profiling
  melanoma progression
    BRAF mutations, 18
    nevi and primary melanoma, 18–19
    nevus and melanoma transition, 19
    primary and metastatic melanoma
      transition, 19–20
    prognostic role, genes, 21
    proliferation, 17–18
    SAM, 18
    transcriptomic profiles, 21–22
  metastatic melanoma, 22–23
  primary melanoma
    biomarkers, 22
    cDNA microarrays, 20
    custom array, 19
    genomic signatures, 20
    genomic signatures, 20
    hierarchical clustering, 19
    immunohistochemical gene analysis, 20
    microarray analysis, 18, 21
    SLN, RFS and DSS status, 21

Melanoma immunotherapy
  cytokine delivery, 333, 334
  interleukin-12/IL-12
    antitumor activity, 335–336
    biological properties, 334–335
    clinical toxicities, 336
    DLTs, 336
    immunohistochemistry, 337
    immunomodulatory cytokine, 338
    intratumoral injection, 338
    maximum tolerated dose, 336
    metastatic melanoma patients, 338
    mice and cynomologus monkey,
      336–337
    PD and SD, 337
    transfection, efficiency, 338
  interleukin-15/IL-15
    biological properties, 344
    GM-CSF, 344–345
    HSV-1, 346
    p53-expressing tumor cells, 345–346
    therapeutic effect, 345
    tumor microenvironment, 345
  interleukin-21/IL-21
    biological properties, 339–340
    cancer immunotherapy, 341–343
    preclinical model, antitumor activity,
      340–341
  novel cytokine, 345–346
  tumor microenvironment, 345
Melanoma vaccines
  cancer specific T Cell responses and
    correlation
    assessment, 219–220
    autologous tumor cells, 221
    cytokine production, 219
    disease protection, 218, 221
    gene expression analysis, 220
    phenotypic and functional analysis, 219
    vaccination, 218–219
  cell based vaccines, 211
  dendritic cell-based vaccines, 215
  gangliosides, 211–212
  immunological tolerance, 217–218
  nucleic acid-based vaccines, 216–217
  peptide and recombinant protein
    autologous dendritic cells, 212
    cancer testis antigens, 214
    CD8$^+$ T cells, 212–213
    DERMA, 214
    GlaxoSmithKline Bio, 214
    gp100$_{209-217-210M}$, 213
    intrinsic immunogenicity, 213

intrinsic poor immunogenicity, 212
long synthetic peptides, 214
metastatic melanoma,
    survival time, 213
recombinant vector-based vaccines,
    215–216
T cell vaccines
    antigen and adjuvant, 208
    CD8 T cell responses, 209, 213
    criteria, adjuvant, 208
    current and future development, 209
    immunological adjuvant, 208
    therapeutic vaccination, 209
Microphthalmia-associated transcription
    factor (MITF), 128
Mixed lymphocyte-tumor cell cultures
    (MLTC), 189
Molecular targets and subtypes
    acral lentiginous melanomas, 4, 6
    acral melanomas, 4
    antihormonal therapy, 4
    BRAF, 5–7
    c-KIT, 9–10
    CML and RCC, 4–5
    GNAQ, 11
    HER2/neu oncogene, 4
    KIT inhibitor imatinib, 10
    lentigo melanoma, 4
    mucosal melanomas, 4, 7
    nevi, 7, 8, 12
    nodular melanoma, 4, 8
    NRAS, 7–8
    PI3K-AKT pathway, 8–9
    PLX4032, 11
    skin cancer, 4
    superficial spreading melanoma, 8
    superficial spreading melanoma, 4
    targeted therapy, 4
    uveal melanoma, 4
mTOR, PI$_3$K, and AKT pathways
    clinical results, 115–117
    combination chemotherapy, 114
    downstream event, transcription control,
        110–111
    everolimus and rapalogs
        temsirolimus, 113
    genetic alteration
        -C1, 107–108
        -C2, 108–109
        pleiotropic activity, 108
    immunosuppression, 119–120
    molecular oncogenesis, 114
    multi-kinase inhibitors, 115

mutations and gene alterations via.
    signaling
    AKT mutation, 111–112
    BRAF mutations, 112
    clinicopathology, 112
    MAPK pathway, 111
    PTEN function loss, 112
    rapalogs drugs, 112–113
    optimal therapeutic index, 114
    patient history, 113
    pharmacodynamics and biomarkers,
        118–119
    rapalogs temsirolimus and everolimus,
        117–118
    upstream effectors, PTEN, PI3K,
        and AKT, 109–110
    VEGFR2 blockade, 115
Myeloid-derived suppressor cells
    (MDSCs), 95

N

National Cancer Institute (NCI), 234
Nonsteroidal antiinflammatory drugs
    (NSAIDs), 83
Notch and β-catenin pathways
    axin composition, 81–82
    cancer
        initiation and progression,
            79–80
        malignant transformation,
            80–81
        solid tumors, 80
        Wnt signaling pathway., 81
    cascade signaling, 78–79
    CK1 and GSK3b, 79, 82
    clinical perspectives, 84
    CTEP, 81
    GSIs, 81
    helix-loop-helix domains, 78
    ligand-receptor interaction, 78
    NSAIDs, 83
    Parkinson's disease, 81
    plasticity, 84
    RO4929097, 81
    therapeutics, 84
    Wnt/b-catenin and cancer, 82–83
NRAS, 7–8

O

O^6-methylguanine methyltransferase
    (MGMT), 34

P
Peripheral blood mononuclear cells
    (PBMCs), 94
PI3K-AKT pathway, 8–9
Platelet-derived growth factor receptor
    (PDGFR), 46

R
Receptor tyrosine kinase (RTK), 44
Retinoblastoma Protein (Rb), 130

S
Sentinel lymph node (SLN), 21
Signal Transducer and Activator of
    Transcription (STAT), 90
Solid human tumors, B7-H1 expression,
    295–296
Squamous cell carcinoma (SCC), 137
STAT3 and src signaling
    angiogenesis and metastasis, 92–94
    dephosphorylation, 90
    EGFR and bFGFR, 91
    immune evasion, 94
    MDSCs, 95
    melanoma tumor cells, 91
    melanoma tumorigenesis, 92
    melanoma via small-molecule inhibitors,
        96–98
    metastasis, tumor, 93
    MMICs and PBMCs, 94
    oncogenesis interaction, 90
    proliferation, 92
    receptor-dependent and independent
        pathway, 90
    survival, tumor cells, 92–93
    targeted therapy, melanoma, 96
    treatment, 96
    tumor-associated immune cells, 94–95
    tumor cell growth regulation, 92
Statistical analysis of microarrays (SAM), 18

T
T cell-extrinsic suppression, 276–277
Therapy
    biologic subsets, 27–28
    chemotherapy, 34
    emerging molecular markers, 36
    GSIs, 30
    kinase mutations and clinical response
        B-Raf, 28–29
        c-kit, 29–30

mechanism-based predictive biomarker,
    34–35
melanoma vaccines, clinical response
    anti-PD-1 mAb, 33
    chemokines, 31
    immune inhibitory mechanisms,
        32–33
    immunotherapeutic intervention, 31
    MAGE3 protein-based vaccine, 32
    MHC-binding epitopes, 32
    tryptophan-catabolizing enzyme
        and IDO, 32
    tumor biopsy, 31
    tumor microenvironment, 33
OncotypeDx, breast cancer, 36
patient-specific therapy, 36–37
PI3 kinase, 30
serum and germline DNA, 35
stabilized b-catenin, 30–31
T lymphocytes, melanoma antigens
    CTL on human melanomas, 198–199
    HLA-loss, 199–200
    immunoaffinity purification, 189
    immunogenic tumors, 188
    immunotherapy, 199
    melanocyte differentiation antigens,
        195–196
    melanoma antigens resulting, 189–190
    melanoma cells, 196–197
    multiple HLA/peptide association, 198
    reverse immunology, 189
    shared tumor-specific antigens
        cancer-germline gene, 190–191
        gene families, 191
        human tumor antigens, 195
        MAGE-A genes, transcript NA17,
            191, 193–194
        pseudogene, 191, 195
        tumor antigens, main genes,
            191–192
    TILs, 188
    tumor-specific T cells, 188–189, 198
    vaccination, 196–197
Tremelimumab, 277–278
Tumor-infiltrating lymphocytes (TIL), 235
    ACT, short-term tumor control, 248
    adoptive therapy, 259–261
    function and persistence, 251–252
Tumor-infiltrating lymphocytes (TILs), 188
Tumor microenvironment modulation
    composition and development
        immune cells, 356–357
        stroma, 355–356
        tumor cells, 354–355

immune cell-mediated suppression, 359–360
immune escape mechanism
  stroma-mediated suppression, 358–359
  tumor cell-mediated suppression, 357–358
immunotherapy
  local immune system, 363–365
  stroma, 362–363
  tumor, 360–362
melanoma antigens, 353–354

milieu, cellular and noncellular components, 354
tumor and immune system interaction, 354
Tumor necrosis factor receptor (TNF), 317
Tyrosine kinase inhibitors (TKIs), 44, 168

V
Vascular disrupting agents (VDAs), 169
Vascular endothelial growth factor (VEGF), 158, 354